D1693034

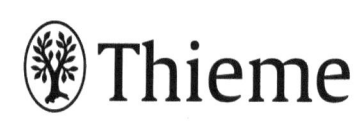

Modern Management of Spinal Deformities

A Theoretical, Practical, and Evidence-based Text

Robert Dickson, ChM, FRCS, DSc
Emeritus Professor of Orthopaedic Surgery
Consultant Spinal Surgeon
University of Leeds
Leeds, UK

Juergen Harms, MD
Professor of Orthopaedic Surgery
Spine Surgery at the Ethianum Clinic
Heidelberg, Germany

935 illustrations

Thieme
Stuttgart • New York • Delhi • Rio de Janeiro

Library of Congress Cataloging-in-Publication Data
Names: Dickson, Robert A., author. | Harms, Jürgen, author.
Title: Modern management of spinal deformities: a theoretical, practical, and evidence-based text / Robert Dickson, Juergen Harms.
Description: Stuttgart; New York: Thieme, [2017] | Includes bibliographical references and index.
Identifiers: LCCN 2017018237 (print) | LCCN 2017018914 (ebook) | ISBN 9783132016415 | ISBN 9783132016316 (hardcover)
Subjects: | MESH: Spinal Diseases–surgery | Spine–abnormalities | Spine–surgery | Evidence-Based Medicine
Classification: LCC RD768 (ebook) | LCC RD768 (print) | NLM WE 727 | DDC 617.5/6059-dc23
LC record available at https://lccn.loc.gov/2017018237

© 2018 by Georg Thieme Verlag KG

Thieme Publishers Stuttgart
Rüdigerstrasse 14, 70469 Stuttgart, Germany
+49 [0]711 8931 421, customerservice@thieme.de

Thieme Publishers New York
333 Seventh Avenue, New York, NY 10001 USA
+1 800 782 3488, customerservice@thieme.com

Thieme Publishers Delhi
A-12, Second Floor, Sector-2, Noida-201301
Uttar Pradesh, India
+91 120 45 566 00, customerservice@thieme.in

Thieme Publishers Rio de Janeiro, Thieme Publicações Ltda.
Edifício Rodolpho de Paoli, 25º andar
Av. Nilo Peçanha, 50 – Sala 2508
Rio de Janeiro 20020-906 Brasil
Tel: +55 21 3172-2297 / +55 21 3172-1896

Cover design: Thieme Publishing Group
Typesetting by DiTech Process Solutions, India

Printed in Germany by CPI, Leck   5 4 3 2 1

ISBN 978-3-13-201631-6

Also available as an e-book:
eISBN 978-3-13-201641-5

Important note: Medicine is an ever-changing science undergoing continual development. Research and clinical experience are continually expanding our knowledge, in particular our knowledge of proper treatment and drug therapy. Insofar as this book mentions any dosage or application, readers may rest assured that the authors, editors, and publishers have made every effort to ensure that such references are in accordance with **the state of knowledge at the time of production of the book.**

Nevertheless, this does not involve, imply, or express any guarantee or responsibility on the part of the publishers in respect to any dosage instructions and forms of applications stated in the book. **Every user is requested to examine carefully** the manufacturers' leaflets accompanying each drug and to check, if necessary in consultation with a physician or specialist, whether the dosage schedules mentioned therein or the contraindications stated by the manufacturers differ from the statements made in the present book. Such examination is particularly important with drugs that are either rarely used or have been newly released on the market. Every dosage schedule or every form of application used is entirely at the user's own risk and responsibility. The authors and publishers request every user to report to the publishers any discrepancies or inaccuracies noticed. If errors in this work are found after publication, errata will be posted at www.thieme.com on the product description page.

Some of the product names, patents, and registered designs referred to in this book are in fact registered trademarks or proprietary names even though specific reference to this fact is not always made in the text. Therefore, the appearance of a name without designation as proprietary is not to be construed as a representation by the publisher that it is in the public domain.

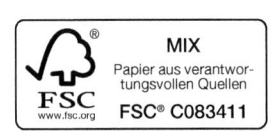

This book, including all parts thereof, is legally protected by copyright. Any use, exploitation, or commercialization outside the narrow limits set by copyright legislation without the publisher's consent is illegal and liable to prosecution. This applies in particular to photostat reproduction, copying, mimeographing or duplication of any kind, translating, preparation of microfilms, and electronic data processing and storage.

We dedicate this text to late Dr. Kenton D. Leatherman, the most distinguished North American spine surgeon of his generation, whose surgical skills and analysis of spinal deformities were at least half a century ahead of his time; a truly great man and the best friend of children with spinal deformities.

Robert Dickson, ChM, FRCS, DSc
Juergen Harms, MD

Contents

Foreword xi

Preface xiii

Acknowledgments xiv

About the Authors xv

1. **The Beginnings of Surgery for Spinal Deformities** 1
   1.1 The Early Days 2
   1.2 Posterior Instrumentation 3
   1.3 Anterior Instrumentation 8
   References 10

2. **Basic Principles** 13
   2.1 Definitions and Terminology 14
      2.1.1 Planes and Deformities 14
      2.1.2 Nonstructural and Structural Deformities 14
   2.2 Curve Characteristics 15
      2.2.1 Named Vertebrae 15
      2.2.2 Curve Size 15
      2.2.3 Vertebral Rotation 16
      2.2.4 Curve Patterns 17
   2.3 Spinal Growth 20
      2.3.1 Indices of Maturity 20
      2.3.2 Measurement of Bone Age 21
      2.3.3 Centile Charts 23
   2.4 Classification of Spinal Deformities 23
   2.5 Primary, Progressive, or Structural Deformities 24
      2.5.1 Idiopathic Deformities 24
      2.5.2 Congenital Deformities 28
      2.5.3 Neuromuscular Deformities 29
      2.5.4 Deformities due to Neurofibromatosis 29
      2.5.5 Miscellaneous Conditions Associated with Spine Deformities 30
      2.5.6 Miscellaneous Conditions in which a Spinal Deformity Is Common 33
   2.6 Secondary, Nonprogressive or Nonstructural Deformities 36
      2.6.1 Pelvic Tilt Scoliosis 36
      2.6.2 Irritative Lesions 36
      2.6.3 Hysterical Scoliosis 36
   References 36

3. **The Etiology of Spinal Deformities** 37
   3.1 Introduction 38
   3.2 The Development of Idiopathic Scoliosis ... 42
   3.3 Experimental Models 47
   3.4 What Pathogenesis Tells Us about Treatment 53
      3.4.1 Surgical Treatment of Spinal Deformities 53
   References 60

4. **Idiopathic Scoliosis** 63
   4.1 Epidemiology of Late-Onset Idiopathic Scoliosis 64
      4.1.1 Scoliosis in the Community 64
   4.2 Screening for Scoliosis 65
      4.2.1 Definitions and Criteria 65
      4.2.2 Natural History 66
   4.3 Late-Onset Idiopathic Scoliosis 68
      4.3.1 Clinical Presentation and Evaluation 68
      4.3.2 Classification 71
      4.3.3 Treatment 75
      4.3.4 Radiological Evaluation 79
      4.3.5 Specific Curve Patterns 80
   4.4 The Adolescent with the Bigger Curve 99
      4.4.1 Intraoperative Traction 101
      4.4.2 Anterior Multiple Diskectomy 102

4.5	**Osteotomies**	102		Case 4: Anterior Instrumentation Only; Lenke 1b	117
4.5.1	Smith-Peterson Osteotomy	102		Case 5: Posterior Instrumentation Only; King 4, Lenke 1	121
4.5.2	Ponte Osteotomies	103		Case 6: Posterior Instrumentation Only; Lenke 1c	122
4.5.3	Pedicle Subtraction Osteotomy	104			
4.5.4	Apical Vertebral Resection	104		Case 7: Combined—Anterior Diskectomy Then Posterior Instrumentation; Lenke 1AL	122
4.6	**Early-Onset Idiopathic Scoliosis**	106		Case 8: Combined—Anterior Diskectomy Then Posterior Instrumentation; Lenke 1AL	124
4.6.1	Clinical Features	106			
4.6.2	EDF Cast Treatment	110		Case 9: Thoracolumbar/Lumbar; Single Lenke 5	124
4.6.3	Operative Treatment	111		Case 10: Double Curves; Lenke 6	127
4.6.4	Other Methods of Growth Modulation	113		Case 11: Double Thoracic/Lumbar; Lenke 3	128
	Case Gallery	115		Case 12	129
	Case 1: The Value of Anterior Multiple Diskectomy	115		**References**	131
	Case 2: Anterior Instrumentation Only; Lenke 1 AR	116			
	Case 3: Anterior Instrumentation Only; Lenke 1b	117			

5. Scheuermann's Disease ... 135

5.1	**Pathogenesis**	136	**5.4**	**Management**	141
5.2	**Clinical Diagnosis**	137	5.4.1	Conservative Treatment	141
			5.4.2	Surgical Treatment	142
5.3	**Radiological Diagnosis**	139		**References**	151

6. Congenital Deformities ... 153

6.1	**Etiology of Congenital Spine Anomalies**	154	**6.7**	**Spinal Dysraphism**	192
6.1.1	Normal Development of Axial Structures	154	6.7.1	Tethered Conus	196
6.1.2	Theories of the Developmental Basis of Deformities	154	**6.8**	**Congenital Spinal Deformity Syndromes**	197
6.1.3	The Pathogenesis of Congenital Vertebral Malformations	156	6.8.1	Klippel-Feil Syndrome	197
			6.8.2	VACTERL Association	198
6.2	**The Clinical Spectrum of Deformity**	159	6.8.3	Thoracic Insufficiency Syndrome	198
			6.8.4	Conditions Associated with Congenital Spine Deformities	199
6.3	**Congenital Bone Anomalies**	159			
6.3.1	Congenital Scoliosis	160		**Case Gallery**	204
6.4	**Practice Point**	176		Case 1: Multiple Hemivertebrae—T1, T8, T11	204
6.4.1	Preoperative	176		Case 2: Hemivertebrae Plus Contralateral Bar	206
6.4.2	Surgical Technique	179		Case 3: Lower Lumbar/Lumbosacral Anomalies	207
6.5	**Congenital Kyphosis**	180		Case 4: Thoracic Meningocele	208
6.5.1	Natural History	181			
6.5.2	Congenital Cord Deformities	187		**References**	211
6.6	**Congenital Lordosis**	191			

7. Neuromuscular Deformities ... 215

7.1	**Introduction**	216	7.2.2	The Spine in Cerebral Palsy	218
7.2	**Cerebral Palsy**	216	**7.3**	**Poliomyelitis**	221
7.2.1	General Orthopaedic Principles	217	7.3.1	The Spine in Poliomyelitis	222

7.4	The True Neuromuscular Diseases of Childhood	224	7.6	Scoliosis in the True Neuromuscular Diseases	228
7.4.1	Spinal Muscular Atrophy	224	7.6.1	Spinal Muscular Atrophy	228
7.5	Peripheral Neuropathies, Friedreich's Ataxia, and Arthrogryposis Multiplex Congenita	225	7.7	The Other True Neuromuscular Diseases	229
			7.8	Duchenne Muscular Dystrophy	229
7.5.1	The Peripheral Neuropathies	225		Case Gallery	232
7.5.2	The Muscular Dystrophies	226		Case 1	232
7.5.3	Congenital Myopathies	227			
7.5.4	Familial Dysautonomia	227		References	233
7.5.5	Malignant Hyperpyrexia	227			

8. Deformities Associated with Neurofibromatosis ... 237

8.1	Introduction	238	8.4.1	Scoliosis	242
			8.4.2	Kyphosis	245
8.2	Axial Skeletal Lesions in Neurofibromatosis	239	8.5	Cervical and Cervicothoracic Spine Deformities	247
8.3	Spinal Deformities in Neurofibromatosis	239			
8.3.1	Pattern of Deformity	239		Case Gallery	249
8.3.2	Neurological Involvement	241		Case 1: Thoracolumbar Kyphosis	249
8.4	Management of Spinal Deformities in Neurofibromatosis	242		References	250

9. Spinal Deformity due to Tumors ... 253

9.1	Intradural Tumors	254	9.2.4	Treatment of the Postlaminectomy Kyphosis in Association with Intradural Tumors	260
9.1.1	Clinical Features	254			
9.1.2	Investigations	255			
9.1.3	Treatment of Intramedullary Tumors	255	9.3	Extradural Tumors	260
9.2	Syringomyelia	256	9.3.1	Osteoid Osteoma and Osteoblastoma	260
			9.3.2	Giant Cell Tumor	263
9.2.1	Spinal Deformity in Association with Intradural Neoplasms and Syringomyelia	257	9.4	Tumor-like Lesions	266
9.2.2	Management of the Scoliosis Associated with Intradural Neoplasms and Syringomyelia	259	9.4.1	Aneurysmal Bone Cyst	266
			9.4.2	Eosinophilic Granuloma	266
9.2.3	Deformities Associated with the Treatment of Intradural Tumors	259		References	266

10. Miscellaneous Conditions Associated with Spine Deformities ... 269

10.1	Heritable Disorders of Connective Tissue	270	10.2	Skeletal Dysplasias	280
10.1.1	Osteogenesis Imperfecta: Brittle Bone Syndrome	270	10.2.1	Achondroplasia	280
10.1.2	Marfan Syndrome	272	10.2.2	Spondyloepiphyseal Dysplasia Tarda	284
10.1.3	Mucopolysaccharidoses	275		References	284
10.1.4	MPS IV: Morquio's Syndrome	275			

11. Spondylolysis and Spondylolisthesis ... 287

11.1	Introduction	288	11.2.2	Isthmic	289
			11.2.3	Degenerative	291
11.2	Etiology and Radiology	288	11.2.4	Traumatic	292
11.2.1	Dysplastic	288	11.2.5	Pathological	292

Contents

11.3	**The Terminology and Measurement of Spondylolisthesis** 293	
11.4	**The Marchetti and Bartolozzi (M-B) Classification** 294	
11.5	**Mac-Thiong and Labelle's Classification** .. 296	
11.6	**Clinical Features and Treatment** 299	
11.6.1	Dysplastic Spondylolisthesis 299	
11.7	**Practice Points** 301	

11.7.1 Reduction, Fixation, and Fusion of Severe Dysplastic Spondylolisthesis 301

11.8 Intertransverse Fusion 302

11.8.1 Spondylolysis 303
11.8.2 Isthmic Spondylolisthesis 305
11.8.3 Degenerative Spondylolisthesis 306
11.8.4 Pathological Spondylolisthesis 307

References 307

Index 311

Foreword

In 1988, in his foreword to Leatherman and Dickson's *The Management of Spinal Deformities*, Robert Owen, the renowned Professor of Orthopaedic Surgery from Liverpool, noted that in medieval times intimate collaboration between master and apprentice was widely understood as required for transferring knowledge and skills to the next generation. He stated that the Leatherman/Dickson text represented this pattern with Kenton Leatherman (Louisville) representing the artist/master craftsman and Dickson serving in the apprentice role (having taken a sabbatical year with the renowned Leatherman in Louisville).

Rather than matching a master and his apprentice, the current text represents the lifetime experience of two masters of "spine thinking" and surgery, Professors Robert Dickson of Leeds, United Kingdom, and Professor Juergen Harms of Germany. As Dickson notes in the preface, he has had a lifelong interest in understanding the three-dimensional nature of spinal deformity, particularly emphasizing what Roaf (Liverpool) and Somerville (Oxford) had described. They appreciated that thoracic scoliosis represents a lordotic pattern rather than the "kyphosis" that had long been incorrectly applied to a typical teenager with scoliosis. It should be noted that parallel studies of the three-dimensional nature of scoliosis were occurring in French centers during the same time frame.

Dickson has devoted his lengthy career toward better understanding the architecture of spinal deformity and its surgical treatment possibilities as well as eloquently describing (in both oral and written methods) the nature of spinal deformity to the "scoliosis community." Dickson's succinct presentations and "floor commentary" at the Scoliosis Research Society over the last three decades have brilliantly illuminated our field.

This text's co-author, Juergen Harms, Professor of Orthopaedic Surgery, Ethianum Clinic Heidelberg, Germany, represents the pinnacle of understanding both spinal deformity and its surgical management. His ability to safely treat even the most severe forms of deformity has drawn visitors and fellows from throughout the world to his center. When I visited other major European teaching hospitals, and was presented with an extreme case, the discussion frequently ended with "we did not know what to do so we sent it to Professor Harms" (with an almost certain positive final outcome). As a result of Harms' immense contributions to the scoliosis world, the world's most esteemed spine surgery outcomes research organization is named after him —"The Harms Study Group."

Masters of an art or craft appreciate a good apprentice, but even more greatly value meeting someone who has a similarly sophisticated understanding of a complex field or problem. Such was the case in 1988, when Dickson first met Harms at a 1988 Portuguese Orthopaedic Association meeting in Oporto. Professor Harms notes that prior to listening to Professor Dickson's talk in Oporto, he did not really understand the new thinking regarding the full understanding of the sagittal profile in scoliosis. He remains indebted to Dickson for opening his eyes to this concept. He considers that he himself was the "apprentice" and Professor Dickson the "mentor" in this case. They subsequently shared a common bond in understanding the true nature of spinal deformity in three dimensions, which led to a strong friendship and professional collaboration. Professors Dickson and Harms have worked together in some capacity in the past, including both of them serving as subeditors of the 2010 Harms Study Group textbook entitled *Idiopathic Scoliosis—The Harms Study Group Treatment Guide* (lead editor Peter Newton). This informative textbook included many subsidiary contributors, thus not allowing full insight into Dickson/Harms "scoliosis thinking."

About a year ago, I heard "through the grapevine" that Dickson and Harms were planning to combine their energy in producing a textbook that would present a combined lifetime experience in understanding and treating spinal deformity. I assumed that this would be a standard "multi-authored, many contributors" treatise that harnesses the energy of one's disciples (contributions by prior fellows, colleagues, etc.) to minimize the workload of the senior authors. I was surprised and delighted to find that Dickson and Harms planned to write a full textbook without contributors.

The 1988 text by Leatherman and Dickson (mentioned above) represented the first comprehensive English language textbook that accurately described the true nature of idiopathic scoliosis deformity. Although read and recognized by the cognoscenti, the text was less widely distributed and appreciated than it deserved considering its keen intellectual content. Fortunately, nearly 30 years later, Dickson reappears (along with Harms) to create this current brilliant synthesis.

During this time period, wonderful new developments in digital production and illustration, which are exemplified in the current text published by Thieme, have evolved. The expressive writing style, clear illustrations, and classic teaching cases make reading the book a pleasant journey.

For example, the use of a vertically positioned and rotated hotel-style coat hanger, demonstrating the need for Stagnara's views to determine true curve severity, brilliantly symbolizes the hundreds of "keys to understanding" found in this book. Each chapter concludes with an "international" bibliography.

The great effort and energy required to create this important work during the closing years of two remarkable careers represents an intellectual gift to the spine community (they could have just enjoyed golf or their horses). Rarely does one experience a combined summation of two masters' "lifetime understanding" of their craft/art. Every spine surgery trainee, fellow, practicing surgeon, and even esteemed "senior professor" will want to read this landmark textbook.

Dennis R. Wenger, MD
Clinical Professor of Orthopaedic Surgery
University of California San Diego
Director, Pediatric Orthopaedic Training Program
Rady Children's Hospital San Diego
San Diego, California, USA

Preface

The wonderful world of the study and treatment of scoliosis and other spinal deformities has attracted an increasing number of orthopaedic surgeons and, indeed, individuals from other disciplines. Accordingly, knowledge has advanced considerably from the turn of the century when the great pioneers began a revolution in their management. The past 10 years in particular have seen an exponential increase in the variety of procedures —and, specially, instrumentations—that can be performed for virtually all types of spinal deformities. Indeed, there can be few branches of orthopaedic surgery where so much development has occurred so quickly. Therefore, in order for the learning spinal surgeon to select safely from this ever-expanding array of metalwork and techniques and, in particular, to understand why one or another treatment should or should not be embarked upon, a sound knowledge of the underlying basic principles and a philosophy of management form an essential infrastructure.

It is the *what*, the *why*, and the *when* rather than the *how* that are the most important factors governing safe and competent practice and so we all the while emphasize these points throughout the text.

The spine surgeon can then complement this firm base with increasing clinical exposure so that the process of experience adds the further important ingredients of clinical responsibility combined with technical ability. We trust therefore that our joint venture, *Modern Management of Spinal Deformities*, reflects this sort of orderly sequence of information.

Robert Dickson, ChM, FRCS, DSc
Juergen Harms, MD

Acknowledgments

We would both give very many thanks to Mrs. Helen Radcliffe, Professor Dickson's personal assistant, who has carefully typed and input every word of the text.

R.D. would like to thank the Trustees of the Yorkshire Children's Spine Foundation (YCSF): Sir James Hill Bt, Mr. Edgar Price FRCS, Mr. Colin Hall, Mr. Robin Lee, Mrs. Susan Burgess, Mr. Chris Coughlin, and Mr. David Sharples. A special thanks to the YCSF for their help in raising thousands of pounds for research into the cause and treatment of spinal deformities in children.

R.D. would also like to thank the research fellows and associates from the Leeds Scoliosis Study Group who have carried out so much research work into spinal deformities in children: Ian Archer, John Lawton, Paul Walker, Phil Deacon, Malcolm Smith, Brian Flood, Rowan Poole, David Dempster, Alistair Stirling, John Cruickshank, Peter Millner, Dr. M. Koike, Dr. D. Tanni, Neil Oxborrow, Frank Howell, Jim Mahood, and Drs. Richard Hall and Ruth Wilcox (now both Professors at the Institute of Medical and Biological Engineering, University of Leeds).

R.D. would like to thank in particular his friend and coauthor Juergen Harms for allowing us to use so many of his excellent scoliosis cases to illustrate this book.

J.H. would like to thank three people in particular who have influenced his understanding of scoliotic deformities: his coauthor and friend, Bob Dickson; Klaus Zielke, who helped him understand the complexity of scoliosis and encouraged him to step into anterior scoliosis correction; and John Hall, who stimulated him to try to understand the complexity of congenital deformities and encouraged him as well to use anterior procedures to treat those.

Robert Dickson, ChM, FRCS, DSc
Juergen Harms, MD

About the Authors

Robert (Bob) Dickson

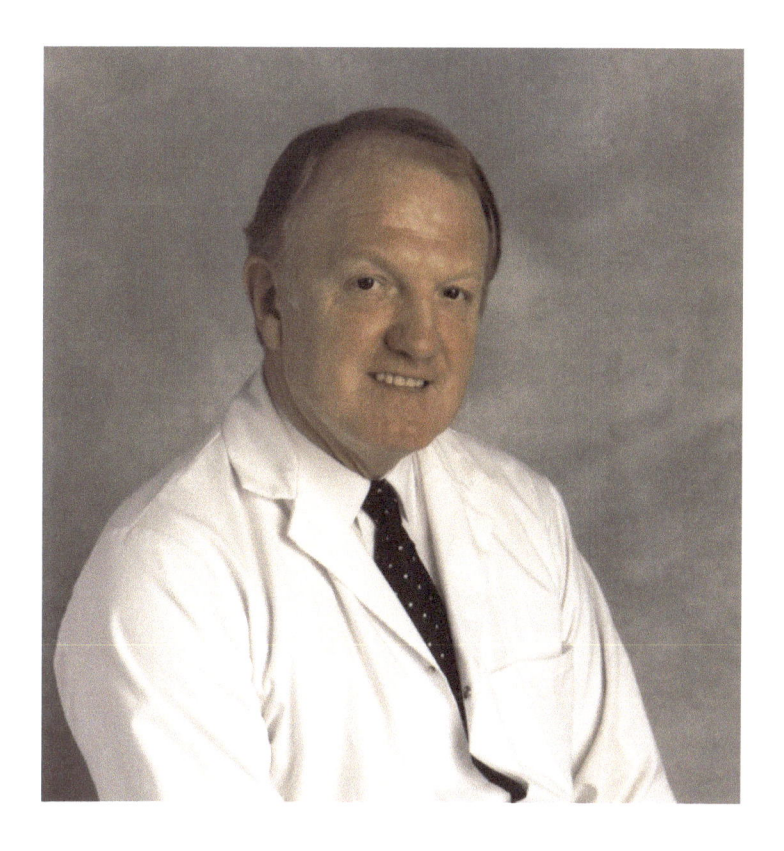

1961–1967	Studied medicine at the University of Edinburgh Medical School.
1967–1968	House surgeon in orthopaedic trauma to Professor J. I. P. James, the Royal Infirmary of Edinburgh.
1968–1969	Assistant lecturer in anatomy, University of Manchester Medical School.
1969–1972	Training in general and plastic surgery, Hammersmith Hospital, London.
1972–1975	Training orthopaedic and trauma surgery, The Nuffield Orthopaedic Centre and the Radcliffe Infirmary, Oxford.
1975–1976	Fellowship in Spine Surgery with Dr. K. D. Leatherman, Louisville, Kentucky.
1976–1980	Clinical Reader and Consultant Orthopaedic Surgeon, The Nuffield Orthopaedic Centre, Oxford.
1989	Appointed Professor of Orthopaedic Surgery, The University of Hong Kong but unfortunately was unable to take up this post.
1991–present	Professor of Orthopaedic Surgery, University of Leeds, Consultant Orthopaedic Spine Surgeon, St. James's University Hospital, Leeds and the Leeds General Infirmary. Bob was attracted to Leeds, which is England's third largest city after London and Birmingham, and St. James's University Hospital, Leeds is the biggest teaching hospital in Europe (Guinness Book of Records). He was told it was one of the happiest environments to work in, and his more than a quarter century of work there readily confirmed that.

Bob eschewed private practice, devoting his nonclinical time to research into spinal deformities, particularly the etiology and pathogenesis of idiopathic scoliosis, upon which he had published more than anyone else, as well as developing novel three-dimensional approaches to treatment. During the latter part of his clinical career and in retirement, Bob could not avoid being Dean of the Faculty of Medicine and Dentistry in the University of Leeds, Chairman of the Professional Conduct Committee of the General Medical Council, and Chairman of the Council of Management at the *Journal of Bone and Joint Surgery*.

About the Authors

Juergen Harms

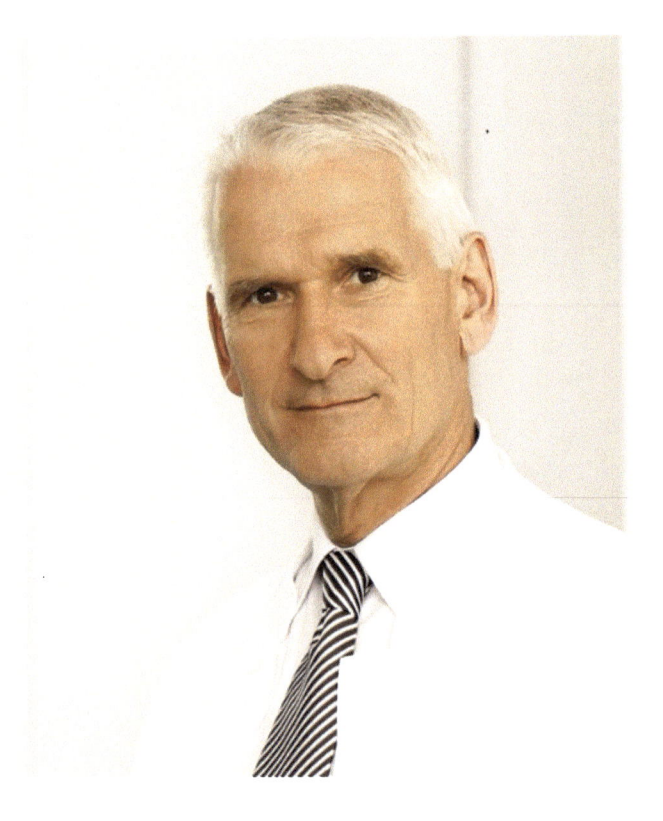

1963–1968	Studied medicine in Frankfurt/M. and Saarbrücken, Germany.
1968–1973	General and trauma surgery and training in Neuburg/Donau and Ludwigshafen, Germany.
1973–1980	Training in orthopaedic and trauma surgery at University Hospital Homburg/Saar.
1978	Professor of Orthopaedic Surgery.
1980–2011	Head of Spine Surgery SRH Klinikum Karlsbad-Langensteinbach. Developed new surgical techniques and implant systems in spine, which became state-of-the-art in spine surgery and remain so till today.
2011–present	Ethianum Clinic Heidelberg, Consultant Spine Surgeon, Heidelberg, Esslingen, Hanover, and Achern.

Juergen has always been active in spinal research throughout his career, developing new surgical techniques and implant systems, many of which have become state-of-the-art in spine surgery today. He is an authority on cervical spine surgery, including transoral cases which now total more than 300. In his "retirement" he sold all his horses and stables and now does even more spinal surgery than he ever did, while his wife plays golf.

The Harms Study Group (HSG) was conceived in the 1990s comprising Juergen and a variety of North American scoliosis surgeons, most already well known, principally to generate new ideas about scoliosis management but also to utilize their collective data so as to maximize patient numbers for some of the different operative procedures and conditions that they all treated. They were administered and generally kept in check by Michelle Marks and Bo Jamieson. Bob was very pleased when the group asked him to become an honorary member to contribute and help edit the HSG textbook on idiopathic scoliosis which was published in 2012. The HSG meetings also offer the opportunity for help and advice about complex cases, particularly from Juergen, and so the activities of the HSG are mutually beneficial to all parties.

Bob and Juergen are the same age and first met when they both gave guest lectures at the Portuguese Orthopaedic Association in Oporto in 1988. They immediately realized that they shared a common bond of understanding spinal deformities in three dimensions, with particular reference to the front of the spine and the important need for anterior spinal procedures in the management of different spinal deformities, as is well demonstrated in this text. A strong bond of friendship developed long before the HSG was established.

Chapter 1

The Beginnings of Surgery for Spinal Deformities

1.1	The Early Days	2
1.2	Posterior Instrumentation	3
1.3	Anterior Instrumentation	8

1 The Beginnings of Surgery for Spinal Deformities

1.1 The Early Days

For more than two millennia various contraptions, casts, and braces have been used in an attempt to correct or improve spinal deformities with no success whatsoever with the exception of serial plaster casts for early-onset (infantile) idiopathic scoliosis and extension braces or casts for Scheuermann's disease. In the fifth century BC Hippocrates described scoliosis for the first time and used a distraction apparatus in an attempt to correct the deformity.[1] In the second century AD Galen coined the terms scoliosis, kyphosis, and lordosis and treated scoliosis by chest binding and spinal jackets.[2] There was no advancement in the Dark Ages (500 to 1000 AD) except that hunch-backed patients were regarded as heretics and, like criminals, were put on the rack.[3] Ambrose Paré used external breast plates while André recommended proper tables and chairs, periods of recumbency, braces, and corsets.[4] The Le Vacher brothers introduced the Minerva cast for the treatment of tuberculosis of the spine and an extension chair with vertical traction and lateral pressure straps for scoliosis.[5] Meanwhile, Venel, in 1780, developed a day brace and traction at night.[6]

Sayre, in 1877, described his technique of suspension casting.[7] He became president of the American Medical Association. Then, in 1876, Adams (of the forward bend test) much more importantly performed careful dissection of cadavers with idiopathic scoliosis thus recognizing the importance of lordosis at the curve apex. This was the most important observation about scoliosis in the entire 19th century if not the 20th as well. He went to the United States with Lister to watch Sayre.[8]

Meanwhile, in the 1940s, Walter Blount in Milwaukee developed the brace that bears the city's name.[9,10] This was specifically to support the poliomyelitis collapsing spine after surgery and to prop up the spine pressure was applied against the occiput and chin above and the pelvis below. It was never designed for any other use but it was soon used as the nonoperative treatment for idiopathic scoliosis. Then an underarm orthosis was devised by John Hall in Boston.[11] Patients were imprisoned in these braces for as many as 23 hours a day for years. This practice continued for the next 20 or 30 years and no one dared challenge this Draconian regimen.[12] Soon, however, retrospective studies[13,14] confirmed that such braces were of no value in mitigating the progression of idiopathic scoliosis. The proponents did not like this one bit.

Then the ravages to the spine of tuberculosis, and poliomyelitis in particular, led to the introduction of surgery for spinal deformities. The first surgical attempts were in the mid to late 19th century and Delpech[15] and Guerin[16] were enthusiasts for the use of tenotomy. Guerin operated on 740 patients using tenotomy and claimed that 358 were completely cured while 287 benefitted. However, 77 did not benefit and 18 died![16] In 1889 Volkmann carried out rib resection and this is thought to be the first known scoliosis surgery on bony structures.[17]

Then, in 1895, Roentgen discovered X-rays[18] and although he won the Nobel Prize it could well be argued that reducing the three-dimensional scoliosis deformity to two dimensions on a radiograph was a major factor in preventing further development of an understanding of the pathogenesis of idiopathic scoliosis despite Adams' original dissection and his subsequent statement that "lordosis plus rotation equals lateral flexion"[8]—a statement continually ignored through the years.

Berthold Hadra first applied implants to the spine in the nature of spinous process wiring in 1891.[19] Then, in 1902, Fritz Lange implanted metal rods attached to the spinous processes with slings of silk.[20] These implants were of course for tuberculosis of the spine. Wreden in Germany was the first to apply metal implants to the spine to treat scoliosis.[21] This treatment consisted of rib resection followed by an extension bed and then the application of metal plates to the spinous processes. Although bone grafts to the skeleton had been applied in 1682 to repair a soldier's skull[22] and in 1878 to rebuild a boy's humeral shaft[23]; the first time that this was done to the spine was by Albee in the United States[24] and De Quervain in Europe in 1911.[25] They both applied cortical struts to the spine to treat tuberculosis. Albee used a tibial strut graft in the curve concavity keying it to the spine with pieces of bone (▶ Fig. 1.1).

Next Russell Hibbs in New York described his subperiosteal dissection of the spine right out to the facet joints and base of the transverse processes and, having excised the facet joints, then raised bone flaps in the process thus conjoining adjacent vertebrae with bone graft.[26] Then, in closing, he put the periosteum back over the fusion area and this technique is precisely the same as that used today. It should always be remembered that spinal fusion is a biological operation and that the addition of metalwork is to obtain and maintain a correction until the fusion has matured. As with skin grafting, for example, it is the recipient area that is all important and so it is with bone grafting. Skin grafts don't "take" on bare cortical bone and nor do bone grafts. Nowadays with the insertion of a profusion

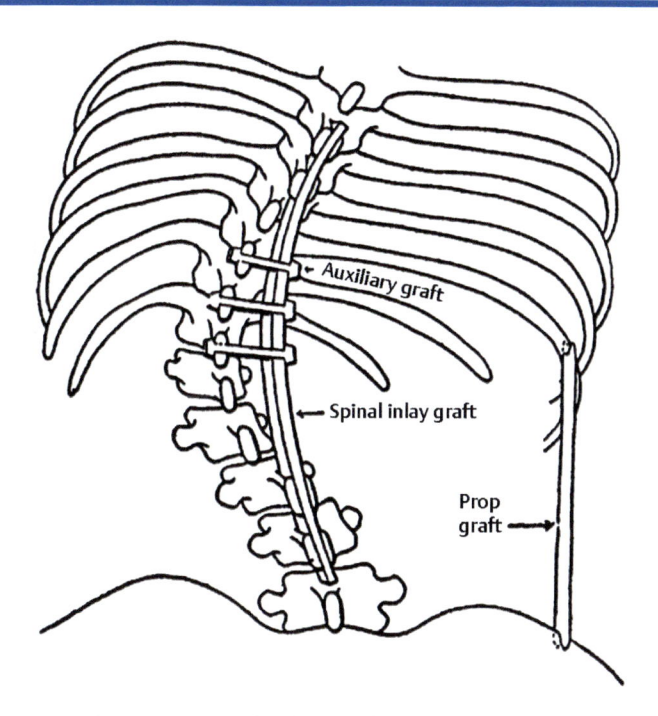

Fig. 1.1 Albee's spinal operation. A bone-distracting cortical graft on the concave side acts like a distraction rod attached to the spine by horizontal bone keys. (Reproduced with permission from Newton P, O'Brien M, Shufflebarger H, et al. Idiopathic Scoliosis: The Harms Study Group Treatment Guide. Stuttgart/New York: Thieme; 2010: 3.)

of metalwork, the biological nature of the procedure tends to be relegated. All non–load-bearing cortical bone (i.e., not supporting metalwork) must be meticulously decorticated out to the tips of the transverse processes so that whatever bone graft material inserted has an optimal chance of being incorporated. Inserting metalwork and then throwing in a handful of bone graft material as an afterthought is not the way to produce a sound spinal fusion. Hibbs stated that "the dissection was in a practically dry field without injury to the muscles." This was carried out between 1914 and 1919 on 59 patients, most of whom were polio patients who had undergone preoperative traction. Extraordinarily, there was only a 2% mortality rate.

Then in 1931 Hibbs, Risser, and Ferguson went on to report on 360 cases treated surgically over a 13-year period.[27] The aim was to prevent progression and this was achieved in almost half the cases with about a third having an increase in deformity because of too short a fusion. Risser along with Hibbs designed a turnbuckle cast which they began to use in 1920 with traction and bending preoperatively. Notwithstanding, all was not good, and in 1929 Steindler gave up spinal fusion because of a 60% pseudarthrosis rate.[28] However, in 1943, Howorth reported 600 cases with only a 14% pseudarthrosis rate.[20] In the early 1950s Risser developed his localizer cast and these were used before surgery with a window cut out of the back of the cast to perform Hibbs' fusion operation.[29]

Then, in 1941, the American Orthopaedic Association reviewed the surgical treatment of scoliosis in 425 cases.[30] There was a 28% pseudarthrosis rate and an even greater rate of complete loss of correction so that the end result was that 70% were rated fair or poor and only 30% good or excellent. Then the great polio epidemics of the mid-20th century yielded many scoliosis cases and in 1952 Cobb reported on 672 patients treated surgically with a 4% pseudarthrosis rate.[31]

1.2 Posterior Instrumentation

Then came the Harrington revolution in 1962 with his two-rod distraction and compression instrumentation which still remains the basis of modern day scoliosis surgery.[32] He first performed his procedure on these polio cases without fusion, with the Milwaukee brace applied postoperatively. Then Moe, in 1966, reported on 173 patients treated by the Harrington technique versus 100 treated by Risser localizer casting and fusion and the achievement of greater correction with the Harrington instrumentation and a similar pseudarthrosis rate but a greater rate of infection.[33] However, results overall were considered to be very good. Harrington continued to improve his results and reported almost 600 cases in 1973 recommending a long fusion from above and below the end vertebrae so that the whole of the structural deformity was included.[34] Unfortunately, because the three-dimensional nature of the deformity was not appreciated, the rotational component (rib or loin hump) was not corrected (▶ Fig. 1.2).

Then segmental instrumentation came into fashion with Resina and Alves in Portugal adding wiring to the Harrington rod.[35] This was followed by the important advance of Luque in Mexico in 1982 with his two L-rod system attached to the spine with sublaminar wires[36] (▶ Fig. 1.3). For paralytic curves that require the pelvis to be stabilized, Alan and Ferguson devised the technique known as the Galveston technique with the short L of the rod passing across the back of the pelvis.[37] However, rather like original Harrington instrumentation, this was applied to the frontal plane of the patient and so the three-dimensional nature of the deformity and in particular the apical lordosis was not addressed although it is the most important part of this three-dimensional deformity.

Then in both France and England came the appreciation of the importance of derotation of the spine rather than addressing the frontal plane. The Leeds group deliberately

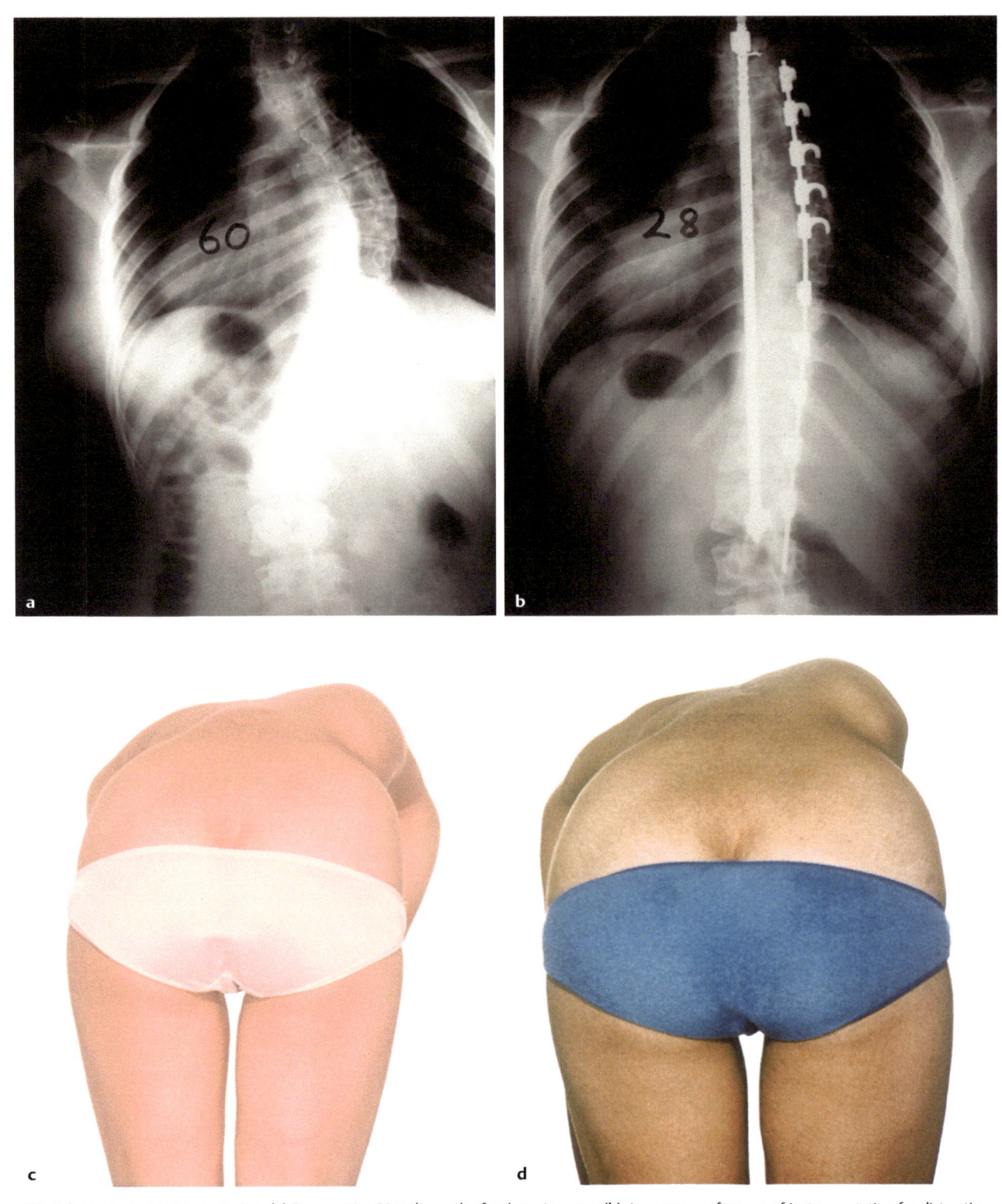

The Beginnings of Surgery for Spinal Deformities

Fig. 1.2 Harrington instrumentation. (a) Preoperative PA radiograph of a thoracic curve. (b) Appearance after use of instrumentation for distraction and compression, showing a significant improvement in the frontal plane. (c) Rib hump before surgery. (d) Rib hump 2 years after surgery, showing that the deformity in the transverse plane has remained unaltered. (Reproduced with permission from Newton P, O'Brien M, Shufflebarger H, et al. Idiopathic Scoliosis: The Harms Study Group Treatment Guide. Stuttgart/New York: Thieme; 2010: 5.)

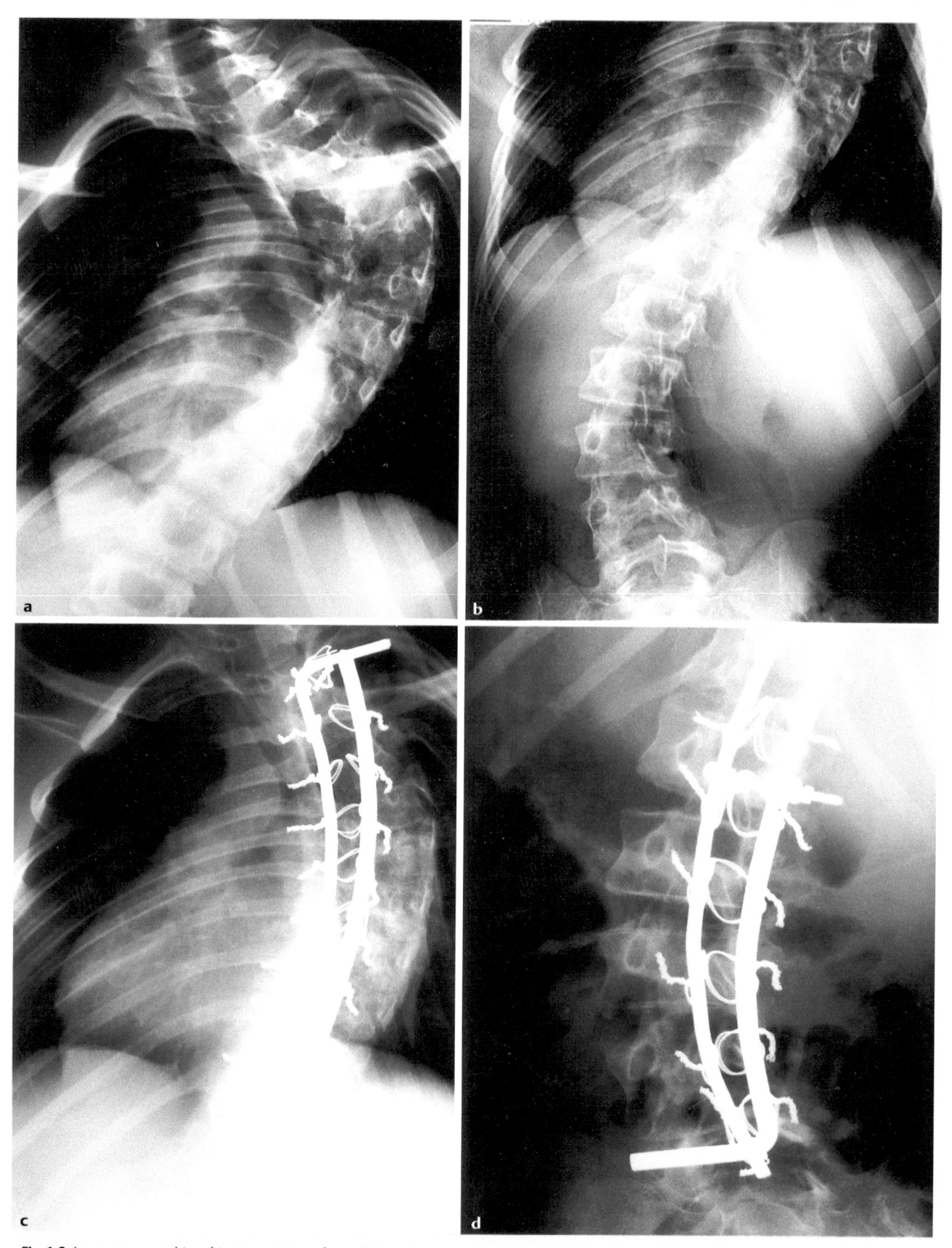

Fig. 1.3 Luque segmental L-rod instrumentation for a child with Friedreich's ataxia. (a,b) PA radiograph before surgery. (c,d) PA radiograph after instrumentation. (Reproduced with permission from Newton P, O'Brien M, Shufflebarger H, et al. Idiopathic Scoliosis: The Harms Study Group Treatment Guide. Stuttgart/New York: Thieme; 2010: 6–7.)

bent the Harrington rod into kyphosis in the thoracic region so that the concave sublaminar wires would lift the depressed apical region[38–40] (▶ Fig. 1.4). Of course this is only applicable to fairly simple, flexible curves with a Cobb angle of, say, less than 50 degrees. The asymmetric apical prisms are not so tightly locked together that they cannot be untwisted with the concave side elevated by the simple application of metalwork. However, the more rigid the deformity becomes—and therefore the more the Cobb angle is beyond 50 degrees—a simple application of posterior metalwork cannot affect the apical region. No correction was possible and so it was quite obvious that space had to

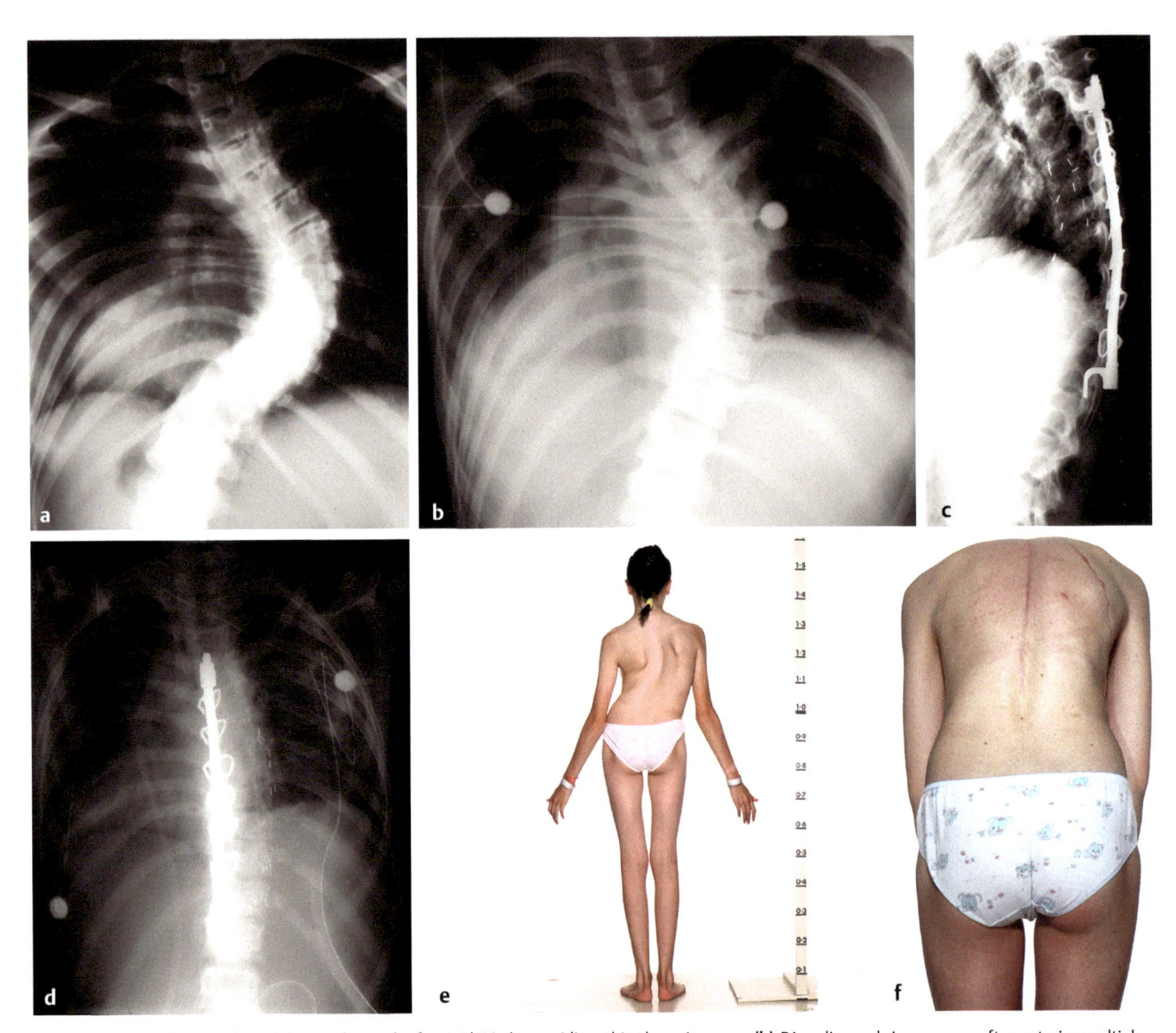

Fig. 1.4 The Leeds procedure. **(a)** PA radiograph of a rigid 90-degree idiopathic thoracic curve. **(b)** PA radiograph in recovery after anterior multiple discectomy (five disks removed). This is not an anterior release but a deliberate lordosis reducing procedure to allow correction of the deformity. There has already been a 70% correction of the Cobb angle simply from spontaneous shortening of the leading edge of the spinal deformity and allowing it to collapse into itself. **(c)** In the second stage of instrumentation, the rod has been prebent to restore kyphosis, and the concave sublaminar wires now pull backward to derotate the spine. **(d)** PA view after instrumentation, showing almost complete restoration of rotation and rib symmetry.
(e) Preoperative PA view of the patient's severe deformity. **(f)** Postoperative appearance, showing virtually complete correction. We had never seen such superb corrections of such severe rigid deformities. (Reproduced with permission from Newton P, O'Brien M, Shufflebarger H, et al. Idiopathic Scoliosis: The Harms Study Group Treatment Guide. Stuttgart/New York: Thieme; 2010: 7–8.)

The Beginnings of Surgery for Spinal Deformities

be made available between the individual vertebrae to produce flexibility and this was achieved by anterior multiple diskectomy in a first stage and now, when followed by posterior instrumentation, the deformity was just as correctable as with the simple, flexible less-than-50-degree curves as was first described by the Leeds group[40] and is the crucially important part of the strategy behind the Leeds procedure. Now corrections of curves up to a 100 degrees or more was obtained and often the associated deformity was completely corrected. The strategy behind the Leeds procedure is further discussed at the end of Chapter 3.

However, in France, a very ingenious method was developed by Yves Cotrel and Jean Dubousset (CD instrumentation)[41] (▶ Fig. 1.5). This was a two-rod system and attached initially to the spine by hooks and then by pedicular screw fixation. The idea was to de-rotate the spine by placing one of the rods into a bit of scoliosis and then rotate the spine in the hooks into the sagittal plane to lift the depressed concavity. This segmental form of instrumentation was the forerunner of the present generation spinal instrumentation. Nowadays for idiopathic scoliosis it is fashionable to use posterior rods with transpedicular fixation at each level, dragging even bigger and more rigid curves into line (▶ Fig. 1.6).

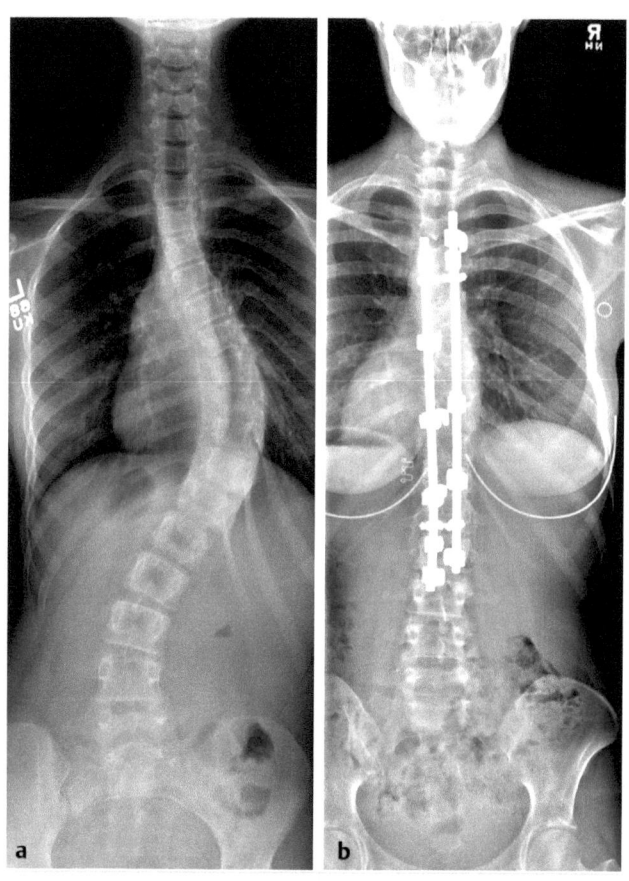

Fig. 1.5 Cotrel-Dubousset instrumentation. **(a)** PA radiograph of a thoracic curve. **(b)** PA radiograph after Cotrel-Dubousset instrumentation. (Reproduced with permission from Newton P, O'Brien M, Shufflebarger H, et al. Idiopathic Scoliosis: The Harms Study Group Treatment Guide. Stuttgart/New York: Thieme; 2010: 9.)

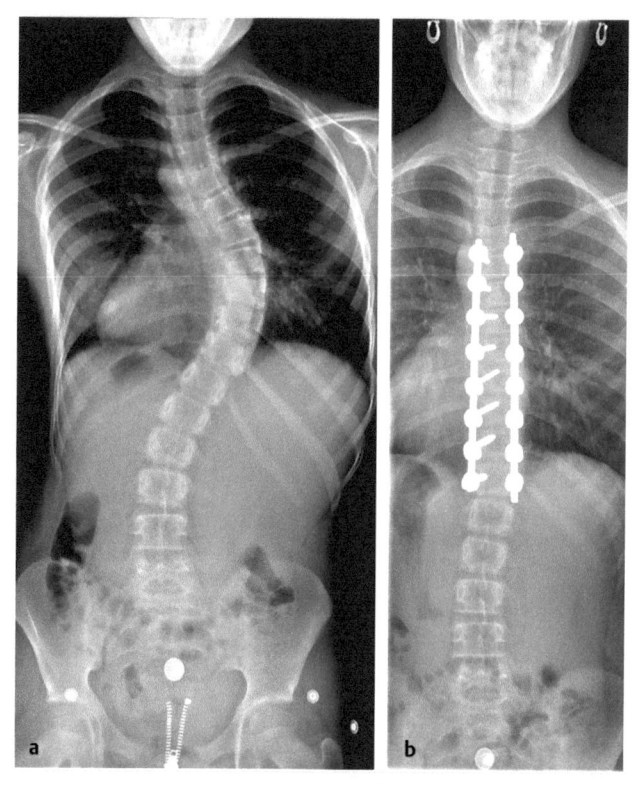

Fig. 1.6 Transpedicular fixation. **(a)** PA radiograph of a thoracic curve. **(b)** Appearance after use of end-vertebra-to-end-vertebra bilateral transpedicular screw instrumentation. (Reproduced with permission from Newton P, O'Brien M, Shufflebarger H, et al. Idiopathic Scoliosis: The Harms Study Group Treatment Guide. Stuttgart/New York: Thieme; 2010: 9.)

The Beginnings of Surgery for Spinal Deformities

1.3 Anterior Instrumentation

Meanwhile, pari passu with the development of posterior approaches for spinal deformity, anterior spinal surgical procedures also were developed and had certain advantages. In 1934 Ito described anterior approaches for tuberculosis of the spine[42] which were then further advanced in Hong Kong by Arthur Hodgson—again, for treating tuberculosis of the spine.[43] The disease was effectively excised and strong strut grafts from the pelvis or rib were inserted to replace the deficit. Then Hodgson[44] turned to scoliosis but his "opening wedge osteotomy" stretched the spinal cord with an unacceptably high rate of paralysis. Anterior resection for congenital vertebral anomalies goes back to 1928 with Royle[45] and then with Von Lackum and Smith[46] and Wiles.[47] Real progress in the management of rigid spinal curves was not made until Leatherman in Louisville, Kentucky, developed a closing wedge osteotomy for spinal curves with great success and minimal neurological complications[48] (▶ Fig. 1.7). Nowadays osteotomies can be done from the back only.[49] However, for tuberculosis or other spinal infections and for secondary metastatic spinal disease, there is no substitute for an anterior approach so as to really thoroughly excise disease, decompress the spinal cord, and rebuild the anterior and middle columns properly.

Anterior instrumentation became very popular with the introduction by Dwyer from Australia of the instrumentation technique that bears his name.[50] The intervertebral disks were first removed across the apex and then transverse screws were passed across the vertebral body, these screws having a hollow head to receive a cable. The cable was shortened by compressing the screw heads so that the anterior length of the spine was reduced and thus the scoliosis corrected (▶ Fig. 1.8). He introduced it for idiopathic thoracolumbar and lumbar scoliosis but most scoliosis surgeons approached this technique with caution and first applied it to neuromuscular disorders. Then Zielke in Germany modified the Dwyer system using a threaded compression rod in place of the braided cable and this was the forerunner of modern anterior systems[51] (▶ Fig. 1.9). It was Harms who promoted the concept of kyphosing the thoracic spine with anterior instrumentation[52] for idiopathic thoracic scoliosis

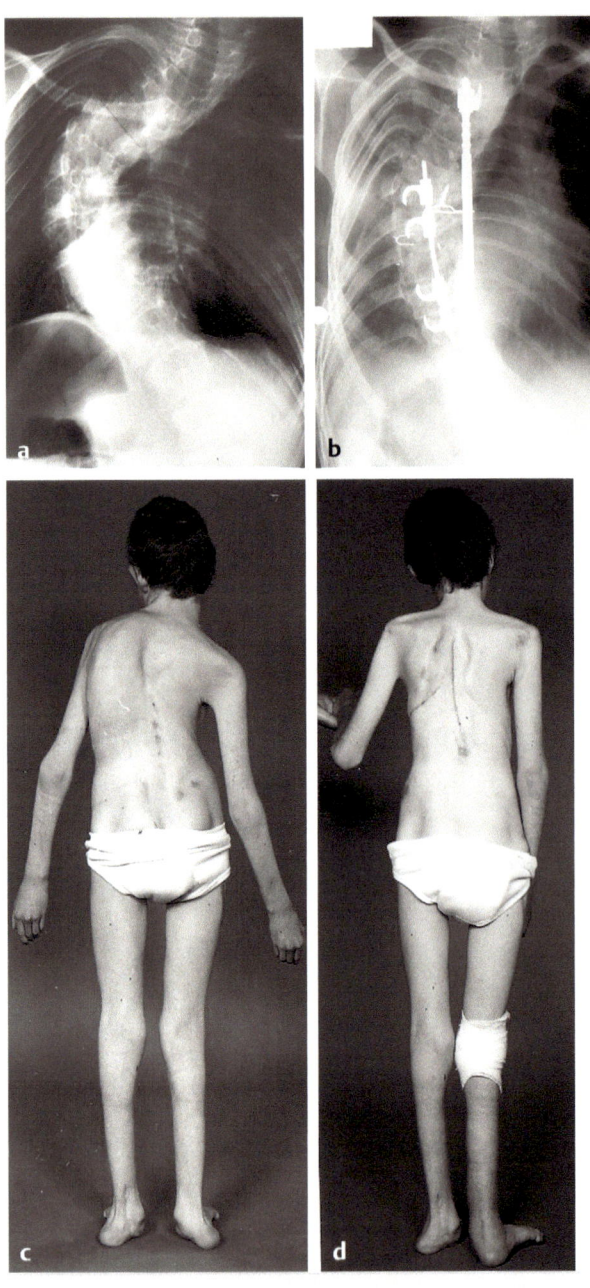

Fig. 1.7 Leatherman two-stage wedge resection. (a) PA radiograph of a severe rigid thoracic curve. (b) PA radiograph after apical wedge resection, the wedge being first closed by the compression system before further stabilization with a distraction rod. (c) Clinical photograph of the patient's severe deformity before surgery. (d) View showing excellent correction after surgery. (Reproduced with permission from Newton P, O'Brien M, Shufflebarger H, et al. Idiopathic Scoliosis: The Harms Study Group Treatment Guide. Stuttgart/New York: Thieme; 2010: 10.)

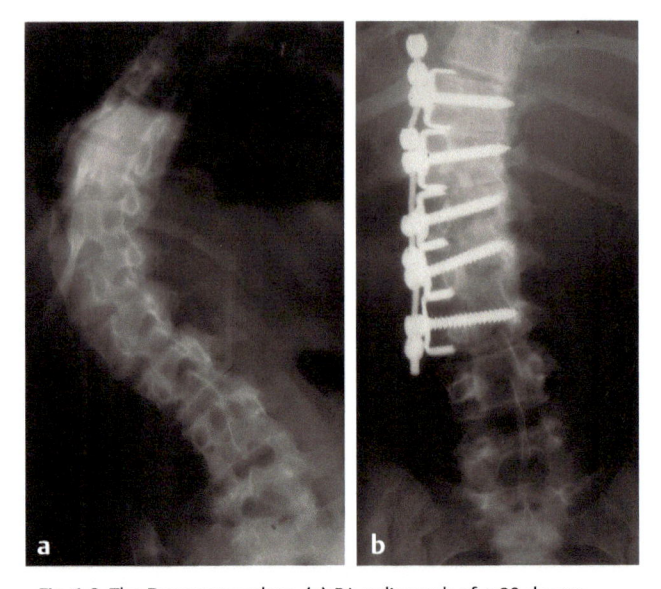

Fig. 1.8 The Dwyer procedure. (a) PA radiograph of a 90-degree thoracolumbar curve. (b) PA radiograph 2 years later, showing excellent correction with only four intervertebral joints fused. (Reproduced with permission from Newton P, O'Brien M, Shufflebarger H, et al. Idiopathic Scoliosis: The Harms Study Group Treatment Guide. Stuttgart/New York: Thieme; 2010: 11.)

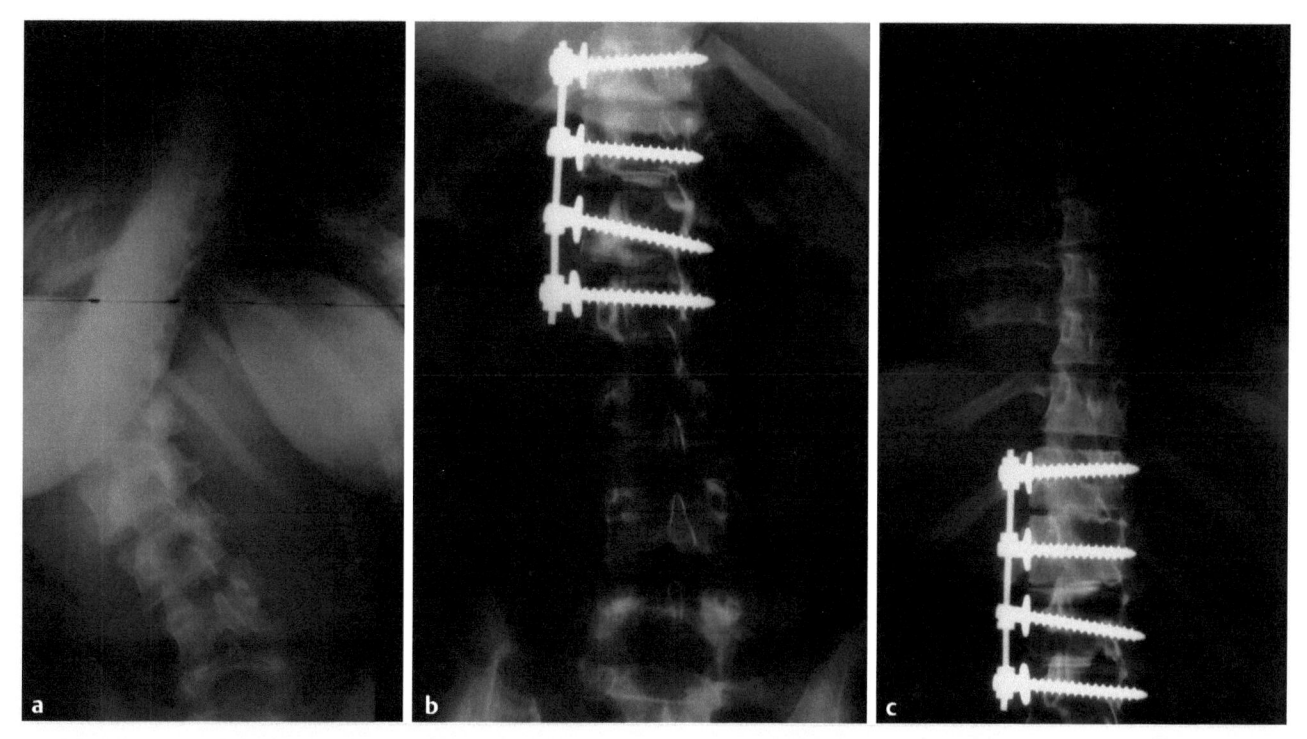

Fig. 1.9 The Zielke procedure. **(a)** PA radiograph of a 70-degree thoracolumbar curve. **(b,c)** PA radiograph 2 years postoperative. The entire thoracolumbar spine has been restacked with the use of only four screws and fusion of only three intervertebral joints. (Reproduced with permission from Newton P, O'Brien M, Shufflebarger H, et al. Idiopathic Scoliosis: The Harms Study Group Treatment Guide. Stuttgart/New York: Thieme; 2010: 12.)

(▶ Fig. 1.10). This of course makes enormous sense because it is the front of the spine in structural scoliosis that is too long and thus by removing disks and shortening the front of the spine the deformity was corrected in all three dimensions.

Using the phrase "anterior release" implies that the true three-dimensional nature of the deformity is still not appreciated. You cannot release the front of the spine in a lordoscoliosis because the front of the spine is too long, not too short. Thus, the rationale for an anterior approach is not to "release" it but to shorten it by multiple diskectomy and then letting it collapse into itself (the Leeds procedure) to re-create kyphosis followed by, if that is the option, anterior instrumentation to fully approximate the vertebrae after diskectomies, and thereby correct the deformity in all planes. This is not just paying lip service to physiological sagittal curves but a deliberate kyphosing strategy so as to correct the deformity in all three planes. Importantly, with removal of the growth plates also, anterior growth over the apical region has been stopped so that recurrence of the deformity is prevented.

Nowadays nearly every deformity, however big and stiff, is dealt with by posterior surgery alone although there are many cases where an anterior approach is clearly the better option. In addition, of course the spine is not easily shortened by posterior surgery and it will be interesting to see reliable neurological complication data, because undue lengthening of the spine was the prime cause of paralysis in the days of Harrington instrumentation and provided the rationale behind the wake up test.[53] If there was a neurological concern then the distraction rod could be detensioned by loosening or removing it completely to allow the best environment for neurological recovery. To put it bluntly, that was precisely why Stagnara introduced the wake up test because if the toes wouldn't wiggle then you only had a few hours to save the situation. Meanwhile, we have not encountered this problem by approaching anteriorly because the spinal cord is not stretched. We now, of course, use electrophysiological monitoring of the cord that tells us how the cord is functioning throughout surgery.[54]

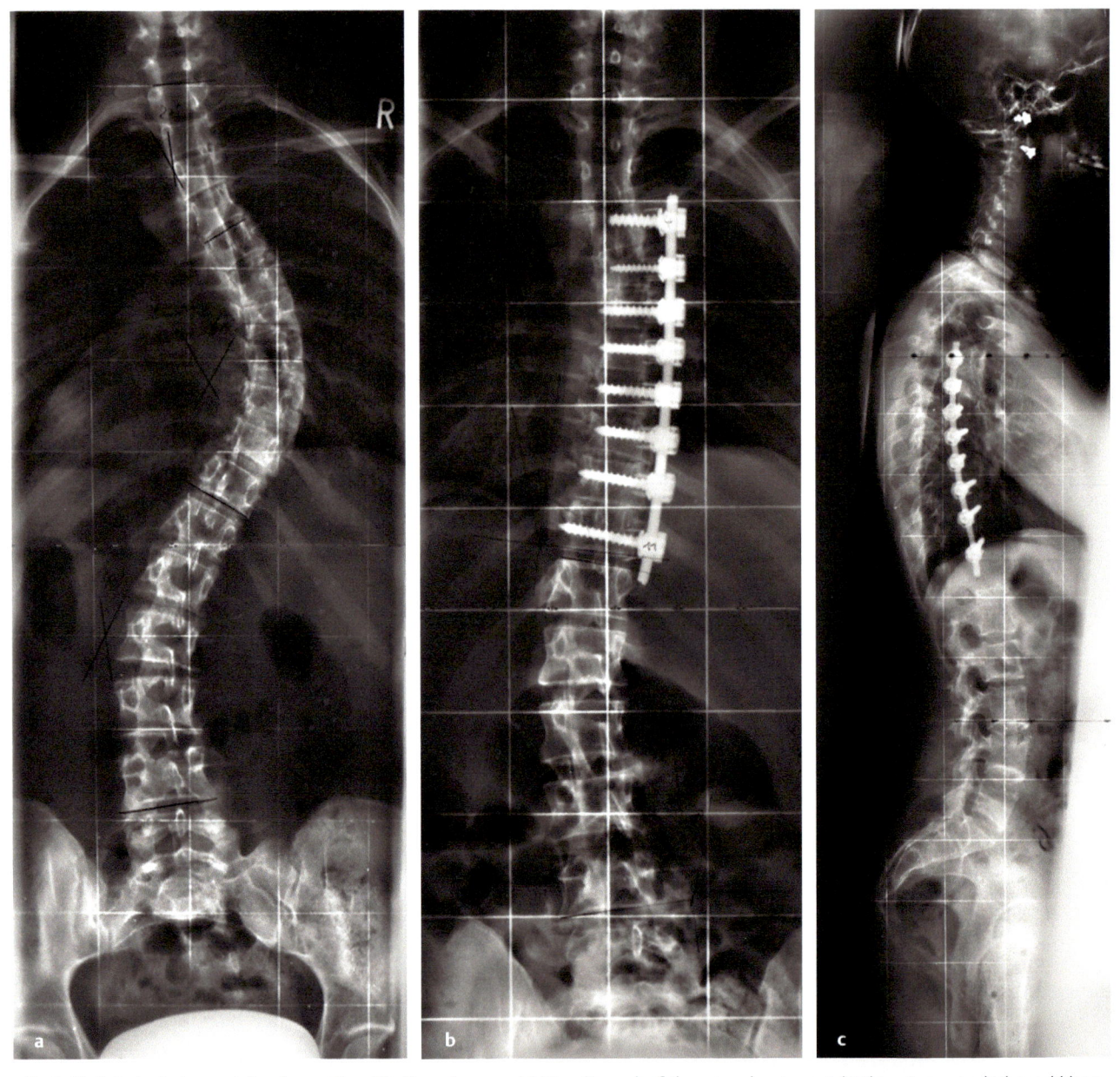

Fig. 1.10 Anterior instrumentation for an idiopathic thoracic curve. (a) PA radiograph of the spine showing a right thoracic curve which would be a Lenke type 1AL curve. (b) PA radiograph after anterior instrumentation of the thoracic curve showing a perfectly balanced mild S-shaped configuration. Note there is no residual rotation of the thoracic curve and prefect rib symmetry indicating a full three-dimensional correction. (c) Lateral radiograph showing restoration of a gentle thoracic kyphosis, a key part of this procedure.

References

Note: References in **bold** are Key References.

[1] Jones WHS. Hippocrates (4 vols). London: Heinemann; 1922–1931
[2] Huebert HT. Scoliosis. A brief history. Manit Med Rev. 1967; 47(8):452–456
[3] Kumar K. Spinal deformity and axial traction. Spine. 1996; 21(5):653–655
[4] Moen KY, Nachemson AL. Treatment of scoliosis. An historical perspective. Spine. 1999; 24(24):2570–2575
[5] **Rang M. The story of orthopaedics. Philadelphia: WB Saunders; 2000**
[6] Böni T, Rüttimann B, Dvorak J, Sandler A. Jean-André Venel. Spine. 1994; 19(17):2007–2011
[7] Sayre JW. Lewis Albert Sayre. Spine. 1995; 20(9):1091–1096
[8] **Adams W. Lectures on the pathology and treatment of lateral and other forms of curvature of the spine. London: Churchill and Sons; 1865**
[9] **Blount WP. Scoliosis and the Milwaukee brace. Bull Hosp Jt Dis. 1958; 19:152–165**
[10] Blount WP, Moe JH. The Milwaukee Brace. Baltimore: Williams & Wilkins; 1973
[11] Watts HG, Hall JE, Stanish W. The Boston brace system for the treatment of low thoracic and lumbar scoliosis by the use of a girdle without superstructure. Clin Orthop Relat Res. 1977(126):87–92
[12] Carr WA, Moe JH, Winter RB, Lonstein JE. Treatment of idiopathic scoliosis in the Milwaukee brace. J Bone Joint Surg Am. 1980; 62(4):599–612
[13] Miller JAA, Nachemson AL, Schultz AB. Effectiveness of braces in mild idiopathic scoliosis. Spine. 1984; 9(6):632–635
[14] Goldberg CJ, Dowling FE, Hall JE, Emans JB. A statistical comparison between natural history of idiopathic scoliosis and brace treatment in skeletally immature adolescent girls. Spine. 1993; 18(7):902–908
[15] Rang M. The story of orthopaedics. Philadelphia: WB Saunders; 2000:334

[16] Rang M. The story of orthopaedics. Philadelphia: WB Saunders; 2000:160
[17] Hall JE. Spinal surgery before and after Paul Harrington. Spine. 1998; 23 (12):1356–1361
[18] Rang M. The story of orthopaedics. Philadelphia: WB Saunders; 2000:22–23
[19] Rang M. The story of orthopaedics. Philadelphia: WB Saunders; 2000:417–421
[20] **Howorth MB. Evolution of spinal fusion. Ann Surg. 1943; 117(2):278–289**
[21] Wreden. Zentralorgan der gesellschaft der gesamten chirurgie und ihrer grenzgebiete. Berlin: J. Springer;1923:434
[22] Rang M. The story of orthopaedics. Philadelphia: WB Saunders; 2000:318
[23] Rang M. The story of orthopaedics. Philadelphia: WB Saunders; 2000: 319–321
[24] Albee F. Transplantation of a portion of the tibia into the spine for Pott's disease: A preliminary report. J Am Med Assoc. 1911; 57:885–886
[25] DeQuervain F, Hoessly H. Operative immobilisation of the spine. Surg Gynecol Obstet. 1917; 24:428–436
[26] Hibbs RA. A report of fifty-nine cases of scoliosis treated by the fusion operation. By Russell A. Hibbs, 1924. Clin Orthop Relat Res. 1988; 229(229):4–19
[27] **Hibbs RA, Risser JC, Ferguson AB. Scoliosis treated by the fusion operation. End-result study of three hundred and sixty cases. J Bone Joint Surg. 1931; 13:91–104**
[28] Steindler A. Diseases and deformities of the spine and thorax. St Louis: CV Mosby; 1929
[29] Risser JC, Lauder CH, Norquist DM, Cruis WA. Three types of body casts. Instr Course Lect. 1953; 10:131–142
[30] Research Committee of the American Orthopaedic Association. End result study of the treatment of idiopathic scoliosis. J Bone Joint Surg Am. 1941; 23:963–977
[31] Cobb JR. Technique, after-treatment, and results of spine fusion for scoliosis. In: Edwards JW, ed. Instructional Course Lectures (vol. 9). Ann Arbor: American Academy of Orthopaedic Surgeons; 1952: 65–70
[32] **Harrington PR. Treatment of scoliosis. Correction and internal fixation by spine instrumentation. J Bone Joint Surg Am. 1962; 44-A:591–610**
[33] Moe JH, Valuska JW. Evaluation of treatment of scoliosis by Harrington instrumentation. J Bone Joint Surg Am. 1966; 48A:1656–1657
[34] Harrington PR, Dickson JH. An eleven-year clinical investigation of Harrington instrumentation. A preliminary report on 578 cases. Clin Orthop Relat Res. 1973(93):113–130
[35] Resina J, Alves AF. A technique of correction and internal fixation for scoliosis. J Bone Joint Surg Br. 1977; 59(2):159–165
[36] **Luque ER. Segmental spinal instrumentation for correction of scoliosis. Clin Orthop Relat Res. 1982(163):192–198**
[37] **Allen BL, Jr, Ferguson RL. The Galveston technique for L rod instrumentation of the scoliotic spine. Spine. 1982; 7(3):276–284**
[38] **Dickson RA, Archer IA, Deacon P. The Surgical Management of Idiopathic Thoracic Scoliosis. J Orthopaedic Surgical Techniques. 1985; 1:23–28**
[39] Archer IA, Deacon P, Dickson RA. Idiopathic scoliosis in Leeds: A management philosophy. J Bone Joint Surg Br. 1986; 68B:670
[40] **Dickson RA, Archer IA. Surgical treatment of late-onset idiopathic thoracic scoliosis. The Leeds procedure. J Bone Joint Surg Br. 1987; 69(5):709–714**
[41] Dubousset J, Graf H, Miladi L, Cotrel Y. Spinal and thoracic derotation with CD instrumentation. Orthop Trans. 1986; 10:36
[42] Ito H, Tsuchiya J, Asami GA. A new radical operation for Pott's disease. J Bone Joint Surg. 1934; 16:499–515
[43] Hodgson AR, Stock FE. Anterior spinal fusion a preliminary communication on the radical treatment of Pott's disease and Pott's paraplegia. Br J Surg. 1956; 44(185):266–275
[44] Hodgson AR. Correction of fixed spinal curves. J Bone Joint Surg 1965; 47: 1221–1227
[45] Royle ND. The operative removal of an accessory vertebra. Med J Aust. 1928; 1:467
[46] Von Lackum HL, Smith A de F. Removal of vertebral bodies in the treatment of scoliosis. Surg Gynecol Obstet. 1933; 53:250–256
[47] Wiles P. Resection of dorsal vertebrae in congenital scoliosis. J Bone Joint Surg Am. 1951; 33 A(1):151–154
[48] Leatherman KD, Dickson RA. Two-stage corrective surgery for congenital deformities of the spine. J Bone Joint Surg Br. 1979; 61-B(3):324–328
[49] Nakamura H, Matsuda H, Konisishi S, Yamano Y. Single-stage excision of hemivertebrae via the posterior approach alone for congenital spine deformity: follow-up period longer than ten years. Spine. 2002; 27:110–115
[50] Dwyer AF, Newton NC, Sherwood AA. An anterior approach to scoliosis. A preliminary report. Clin Orthop Relat Res. 1969; 62(62):192–202
[51] Zielke K, Berthet A. [VDS—ventral derotation spondylodesis—preliminary report on 58 cases]. Beitr Orthop Traumatol. 1978; 25(2):85–103
[52] Betz RR, Harms J, Clements DH, III, et al. Comparison of anterior and posterior instrumentation for correction of adolescent thoracic idiopathic scoliosis. Spine. 1999; 24(3):225–239
[53] Vauzelle C, Stagnara P, Jouvinroux P. Functional monitoring of spinal cord activity during spinal surgery. Clin Orthop Relat Res. 1973(93):173–178
[54] Devlin VJ, Schwartz DM. Intraoperative neurophysiologic monitoring during spinal surgery. J Am Acad Orthop Surg. 2007; 15(9):549–560

Chapter 2

Basic Principles

2.1	Definitions and Terminology	*14*
2.2	Curve Characteristics	*15*
2.3	Spinal Growth	*20*
2.4	Classification of Spinal Deformities	*23*
2.5	Primary, Progressive, or Structural Deformities	*24*
2.6	Secondary, Nonprogressive or Nonstructural Deformities	*36*

2 Basic Principles

2.1 Definitions and Terminology

Over the last several decades a spinal deformity language has evolved with which we all need to be familiar so that we can communicate with each other either by written or spoken word. This is based on the excellent work of the Scoliosis Research Society.[1] Some of the terms we have come to use have no obvious meaning, such as "nonstructural" scoliosis, and, indeed, we should probably look at many of these different terms and consider a better use of words.

2.1.1 Planes and Deformities

The spine has three planes: the frontal or coronal plane, the sagittal or lateral plane, and the transverse or axial plane (▶ Fig. 2.1). In the coronal plane the spine should be straight and if it is not then a scoliosis (lateral spinal curvature) is present (▶ Fig. 2.2). Meanwhile, in the sagittal plane there are four natural curvatures (▶ Fig. 2.2): cervical and lumbar lordoses (curvatures convex anteriorly) and thoracic and sacral kyphoses (curvatures convex posteriorly) (▶ Fig. 2.3). These curvatures in the sagittal plane develop in the early years of life. The cervical lordosis develops as infants raise their heads when they begin to look around their environment whereas the lumbar lordosis develops later when they start sitting and standing up. In the transverse plane, the vertebrae should be symmetrical but are not, even in the so-called "normal" spine.

2.1.2 Nonstructural and Structural Deformities

These terms do not describe the deformities that bear their name in any meaningful way. Nonstructural deformities would include those secondary to a leg length inequality, or secondary to muscle spasm provided by a painful focus in the spine (e.g., osteoid osteoma or adolescent disk hernia) (▶ Fig. 2.4). Structural spinal deformities are due primarily to a spinal problem and the etiological classification described later lists all the conditions associated with structural deformities. Perhaps structural deformities could be termed "primary" spinal deformities and nonstructural deformities "secondary" to some other pathological problem. There is another rather poor differentiation between nonstructural and structural deformities. Structural deformities are regarded as having a rotational component in addition to the lateral curvature and nonstructural deformities do not—however, this is often not so. Whereas structural deformities due to idiopathic scoliosis do have rotation (▶ Fig. 2.5), those with a congenital hemivertebra as the keystone to the curvature are often not associated with rotation (▶ Fig. 2.6) while leg length inequality produces a secondary nonstructural scoliosis in the lumbar spine where there is already a natural lordosis and so there is obligatory spinal rotation[2] (▶ Fig. 2.4a) (biplanar asymmetry).[3]

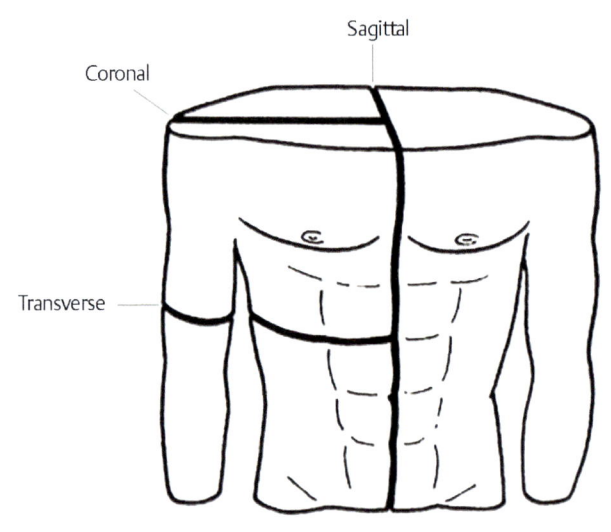

Fig. 2.1 The planes of the body. (Reproduced with permission from Newton P, O'Brien M, Shufflebarger H, et al. Idiopathic Scoliosis: The Harms Study Group Treatment Guide. Stuttgart/New York: Thieme; 2010: 17.)

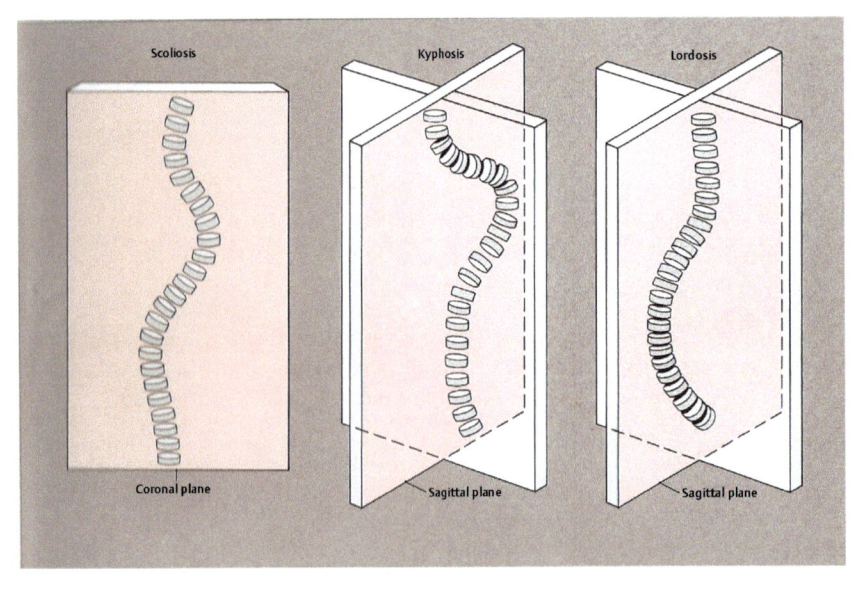

Fig. 2.2 Diagrammatic representation of deformities in the coronal and sagittal planes. (Reproduced with permission from Greenspan A. Scoliosis and anomalies with general effect on the skeleton. In: Orthopaedic Radiology. A Practical Approach. 2nd ed. London: Gower Medical Publishing; 1992: Figure 28.3.)

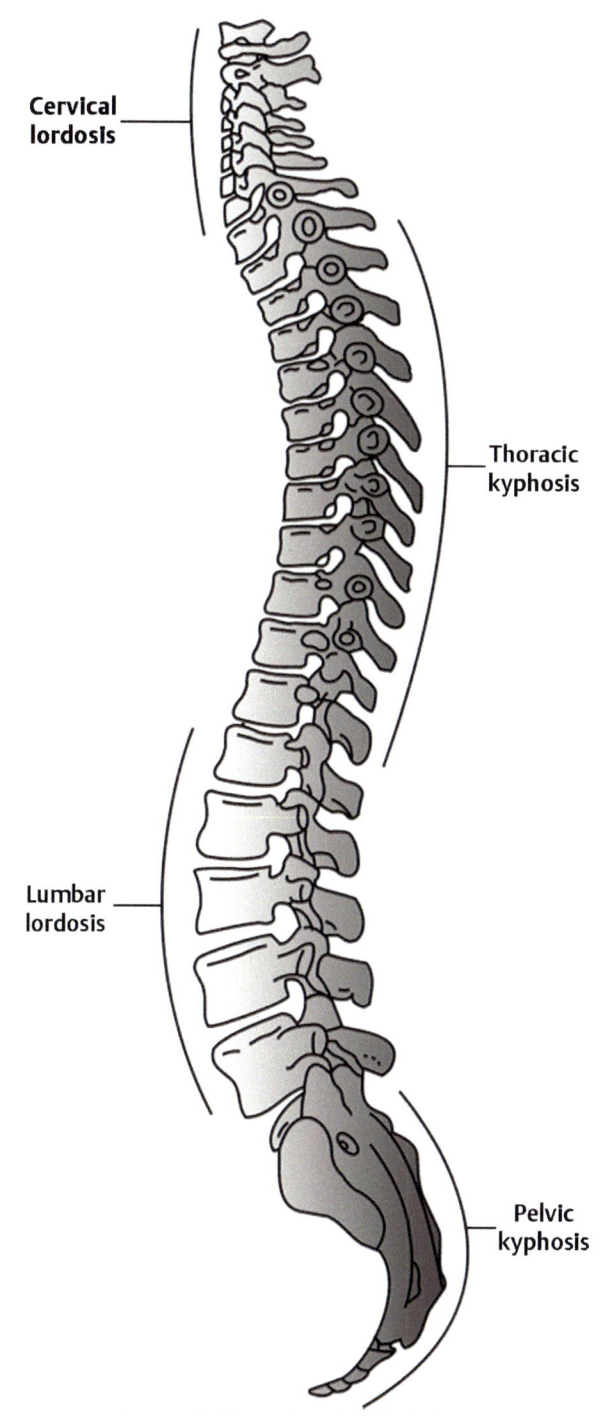

Fig. 2.3 The four natural curvatures of the spine in the sagittal plane: cervical and lumbar lordoses and thoracic and pelvic kyphoses. (Reproduced with permission from Newton P, O'Brien M, Shufflebarger H, et al. Idiopathic Scoliosis: The Harms Study Group Treatment Guide. Stuttgart/New York: Thieme; 2010: 17.)

2.2 Curve Characteristics

2.2.1 Named Vertebrae

▶ Fig. 2.7 shows the typical appearances of a moderate idiopathic thoracic scoliosis. It is customary to look at posteroanterior (PA) X-rays as we look at our patients mainly from the back (which, incidentally, reduces the radiation dosage to the developing breast and thyroid in females by first travelling through the thickness of the neck and torso[4]). The vertebrae maximally tilted at each end of the curvature are referred to as the end vertebrae, in this case T5 above and T11 below, whereas the apical vertebra is that at the center of the scoliotic curve, in this case T8. If there happens to be an even number of vertebrae in the curve then the two central vertebrae are both apical; if there is an odd number of vertebrae then there is one apical vertebra at the center of the curvature, as in this case. However, the true structural curvature extends from the first neutral (nonrotated) vertebra above to the first neutral vertebra below and these are above and below the upper and lower end vertebrae, respectively, in this case T3 above and T12 below.

2.2.2 Curve Size

Although there is more than one method of measuring curve size —such as the Ferguson[5] method of drawing longitudinal lines at the top and bottom of the curve and measuring the angle of intersection—the universal method of measuring curve size is that of Cobb.[6] Lines are drawn along the upper end plate of the upper end vertebra and the lower end plate of the lower end vertebra and these lines are then produced until they intersect and that is the Cobb angle (▶ Fig. 2.8). Of course, with mild to moderate curves these lines do not intersect on the X-ray film and thus it has been traditional to drop perpendiculars and measure the angle of intersection in that way. But it is quite unnecessary to do that and possibly damages the X-ray emulsion and so a Cobbometer is strongly recommended (based upon the Oxford Orthopaedic Engineering Centre Cobbometer, you can construct one yourself)[7] (▶ Fig. 2.9). You should have one in your pocket to measure curve size in clinic. It is not necessary to draw any lines on the X-ray film itself. Furthermore, it is far more accurate than when measurements are made drawing lines and then applying a protractor. However, nowadays, using the Picture Archiving and Communications System (PACS) or alternative X-ray system technique, there are tools available to make all the measurements which simplifies matters greatly with considerable precision.

Of course these measurements are made on a PA radiograph of the patient with each vertebra progressively more rotated toward the apex. This clearly means that the curve has rotated out of the frontal plane, mostly at the apex. The less the curve size, the closer it is to the frontal plane and the less the amount of apical rotation. A curve of 60 degrees is therefore much more than twice as big as a curve of 30 degrees because it is seen less en face. Stagnara realized this and in his scoliosis series of X-rays the really important ones were the true plan d'élection views[8] (▶ Fig. 2.10). If the apical region is rotated, say, 30 degrees from the frontal plane, then the patient is turned or the X-ray beam is turned 30 degrees so that a true AP plan d'élection view is taken. Similarly, a lateral view of the patient is not a true lateral projection and the patient or X-ray beam must now be rotated 90 degrees to the AP plan d'élection view to obtain the true lateral. Lateral views of the patient therefore appear to be more and more kyphotic with increasing curve size when of course there is no such thing as kyphoscoliosis as we shall see again later. Rotating a coat hanger and looking at it or taking photographs is a useful way of understanding the problems of spinal rotation (▶ Fig. 2.11). In simple terms the

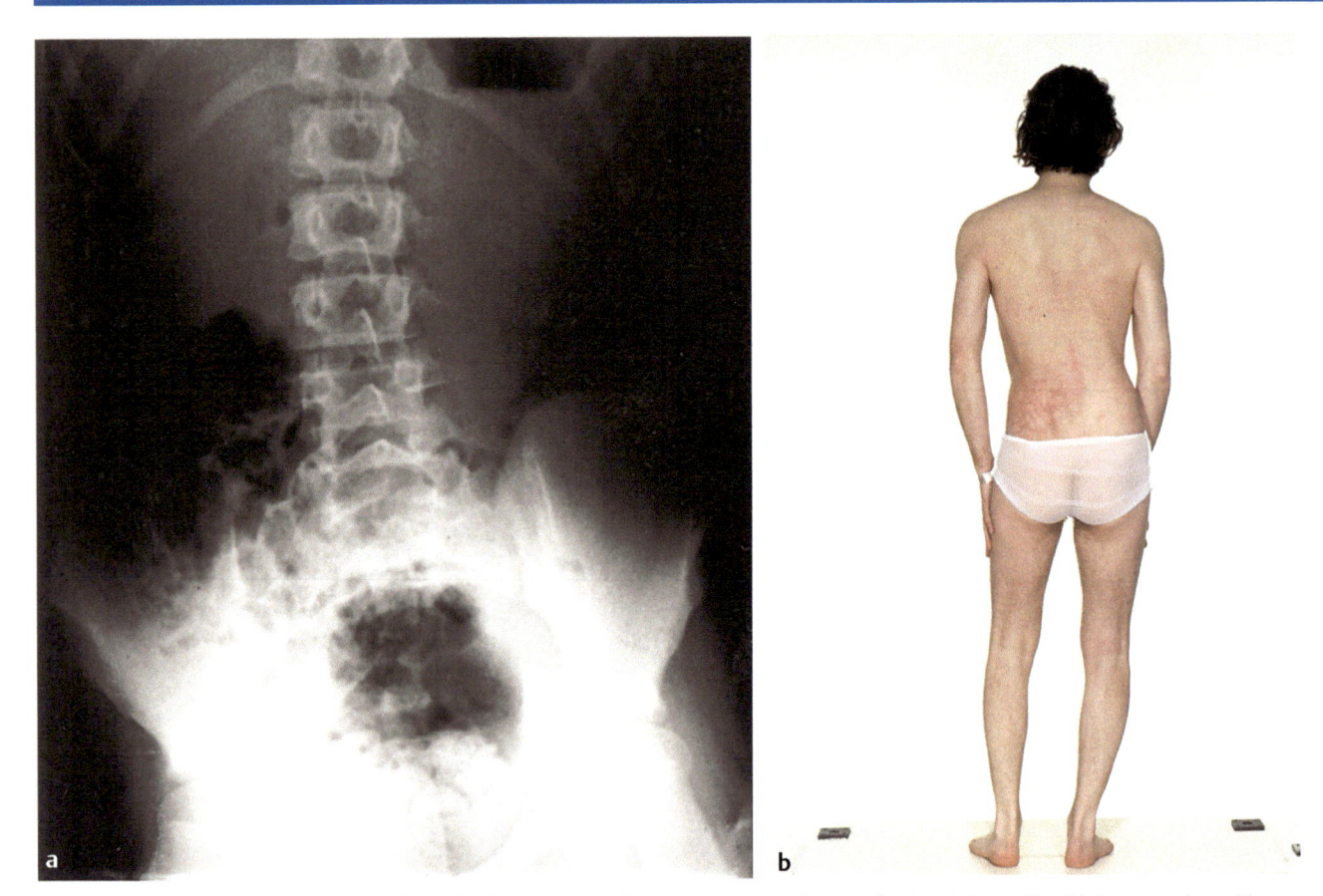

Fig. 2.4 Nonstructural scoliosis. **(a)** PA radiograph of a nonstructural lumbar curve secondary to a leg-length inequality. **(b)** A teenage boy with a nonstructural lumbar scoliosis caused by muscle spasm from an adolescent disk hernia. Note the erythema ab igne from the use of heat pads because of severe left lumbar pain. (Reproduced with permission from Newton P, O'Brien M, Shufflebarger H, et al. Idiopathic Scoliosis: The Harms Study Group Treatment Guide. Stuttgart/New York: Thieme; 2010: 18.)

Cobb angle changes its apparent magnitude simply by changing the plane of projection. Notwithstanding, inevitably, all publications about the size of a scoliosis before and after treatment use arithmetic data, means, and percentage changes that, because of the effect of rotation, are effectively meaningless. A curve that changes from 60 to 30 degrees as a result of treatment represents much more than a 50% improvement.

2.2.3 Vertebral Rotation

This is an important measurement because it provides useful information as to the severity of the deformity particularly in terms of its flexibility and thus correctability. A thoracic curve of 40 degrees with a lot of apical rotation is a much more severe clinical deformity in terms of rib hump and stiffness than a 40-degree curve with less rotation.

The method of Nash and Moe was an early technique described for recording apical vertebral rotation[9] (▶ Fig. 2.12). It is still useful and probably the best method of measuring rotation other than on three-dimensional (3D) magnetic resonance imaging (MRI) or low dose computed tomography (CT) scans using the measurement tools available on the machine. If a vertebra is not rotated, then the pedicles will be equidistant from the sides of the vertebral body. Rotation with a lordoscoliosis always occurs with the posterior elements turning toward the concavity of the curve (concordant rotation) (▶ Fig. 2.5) and therefore the convex pedicle moves farther away from the side of the vertebral body while the concave pedicle is seen progressively less well—rather like an eclipse of the sun. Nash and Moe's method is to grade the amount of rotation in pluses but it is more precise to measure the distance between the lateral side of the convex pedicle and the convex side of the vertebral body and express it as a percentage of the total width of the vertebral body.[1]

Another method of measuring rotation is using the protractor devised by Perdriolle[10] (▶ Fig. 2.13). There are a number of longitudinal lines on the protractor and the line that bisects the convex pedicle indicates the degree of rotation of that vertebra when read off from the bottom of the protractor. It has not been validated for the whole length of the spine indicating that Nash and Moe's method is preferred. Nowadays rotation can be readily measured by MRI scanning using the inbuilt measuring tools (▶ Fig. 2.14).

Another method of measuring rotation is that described by Min Mehta many years ago and is really only applicable to early onset (infantile) idiopathic scoliosis[11] (▶ Fig. 2.15). At the curve apex, the angle of the neck of the ribs subtended against a line along the vertical axis of the vertebra is measured on each side. These are referred to as the rib vertebra angles (RVAs). On the convex side the ribs droop more and thus the convex RVA is smaller than on the concave one. If the difference in the angles (the rib vertebra angle difference [RVAD]) is bigger than 20 degrees, this suggests the likelihood of a progressive curve, along with a bigger Cobb angle. This is in no way surprising, the

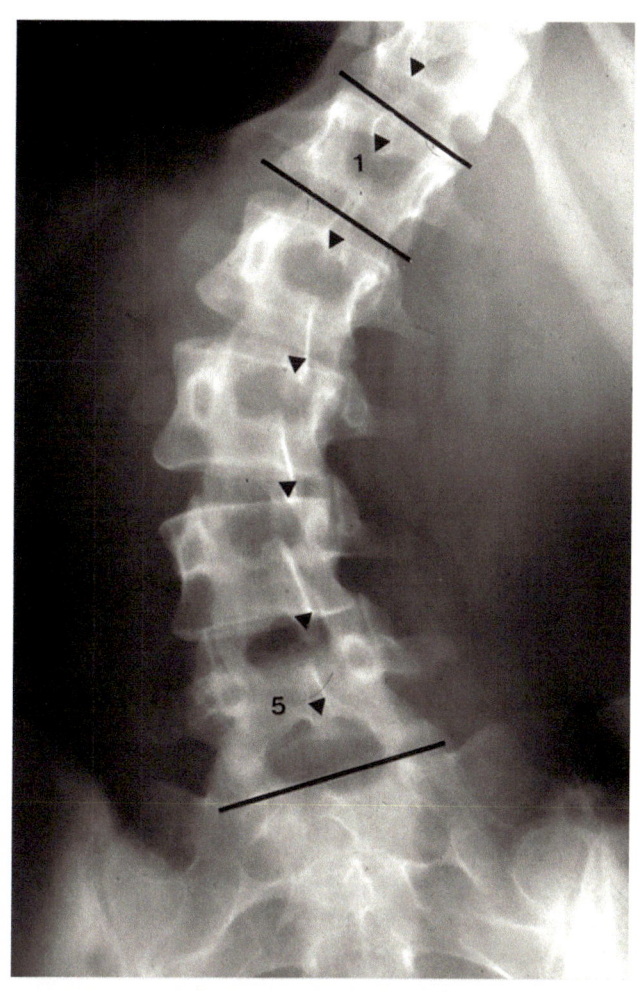

Fig. 2.5 PA radiograph of an idiopathic lumbar curve. The spinous processes have been labelled with *black triangles*, and it can be clearly seen that they rotate toward the concavity of the curve, as is always the case with structural scoliosis. The back of the spine is therefore shorter than the front and so all structural scolioses are lordoscolioses. (Reproduced with permission from Newton P, O'Brien M, Shufflebarger H, et al. Idiopathic Scoliosis: The Harms Study Group Treatment Guide. Stuttgart/New York: Thieme; 2010: 18.)

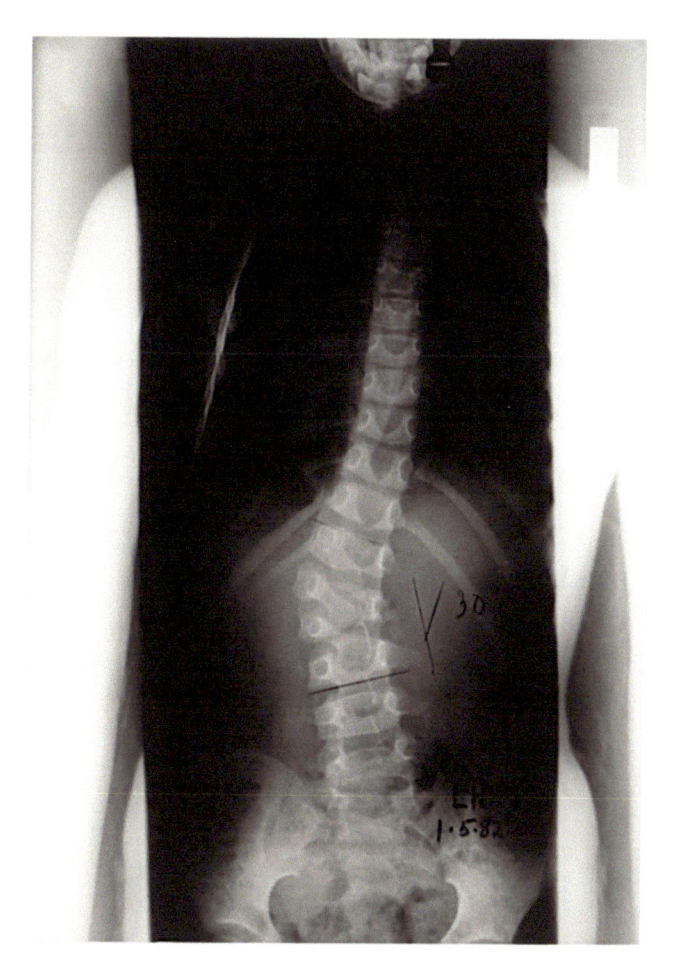

Fig. 2.6 Scoliosis due to a hemivertebra showing no rotation.

bigger the curve and the more rotation then the more likely the deformity will worsen. However, double structural infantile curves are always progressive as in ▶ Fig. 2.15c,d.

Going back to late-onset (adolescent) idiopathic scoliosis, another method of perceiving the amount of rotation is to measure the degree of *pseudokyphosis* on the lateral radiograph of the patient. As soon as the lordotic area at the apex of the curve moves out of the frontal plane it points progressively farther backward and gives the spurious appearance of kyphosis when the lateral X-ray of the patient is viewed (▶ Fig. 2.10c). It should be remembered that kyphosis means that the back of the spine points backward and in structural scoliosis it is the front of the spine moving progressively more backward as the lordosis twists out of the frontal plane. It can be readily appreciated that curves with a bigger Cobb angle have a bigger pseudokyphosis on the lateral X-ray of the patient. Thus, the lateral view of the patient is an index of the amount of scoliosis and rotation. If the PA Cobb angle is, say, 40 degrees and the amount of apical rotation 10 degrees versus a Cobb angle of 40 degrees and apical rotation of 20 degrees then the one with the apical rotation of 20 degrees will have a much bigger pseudokyphosis on the lateral X-ray of the patient and a bigger rib hump if the curve is thoracic. Thus when the Lenke classification brings in the amount of so-called kyphosis it loses its objectivity and much of its value.[12]

2.2.4 Curve Patterns

There are single, double, and multiple curve patterns (▶ Fig. 2.16). With idiopathic scoliosis it is commonly thought that the right thoracic single curve pattern is the most common but on inspection of the radiographs this is not so with vertebrae above and below the so-called major curve being rotated in the opposite direction indicating the presence of a double or multiple curve pattern. The paper by Cruickshank et al. on this subject is well worth studying.[13] If the apex of the curve is in the thoracic region (T2 to T11) then it is described as a thoracic curve. It is nearly always at T7 to 9. Thoracolumbar curves have the apex at T12 or L1 whereas cervicothoracic curves have their apex at C7 or T1. Lumbar curves are apical from L2 to L4 (nearly always at L2) and the unusual lumbosacral curve is apical at L5 or S1. Double curves tend to be thoracic and thoracolumbar/lumbar whereas the common classic thoracic double major is a double curve with a thoracic curve and a cervicothoracic curve

Basic Principles

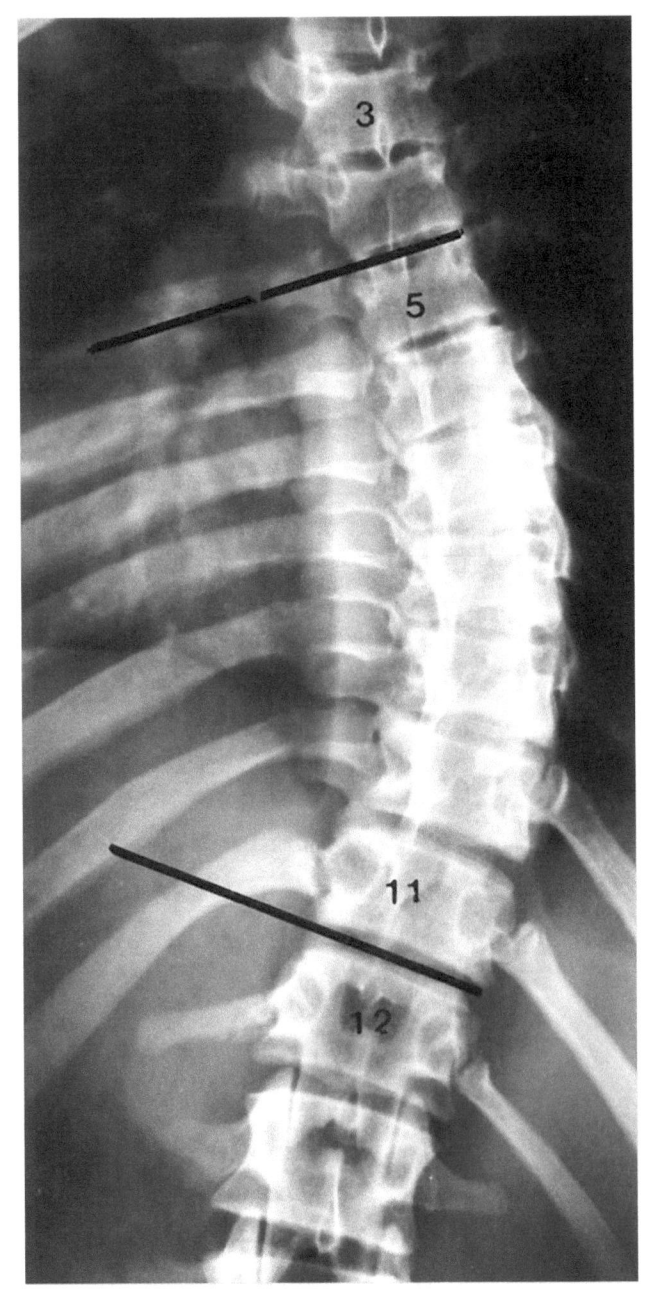

Fig. 2.7 PA radiograph of an idiopathic thoracic curve. Again, being a structural curve, there is rotation with the spinous processes turning toward the curve concavity. The end vertebrae for Cobb angle measurement (the most tilted vertebrae at the top and bottom of the curve) are T5 above and T11 below. The first neutral vertebra above is T3, two above the upper end vertebra; T12 is the lower neutral vertebra. The apical vertebra is T8. (Reproduced with permission from Newton P, O'Brien M, Shufflebarger H, et al. Idiopathic Scoliosis: The Harms Study Group Treatment Guide. Stuttgart/New York: Thieme; 2010: 19.)

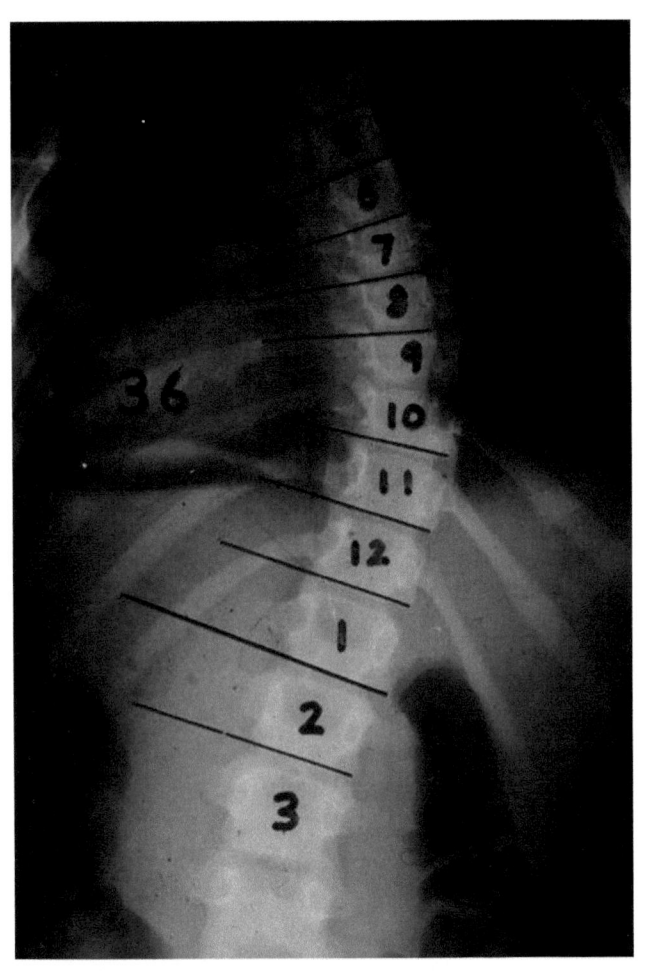

Fig. 2.8 PA radiograph of a right thoracic curve with lines drawn along the lower borders of the vertebrae below the apex and the upper borders of the vertebrae above the apex showing that it is easy to pick out maximally tilted end vertebrae, namely T6 and L1.

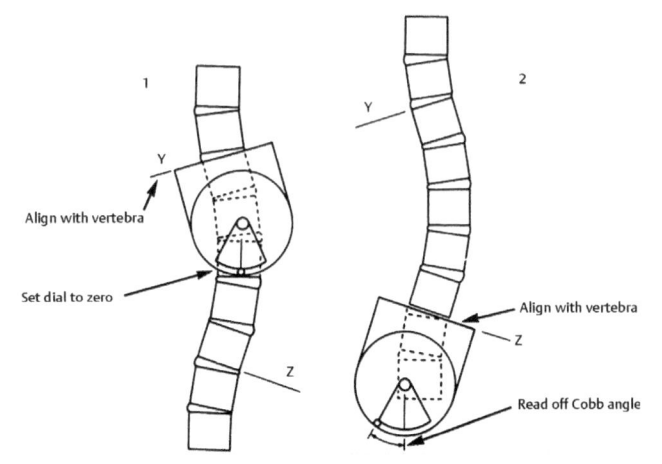

Fig. 2.9 Measuring the Cobb angle with the Oxford Cobbometer (a protractor with a vertical free hanging needle). The upper border of the instrument is first aligned with the upper surface of the upper end vertebra, and the protractor dial is set to zero. When the upper border of the instrument is then aligned with the lower surface of the lower end vertebra, the needle gives the Cobb angle. (Reproduced with permission from Newton P, O'Brien M, Shufflebarger H, et al. Idiopathic Scoliosis: The Harms Study Group Treatment Guide. Stuttgart/New York: Thieme; 2010: 19.)

above[14] (▶ Fig. 2.17). Moe was the first to describe the importance of this curve because if there is a right thoracic curve as the major curve and a cervicothoracic above this in the opposite direction then the shoulders will be tilted with the left shoulder higher than the right (the signe d'épaule[15]). It would be inappropriate just to deal with the thoracic curve surgically and, thus, by improving that only, there would necessarily be further

Basic Principles

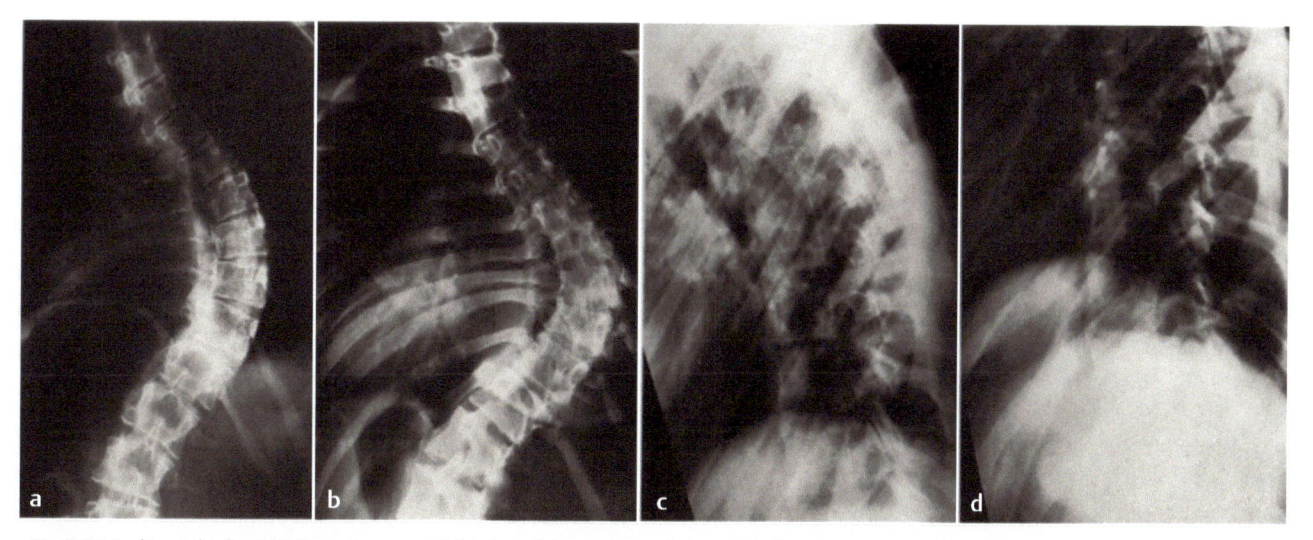

Fig. 2.10 Radiograph of a right thoracic curve. **(a)** PA view of the patient. **(b)** A true PA plan d'élection view showing a much bigger curve. **(c)** Lateral view of the patient showing the spurious appearance of kyphosis. **(d)** True lateral view, showing the essential lordosis. These are all views of the same deformity! (Reproduced with permission from Newton P, O'Brien M, Shufflebarger H, et al. Idiopathic Scoliosis: The Harms Study Group Treatment Guide. Stuttgart/New York: Thieme; 2010: 20.)

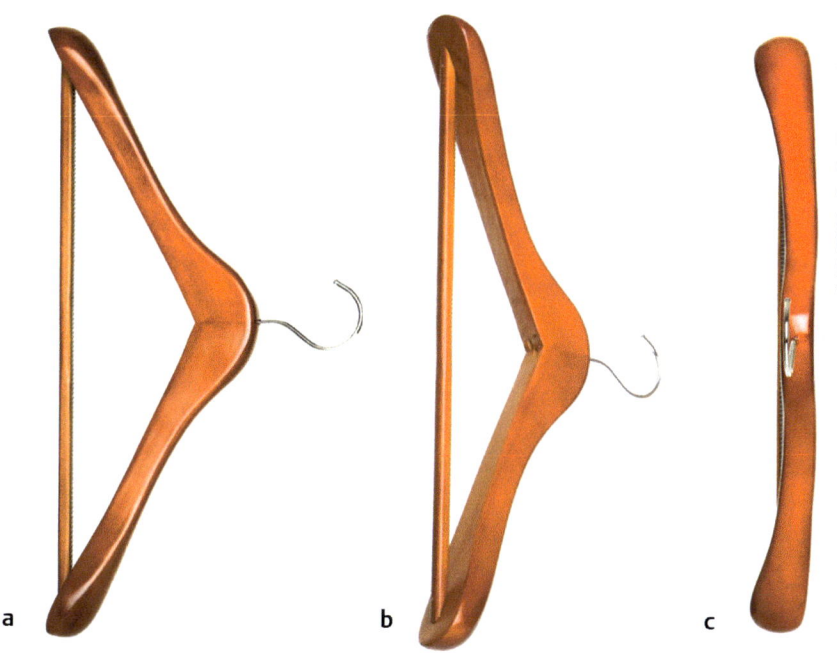

Fig. 2.11 **(a)** PA view of a coat hanger, showing an angle of 60 degrees. **(b)** The coat hanger has been rotated 45 degrees and now the Cobb angle registers only 30 degrees because the coat hanger is not being seen en face as it is in **(a)**. **(c)** When the coat hanger is turned a further 45 degrees there is no angle at all, (Reproduced with permission from Newton P, O'Brien M, Shufflebarger H, et al. Idiopathic Scoliosis: The Harms Study Group Treatment Guide. Stuttgart/New York: Thieme; 2010: 21.)

tilting of the cervicothoracic curve above, and an ugly higher left shoulder.

The direction of a curve is described according to its convexity. Thus right thoracic curves or left thoracolumbar or lumbar curves are common.

Spinal balance (compensation) can be easily appreciated if there is a single curve—say, a single right thoracic curve. Above and below this are compensatory curves bringing the head up straight and the lumbar spine and pelvis straight down below so that the head is centered over of the pelvis. This can be assessed using a plumb line dropped down from the vertebra prominens and see whether it cuts through the middle of the natal cleft. Perhaps a more precise method can be done radiologically[16] (▶ Fig. 2.18). For spinal balance, the upper and lower compensatory curves should have the same magnitude; if the lower one is bigger than the upper one, then spinal balance has been lost and this is referred to as decompensation (▶ Fig. 2.19).

It is worth exploring these compensatory curves in a little more detail.[13] For example, a radiograph of a right thoracolumbar curve shows that a vertebra or two above and below the major curve are still rotated in the direction of the concavity of the major curve. It is much easier to demonstrate this illustratively using a thoracolumbar or lumbar curve because the background air and abdominal gases provide much better contrast to the bony anatomy (▶ Fig. 2.20). The

Basic Principles

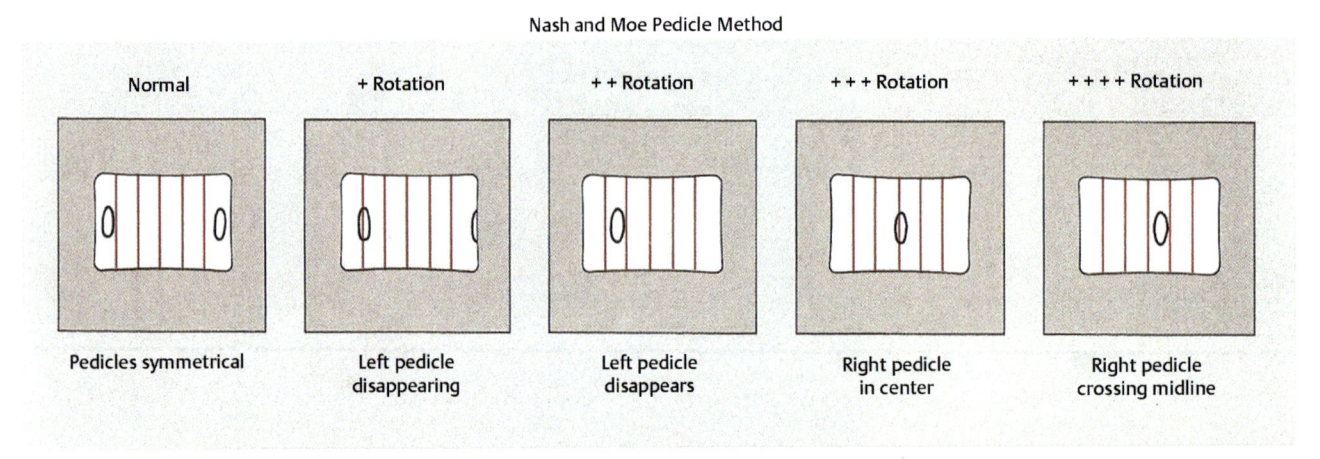

Nash and Moe Pedicle Method

Normal	+ Rotation	+ + Rotation	+ + + Rotation	+ + + + Rotation
Pedicles symmetrical	Left pedicle disappearing	Left pedicle disappears	Right pedicle in center	Right pedicle crossing midline

Fig. 2.12 Nash-Moe method of measuring vertebral rotation. The distance that the convex pedicle has moved from the convex side of the vertebral body is graded from 0 to 4 (0, normal; 1, +; 2, ++; 3, +++; 4, ++++). (Reproduced with permission from Greenspan A. Scoliosis and anomalies with general effect on the skeleton. In: Orthopaedic Radiology. A Practical Approach. 2nd ed. London: Gower Medical Publishing; 1992: Figure 28.14.)

lower end vertebra is L3 and clearly below L3 is the compensatory curve. It can, however, be seen that in the major structural curve to the left the spinous processes are of course rotated toward the right, as with concordant rotation. But, as we go into the lower compensatory curve, the spinous processes are still rotated to the right and yet these compensatory curves are convex to the right and not the left. Therefore, there is discordant rotation at the beginnings of the upper and lower compensatory curves indicating that these, at least to begin with, are kyphoses (direction of rotation in the same direction as that of tilt). This is best shown with the lower compensatory curve where L4 at the beginning of the lower compensatory curve is clearly seen to be rotated to the right and indeed the L5 vertebra is to a much lesser extent. These compensatory curves are therefore kyphoscolioses in contradistinction to the structural curve which is a lordoscoliosis. Indeed, for 3D balance of the spine, the central lordoscoliosis must be balanced by kyphoscolioses above and below. We shall deal with this in more detail in the next chapter where there are important "must know" concepts.

If a PA radiograph of the common thoracic and lumbar double structural pattern is inspected (▶ Fig. 2.21) then it can be seen that there may be a vertebra in between the two curves that is not rotated (i.e., neutral), in this case T9, and that the curve immediately below the thoracic curve is rotated to the right—the beginning of the lower lordoscoliosis. This means that with any double structural curve pattern all the vertebrae are lordotic or at the most the junctional vertebra is neutral but there is no junctional kyphosis. On a lateral radiograph of the patient it may look as if there is a kyphosis but this appearance again is spurious—the junctional area being just less lordotic than the areas above and below. It can also be seen on a lateral radiograph of a patient with a thoracic and thoracolumbar or lumbar double structural curve pattern that the lateral profile is extremely flat, being of course lordotic all the way down (▶ Fig. 2.22). All this is quite important bearing in mind that the surgeon should be trying to correct the deformity in all three planes. Unfortunately, despite the fact that these structural curves are lordotic and not kyphotic, the lateral X-ray of the patient is still believed to show kyphosis.[12] It is difficult/impossible in these circumstances to plan the proper surgical strategy unless the true 3D nature of the deformity is fully understood.

2.3 Spinal Growth

This is another important area where confusion also exists. Because scoliotic deformities in children have the potential to progress during growth it is very important to assess this risk accurately and this means repeat measurements regularly to see how children travel through their adolescence.

2.3.1 Indices of Maturity

To assess growth velocity there are a certain number of useful variables that can be quite easily measured. Radiologically, there are two traditional methods of assessing progression of a scoliosis and that is to determine the status of ossification of the iliac crest and the vertebral ring apophyses. Unfortunately, the vertebral ring apophyses are progressively less visible as the patient gets toward maturity but the iliac crest is visible on standard scoliosis X-rays and so no additional films for this purpose are required. Using this method of assessing the growth of the iliac crest apophysis is attributable to Risser (Risser sign) and there are six stages, 0 to 5 (▶ Fig. 2.23).[17] The iliac crest apophysis first appears posterolaterally and then moves medially around the iliac crest until finally the apophysis fuses to the rest of the pelvis at pelvic maturity, Risser 5. Thus 0 is when the apophysis hasn't appeared radiographically and 1, 2, 3, and 4 are arbitrary divisions of the perimeter of the apophysis divided into four quarters. It is easy therefore to go from 0 to 5 on plain films.

The only problem with this is that the spine continues to grow for several years after maturity of the pelvis and thus Risser 5 is not the end of spinal growth.[18,19] It has clearly been shown that the spine can and usually does grow into the early mid-twenties or beyond.[20,21]

Basic Principles

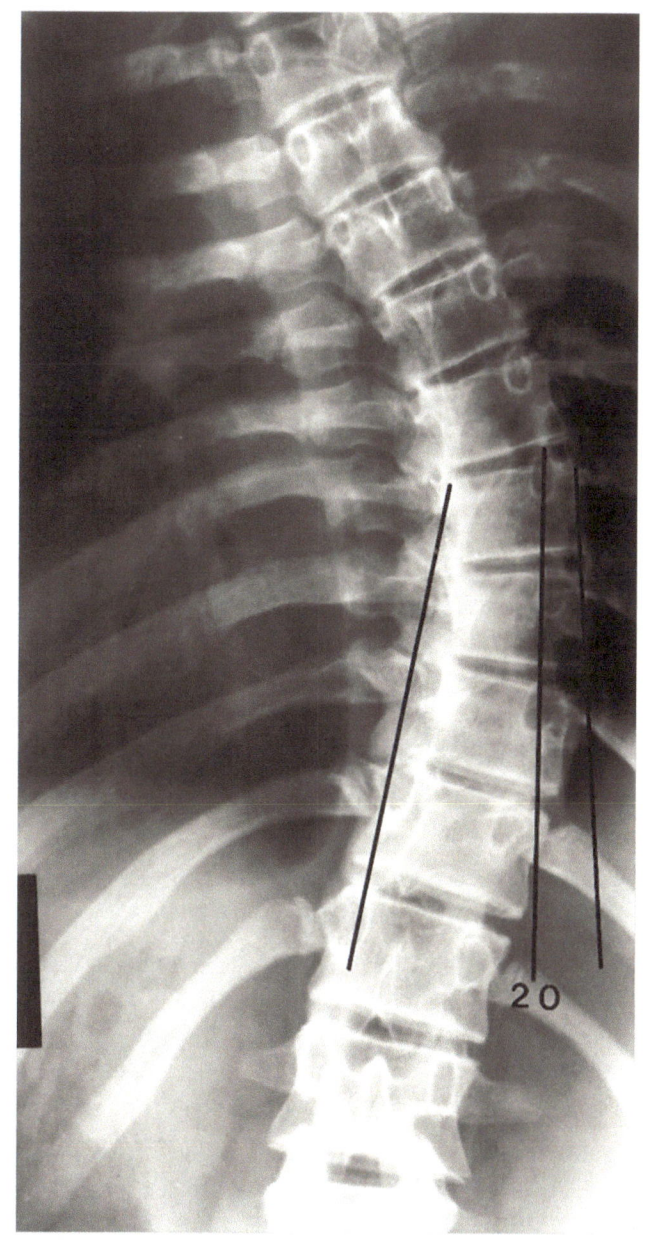

Fig. 2.13 Measuring rotation using Perdriolle's protractor. The protractor comprises diverging lines and is laid over the PA radiograph, with the side lines of the protractor aligned with the sides of the vertebral body. The line that bisects the convex pedicle indicates the degree of rotation of that vertebra. (Reproduced with permission from Newton P, O'Brien M, Shufflebarger H, et al. Idiopathic Scoliosis: The Harms Study Group Treatment Guide. Stuttgart/New York: Thieme; 2010: 21.)

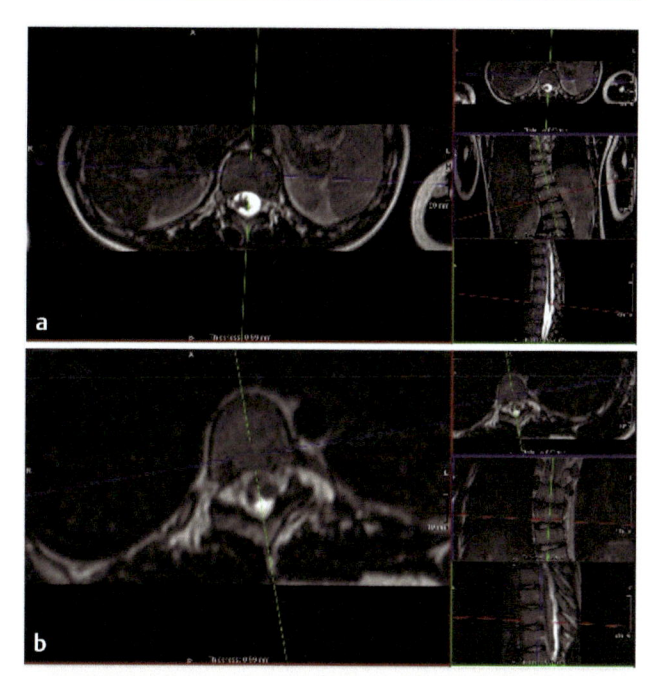

Fig. 2.14 Measuring vertebral rotation by MRI scanning. (a) Measuring the rotation of the upper end vertebra. This is the reference plane to measure apical rotation. (b) Measuring the rotation of the apical vertebra; the lines are drawn by the MRI software which will also calculate the angle of apical rotation—in this case, 10 degrees. Remember that this is measured in the supine position whereas Nash and Moe can be measured on any PA radiographs, erect or supine, lateral bending, or maximum stretch films. (With thanks to Dr. J Rankine, Consultant Spine Radiologist, The Leeds Hospitals.)

This accounts for why there were publications at Risser 5 of the size of the scoliosis then later in life showing a bigger Cobb angle and thus it was guesstimated perhaps due to female hormones that a scoliosis could increase in size by one or two degrees per year. The Leeds Group demonstrated that adolescents grow all of 2 cm after maturation of the pelvis (increasing length of the torso, sitting height and not standing).[20] If therefore Cobb angles are measured at Risser 5 and then measured at the age of 25 there certainly would be an increase—as would be expected—with a spine continuing to grow and so looking at X-rays taken in later adult life should not give the impression that the spine is continuing to grow all the while.

Weinstein has, however, produced some interesting data about curve progression in adult life[22] and we shall look at this in more detail in Chapter 4.

Meanwhile, at the other end of the age spectrum, Dimeglio has studied spinal growth and shown that vertebrae are about half adult size by the age of 2 and not short of full adult size before teenage.[23]

2.3.2 Measurement of Bone Age

In general pediatric practice, and particularly in children who do have overall growth disturbances, it has long been traditional to measure bone age by X-raying the left hand and wrist (left only by convention) and, by comparing the size and status of ossification of the carpal bones and the radius and ulna with atlases, it is possible to derive a bone age which often differs appreciably from chronological age. One of the first atlases that was used was the *Greulich and Pyle Atlas* and this was based upon well advanced upper class children in Cleveland, Ohio, in the 1930s.[24] A much more up-to-date and precise atlas is that by Tanner and Whitehouse (Second Method), which can permit measurement of bone age to one decimal place.[25] It is much more important to know what skeletal age is rather than chronological age and thus you can see rate of skeletal growth. Curves of course tend to progress in particular during phases of increased growth velocity.

Basic Principles

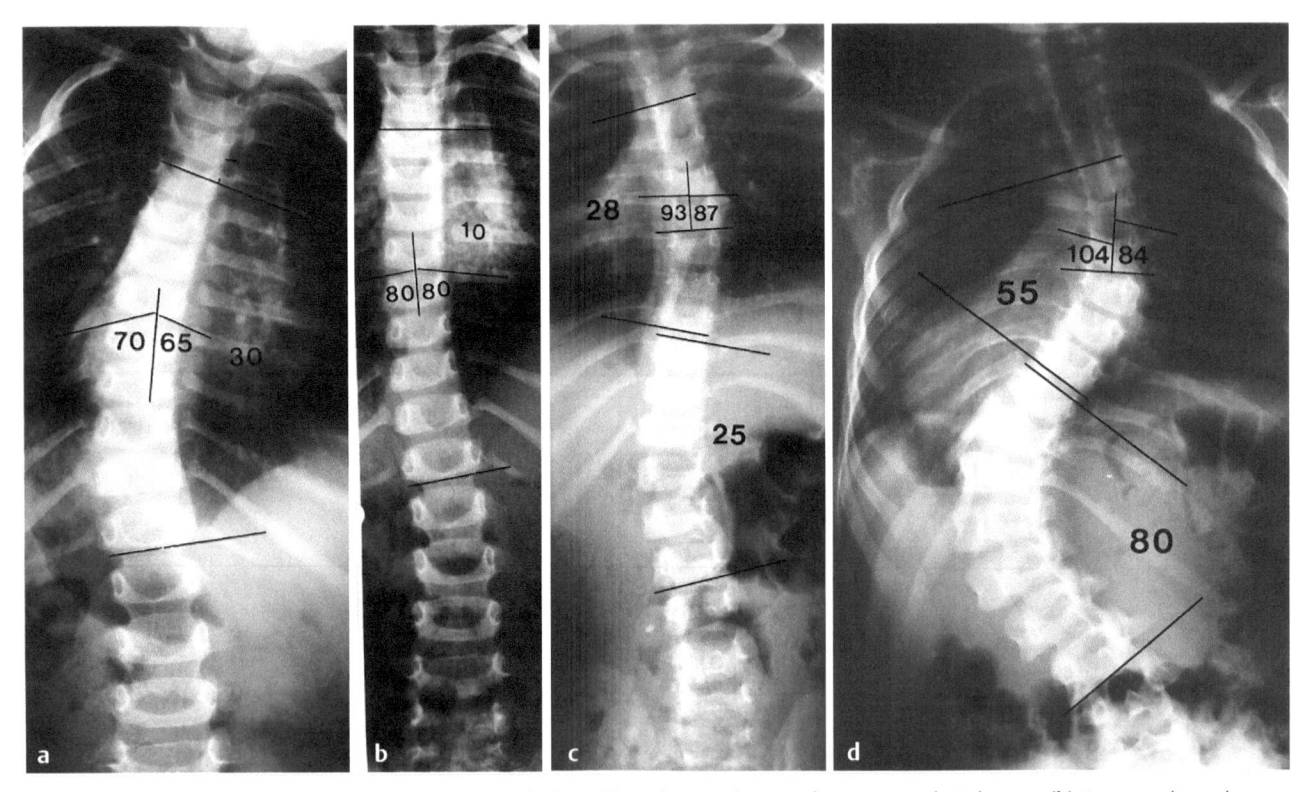

Fig. 2.15 (a) Infantile idiopathic thoracic scoliosis. Although the Cobb angle is 30 degrees, the RVAD is only 5 degrees. (b) Two years later, the deformity has almost resolved. (c) Infantile idiopathic double-structural scoliosis to the right in the thoracic region and to the left in the thoracolumbar region. Although the Cobb angles measure only 28 and 25 degrees, respectively, and the RVAD of the thoracic curve measures only 6 degrees, infantile double-structural curves are always progressive unless treated. (d) One year later both curves have increased significantly, particularly the lower one. Unfortunately, no therapeutic action was taken in the interim. (Reproduced with permission from Newton P, O'Brien M, Shufflebarger H, et al. Idiopathic Scoliosis: The Harms Study Group Treatment Guide. Stuttgart/New York: Thieme; 2010: 22.)

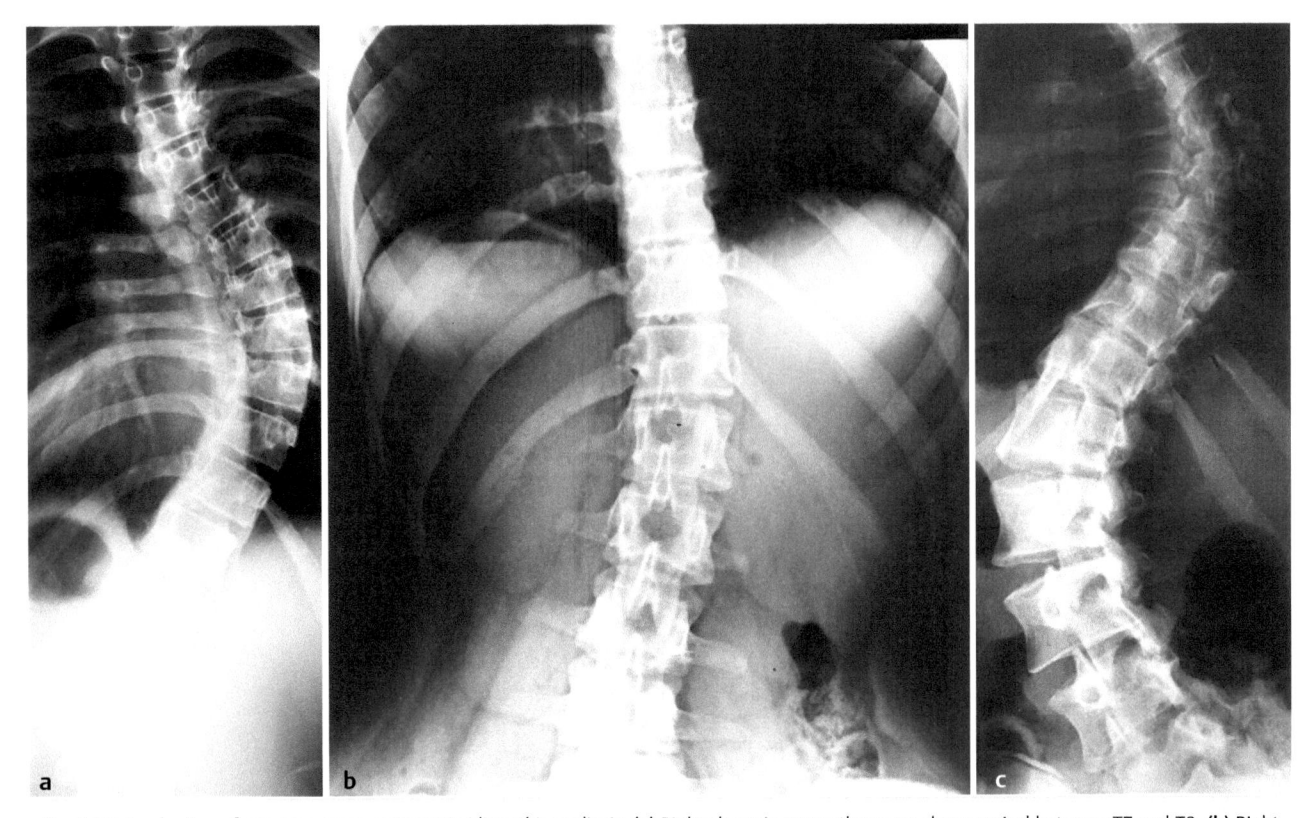

Fig. 2.16 A selection of common curve patterns in idiopathic scoliosis. (a) Right thoracic curve; these are always apical between T7 and T9. (b) Right thoracolumbar curve: these are apical at T12 or L1. (c) Right thoracic and left lumbar double-structural curve; lumbar curves are always apical at L2. (Reproduced with permission from Newton P, O'Brien M, Shufflebarger H, et al. Idiopathic Scoliosis: The Harms Study Group Treatment Guide. Stuttgart/New York: Thieme; 2010: 23.)

Basic Principles

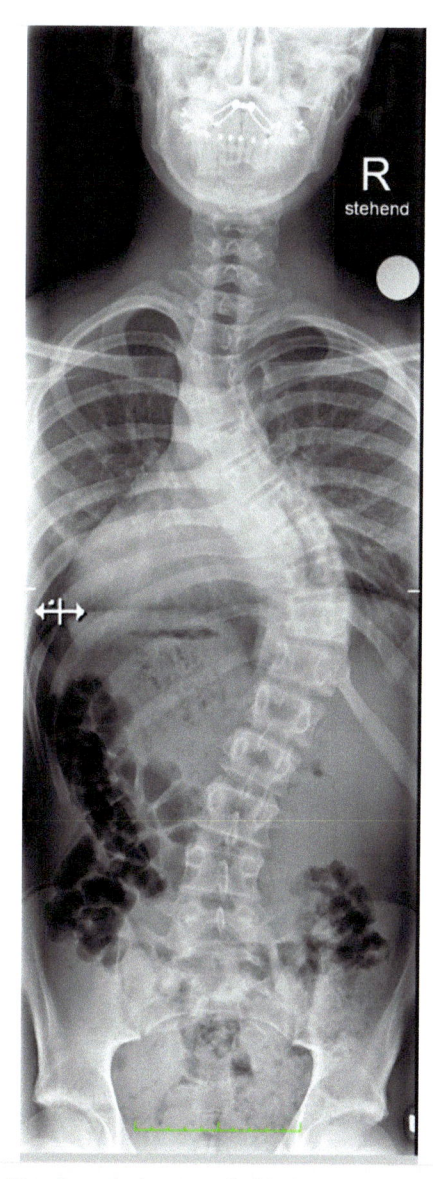

Fig. 2.17 PA radiograph showing a double thoracic curve. There is a right thoracic curve and then above it a left cervicothoracic curve so that the left shoulder is higher than the right (the signe d'épaule). The Lenke classification of this pattern of curvature is Type 2 AN.

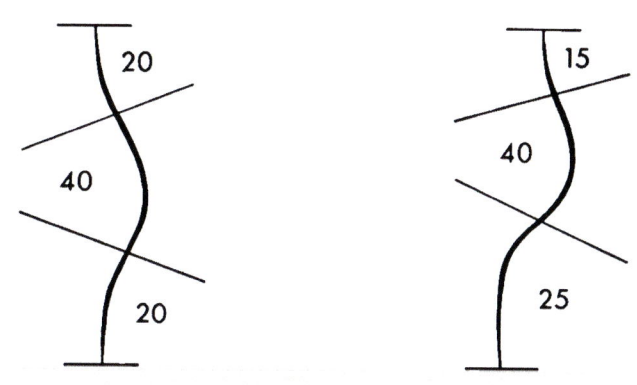

Fig. 2.18 Measuring spinal balance (compensation). The sum of the upper and lower compensatory curves is always equal to the size of the structural curve. (Left) When the spine is in perfect balance, the upper and lower compensatory curves are of equal magnitude. (Right) When the spine lists to the side of the convexity of the curve (decompression), it does so because the lower compensatory curve is bigger than the upper compensatory curve. In this case, the spine is decompensated by 10 degrees. (Reproduced with permission from Newton P, O'Brien M, Shufflebarger H, et al. Idiopathic Scoliosis: The Harms Study Group Treatment Guide. Stuttgart/New York: Thieme; 2010: 23.)

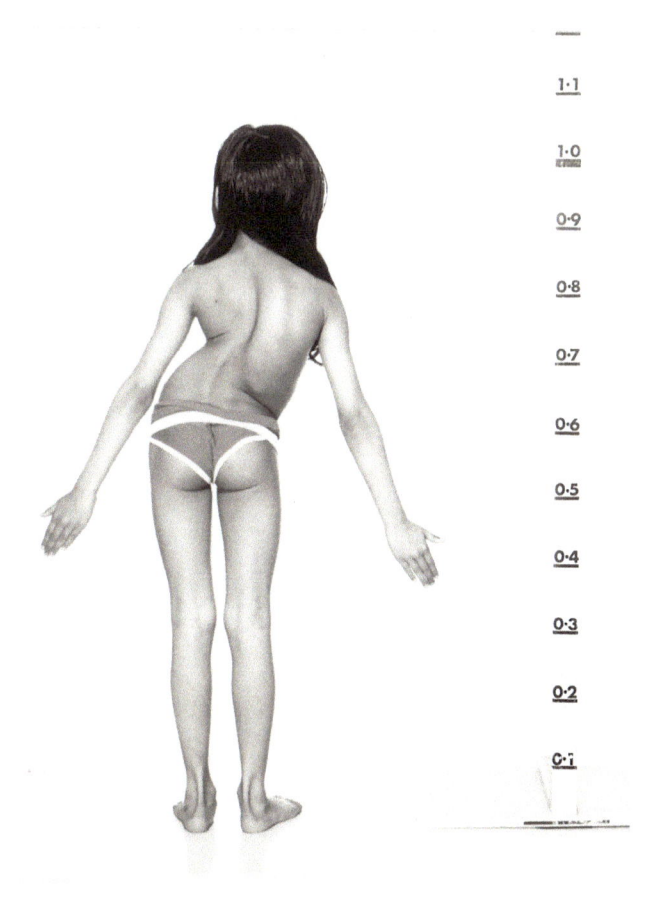

Fig. 2.19 Decompensation. There is a marked list of the torso to the side of the convexity of the curve.

2.3.3 Centile Charts

There are a number of anthropometric and other measurements that can be made but standing and sitting height are easily measured in the outpatient clinic on a calibrated stadiometer. These can be simply compared to measures of bone age and charts can be filled in at each visit and be in the outpatient notes (▶ Fig. 2.24).

2.4 Classification of Spinal Deformities

This is a classification by etiology and it is an extremely good classification.[26] It is one that all scoliosis surgeons work with. The important thing about a classification is that it is not too complex and is at least straightforward and memorable! We have made a few minor alterations, for example in the idiopathic scoliosis and the

Basic Principles

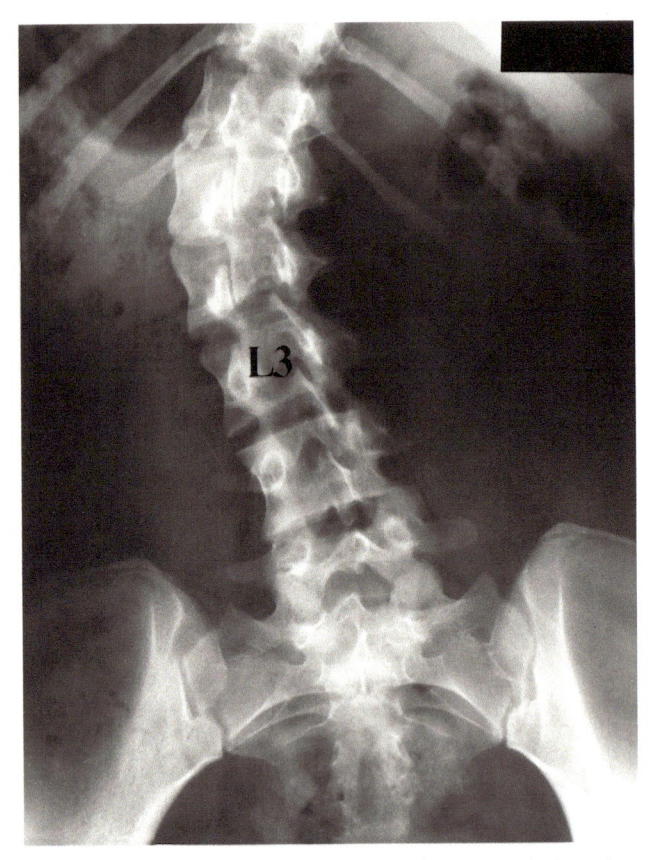

Fig. 2.20 The lower part of a left thoracolumbar curve with the end vertebra at L3 and L4 and L5 still rotated in the same direction as the structural curve.

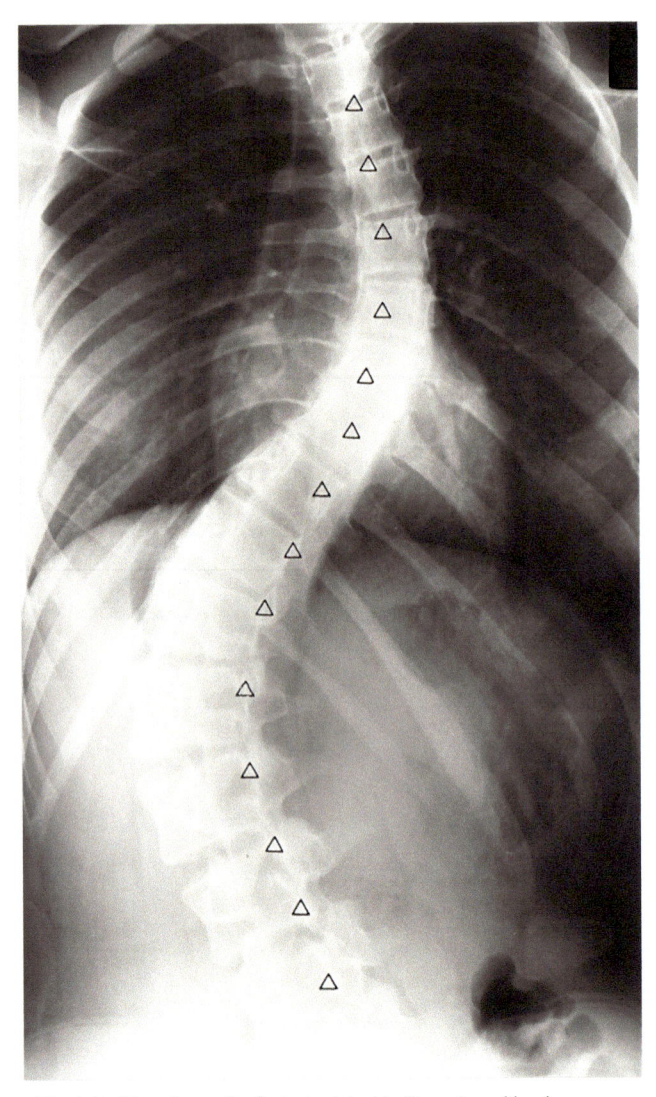

Fig. 2.21 PA radiograph of a typical double thoracic and lumbar curve. The tips of the spinous processes are marked with triangles. T9 is the neutral vertebra between the two lordoscolioses and therefore cannot be kyphotic.

spondylolisthesis sections, but the rest stays the same. ▶ Table 2.1 shows the short, simple classification and ▶ Table 2.2 is the classification in much more detail—really, for reference purposes.

2.5 Primary, Progressive, or Structural Deformities

2.5.1 Idiopathic Deformities

Idiopathic Scoliosis

This is defined as a lateral curvature of the spine with rotation in the absence of any congenital spinal anomaly or associated musculoskeletal condition. It is always a lordoscoliosis, the most common type of spinal deformity, and, as will be seen, idiopathic kyphoscoliosis cannot and does not exist. The same type of lordoscoliosis is also commonly seen, for example, with mild von Recklinghausen's disease, Marfan syndrome, congenital heart disease, and some congenital spine deformities. It was traditionally divided into three categories according to age of onset[27]—infantile, juvenile, adolescent—although this subdivision is commonly transgressed (referring to a child of 10 with a 100-degree curve as having adolescent idiopathic scoliosis when the deformity must have started much earlier). However, it is not at all clear whether juvenile idiopathic scoliosis actually exists. James himself couldn't be sure, and, if it does, then its prevalence rate may not justify a separate juvenile category. The really important groups are the early-onset and late-onset varieties and thus it is more rational to refer to two categories only—early-onset idiopathic scoliosis (EOIS; onset before the age of 5 years) and late-onset idiopathic scoliosis (LOIS; onset after the age of 5 years)[28] (▶ Fig. 2.25).

Early-onset Idiopathic Scoliosis (EOIS)

The onset is between birth and 5 years of age. Although idiopathic by definition, it may be a problem of pressure moulding. Approximately 90% resolve spontaneously (▶ Fig. 2.15), while 10% are static or progressive, some of which can later become serious, life-threatening problems (▶ Fig. 2.25a). It may be that the static variety is erroneously considered to be the formerly named juvenile idiopathic scoliosis. It may also be that the early onset static case sometimes forms the template for subsequent progression during the adolescent growth spurt.

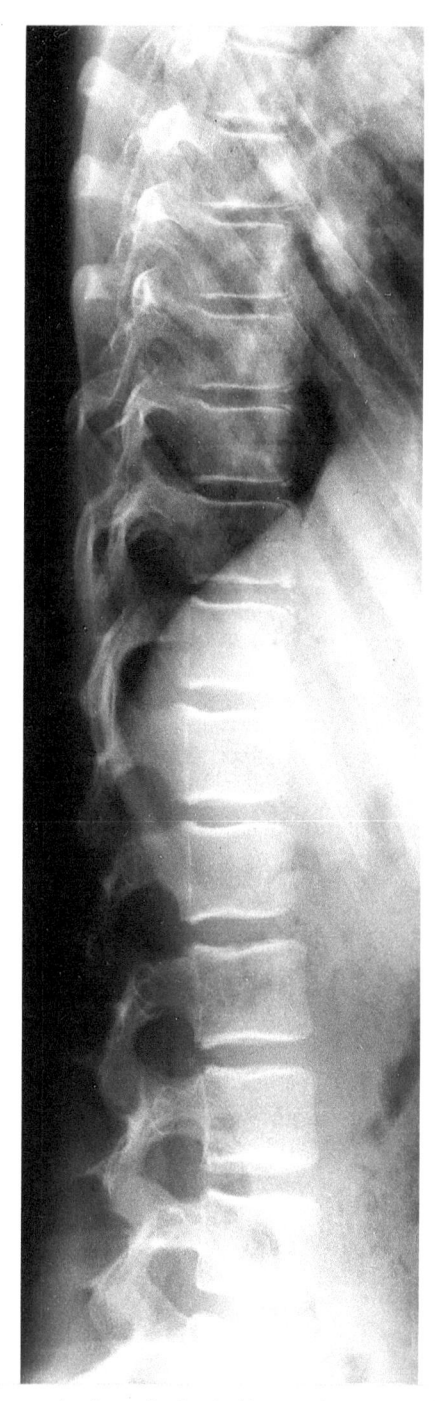

Fig. 2.22 Lateral radiograph of a double curve looking very flat because it is lordotic throughout.

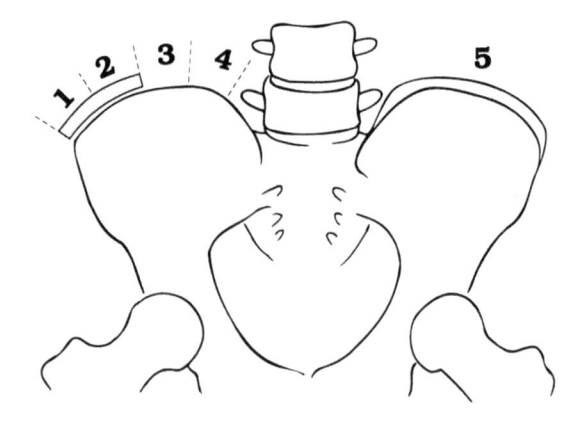

Fig. 2.23 Risser sign. The iliac crest apophysis appears first anteriorly and then moves round the iliac crest to end posteriorly. This is divided into sixths, with Risser 5 occurring when the iliac crest apophysis fuses with the pelvis. Accordingly, patients' maturity can be rated from Risser 0 through Risser 5. (Reproduced with permission from Newton P, O'Brien M, Shufflebarger H, et al. Idiopathic Scoliosis: The Harms Study Group Treatment Guide. Stuttgart/New York: Thieme; 2010: 24.)

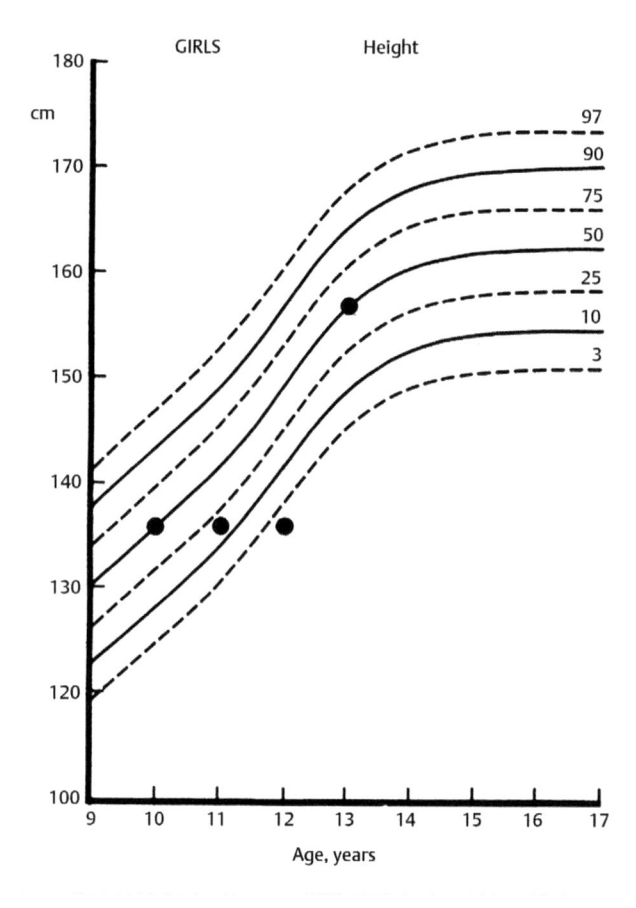

Fig. 2.24 The 1975 Tanner and Whitehouse centile chart for the height of girls. On this chart is plotted the height of a 10-year-old who does not grow for the next 2 years. Between the ages of 12 and 13, however, she has put in 3 years' growth to get back to the 50th centile and therefore during this period her growth velocity is excessive. (Reproduced with permission from Newton P, O'Brien M, Shufflebarger H, et al. Idiopathic Scoliosis: The Harms Study Group Treatment Guide. Stuttgart/New York: Thieme; 2010: 25.)

Late-onset Idiopathic Scoliosis (LOIS)

The onset is from 6 years of age to maturity (▶ Fig. 2.25b). Although this is the most prevalent type of idiopathic scoliosis this age of onset implies a more benign course compared with the early-onset progressive cases. The great majority of, if not all, cases that start in this phase of growth do so during late childhood and early adolescence. The important point to appreciate is that it is the early-onset progressive case that produces the cardiopulmonary notoriety of idiopathic scoliosis because it

Basic Principles

Table 2.1 Basic etiological classification of spinal deformities

Primary, progressive, or structural deformities
Idiopathic deformities
1. Idiopathic scoliosis
    a) Early-onset
    b) Late-onset
2. Idiopathic kyphosis
    a) Type I – classical Scheuermann's disease
    b) Type II – 'apprentice's spine'

Congenital deformities
1. Bone deformities
    a) Scoliosis
        i. Failure of formation
        ii. Failure of segmentation
        iii. Mixed
    b) Kyphosis
    c) Lordosis
2. Cord deformities
    a) Myelodysplasia scoliosis
    b) Myelodysplasia kyphosis
    c) Myelodysplasia lordosis
3. Bone and cord deformities
4. Syndromes in which congenital spine deformities are prevalent

Neuromuscular deformities
1. Cerebral palsy
2. Poliomyelitis
3. True neuromuscular disorders
4. Familial dysautonomia
5. Malignant hyperpyrexia

Deformities in association with neurofibromatosis
1. Dystrophic deformities
2. Idiopathic-type deformities

Mesenchymal deformities
1. Heritable disorders of connective tissue
2. Mucopolysaccharidoses
3. Bone dysplasias
4. Metabolic bone disease
5. Endocrine disorders

Traumatic deformities
1. Vertebral
2. Extravertebral

Deformity due to infection
1. Pyogenic infection
2. Tuberculosis

Deformity due to tumors
1. Intradural tumors
2. Syringomyelia
3. Paravertebral childhood tumors
4. Primary extradural tumors
5. Metastatic spinal disease

Miscellaneous conditions
Spinal deformity in adults
1. True adult deformities
2. Adult-presenting deformities

Spondylolisthesis
1. Dysplastic
2. Isthmic
3. Degenerative
4. Traumatic
5. Pathological

Secondary, nonprogressive or nonstructural deformities
Pelvic tilt scoliosis
Irritative lesions
Hysterical scoliosis

Table 2.2 Etiological classification in detail

Primary, progressive, or structural deformities
Idiopathic deformities
1. Idiopathic scoliosis
    a) Early-onset – before 5 years of age
    b) Late-onset – after 5 years of age
2. Idiopathic kyphosis
    a) Type I – classical Scheuermann's disease – thoracic
    b) Type II – 'apprentice's spine' – thoracolumbar or lumbar

Congenital deformities
1. Bone deformities
    a) Scoliosis
        - Failure of formation
            Complete unilateral – hemivertebra
            Partial unilateral – wedge vertebra
        - Failure of segmentation
            Complete or bilateral – 'bloc'
            Partial or unilateral – 'bar'
        - Mixed formation and segmentation anomalies
    b) Kyphosis
        - Failure of formation
        - Failure of segmentation
        - Mixed
    c) Lordosis
2. Cord deformities
    a) Myelodysplasia scoliosis
    b) Myelodysplasia kyphosis (the congenital kyphosis of myelomeningocele)
    c) Myelodysplasia lordosis
3. Bone and cord deformities
    a) Formation/segmentation anomalies above myelodysplasia scoliosis
4. Syndromes in which congenital spine deformities are prevalent
    a) Klippel-Feil syndrome
    b) Pterygium syndrome
    c) Holt-Oram syndrome
    d) Goldenhar syndrome
    e) Treacher Collins syndrome
    f) Apert's syndrome
    g) Crouzon's syndrome
    h) Jarcho-Levin syndrome
    i) Larsen's syndrome
    j) Silver's syndrome
    k) Freeman-Sheldon syndrome

Neuromuscular deformities
1. Cerebral palsy
2. Poliomyelitis
3. True 'neuromuscular disorders'
    a) Spinal muscular atrophy
    b) Peripheral neuropathies
        - Peroneal muscular atrophy
        - Hypertrophic polyneuritis
    c) Friedreich's ataxia
    d) Arthrogryposis
    e) The muscular dystrophies
        - Duchenne dystrophy
        - Other dystrophies
        - Congenital myopathies
4. Familial dysautonomia (Riley-Day Syndrome)
5. Malignant hyperpyrexia

Deformities in association with neurofibromatosis
1. Dystrophic deformities
    a) Lordoscoliosis
    b) Kyphosis
2. Idiopathic-type deformities
    a) Lordoscoliosis
    b) Kyphosis

Mesenchymal deformities
1. Heritable disorders of connective tissue

Table 2.2 Etiological classification in detail (*continued*)

    a) Skeletal—osteogenesis imperfecta
    b) Extraskeletal
- Marfan syndrome
- Homocystinuria
- Congenital contractural arachnodactyly
- Ehlers-Danlos syndrome

2. Mucopolysaccharidoses
    a) Hurler's syndrome
    b) Hunter's syndrome
    c) Morquio's syndrome
    d) Maroteaux-Lamy syndrome
3. Bone dysplasias
    a) Predominantly epiphyseal
- Multiple epiphyseal dysplasia
- Chondrodysplasia punctata
- Hereditary progressive arthro-ophthalmopathy

    b) Predominantly metaphyseal
- Achondroplasia
- Hypochondroplasia

    c) Vertebral only
- Brachyolmia

    d) Predominantly vertebral and epiphyseal
- Spondyloepiphyseal dysplasia tarda

    e) Vertebral and metaphyseal
- Spondylometaphyseal dysplasia

    f) Vertebral, epiphyseal and metaphyseal
- Pseudo-achondroplasia
- Spondyloepiphyseal dysplasia congenita
- Metatropic dwarfism
- Kniest disease
- Diastrophic dwarfism

    g) With decreased bone density
- Idiopathic juvenile osteoporosis

    h) With increased bone density
- Frontometaphyseal dysplasia
- The hyperphosphatasias

    i) Other dysplasias
- Cleidocranial dysplasia
- Progeria
- Smith-Lemli-Opitz syndrome

4. Metabolic bone disease
    a) Rickets
5. Endocrine disorders
    a) Pituitary disorders
    b) Thyroid disorders
    c) Adrenal disorders

Traumatic deformities
1. Vertebral
    a) Local spine deformities
    b) Paralytic deformities
2. Extravertebral
    a) Thoracic surgery
- Thoracoplasty
- Thoracotomy

    b) Soft tissue scarring
- Burns to the torso
- Thecoperitoneal shunt syndrome
- Retroperitoneal fibrosis

Deformity due to infection
1. Pyogenic infection
2. Tuberculosis

Deformity due to tumors
1. Intradural tumors
2. Syringomyelia
3. Paravertebral childhood tumors
    a) Wilms' tumors
    b) Neuroblastoma

4. Primary extradural tumors
    a) Bone-forming tumors
- Osteoma
- Osteoid osteoma and benign osteoblastoma
- Osteosarcoma

    b) Cartilage-forming tumors
- Chondroma
- Osteochondroma
- Chondroblastoma
- Chondrosarcoma

    c) Giant cell tumour
    d) Marrow tumors
- Ewing's sarcoma
- The malignant lymphomas

    e) Vascular tumors
- Hemangioma
- Hemangio-endothelioma

    f) Other tumors
- Chordoma

    g) Tumour-like lesions
- Aneurysmal bone cyst
- Eosinophilic granuloma

5. Metastatic spinal disease

Miscellaneous conditions in which a spinal deformity is common
1. Congenital heart disease
2. Juvenile rheumatoid arthritis
3. Ocular and visual problems
    a) Blind children
    b) Ophthalmoplegia
    c) Congenital strabismus
4. Congenital anomalies of the upper extremity

Spinal deformity in adults
1. True adult deformities
    a) Paget's disease
    b) Ankylosing spondylitis
    c) Osteoporosis
    d) Osteomalacia
2. Adult-presenting deformities

Spondylolisthesis
1. Dysplastic
2. Isthmic
    a) Fatigue fracture of pars
    b) Elongated pars
    c) Acute fracture of pars
3. Degenerative
4. Traumatic
5. Pathological

Secondary, nonprogressive or nonstructural deformities

Pelvic tilt scoliosis
1. Leg-length inequality
2. Pelvic asymmetry
3. Both

Irritative lesions
1. Intervertebral disk prolapse
2. Intervertebral diskitis
3. Osteoid osteoma or osteoblastoma

Hysterical scoliosis

is only in the first 3 years of life that the pulmonary alveolar tree re-duplicates (▶ Fig. 2.26). Whereas the late-onset case is a question of disfigurement only, the bigger the deformity the more obvious is the social and psychological upset (more in Chapter 4).

Basic Principles

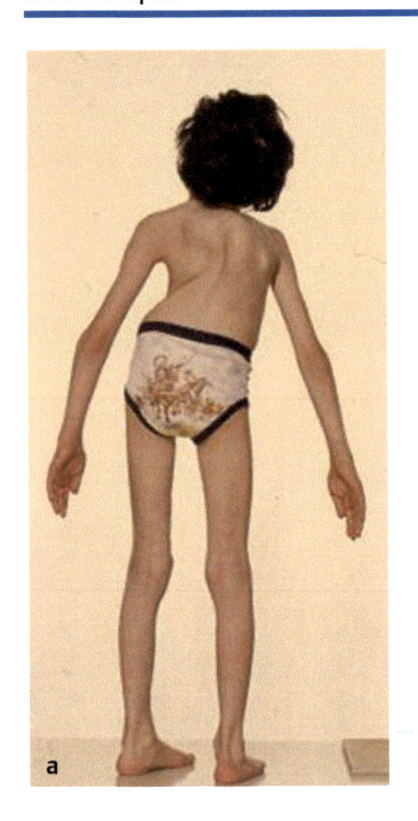

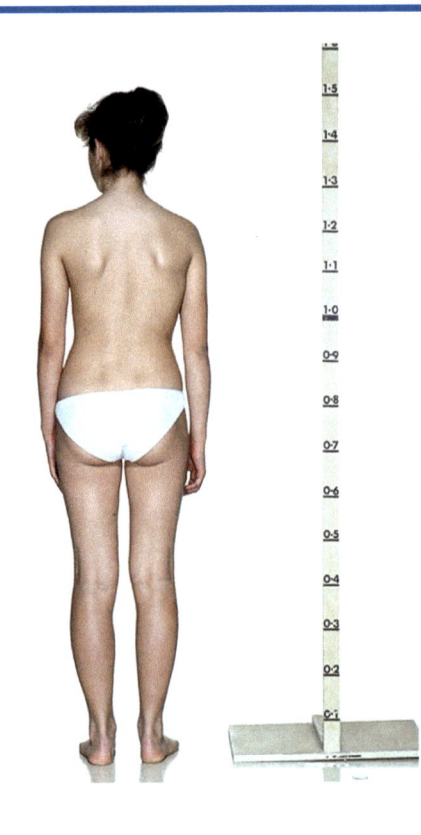

Fig. 2.25 The two fundamental types of idiopathic scoliosis according to age of onset. **(a)** Early onset, a matter of organic health. **(b)** Late onset, a matter of deformity only. (Reproduced with permission from Newton P, O'Brien M, Shufflebarger H, et al. Idiopathic Scoliosis: The Harms Study Group Treatment Guide. Stuttgart/New York: Thieme; 2010: 26.)

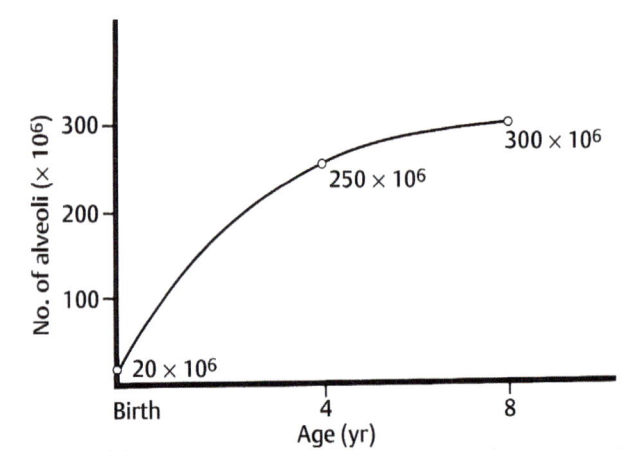

Fig. 2.26 Graph demonstrating the rate of development of pulmonary alveoli. A maximum is reached at the age of 8 years with five-sixths of alveoli being developed by the age of 4 and half by the age of 1 year. (Reproduced with permission from Newton P, O'Brien M, Shufflebarger H, et al. Idiopathic Scoliosis: The Harms Study Group Treatment Guide. Stuttgart/New York: Thieme; 2010: 25.)

Idiopathic Kyphosis

This is Scheuermann's disease, a rigid kyphosis, usually in the mid-lower thoracic region (Type I), with vertebral wedging and end plate irregularity. It is the opposite pathological deformity to idiopathic scoliosis (see Chapter 3) (▶ Fig. 2.27). If this wedging process occurs more on one side of the spine than the other, then a modest scoliosis may also develop but significant progressive rotation does not ensue. Above and below the area of kyphosis there are compensatory lordoses that can rotate to produce an idiopathic scoliosis (which indeed is exactly what it is), but careful inspection reveals that such a curve is not apical in the region of the kyphosis but several segments below.[29]

Less commonly the vertebral wedging occurs at the thoracolumbar junction or upper lumbar region and the wedging is much less dramatic (Type II). It is much more common in older boys/young men and is thought to be the response to vigorous activity, hence its original name of apprentices' spine (▶ Fig. 2.28).

2.5.2 Congenital Deformities

These are due to either abnormal bone development or abnormal spinal cord development, or both. Deformities due to abnormal bone development are then subdivided according to direction of deformity and these are due to either failures of formation or failures of segmentation, which may be complete or partial (▶ Fig. 2.29).

Although this classification gathers all deformities sharing a congenital origin, the individual deformities behave very differently.[30] Solitary lateral hemivertebrae tend to produce purely coronal plane curves often not with any great progression potential although they may throw off secondary curves above and below, whereas extensive lateral segmentation defects can be very progressive rotational deformities and are therefore lordoscolioses. Dorsal hemivertebrae produce progressive kyphoses often with neurological sequelae (▶ Fig. 2.30).

Congenital cord abnormalities (spina bifida) are associated with a collapsing paralytic lordoscoliosis below and less commonly with a pure kyphosis, and at the apex of the latter the vertebrae are congenitally wedged (▶ Fig. 2.31). Completing the

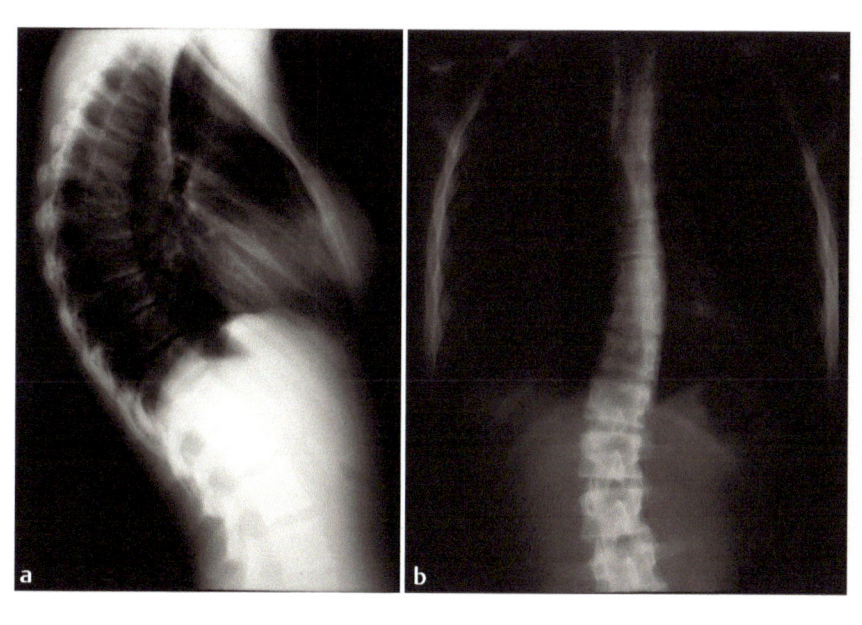

Fig. 2.27 (a) Lateral radiograph of a boy with Scheuermann's disease. (b) PA radiograph showing that the compensatory lumbar hyperlordosis has buckled to produce idiopathic scoliosis below the area of Scheuermann's disease. A perfect human model of the development of idiopathic scoliosis from a primary lordosis.

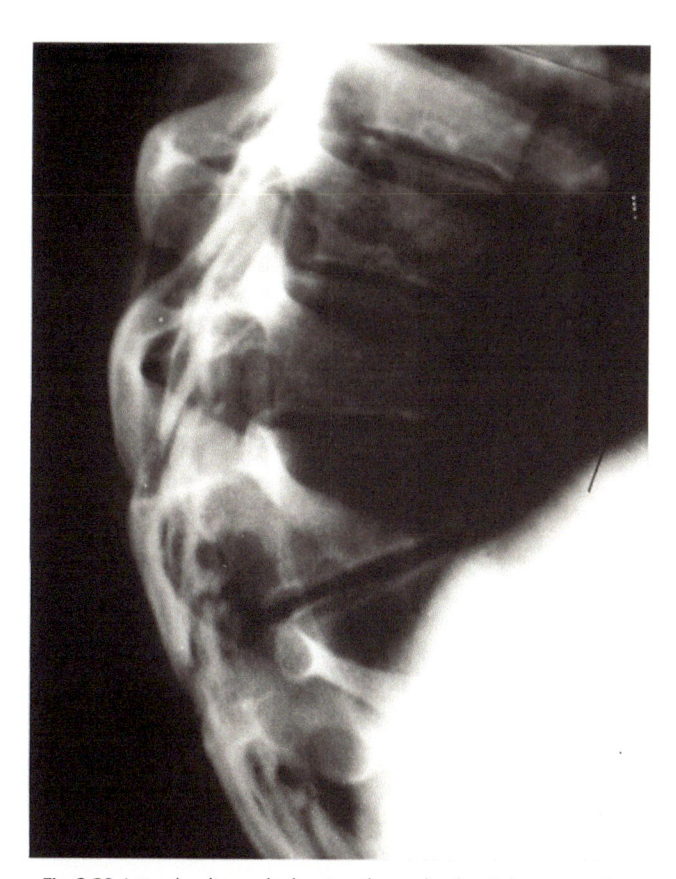

Fig. 2.28 Lateral radiograph showing thoracolumbar Scheuermann's disease (Apprentice's spine). It can sometimes be difficult to differentiate from a minor degree of anterior wedge compression fracture but, of course, there is no history of trauma and the deformity develops gradually.

congenital collection are a number of uncommon syndromes in which congenital bony deformities are prevalent.

2.5.3 Neuromuscular Deformities

These are subdivided into those associated with cerebral palsy, poliomyelitis, or the true neuromuscular disorders such as spinal muscle atrophy, the peripheral neuropathies, Friedreich's ataxia, arthrogryposis, and the muscular dystrophies. In addition, familial dysautonomia and malignant hyperpyrexia are best grouped with the neuromuscular deformities. Here the underlying condition is particularly important as regards management. Duchenne dystrophy curtails life toward the end of the second decade, while cerebral palsy is often associated with significant central and/or sensory impairment. With severe cerebral palsy the deformity is typically a collapsing paralytic lordoscoliosis with pelvic obliquity (▶ Fig. 2.32), although a single thoracic curve associated with intercostal nerve paralysis is common in poliomyelitis.

2.5.4 Deformities due to Neurofibromatosis

There are two distinct progressive scolioses: (1) a short, sharp, angular dystrophic curve which is relentlessly progressive and (2) a milder idiopathic-type curve. The idiopathic-type curve is the more prevalent, but the sharp angular curve has a very serious prognosis (▶ Fig. 2.33). Both are lordoscolioses. The structural deformity in neurofibromatosis can also be a kyphosis, usually thoracic or sometimes cervical and often severe and angular, and may occur in association with a lordoscoliosis above or below it. The more dystrophic the vertebrae, the more severe and progressive the deformity. A nonprogressive lumbar curve secondary to a leg-length inequality is also common in von Recklinghausen's disease due to hemihypertrophy or local gigantism.

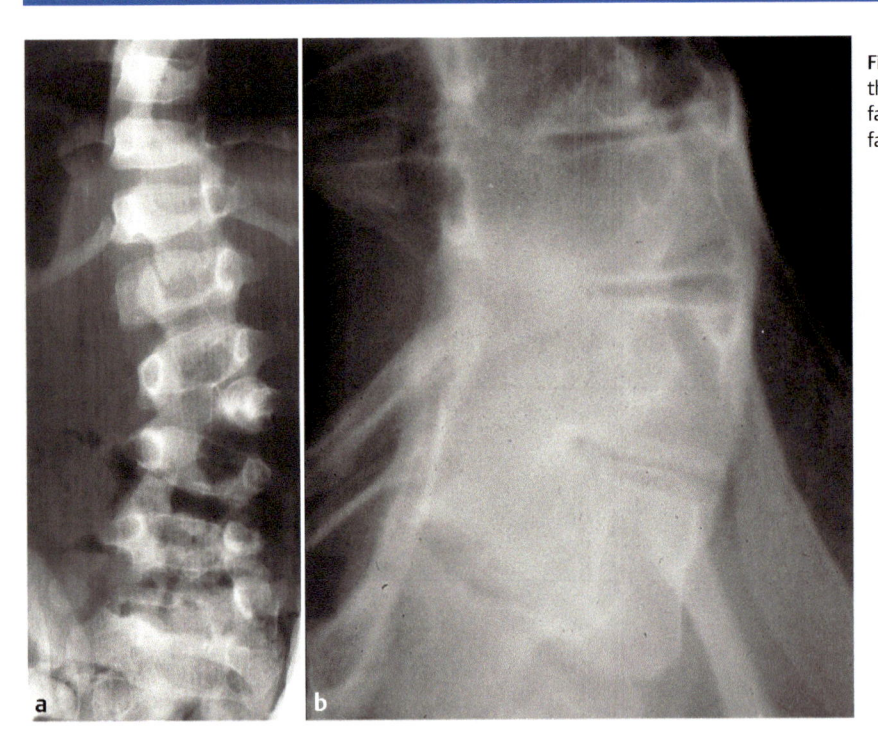

Fig. 2.29 The two basic congenital anomalies that give rise to a spinal deformity. (a) Unilateral failure of formation (hemivertebra). (b) Unilateral failure of segmentation (unilateral bar).

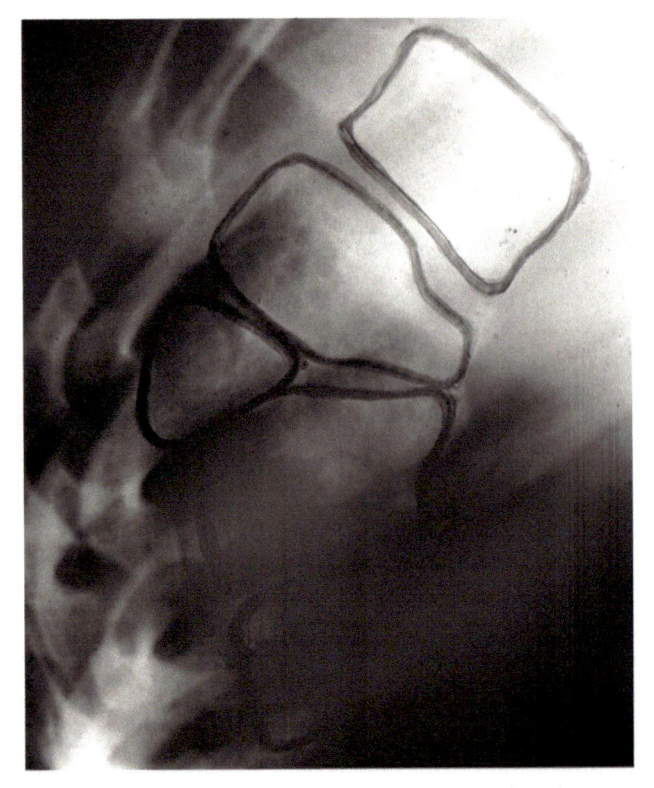

Fig. 2.30 Lateral radiograph showing a dorsal hemivertebra. These produce local angular kyphoses, often with neurological compression.

2.5.5 Miscellaneous Conditions Associated with Spine Deformities

Mesenchymal Disorders

This not very satisfactory term includes connective tissue disorders, mucopolysaccharidoses, bone dysplasias, metabolic, and endocrine disorders. Heritable disorders of connective tissue are problems of collagen formation whose features are either mainly skeletal, as in osteogenesis imperfecta, or extraskeletal, as in Marfan syndrome (▶ Fig. 2.34), Ehlers-Danlos syndrome, and homocystinuria. Osteogenesis imperfecta (the brittle bone syndrome) can be divided into a severe lethal sporadic congenita form and a milder, dominantly inherited tarda form. The mucopolysaccharidoses are problems of breakdown of glycosaminoglycans, and four varieties (Hurler's, Hunter's, Morquio's, and Maroteaux-Lamy syndromes) are associated with a spinal deformity. The bone dysplasias (e.g., achondroplasia, spondyloepiphyseal dysplasia, multiple epiphyseal dysplasia, metatropic dwarfism, diastrophic dwarfism) are associated with short stature and spinal deformity which is in the sagittal plane in the nature of flattened vertebrae (platyspondyly), often with a thoracolumbar bullet-shaped vertebra (▶ Fig. 2.35).

Deformities due to Trauma

This group is subdivided into vertebral or extravertebral deformities. Most vertebral injuries are in the nature of vertical loading in flexion and therefore an angular kyphosis is

Basic Principles

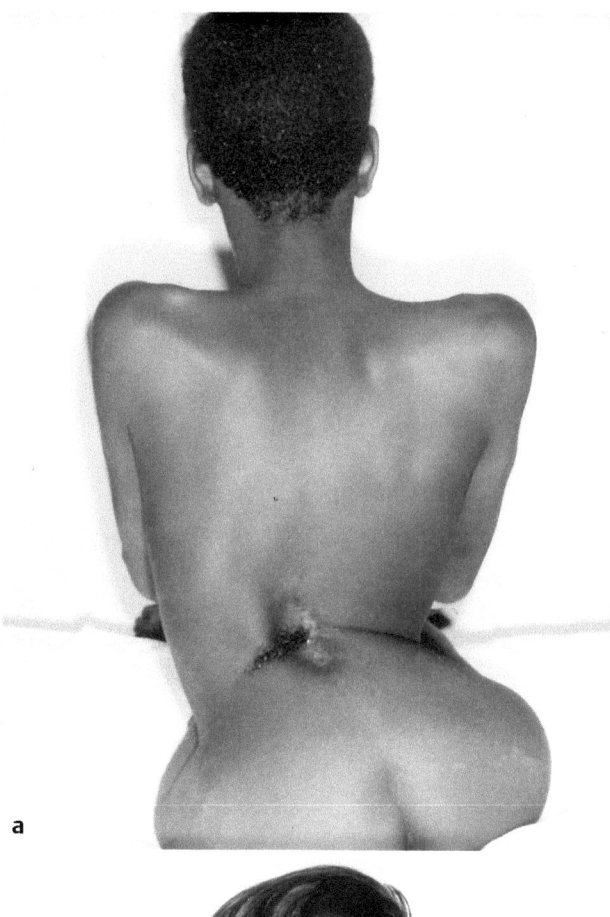

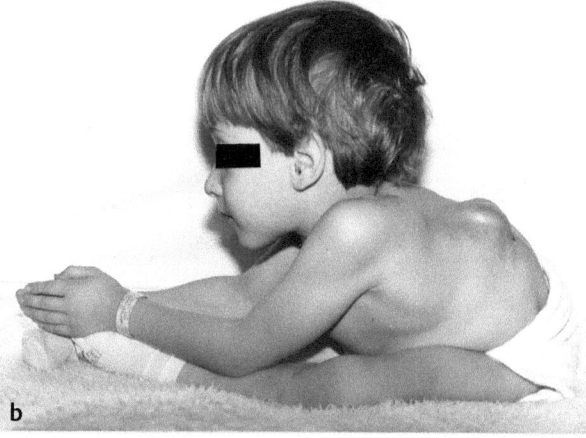

Fig. 2.31 The two types of deformity encountered in myelodysplasia. (a) The collapsing lordoscoliosis with pelvic obliquity. (b) The congenital kyphosis of myelomeningocele.

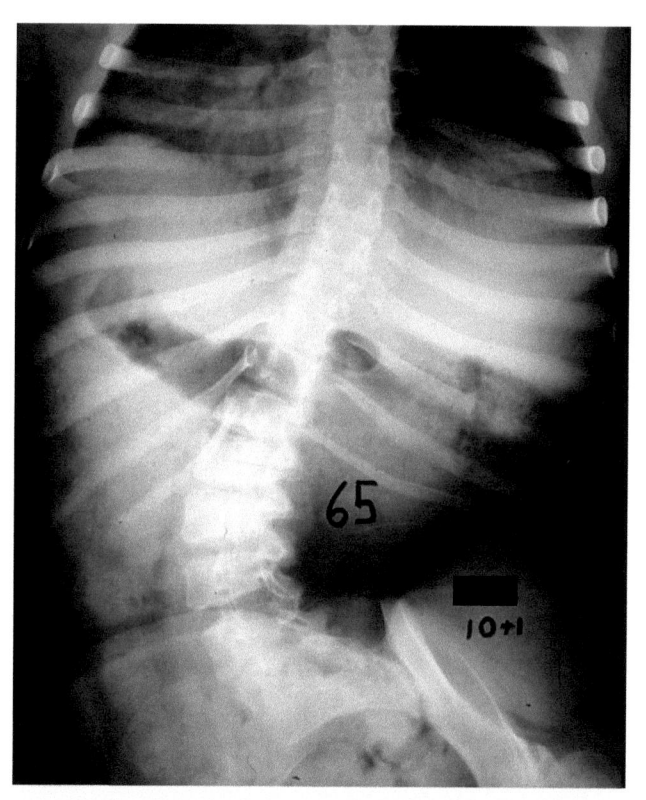

Fig. 2.32 The collapsing lordoscoliosis with pelvic obliquity of poliomyelitis. The spine has mechanically failed at the neuromuscular level.

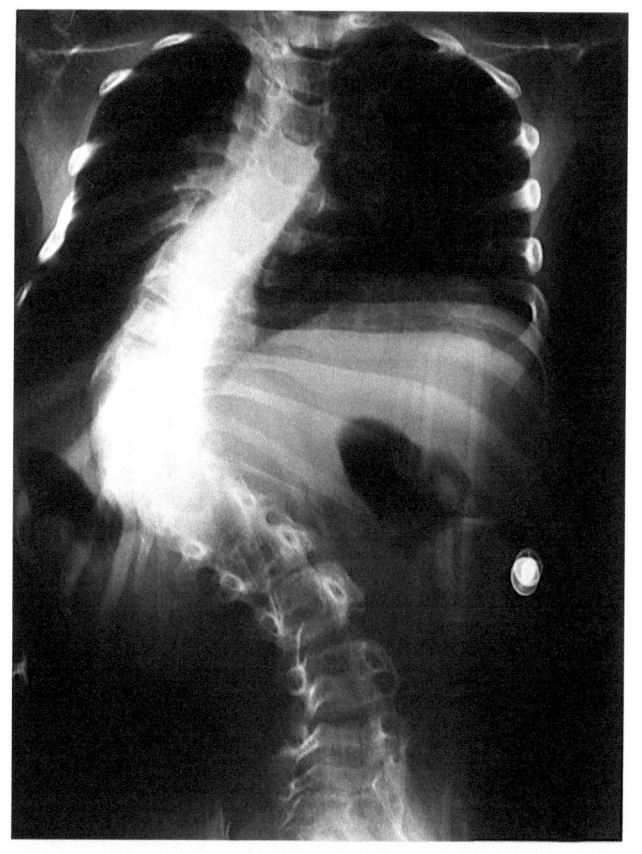

Fig. 2.33 Characteristic short angular curve of dystrophic von Recklinghausen's disease. The spine has mechanically failed at bone level.

produced, sometimes compounded by cord damage. There may therefore be a collapsing paralytic lordoscoliosis below this. However, they are frequently compounded by laminectomy, which is a very serious iatrogenic insult to the growing spine, with a progressive angular kyphosis often giving rise to its own neurological problems. Another iatrogenic cause of spinal deformities is after laminectomy for the treatment of intradural tumors if concomitant spinal fixation and fusion is not carried out (▶ Fig. 2.36). It is so much more difficult to salvage the post-laminectomy kyphosis than to prevent its occurrence in the first place. Extravertebral

Basic Principles

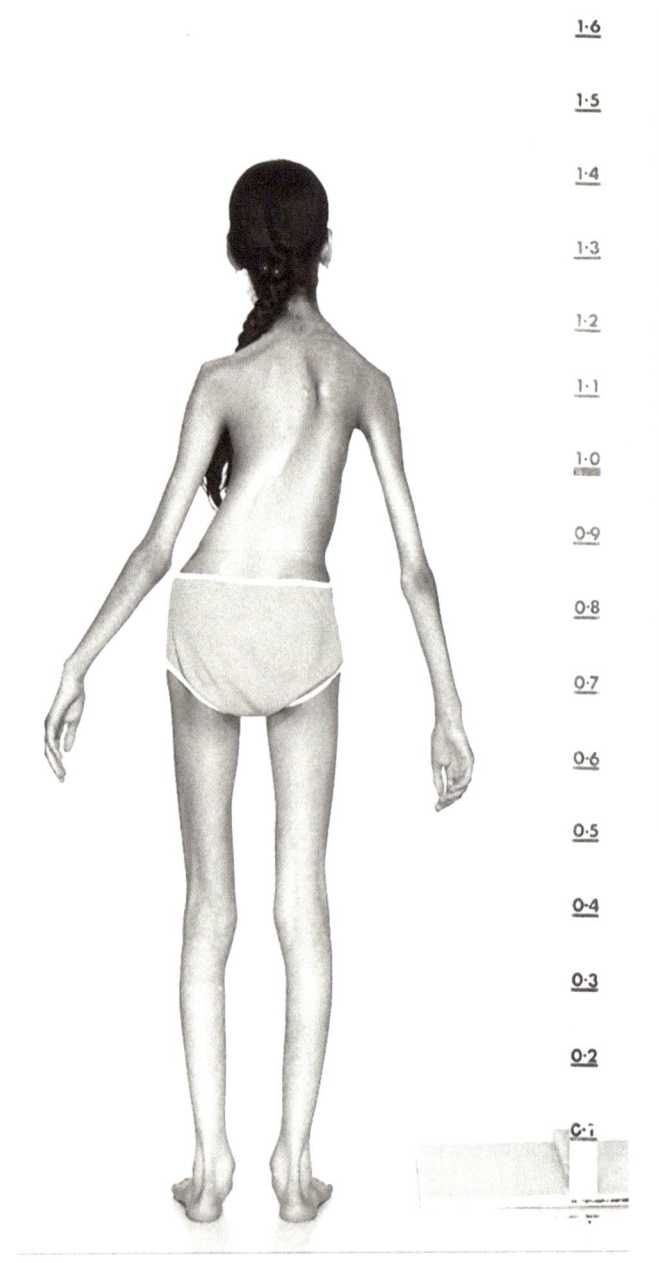

Fig. 2.34 The idiopathic-type curve of Marfan syndrome; the spine has failed at soft tissue level. (Reproduced with permission from Newton P, O'Brien M, Shufflebarger H, et al. Idiopathic Scoliosis: The Harms Study Group Treatment Guide. Stuttgart/New York: Thieme; 2010: 38.)

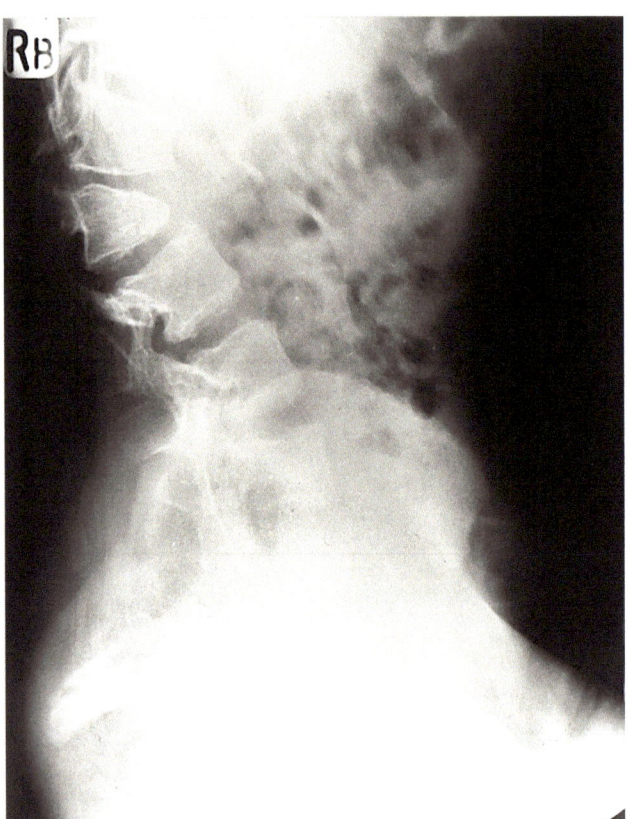

Fig. 2.35 The typical bullet-shaped vertebra of a bone dysplasia.

causes include thoracotomy which can be associated with an idiopathic-type scoliosis and thoracoplasty which may produce a deformity with a rotational prominence, but only if multiple ribs are excised. Soft tissue scarring (burns to the torso, thecoperitoneal shunt syndrome, retroperitoneal fibrosis) can tether the spine into deformity.

Deformities due to Infection

This can produce an angular kyphosis due to destruction of the intervertebral disk and the contiguous margins of the adjacent vertebral bodies. If the deformity is severe enough, or compounded by abscess formation, then the function of the spinal cord can be jeopardized (▶ Fig. 2.37).

Deformities due to Tumors

Intradural tumors and syringomyelia produce idiopathic-type lordoscolioses; indeed, the latter may be the first manifestation of the underlying pathology (▶ Fig. 2.38). The paravertebral childhood tumors (Wilms' tumor and neuroblastoma) produce their deformities by way of the necessary radiation therapy which leads to a reduction in rate of vertebral growth on the side of the spine concave to the lesion. Extradural tumors tend to produce a local kyphotic deformity when the vertebral body collapses. There is a wide variety of primary extradural vertebral body tumors that tend to occur in a young age group, whereas in older individuals metastatic spinal disease is much more likely.

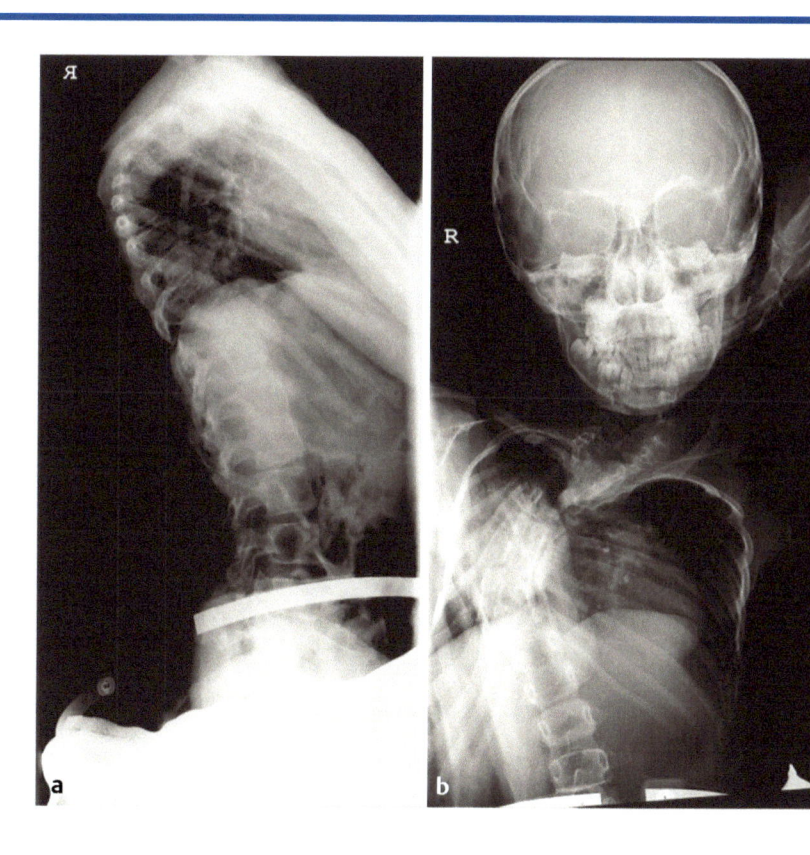

Fig. 2.36 (a) Lateral radiograph showing an angular kyphosis with vertebral wedging due to two tumor resections with multiple segment laminectomy for a high thoracic intramedullary glioma 2 years previously in a 10-year-old girl. Despite laminoplasty, a severe kyphosis has developed. (b) PA radiograph showing that the kyphotic process has been asymmetric thus giving rise to a concomitant scoliosis. This case could have been classified in the spinal tumor category but we thought it such a good example of an iatrogenic insult to the spine when posterior spinal support is destroyed in the growing child.

2.5.6 Miscellaneous Conditions in which a Spinal Deformity Is Common

In congenital heart disease, usually seen in those of the cyanotic variety, there is a much higher prevalence rate of idiopathic-type lordoscolioses. There is also a higher prevalence rate of idiopathic-type deformities in juvenile rheumatoid arthritis, presumably because, in addition to facet joint disease, the relative osteoporosis favors structural vertebral change. For reasons that are not abundantly clear, ocular and visual problems and congenital anomalies of the upper extremity are also associated

Basic Principles

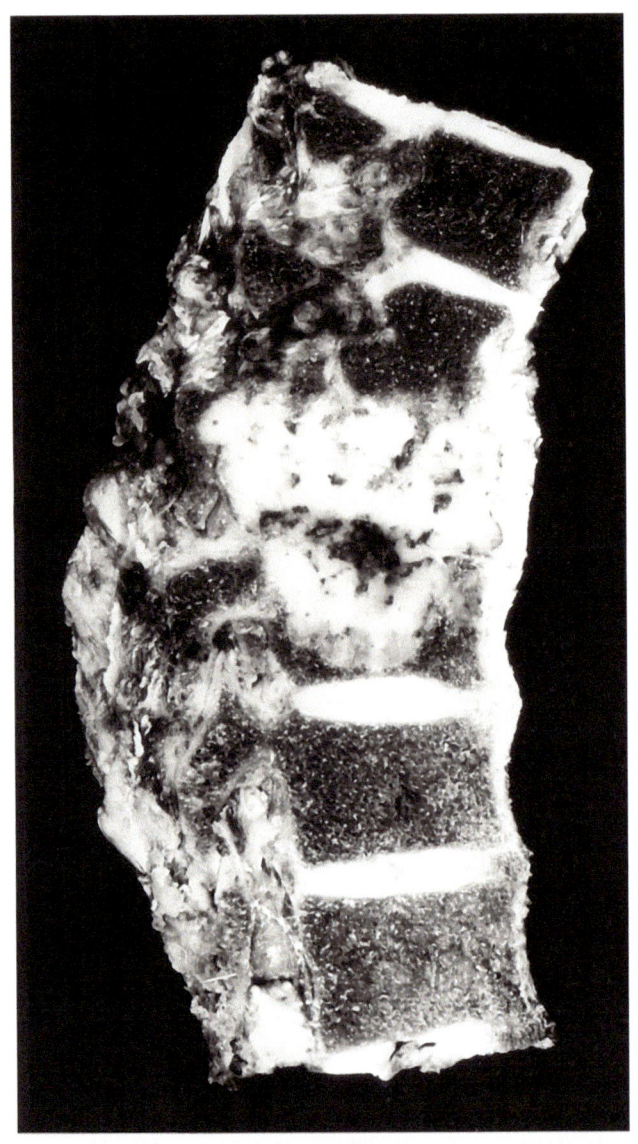

Fig. 2.37 Pathological specimen of the spine of a 50-year-old man with tuberculosis of the T9 and 10 vertebral bodies with caseous material pressing back into the canal.

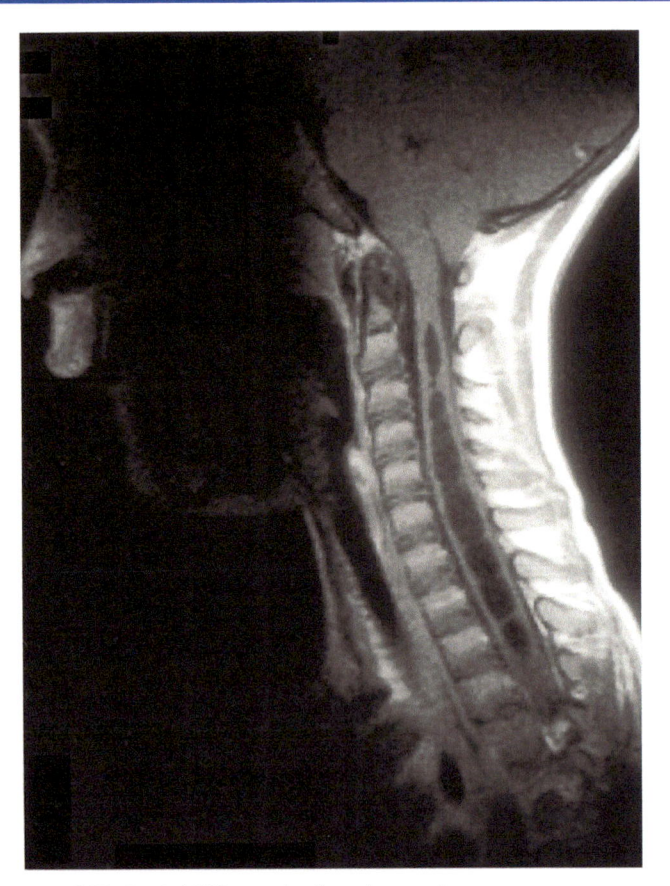

Fig. 2.38 Cervical MRI scan showing a large syrinx.

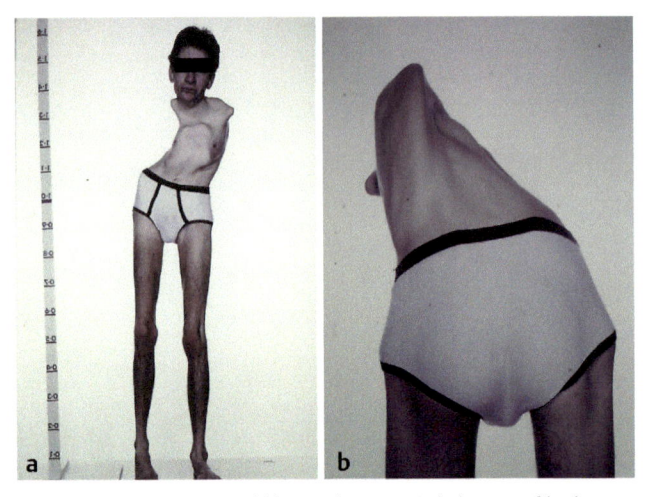

Fig. 2.39 (a) An 18-year-old boy with congenital absence of both upper extremities, four quarter absence on the left, and loss through the glenohumeral joint on the right. **(b)** Forward bending view showing a severe rotated lordoscoliosis with a razor-back appearance. This is the classical appearance of a pseudokyphosis. The most prominent apex of the ridge back are the vertebral bodies themselves, the lordosis having rotated all the way round so that it points directly backward. Despite all these problems, this young man was a terrific chap who was at university, was perfectly well-adjusted, entirely independent and self-sufficient, drove his own car, could write with his foot, could play the piano with his feet, and had no significant respiratory problems. All-in-all, an incredible young man.

with a higher than usual prevalence rate of idiopathic-type deformities (▶ Fig. 2.39).

Spinal Deformity in Adults

Paget's disease, ankylosing spondylitis (▶ Fig. 2.40), osteoporosis (▶ Fig. 2.41), and osteomalacia are deformities that develop after the attainment of spinal maturity and are thus true adult deformities.

Spondylolisthesis

This interesting condition of one vertebra, and the spine above, slipping forward on the one below is very different from the other conditions described in this volume and indeed seldom gives rise to a spinal deformity except with the particularly severe dysplastic variety. Significant degrees of dysplastic slip

Basic Principles

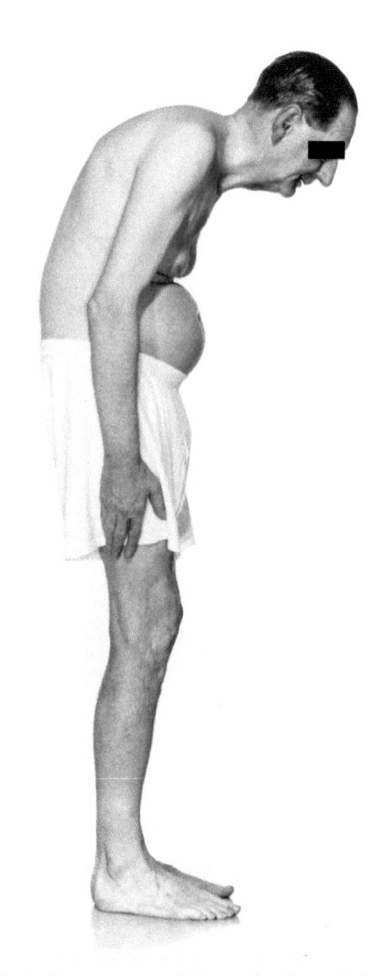

Fig. 2.40 The typical appearance of thoracolumbar ankylosing spondylitis.

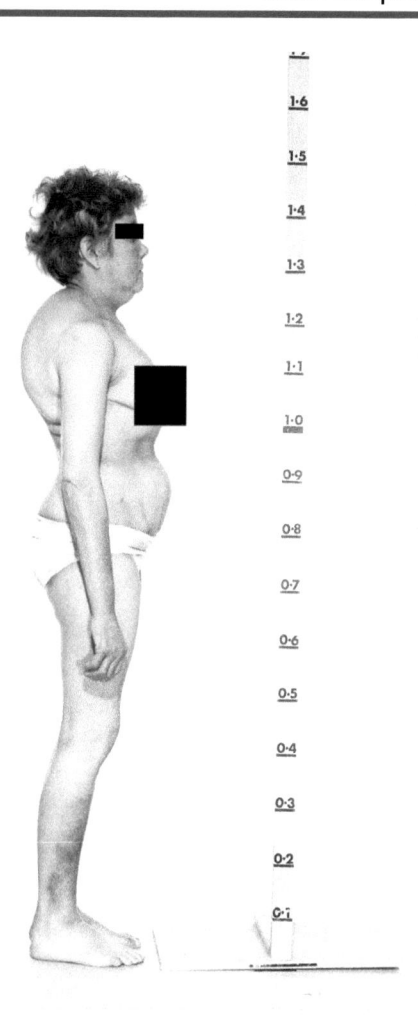

Fig. 2.41 The collapsing kyphosis in a postmenopausal woman with both osteoporosis and osteomalacia.

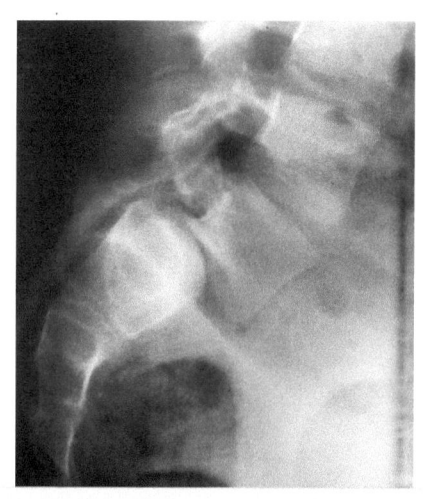

Fig. 2.42 Dysplastic spondylolisthesis. Lateral radiograph of lumbosacral region showing the excessive degree of slip but also the marked lumbosacral kyphosis.

at the L5/S1 level are, in effect, lumbosacral kyphoses with a posteriorly angulated lower lumbar region slipping forward off an anteriorly angulated pelvis (▶ Fig. 2.42). There are several causes of spondylolisthesis. In the dysplastic form congenital abnormalities of the back of L5 or S1 allow the slip to occur. In the isthmic variety the problem lies in the pars interarticularis and traditionally this has been described as a fatigue fracture, an elongated but intact pars, or an acute fracture. In actual fact an elongated pars only occurs with dysplastic spondylolisthesis while an acute pars fracture does not occur on its own but is always part of a more complex vertebral fracture pattern. The degenerative form is due to degenerative facet joints becoming mechanically incompetent at the L4/5 level favoring local slipping. The traumatic variety is due to a fracture in any area other than the pars, and the pathological variety is due to loss of the bony hook mechanism due to local or generalized bone disease.

2.6 Secondary, Nonprogressive or Nonstructural Deformities

2.6.1 Pelvic Tilt Scoliosis

A pelvic tilt and compensatory lumbar or thoracolumbar scoliosis above is produced usually by a leg-length inequality (▶ Fig. 2.4a).

2.6.2 Irritative Lesions

Painful paravertebral muscle spasm causes these nonstructural deformities that resolve when the underlying condition has been dealt with (▶ Fig. 2.4b). Diskitis, disk prolapse, or the benign osteoid osteoma or osteoblastoma are the usual causes.

2.6.3 Hysterical Scoliosis

This is an unusual, unpredictable, and inconsequential deformity that frequently disappears when the patient is lying down or sleeping.

References

Note: References in **bold** are Key References.

[1] **Terminology Committee of the Scoliosis Research Society. A glossary of scoliosis terms. Spine. 1976; 1:57–58**
[2] Walker AP, Dickson RA. School screening and pelvic tilt scoliosis. Lancet. 1984; 2(8395):152–153
[3] **Dickson RA, Lawton JO, Archer IA, Butt WP. The pathogenesis of idiopathic scoliosis. Biplanar spinal asymmetry. J Bone Joint Surg Br. 1984; 66(1):8–15**
[4] Ardran GM, Coates R, Dickson RA, Dixon-Brown A, Harding FM. Assessment of scoliosis in children: low dose radiographic technique. Br J Radiol. 1980; 53(626):146–147
[5] Ferguson AB. The study and treatment of scoliosis. South Med J. 1930; 23:116–120
[6] Cobb JR. Outline for the study of scoliosis. Instr Course Lect. 1948; 5:261–275
[7] Whittle MW, Evans M. Instrument for measuring the Cobb angle in scoliosis. Lancet. 1979; 1(8113):414
[8] du Peloux J, Fauchet R, Foucon B, Stagnara P. Le plan d'election pour l'examen radiologique des cyphoscolioses. Rev Chir Orthop Repar Appar Mot. 1965; 51:517–524
[9] Nash CL, Jr, Moe JH. A study of vertebral rotation. J Bone Joint Surg Am. 1969; 51(2):223–229
[10] Perdriolle R. La Scoliose: Son Etude Tridimensionnelle. Paris: Maloine; 1979
[11] **Mehta MH. The rib-vertebra angle in the early diagnosis between resolving and progressive infantile scoliosis. J Bone Joint Surg Br. 1972; 54(2):230–243**
[12] **Lenke LG, Betz RR, Harms J, et al. Adolescent idiopathic scoliosis: a new classification to determine extent of spinal arthrodesis. J Bone Joint Surg Am. 2001; 83-A(8):1169–1181**
[13] **Cruickshank JL, Koike M, Dickson RA. Curve patterns in idiopathic scoliosis. A clinical and radiographic study. J Bone Joint Surg Br. 1989; 71(2):259–263**
[14] Moe JH. A critical analysis of methods of fusion for scoliosis; an evaluation in two hundred and sixty-six patients. J Bone Joint Surg Am. 1958; 40-A (3):529–554, passim
[15] Dubousset J. Personal communication. The Signe d'epaule was taught by Dr Pierre Queneau, one of his previous mentors
[16] **Leatherman KD, Dickson RA. The Management of Spinal Deformities. London: Wright; 1988:6**
[17] **Risser JC. The Iliac apophysis; an invaluable sign in the management of scoliosis. Clin Orthop. 1958; 11(11):111–119**
[18] Bick EM, Copel JW. The ring apophysis of the human vertebra; contribution to human osteogeny. II. J Bone Joint Surg Am. 1951; 33-A(3):783–787
[19] Bernick S, Cailliet R. Vertebral end-plate changes with aging of human vertebrae. Spine. 1982; 7(2):97–102
[20] **Howell FR, Mahood JK, Dickson RA. Growth beyond skeletal maturity. Spine. 1992; 17(4):437–440**
[21] Weinstein SL. Natural history. Spine. 1999; 24(24):2592–2600
[22] **Weinstein SL, Ponseti IV. Curve progression in idiopathic scoliosis. J Bone Joint Surg Am. 1983; 65(4):447–455**
[23] **Dimeglio A. Growth in pediatric orthopaedics. J Pediatr Orthop. 2001; 21 (4):549–555**
[24] Gruelich WW, Pyle SI. Radiographic Atlas of Skeletal Development of the Hand and Wrist. 2nd ed. Stanford: Stanford University Press; London: Oxford University Press; 1959
[25] **Tanner JM, Whitehouse RH. Atlas of Children's Growth. New York: Academic Press; 1982**
[26] **Goldstein LA, Waugh TR. Classification and terminology of scoliosis. Clin Orthop Relat Res. 1973(93):10–22**
[27] James JIP. Idiopathic scoliosis; the prognosis, diagnosis, and operative indications related to curve patterns and the age at onset. J Bone Joint Surg Br. 1954; 36-B(1):36–49
[28] **Dickson RA. Conservative treatment for idiopathic scoliosis. J Bone Joint Surg Br. 1985; 67(2):176–181**
[29] **Deacon P, Berkin CR, Dickson RA. Combined idiopathic kyphosis and scoliosis. An analysis of the lateral spinal curvatures associated with Scheuermann's disease. J Bone Joint Surg Br. 1985; 67(2):189–192**
[30] **McMaster MJ, Ohtsuka K. The natural history of congenital scoliosis. A study of two hundred and fifty-one patients. J Bone Joint Surg Am. 1982; 64(8):1128–1147**

Chapter 3

The Etiology of Spinal Deformities

3.1	Introduction	38
3.2	The Development of Idiopathic Scoliosis	42
3.3	Experimental Models	47
3.4	What Pathogenesis Tells Us about Treatment	53

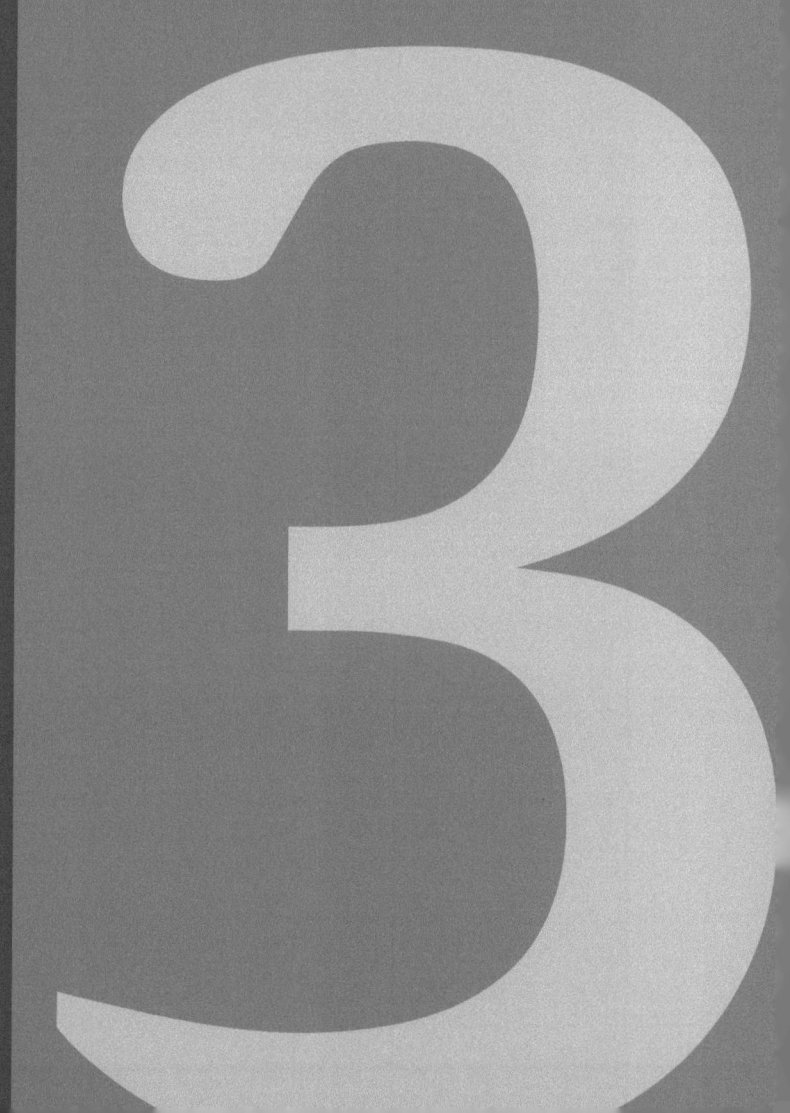

3 The Etiology of Spinal Deformities

3.1 Introduction

It is probably best to start with the etiology of idiopathic scoliosis and then to go on to discuss the etiology of the other spinal deformities in the classification. For whatever reason right–left asymmetry has attracted an illogical proportion of research effort. Nonstructural scoliosis, for example, secondary to a leg length inequality (see ▶ Fig. 2.4a), is indeed a problem of right–left asymmetry and so for that matter is a single congenital hemivertebra (see ▶ Fig. 2.6) that exists only in the coronal plane. However, structural scoliosis (scoliosis with torsion) is a complex deformity involving all three planes.

The deformity of idiopathic scoliosis is three-dimensional resulting from viscoelastic buckling of the spine in both the coronal (producing a lateral bend) and the transverse planes (an axial rotation or torsional buckling) to an approximation of Euler's laws.[1] Euler's laws can be summarized using a rather simplified formula. Euler's laws dictate how engineers' beams or columns fail mechanically and this is in two principal ways: simple angular collapse when a stick bends and breaks, for example, and that would be angular kyphosis; or beam buckling whereby the column fails by twisting deformation (buckling) (▶ Fig. 3.1). From a biomechanical standpoint, the critical buckling point is expressed by the formula:

$$P_{cr} = \frac{N \times EI}{L^2}$$

where P is the critical buckling load, N = a constant for end conditions, E = Young's modulus, I = moment of inertia, and L = effective length of the column. (For nonlinear cases exhibiting anisotropism, appropriate corrections can be made using the tangent modulus and secant modulus theories). It is recognized that Euler's theory provides only a simplistic explanation for spinal instability, since the plastic deformations that occur in a curved column like the spine are more complex. We will develop Euler's laws further as we go through this chapter. While this buckling process is essentially physical, for a progressive deformity to ensue, it is a requirement that the buckling process occurs during the phase of spinal growth, thus the product of spinal buckling can be seen as progressive three-dimensional shape deformation. Observation of this deformation process facilitates an understanding of pathogenesis as well as treatment. Therefore, both biomechanical and biological factors are the critically important issues to consider.[2]

It would be sensible to begin by describing normal spinal shape and then we can see how this shape buckles to produce structural scoliosis. The common characteristics of the normal human spine can be summarized as follows. It is a moderately slender tapered column and in cross-section it can be regarded as a prism of variable orientation.[3] The broad side-to-side width of the cervical and lumbar vertebrae dictates that the bases of the prisms are situated anteriorly while the apices are posterior. By contrast the thoracic vertebral bodies are heart-shaped with a greater length from front to back and are thus prismatic with the apices anterior and the bases posterior. Furthermore, the thoracic prisms are asymmetric with the apices slightly to the right of the midline as a result of the lateral force (or lateral restraint) imposed by the thoracic aorta (▶ Fig. 3.2 and ▶ Fig. 3.3). The spinal column or beam does not have to be prismatic in cross-section to buckle, rather prismatic shape does help the buckling process and its appreciation.[3] In addition in the coronal plane a very small lateral curvature exists in the thoracic region (convex to the right usually, secondary to the "aortic force"), and this is an almost invariable finding described by anatomists centuries ago.[4] To confirm this tendency for right-sided thoracic direction it is the opposite (i.e., to the left) with situs inversus[5,6] (▶ Fig. 3.3b). In this beautiful study utilizing both computed tomography (CT) and magnetic resonance imaging (MRI), the preexisting rotation of the vertebrae from top to bottom in the normal and situs inversus spine is clearly shown. The right-sided preponderance from T6 to T10 to the right in the normal spine and to the left in the situs inversus spine does achieve statistical significance at the 1% level. This nicely demonstrates that just where idiopathic thoracic scoliosis is apical, namely the mid-lower thoracic region; it is predestined to favor the right side. This effect is static dependent upon vertebral shape in the transverse plane. In the lumbar region there is no static predisposition to the left; rather, it is the presence of the abdominal aorta on the left side that produces its effect dynamically, being a pulsatile mass just next to the spine (▶ Fig. 3.3c).

There are also curvatures in the sagittal plane in the ambulant human spine and there are four primary curves: lordoses in the cervical and lumbar regions and kyphoses in the thoracic spine

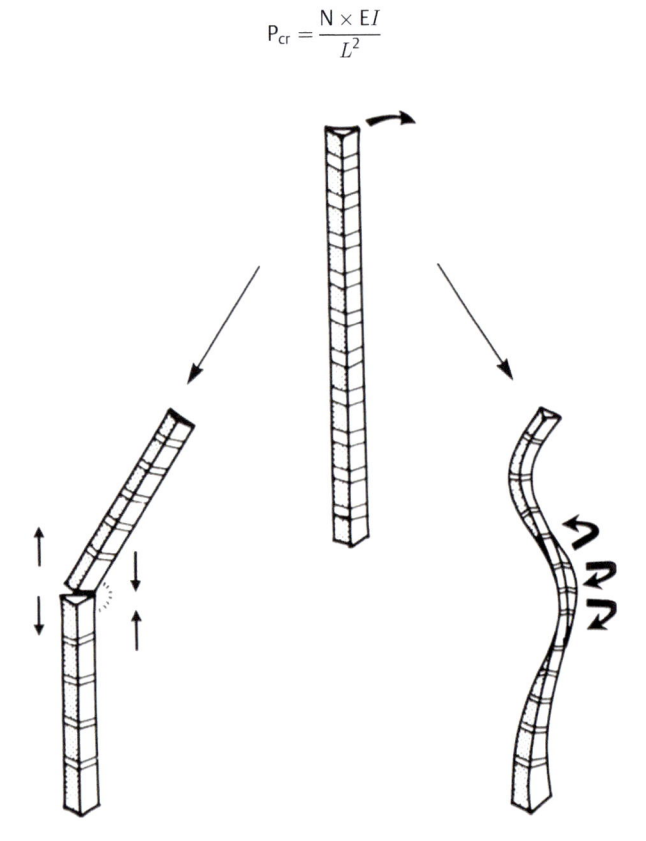

Fig. 3.1 A column or beam can fail in only two ways: left angular collapse (kyphosis) or right beam buckling (lordoscoliosis). (Reproduced with permission from Newton P, O'Brien M, Shufflebarger H, et al. Idiopathic Scoliosis: The Harms Study Group Treatment Guide. Stuttgart/New York: Thieme; 2010: 38.)

The Etiology of Spinal Deformities

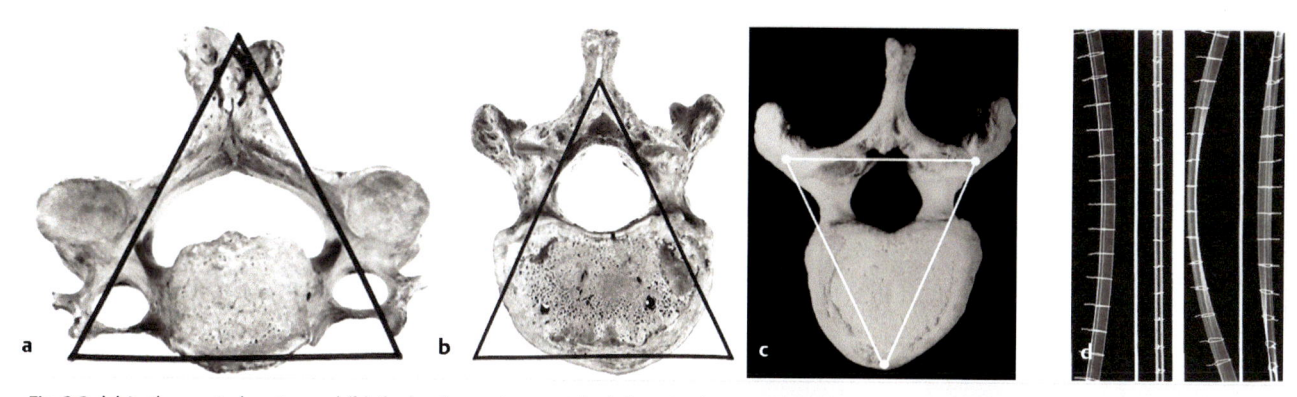

Fig. 3.2 (a) In the cervical region and (b) the lumbar region, vertebral shape in the transverse plane resembles a prism with its base facing anteriorly. (c) In the thoracic region, however, the shape of the transverse plane resembles a prism with its apex pointing anteriorly, which is a much more unstable configuration. ([a–c] Reproduced with permission from Newton P, O'Brien M, Shufflebarger H, et al. Idiopathic Scoliosis: The Harms Study Group Treatment Guide. Stuttgart/New York: Thieme; 2010: 41.) (d) Radiographs of a prismatic spinal model (plastic material) during flexion. In each pair the right picture is an AP projection and on the left the lateral projection. The pair on the left show flexion of the prism toward its base showing no rotation while the pair on the right show a marked degree of rotation when the prism is flexed toward its apex.

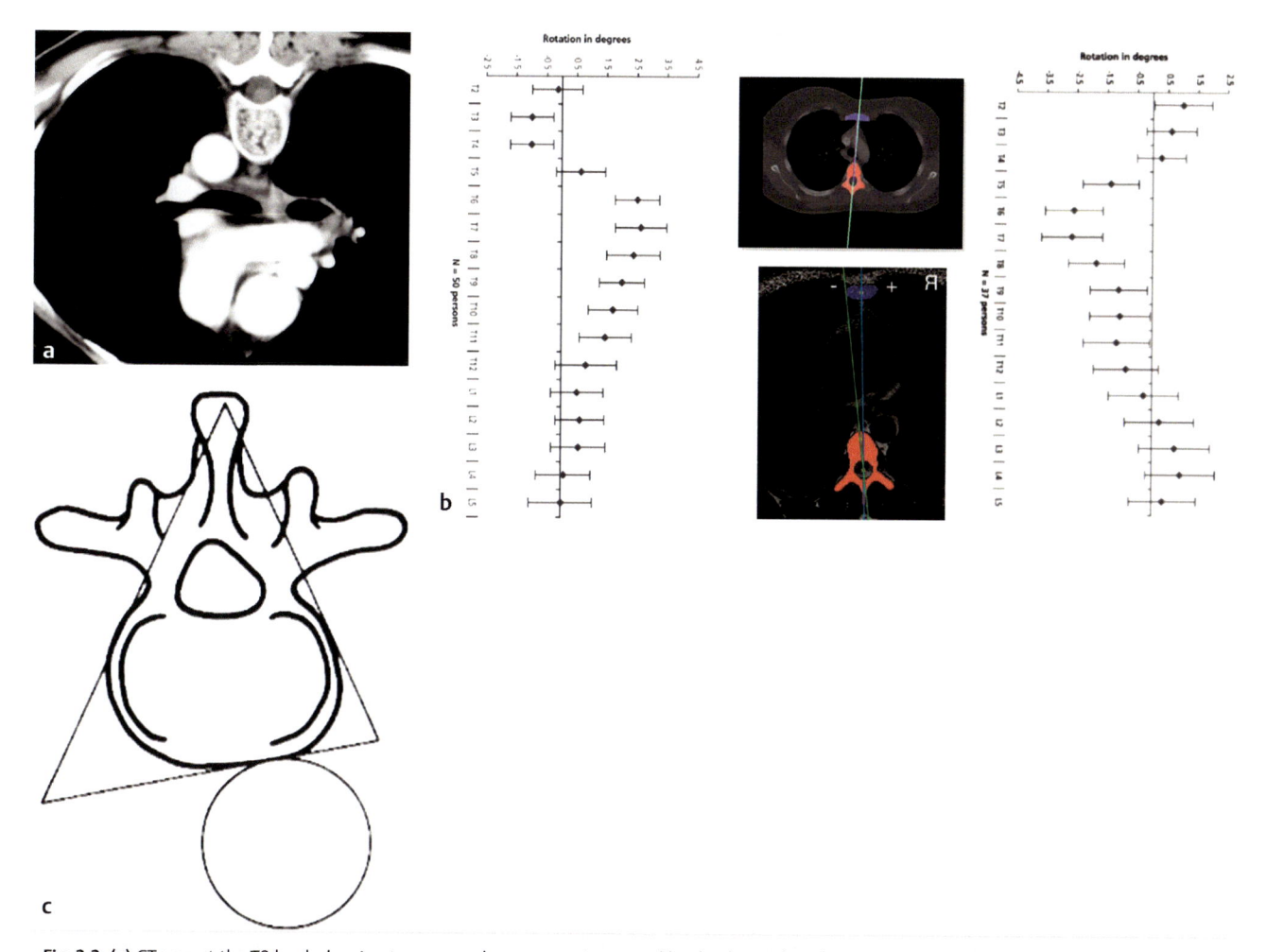

Fig. 3.3 (a) CT scan at the T8 level, showing transverse plane asymmetry caused by the descending thoracic aorta. (b) When there is situs inversus, the rotation is in precisely the opposite direction to the normal anatomy (Levocardia). (Diagram kindly supplied by Dr. Rene Castelein, Head of the Department of Orthopaedic Surgery in Utrecht.) (c) In the lumbar region the abdominal aorta is to the left of the midline and thus rests against the left side of the base of the lumbar prism, favoring left-sided rotation in the lumbar spine. ([a,c] Reproduced with permission from Newton P, O'Brien M, Shufflebarger H, et al. Idiopathic Scoliosis: The Harms Study Group Treatment Guide. Stuttgart/New York: Thieme; 2010: 42.)

The Etiology of Spinal Deformities

and the sacrum. Therefore, it can be seen that the "normal" human spine is not symmetrical in any of its three planes and that the nature of this asymmetry varies along the length of the column. Flexion in the thoracic spine is limited by the relatively reduced disk height and with the rib cage imparting marked rigidity. The presence of a kyphosis indicates that the axis of longitudinal rotation in the thoracic spine is located in front of the spine and thus protects the otherwise rotationally unstable prismatic transverse plane shape from rotation on flexion or compressive loading (▶ Fig. 3.4 and ▶ Fig. 3.5). The thoracic spine is thus normally under tension and not compression.

In idiopathic scoliosis, however, the back of the spinal column rotates toward the curve concavity (concordant rotation) as inspection of every radiograph will confirm (▶ Fig. 3.5), thus indicating that the spinal column is shorter at the back than the front (the back of the spine is running the 200 m on the inside lane) and thus confirms the presence of lordosis in every case (▶ Fig. 3.6).[7] Meanwhile, with a kyphotic thoracic spine compressed to failure, the spinous processes buckle toward the curve convexity and this can be seen in virtually every case of Scheuermann's disease of any degree when there is quite often a mild coronal plane curvature with either no rotation or rotation toward the convexity[8] (discordant rotation) (see Chapter 5). Cervical and lumbar vertebrae with their axes of rotation lying behind the vertebral bodies because of their lordotic sagittal shape are inherently rotationally unstable on flexion but are protected by three factors: (1) low flexural stiffness as a result of the anteriorly based prismatic shape and increased disk height permitting considerable flexion; (2) powerful posterior musculoligamentous structures; and (3) lumbar facet joints with virtually sagittal plane orientation although the lower two lumbar facet joints permit a small amount of rotation. As a result of the natural three-dimensional spinal asymmetry we can regard any axial load as having eccentricity and the spine as a whole as being prebuckled, theoretically reducing the critical load requirements as compared to a straight or single curved column.

Along with restraints imposed by the intervertebral disks, ligaments, and facet joints, the sagittal curvatures of the spine determine the centroidal axes of rotation of any given motion segment in any plane (anterior in the thoracic spine and posterior in the cervical and lumbar spines). The spine exhibits variable stiffness (flexural, torsional, and shear rigidity) throughout its length and at different magnitudes of loading and direction of loading—that is, it is anisotropic, nonlinear, and inhomogeneous.[2]

Motion segments display coupling of rotations and translations such as the thoracic spine axial torque producing a primary axial rotation motion and a secondary frontal rotation (lateral bend) about a helical axis of rotation; the direction to which the posterior elements point is constant, toward the convexity of the curve for the kyphotic thoracic spine. This contrasts with the invariable concave side posterior rotation seen in idiopathic scoliosis. As an aside, the apparent coupling of lateral flexion that accompanies forward flexion in scoliotic spines is no more than true forward flexion of a segment rotated about its longitudinal axis, the local plane of flexion/extension now pointing laterally. It can be seen straightaway that if lateral flexion occurs in the kyphotic thoracic spine it does not produce the natural scoliotic spinous process rotation toward the

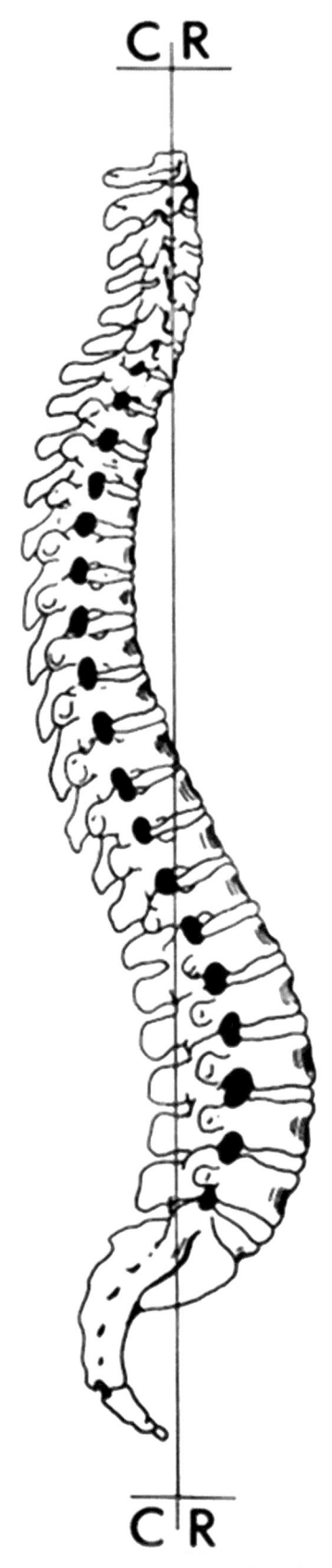

Fig. 3.4 The axis of spinal column rotation. This is determined by the orientation of the posterior facet joints at each level. (Reproduced with permission from Newton P, O'Brien M, Shufflebarger H, et al. Idiopathic Scoliosis: The Harms Study Group Treatment Guide. Stuttgart/New York: Thieme; 2010: 35.)

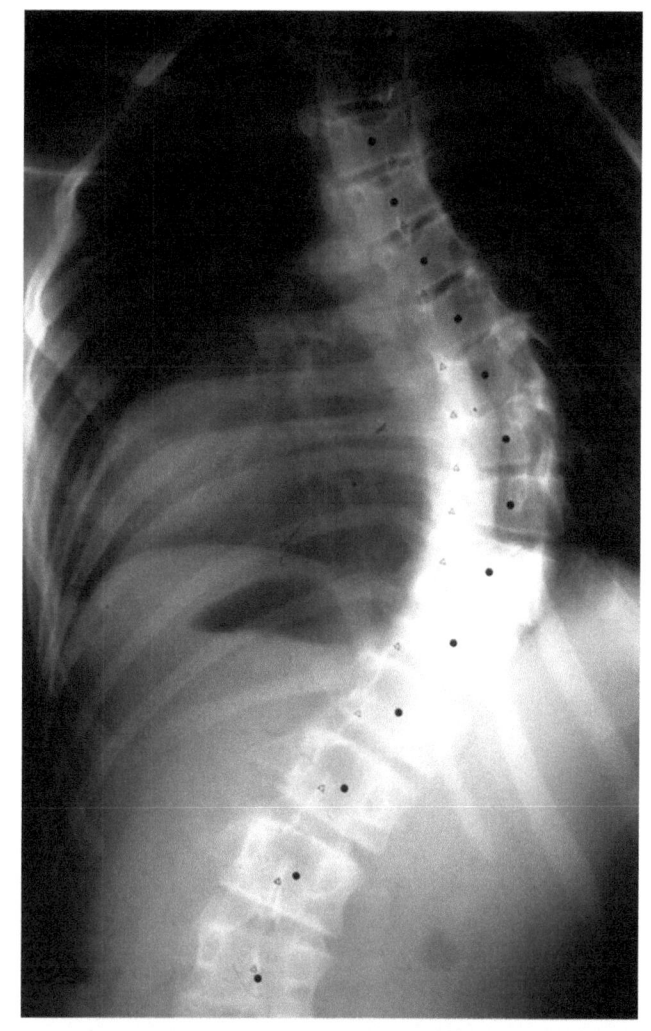

Fig. 3.5 PA radiograph of a thoracic idiopathic scoliosis with the tips of the spinous processes marked with triangles and the middle of the vertebral bodies with dots. It can be seen that the distance down the back of the spine is shorter than the distance down the front, confirming that all structural scolioses are lordotic. (Reproduced with permission from Newton P, O'Brien M, Shufflebarger H, et al. Idiopathic Scoliosis: The Harms Study Group Treatment Guide. Stuttgart/New York: Thieme; 2010: 32.)

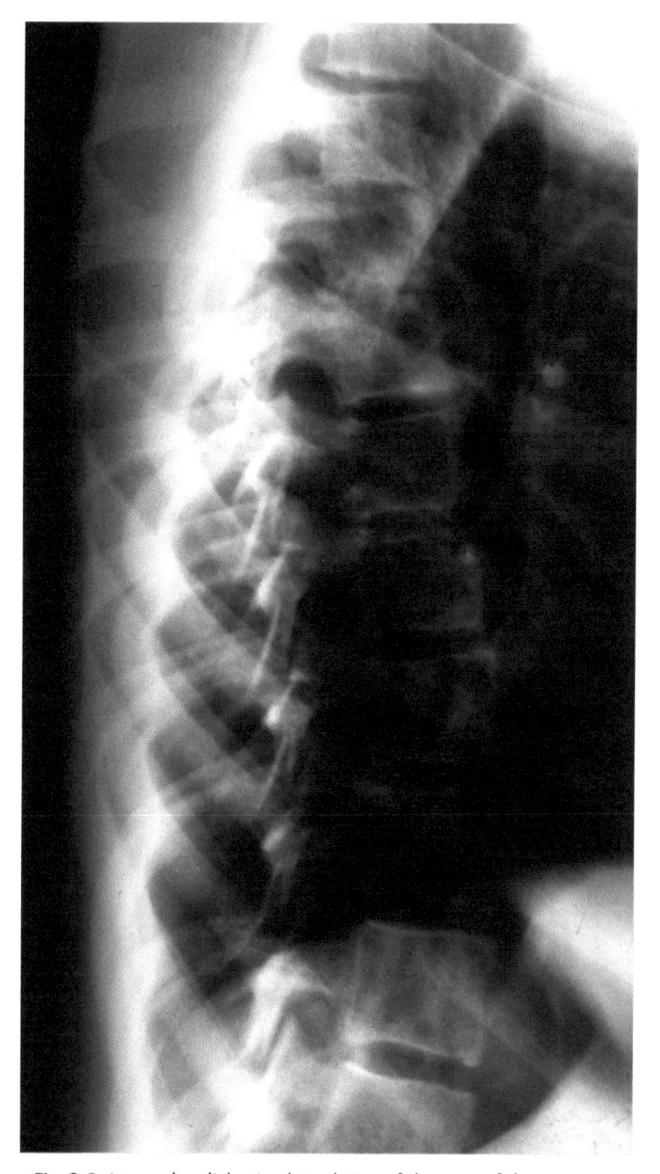

Fig. 3.6 A true plan d'election lateral view of the apex of the curvature shown in ▶ Fig. 3.5, demonstrating the lordosis. (Reproduced with permission from Newton P, O'Brien M, Shufflebarger H, et al. Idiopathic Scoliosis: The Harms Study Group Treatment Guide. Stuttgart/New York: Thieme; 2010: 32.)

curve concavity and therefore efforts at trying to produce experimentally right–left asymmetry, where most attention has been directed, will naturally be fruitless—lateral flexion doesn't occur first.

In terms of the end restraints of the spinal column, the spine can be thought of as permitting translations and rotations only in the sagittal plane, since it is a requirement that the eyes are level and face forward and the pelvis is similarly constrained; the presence of the thoracic aorta may be imagined as perhaps a lateral restraint or a laterally deflecting force.

The structural complexity of the spine in terms of its myriad components is not only complicated by the inconveniences of creep, relaxation, anisotropism, and nonlinearity, but by additional, self-generating deforming forces consequent upon growth. Bone obeys the Hueter[1]-Volkmann[2] law as well as Wolff's[3] law and the vertebral bodies exhibit dynamic deformation as a result of tensile and compressive forces that result in stimulating and inhibiting bone growth, respectively, and further three-dimensional asymmetry—only, of course, during spinal growth (not just at the age of 15 when the pelvis matures

---

[1] **Carl Hueter** (1838–1882), German surgeon who, with Volkmann, noted that compressive forces inhibit growth and tensile forces stimulate growth and now an orthopaedic rule regarding bone growth referred to as the Hueter-Volkmann law. He was Professor of Surgery at Greifswald.
[2] **Richard von Volkmann** (1830–1889), of Volkmann ischemic contracture, was Professor of Surgery at Halle.
[3] **Julius Wolff** (1836–1902), German anatomist. Wolff's law—a bone, normal or abnormal, develops a structure most suited to resist the forces acting upon it.

but up to possibly the age of 25[9]), and then afterward not until osteoporotic or osteoarthritic old age. The more that growth makes the vertebrae asymmetric, the more the spinal column becomes less easy to straighten and requires alternative treatment strategies (see Chapter 4).

3.2 The Development of Idiopathic Scoliosis

Now let's get away from biomechanics for a while to more clinical matters. From the foregoing it would not seem to require much more effort to figure out how idiopathic scoliosis develops especially as the information has been in the literature for decades, if not centuries. The concept of the essential lesion in idiopathic scoliosis as being a relatively fixed lordotic area that, under the influence of transverse or coronal plane asymmetry, rotates to the side and gives rise to a lateral curvature has consistently been put forward as the prime etiology.[10–12] Adams' work in 1865 describes his dissections of bodies with scoliotic spines 40 years before X-rays were invented. He showed quite clearly in his dissections that there was always a lordosis at the apex of the curve in structural scoliosis.[10] Unfortunately, Adams seems to have been relegated to the "forward bend test" but his work really should be read fully by all interested scoliosis surgeons. Another intellectual giant in scoliosis research was Robert Roaf in Liverpool, an individual of the utmost brilliance while at the same time being incredibly pleasant and having the time to help young surgeons, for example, R.A.D., with an interest in scoliosis surgery. As we shall see he also made a considerable contribution to the treatment of spinal deformities.[12] However he told us all about the cause of structural scoliosis although it seems that his papers have gone largely unread by the non-UK scoliosis world. His classic "The Basic Anatomy of Scoliosis"[11] clearly explained how the deformity of idiopathic scoliosis develops and all the Leeds Scoliosis Study Group has done subsequently is to add a little more detail. He pointed out that under the restraining influence of the anterior chest and abdominal wall increased length of the anterior elements can be accommodated only by lateral deviation and rotation of the vertebral bodies and that the degree of torsion varies with relative lengthening of the anterior elements. ▶ Fig. 3.7, an interpretation of one of his figures, represents how this is accomplished with reference in particular to the line of the anterior longitudinal ligament and the line of the interspinous ligaments. He stated that "simple three-dimensional geometry shows that if the vertebral bodies are rotated farther from the midline than the spinous processes there must be lordosis - that is relative lengthening of the anterior longitudinal ligament" (note the use of the word "simple").

He then went on to measure the anterior and posterior spinal lengths from T1 to L5 in both normal and scoliotic spines confirming the relative shortness of the back of the spine with scoliosis (▶ Table 3.1). He then described how a scoliotic spine can be divided into five regions, as shown in ▶ Fig. 3.8. Then for those still struggling with this concept of lordosis as the essential lesion, ▶ Fig. 3.9 shows how lordosis behaves when flexed and the only methods by which it can be corrected. This is of

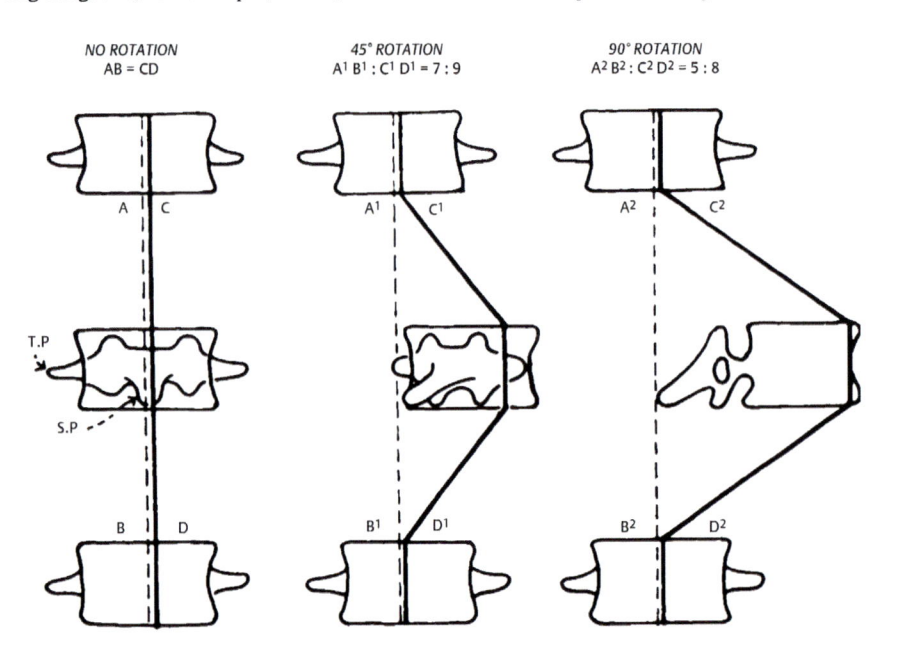

NO ROTATION
AB = CD

45° ROTATION
$A^1B^1 : C^1D^1 = 7 : 9$

90° ROTATION
$A^2B^2 : C^2D^2 = 5 : 8$

CD, C^1D^1, C^2D^2 = Line of anterior longitudinal ligament

AB, A^1B^1, A^2B^2 = Line of interspinous ligament

Fig. 3.7 This diagram is really self-explanatory but as you go from the PA projection on the left to the lateral on the right so, necessarily, the front of the spine over the apical area is longer than the back. Reproduced with permission and copyright © of the British Editorial Society of Bone and Joint Surgery, Roaf R, The basic anatomy of scoliosis. J Bone Joint Surg (Br) 1966; 48B: 786–792, Figure 1.

The Etiology of Spinal Deformities

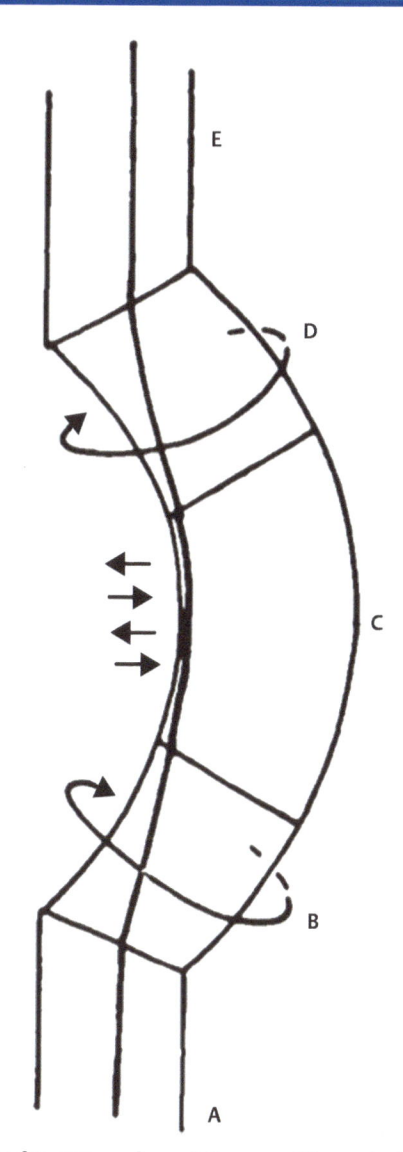

Fig. 3.8 The five regions of a scoliotic curve: **(A)** pure lordosis, **(B)** lordosis and rotation, **(C)** lateral flexion, **(D)** counter rotation, and **(E)** lordosis. Reproduced with permission and copyright © of the British Editorial Society of Bone and Joint Surgery, Roaf R, The basic anatomy of scoliosis. J Bone Joint Surg (Br) 1966; 48B: 786–792, Figure 5.

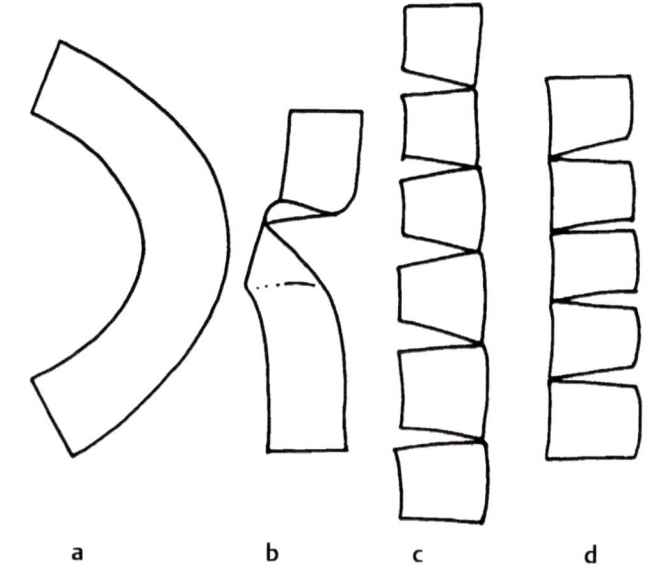

Fig. 3.9 (a) C-shaped piece of cardboard viewed from the side. The long edge represents the anterior longitudinal ligament. If it is straightened, that is, the lordosis corrected by making the upper and lower ends parallel to each other, the longer (or anterior) edge bends and twists sideways **(b)**. This could only be prevented if discrepancies between the anterior and posterior edges are corrected either by lengthening the posterior edge **(c)** or by shortening the anterior edge **(d)**. Reproduced with permission and copyright © of the British Editorial Society of Bone and Joint Surgery, Roaf R, The basic anatomy of scoliosis. J Bone Joint Surg (Br) 1966; 48B: 786–792, Figure 9.

Table 3.1 Anterior and posterior spinal lengths from T1 to L5 in normal and scoliotic spines

	Adult erect		Adult flexed	
	Anterior	Posterior	Anterior	Posterior
Normal spine (in cm)				
Thoracic	25.6	29.8	21.9	31.7
Lumbar	17.6	15	16.7	16.6
Total	43.2	44.8	38.6	48.3
Scoliotic spine (in cm)				
Thoracic	27.8	26.1	25.5	19.7
Lumbar	16.8	12	20.4	10.5
Total	44.6	38.1	45.9	30.2

fundamental importance because it indicates precisely how and why, having understood how the deformity develops, you can correct it logically.[11] This is why in Leeds, particularly for larger more stiff curves, we introduced the concept of shortening the front of the spine (anterior multiple diskectomy), the Leeds Procedure.[13] Perhaps we should have called it Roaf's procedure but we wanted to draw attention to all the work on the pathogenesis of idiopathic scoliosis that we have done in Leeds over the years. We felt that to understand how this three-dimensional deformity develops would be an essential prerequisite for understanding how it can be corrected.

In Leeds we borrowed 11 articulated skeletons with idiopathic scoliosis from the Royal College of Surgeons of Edinburgh Museum (courtesy of Professor D. C. Mekie, the curator) and studied them every which way including carrying out the same anterior and posterior vertebral body height measurements as Roaf had done. We found precisely the same results, namely

The Etiology of Spinal Deformities

over the apical region, the anterior vertebral body heights were significantly bigger than the posterior (▶ Table 3.2).[14]

Another great was Edgar Somerville from Oxford who probably carried out the first sensible experiments to produce structural scoliosis (in rabbits)[15] (▶ Fig. 3.10). Indeed, the title of his seminal paper was "Rotational Lordosis: the development of the single curve." He felt the concept of lordosis as being the essential lesion was so straightforward that he spent the rest of his professional life looking after children with developmental hip dysplasia! It was really he that inspired the Leeds Group to go on and do all the work they did and he was a frequent and most welcome visitor and advisor to the Leeds Unit.

Table 3.2 Mean vertebral body heights

Structural curve (in cm)		
Anterior	Posterior	Difference
1.108	1.063	−0.045
1.107	1.118	−0.011
1.052	0.985	+0.067
1.151	0.919	+0.232; $p < 0.02$
1.152	0.978	+0.174; $p < 0.04$
1.200	1.160	+0.040
1.254	1.281	−0.027
1.280	1.345	−0.065

That the prime lesion in structural scoliosis is an apical lordosis is best appreciated in the thoracic spine which is normally kyphotic and therefore the presence of lordosis would indicate a fairly radical departure from normal sagittal shape. The presence of the essential thoracic lordosis in idiopathic thoracic scoliosis can always be verified; but, with increasing degrees of apical rotation, the more increasingly oblique the lateral spinal radiograph is, which spuriously gives the impression of kyphosis when of course it is just another oblique view of the same lordo-scoliosis.[16] This is precisely why publications and presentations continue to look at and measure lateral radiographs of the patient. It was, for instance, thought that more than 60 degrees of kyphosis on a lateral view, of say a neurofibromatosis patient, was the critical level beyond which anterior surgery was mandated.[17] All this means is that the scoliosis has got a lot bigger and so has the degree of rotation. It is nothing whatever to do with kyphosis. In recent classifications of idiopathic scoliosis, the concept of kyphosis still appears and is thought to be critical in the classification.[18] Of course it is quite right that the more the rotation the more the need for anterior surgery. Because the bigger the Cobb angle and the more rotation the stiffer the curve is and requires an anterior space-making procedure (anterior multiple diskectomy) to allow metalwork to adequately correct the deformity.[13]

It was Stagnara who showed that true views of the scoliosis can be taken when the patient or X-ray beam is rotated to the amount of apical rotation and then true plan d'election views were obtained (see ▶ Fig. 2.10).[7] On the anteroposterior (AP) view when the deformity is seen en face, the Cobb angle is much greater; but, more importantly, when a true lateral is taken of the curve apex, that is, 90 degrees to the true plan d'election AP, the lordosis is unmasked (▶ Fig. 3.6). The lordosis is still present on

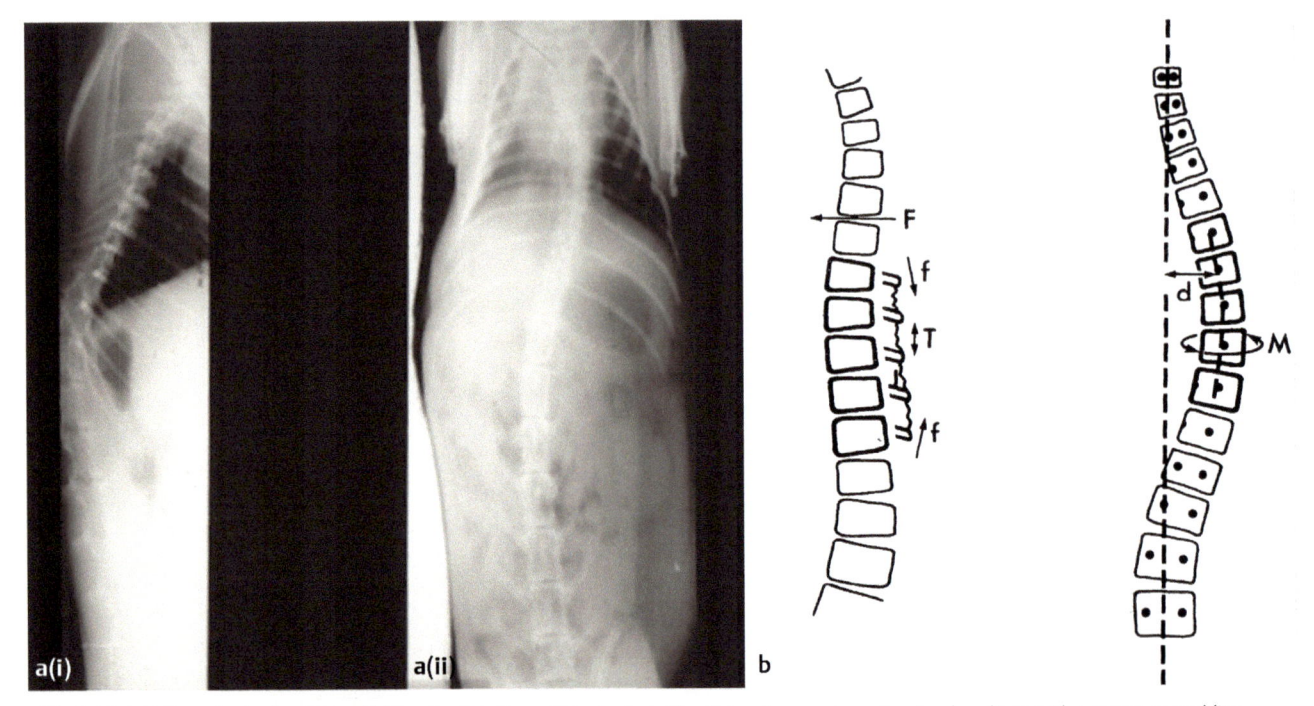

Fig. 3.10 (a) When the back of the rabbit's spine is tethered into lordosis (i) within a few weeks a structural scoliosis with rotation resembling idiopathic scoliosis develops (ii). (b) Simplified theoretical model of biplanar spinal asymmetry. Lateral profile with lower thoracic lordosis (left); anteroposterior view of coronal plane asymmetry (right). $M, \propto, f.d.$ where F = force of forward flexion; T = tightening of posterior structures; f = reactive force; d = distance of coronal plane asymmetry from midline; and M = spinning moment.

true lateral views of the curve apex even in very big curves. However, of course, the degree of apical lordosis does not increase pari passu with the lateral curvature because the farther the lordosis moves from the sagittal plane then the less it is compressed. While a number of possible etiological factors other than an abnormality in the sagittal plane, particularly neuromuscular factors, have their proponents as causative in idiopathic scoliosis,[19-29] it has to be said that the presence of such factors (e.g., proprioception and equilibral dysfunction) have in the main been demonstrated by comparing scoliotic patients with straight-backed controls. The finding of a marginally and sometimes significantly increased prevalence, but not a consistent presence, in the scoliotic population has perversely demonstrated that such factors cannot be etiological as they are not present in all cases* and indeed are not uncommon in straight backed controls. The only consistently present abnormality in all children with idiopathic scoliosis is an abnormality of spinal shape in the sagittal plane. Crucially, as we shall see in the next chapter, a painstaking 6-year prospective epidemiological survey involving 16,000 schoolchildren demonstrated that the lordosis developed before the scoliosis, confirming that it was the primary abnormality.[30]

Quite why the search for the cause of idiopathic scoliosis should continue is barely explicable unless the work of Adams, Roaf, and Somerville, let alone the Leeds Scoliosis Study Group, is either unfamiliar or for whatever reason disregarded. Of course publications from England do not seem to travel well!

The development of single structural curves at other sites and other curve patterns such as double or multiple curves is perhaps less easy to visualize. However, again, the essential lesion lies in the sagittal plane. Looking first at a single curve, usually only the central three or four vertebrae or so are truly lordotic. Inspect a posteroanterior (PA) radiograph of a left thoracolumbar curve (see ▶ Fig. 2.20). Lordotic vertebrae are defined as those that are laterally displaced to the convex side with the spinous processes rotated back toward the curve concavity (concordant rotation). The apical vertebrae will be confirmed as being so orientated but above and below these vertebrae will be neutral vertebrae with the spinous process in the center and beyond that, convex to the left, will be vertebrae whose spinous processes have remained rotated to the left, that is, lateral spinal curvatures with rotation to the convex side (discordant rotation).[31] Therefore, the compensatory curves above and below the structural curve are now kyphoscolioses. That of course must be the case because the central lordoscoliosis must be balanced above and below by asymmetric kyphoses to maintain overall three-dimensional balance in the spine. Moreover, the apex of a single thoracic curve is invariably located at T8 or T9. Should this lordotic area extend slightly lower or slightly higher than usual then there is insufficient "room" to fit in an asymmetric kyphosis before the spine meets the midline. A contralateral lordoscoliosis is therefore produced for balance purposes with the development of a typical double structural curve (see ▶ Fig. 2.16c). This can be seen on any PA radiograph of a double curve. If the upper end of a structural thoracic curve has the same problem, then a contralateral lordoscoliosis is produced above with the production of the typical thoracic double major as described by Moe[32] (see ▶ Fig. 2.17). For single curves the lordotic apex never extends below L2 and so apical at T12/L1 is the thoracolumbar curve and apical at L2 is the lumbar curve. A thoracolumbar or lumbar single curve must therefore be either more lordotic or have greater flexural stiffness and there is evidence of both.

It is recognized that Euler's theory provides only a simplistic explanation for spinal instability since the plastic deformations that occur in a curved column like the spine do not occur at the elastic buckling load (except in the case of a straight beam-column), and are not strictly analogous with a sudden deflection and collapse that occurs at critical load in a true elastic beam column. However, in all age groups, girls with scoliosis, even with curvatures uncoiled, are significantly taller than straight-backed counterparts.[33,34] Furthermore, the finding that girls have more slender spines than boys at any given age would suggest that they have greater effective column length, L, in the Euler equation, a significant mechanism by which the spines of girls have a greater propensity to buckle under load, apart from any other difference there may be in flexural stiffness, EI, in such individuals.

Now we have to add in the effect of biological growth and then the scene is set for the development of the progressive deformity. Careful studies of sagittal profile during growth in normal children have demonstrated that the thoracic kyphosis gradually diminishes becoming minimal in the preadolescent growth period in both boys and girls (▶ Fig. 3.11).[35,36] At this time girls are growing and developing quickly thus magnifying any trend toward flattening of the normal thoracic kyphosis.[33,37] Boys, meanwhile, do not regain their normal thoracic kyphosis until 2 or 3 years later when they are going through their peak adolescent growth velocity. This accounts for the greater preponderance of the opposite deformity (Scheuermann's disease) in boys.[38,39]

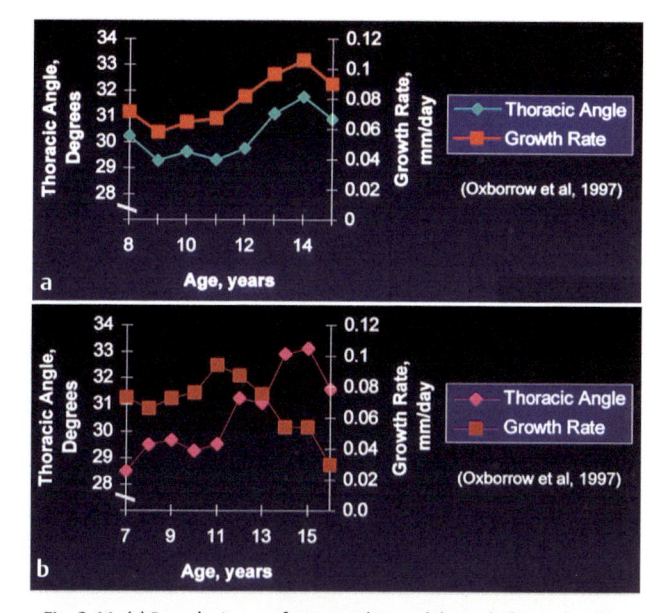

Fig. 3.11 (a) Boys don't grow fastest until toward the end of growth, when the thoracic kyphosis is maximal. (b) The thoracic kyphosis is at its minimum when girls grow fastest. (Reproduced with permission from Newton P, O'Brien M, Shufflebarger H, et al. Idiopathic Scoliosis: The Harms Study Group Treatment Guide. Stuttgart/New York: Thieme; 2010: 39–40.)

---

* **Robert Koch** (1843–1910), German bacteriologist. Laid down four necessary criteria for a diagnosis, Koch's postulates, of which the first has been generalized to all conditions ... "the causative agent must be observed in all cases of the condition".

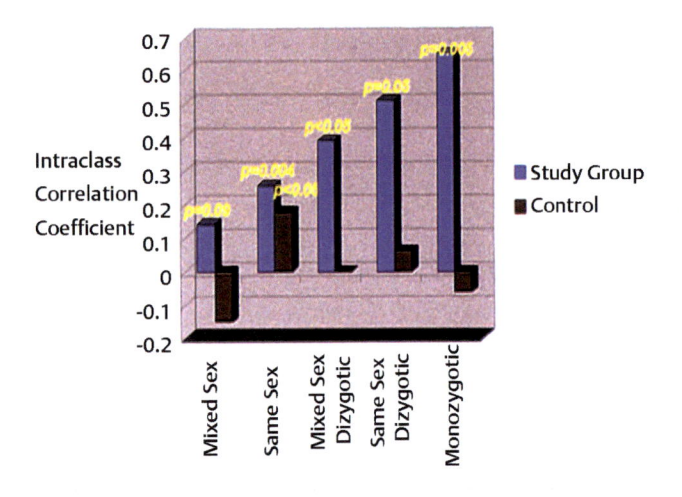

Fig. 3.12 Lateral spinal profile measured in children in a school screening program with a surface-shape computer. This histogram of correlation coefficients demonstrates that as one passes from mixed-sex siblings through same-sex, mixed-sex dizygotic, and same-sex dizygotic to monozygotic siblings (from left to right), the correlation coefficients steadily increase in magnitude, indicating ever closer correspondence between lateral spinal profiles until with identical twins the lateral spinal profiles are virtually the same. This is a very important genetic element in the pathogenesis of idiopathic scoliosis. (Reproduced with permission from Newton P, O'Brien M, Shufflebarger H, et al. Idiopathic Scoliosis: The Harms Study Group Treatment Guide. Stuttgart/New York: Thieme; 2010: 31.)

Interestingly, the pattern of growth and development during adolescence does have a distinctly familial trend[40–42] and of course several studies have shown that idiopathic scoliosis is a strongly familial condition.[41,43–48] Thus many of the factors that might disadvantage the stability of the spinal column are biological ones that would be expected to have similar genetic expression in family members. Therefore, there are a host of genes active in the spine at this time that would very much go against the rather simplistic notion that there can be a single gene for idiopathic scoliosis. Importantly, the suggestion that normal spinal shape might be a familial matter[49] has been proven in our three-dimensional shape study of twins/siblings during growth. Using surface topography measurement in schools but also at the Annual British Twin Conference it was shown that correspondence in lateral profile rose from being insignificant in unrelated children through mixed-sex siblings, same sex siblings, mixed sex dizygotic twins, same sex dizygotic twins, through to monozygotic twins the correlation coefficients steadily increased in magnitude indicating ever closer correspondence so that with identical twins the lateral spinal profiles were virtually the same (▶ Fig. 3.12).[50] Lateral spinal profile is therefore a very important genetic element in the pathogenesis of idiopathic scoliosis.

If we now look at vertebral body shape in the sagittal plane in the thoracic spine it has been suggested that the normal thoracic profile would vary between about 20 degrees and probably a bit less than 40 degrees.[33,36] In addition the upper two thoracic vertebrae and indeed the lower two thoracic vertebrae are either straight or belong to the cervical and lumbar lordoses, respectively. Thus, if we say that the normal thoracic kyphosis from T3 down to T10, eight consecutive vertebrae, would be of the order of 24 degrees (to ease the arithmetic) then an average thoracic vertebral body would be kyphotically shaped by about 3

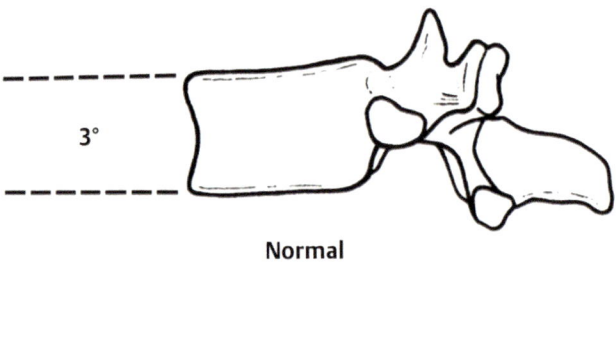

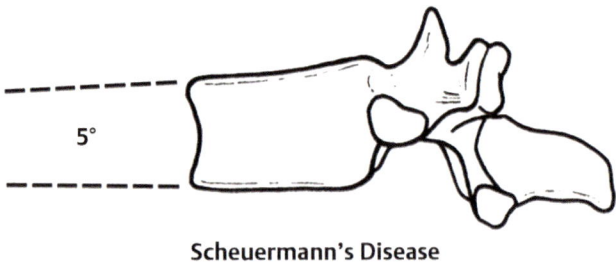

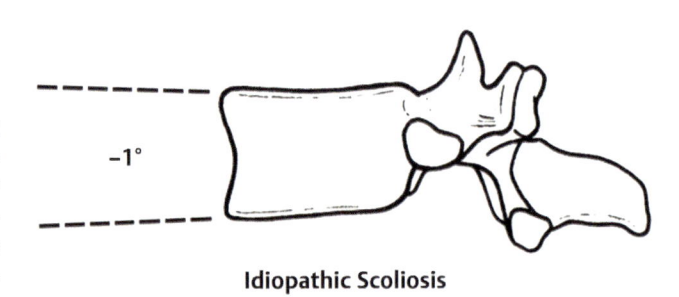

Fig. 3.13 Sagittal vertebral body shape is a delicate matter. (a) Three degrees of kyphosis would be about normal. (b) An increase by 2 degrees over three levels is Sorenson's definition of Scheuermann's disease. (c) Loss of just over 3 degrees of kyphosis renders the spinal column vulnerable to buckling. (Reproduced with permission from Newton P, O'Brien M, Shufflebarger H, et al. Idiopathic Scoliosis: The Harms Study Group Treatment Guide. Stuttgart/New York: Thieme; 2010: 39.)

degrees.[2] It only requires two further degrees to 5 degrees over three consecutive vertebrae to satisfy the definition of Scheuermann's disease. Meanwhile only 3 degrees and a bit more have to be lost to have a lordotic-shaped thoracic vertebra so it can be seen that only very, very small changes are required in sagittal vertebral shape to produce a spinal deformity (▶ Fig. 3.13). It would appear also that spinal shape approximates to a Gaussian distribution[36] (▶ Fig. 3.14) and this will be another familial trend, round-backed children coming from round-backed families and straight-backed children coming from straight-backed families.[49,50] There must be therefore a myriad of genetic effects coming into the equation here.

Because these changes are so subtle it should not be any surprise that school screening programs have demonstrated that 2.2% of girls aged 12 to 14 years have idiopathic scoliosis (a lateral curvature in excess of 10 degrees with concordant rotation).[30] The changes in lateral profile with growth have been demonstrated not only by the Leeds Group but also by Willner and Johnsson in Sweden.[35]

The Leeds epidemiological survey conclusively showed that a thoracic lordosis is the primary event in the generation of idiopathic thoracic scoliosi.[30] A sensitive positive test of an angle of trunk inclination of 5 degrees or more was the criterion for admission to the study, and of the 16,000 Leeds schoolchildren surveyed, 1,000 were harvested and subsequently radiographed on an annual basis for 6 years with AP and lateral low dose films. With such a sensitive entry criterion many children had straight backs to begin with but some developed true idiopathic scoliosis during the course of the study. This afforded the opportunity of going back to look at the lateral profile when the spine was straight in the frontal plane, and children who developed idiopathic scoliosis already had a flat thoracic spine with an apical lordosis (▶ Fig. 3.15).

Going back to Eulerian theory, the critical load is decreased by (1) increased curvature, (2) increased length, and (3) increased intrinsic load. The greater the curve becomes, the more likely it will progress as indeed natural history studies of idiopathic scoliosis have clearly shown (the further the Leaning Tower of Pisa leans, the more it will be likely to fall down hence the recent stabilizing measures). We have already mentioned the increased length of the spinal column in girls[33,34] as well as the increased intrinsic load which is why weaker columns such as those where bone is weaker, such as, dystrophic neurofibromatosis 1 (NF1) (▶ Fig. 2.33) and osteogenesis imperfecta, and where soft tissue support is weak, such as, Marfan syndrome (▶ Fig. 2.34) and Ehlers Danlos syndrome, which are prone to buckling. It is quite clear to see why and where many of these conditions in the etiological classification of structural spinal deformities take their place.

3.3 Experimental Models

In vivo experimentation in human beings would appear to be impractical (although it has been inadvertently and not very intelligently performed). The practice of carrying out a posterior fusion in situ for progressive scoliosis at a very young age[51] is about as logical as carrying out a posteromedial fusion for club foot! We then encountered the horrific short back of the spine tethered in bone with of course continued anterior growth[12] and this was prevalent long before the expression "Crankshaft phenomenon" came into fashion.[52] ▶ Fig. 3.16a is a PA view of

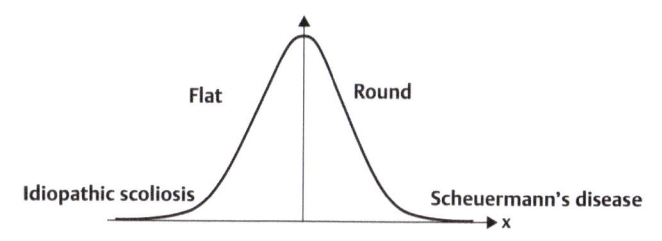

Fig. 3.14 Gaussian distribution. There seems to be a fairly normal distribution of lateral profile in children.[35,36]

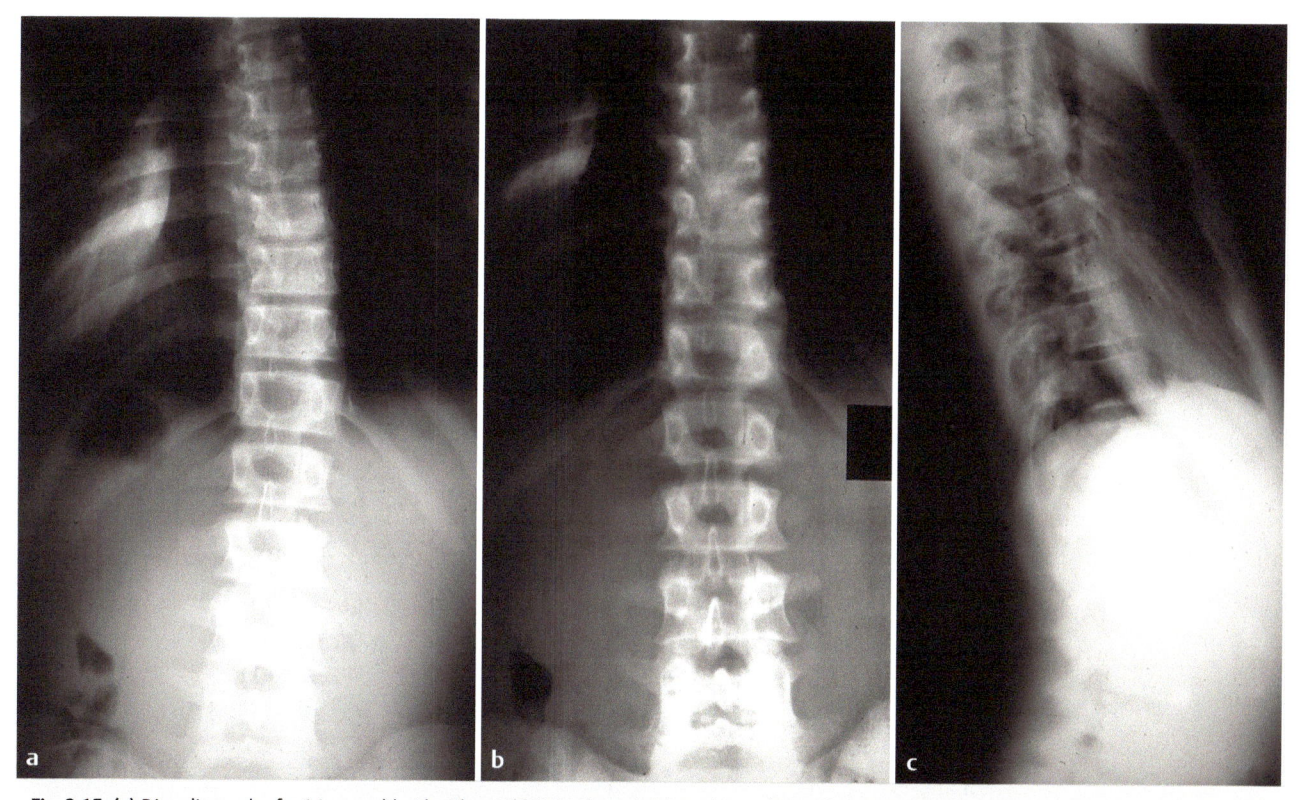

Fig. 3.15 (a) PA radiograph of a 14-year-old girl with a mild right thoracic idiopathic scoliosis. She was part of the Leeds longitudinal epidemiological survey. (b) PA radiograph taken years earlier, when the patient's spine was straight. (c) Lateral radiograph made years earlier, showing the dangerous lateral profile that preceded the development of the patient's curve. (Reproduced with permission from Newton P, O'Brien M, Shufflebarger H, et al. Idiopathic Scoliosis: The Harms Study Group Treatment Guide. Stuttgart/New York: Thieme; 2010: 40.)

The Etiology of Spinal Deformities

a rather immature 12-year-old boy yet to go through his adolescent growth spurt with an early onset idiopathic scoliosis (EOIS) measuring 102 degrees. ▶ Fig. 3.16b is the lateral view showing a pseudokyphosis measuring 100 degrees. The degree of rotation is so bad that the AP and lateral views of the patient have virtually the same magnitude. The surgeon elected to do a posterior fusion with a single Harrington rod (▶ Fig. 3.16c). At follow-up 4 years later the Cobb angle now registers 80 degrees. This is because the spine has rotated so far that now the Cobb angle is getting better (▶ Fig. 3.16d).

▶ Fig. 3.16e confirms that the spinal column (not the front of the spine) is now pointing much more backward. Note the longitudinal scar on the concave side of the spinal column over the lordosis and also note the scar over the right hemipelvis from bone graft retrieval. It is now the front of the spine that is pointing backward. What a dreadful deformity. He would have been better if nothing was done. Leatherman[53] and Roaf[12] were preaching the dangers of posterior fusion in situ more than four decades ago. Progressive scoliosis in a very young spine must be tackled anteriorly or at the very least not tethered posteriorly.

However, there are a host of examples in the everyday world of the basic problem of structural scoliosis. ▶ Fig. 3.17 is a banister rail in St James's University Hospital, Leeds, outside the operating theater and it makes a lordosis at each floor level causing the

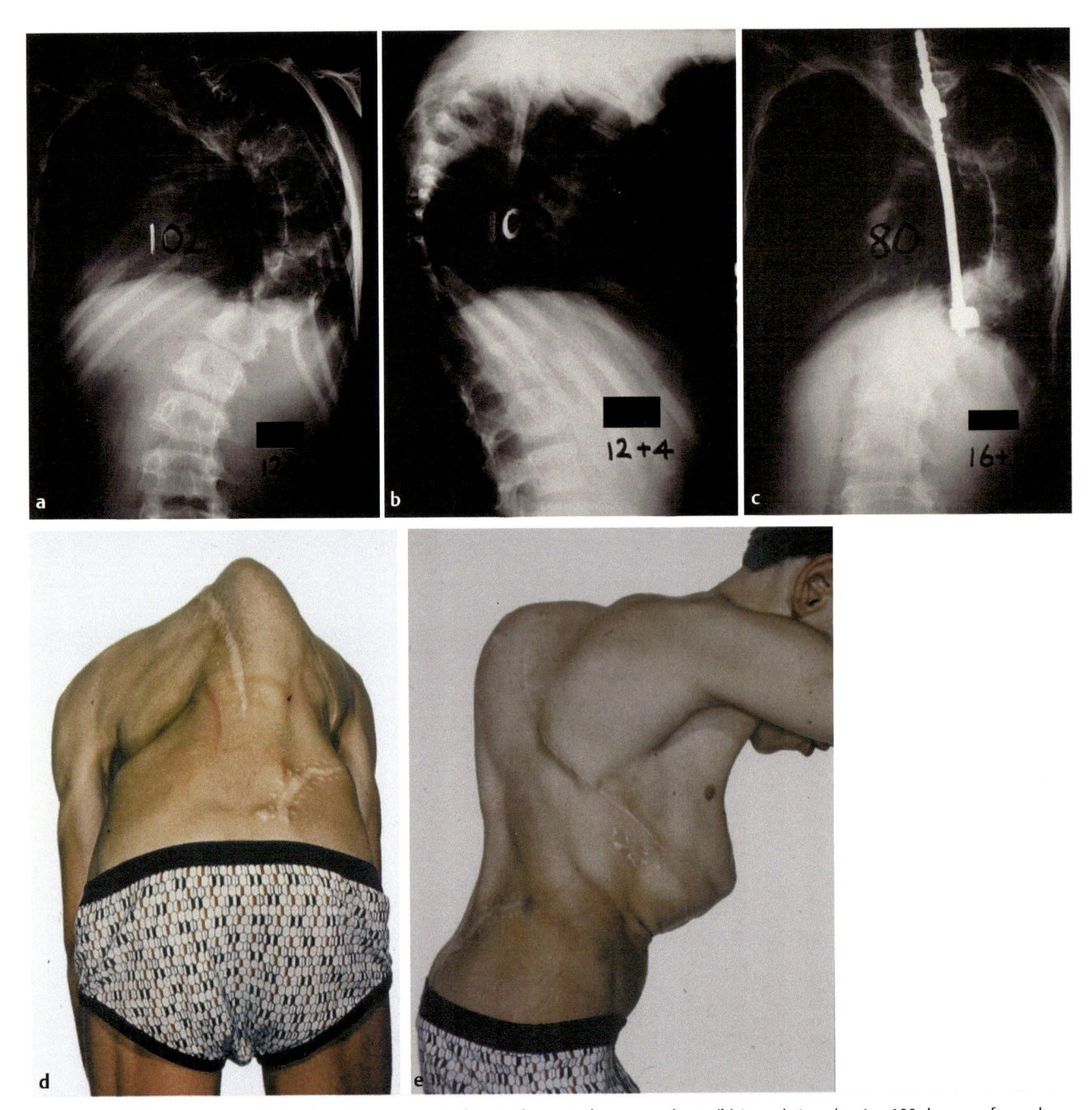

Fig. 3.16 How not to treat idiopathic scoliosis. (a) PA view of a 100-degree early onset scoliosis. (b) Lateral view showing 100 degrees of pseudo pseudokyphosis—in other words, AP and lateral views of the patient show the same deformity. (c) A Harrington rod distraction and posterior fusion was carried out and 4 years later the deformity now measures 80 degrees; the deformity is now so bad that it has swung round to point backward and so the frontal plane view shows improvement. (d) PA appearance of the patient showing the horrendous deformity pointing more backward than sideways. (e) Lateral view of the patient showing the scoliosis is now worse from the side than from the back.

The Etiology of Spinal Deformities

black plastic covering to buckle. This is why your bacon sizzling away in the frying pan curls up and the leading edge may require relief incisions to keep it flat in the frying pan (▶ Fig. 3.9).

As regards biological models there is an appreciable literature about experimental scoliosis in animals and it would be good to read the papers published by Smith on the subject first,[54–56] following earlier Leeds work.[57] In essence, animals, usually New Zealand white rabbits, have been attacked from more or less every direction in an effort to produce progressive structural scoliosis akin to idiopathic scoliosis in the human, spectacularly unsuccessfully. In these cases, there never was an initial hypothesis, rather another go at left–right asymmetry. Attempts at tethering bone or soft tissue on one or other side of the spine failed to produce a spinal deformity at all or caused a minor nonprogressive nonstructural tilt in the spine in the coronal plane only.[58–66] The administration of mutagenic agents to pregnant animals causing a congenital spinal deformity[67,68] and the postnatal induction of rickets[69] and lathyrism[70] produced the expected results but say little about the development of idiopathic scoliosis in humans. Meanwhile the infliction of neurological damage at either spinal cord or nerve root level might be expected to produce a paralytic scoliosis,[65,71–75] which indeed it does, animals tending to wake up from the anesthetic with an appreciable scoliosis.

The work initially undertaken by Langenskiold and Michelsson[22,76] producing scoliosis by excision of rib head or division of costotransverse ligament for many years appeared to be inexplicable until De Salis et al. inadvertently showed that unlike humans, with their artery of Adamkiewicz, the rabbit needs segmental arterial supply to the spinal cord at each level (▶ Fig. 3.18).[21] The rib head and costotransverse ligament are adjacent to the segmental artery and therefore what

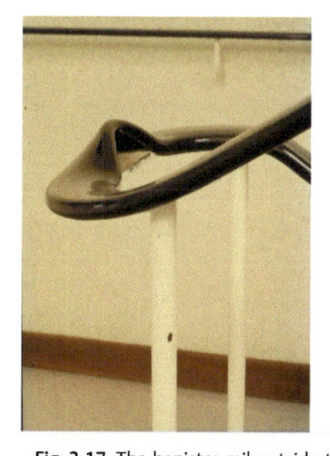

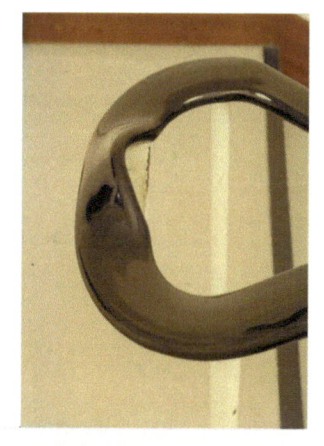

Fig. 3.17 The banister rail outside the operating theatre in St. James's University Hospital, Leeds. The banister rail makes a lordosis at each floor level, causing the black plastic handrail to buckle. (Reproduced with permission from Newton P, O'Brien M, Shufflebarger H, et al. Idiopathic Scoliosis: The Harms Study Group Treatment Guide. Stuttgart/New York: Thieme; 2010: 36.)

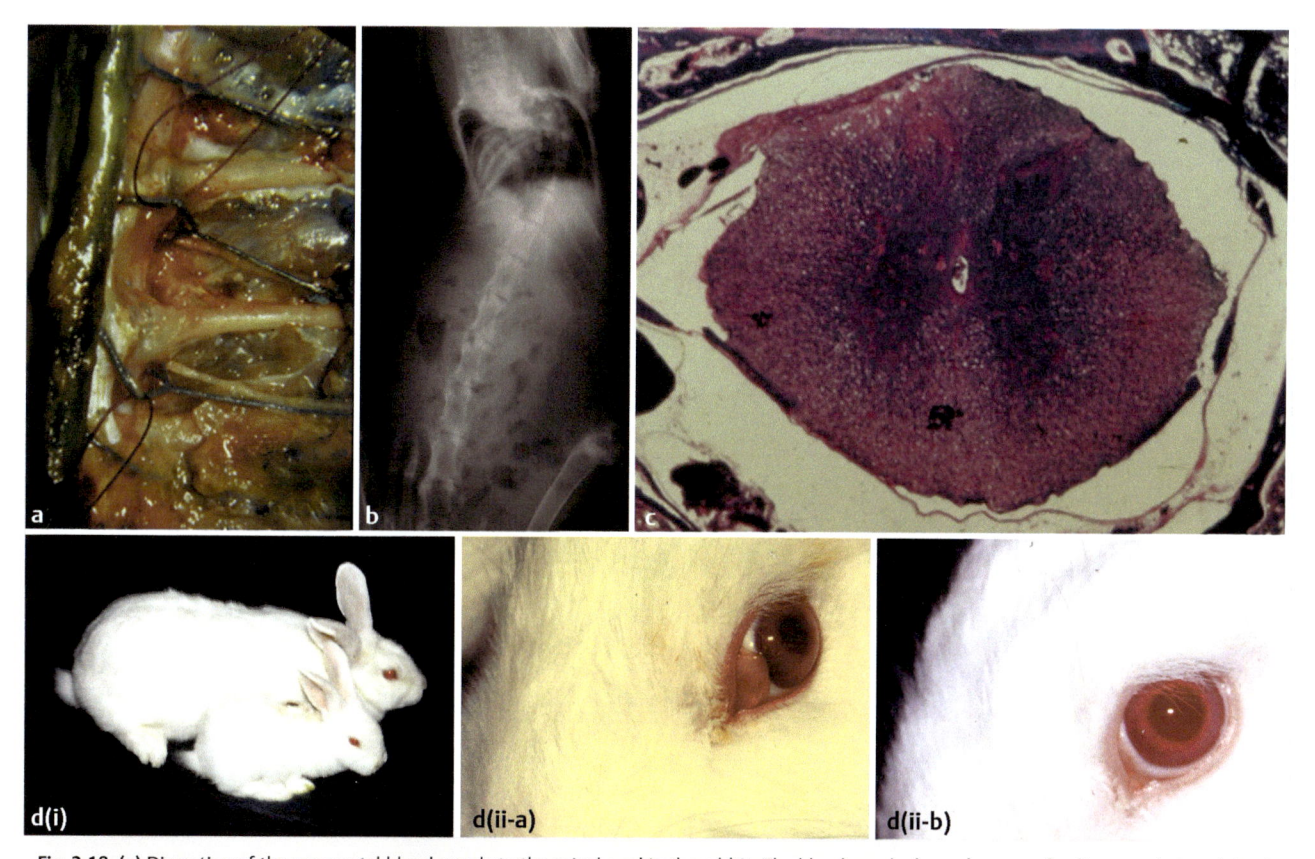

Fig. 3.18 (a) Dissection of the segmental blood supply to the spinal cord in the rabbit. The blood supply depends upon a feeding vessel at each level. (b) When the costotransverse ligament is resected and the segmental artery damaged an immediate severe paralytic-type scoliosis is produced. (c) A cross-section of the spinal cord locally indicates that an infarct has been produced. (d) Two rabbits, one normal and the other with severe scoliosis, in (b) with failure to thrive (i) and cyanosis (ii). ([d(ii-a) and d(ii-b)] Reproduced with permission from Newton P, O'Brien M, Shufflebarger H, et al. Idiopathic Scoliosis: The Harms Study Group Treatment Guide. Stuttgart/New York: Thieme; 2010: 46.)

The Etiology of Spinal Deformities

Langenskiold and Michelsson were doing was to produce a local cord infarct and a rapidly developing neuromuscular type of scoliosis.[54] Rather like severe EOIS with cardiopulmonary problems, these rabbits failed to thrive and developed cyanosis. It was Smith who made this crucial observation[54] explaining Langenskiold and Michelsson's results on the basis of De Salis' work.[21]

The rabbit spine is normally gently kyphotic in the sagittal plane, but if it is tethered into lordosis, without producing spinal cord damage, then they develop the typical lordoscoliosis with growth that we see in idiopathic scoliosis (▶ Fig. 3.10a and ▶ Fig. 3.19). This is really the work of Somerville,[14] extended by the Leeds Group.[54-57] The scoliosis so produced by tethering the back of the rabbit resembles geometrically the human condition in every respect. If the tether is released while the deformity is

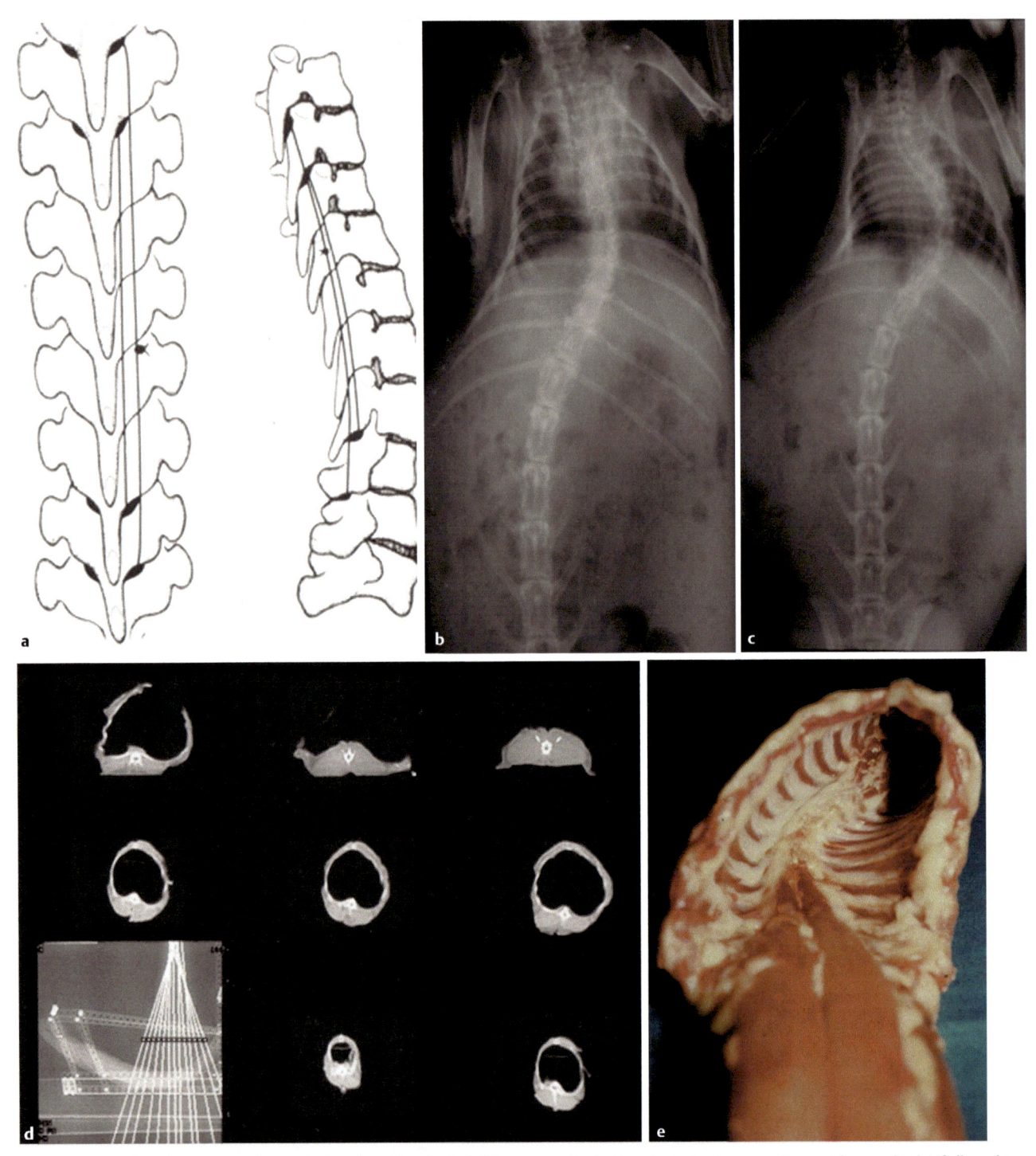

Fig. 3.19 (a) When the growing rabbit spine is tethered into lordosis (b) a progressive lordoscoliosis develops over the next few weeks. (c) If allowed to continue, the lordoscoliosis continues to progress. (d) CT scan showing the same sort of rotation as in the human. (e) Looking inside the chest this resembles closely the appearance at thoracotomy of an idiopathic thoracic curve.

The Etiology of Spinal Deformities

mild then the spine grows straight, a key to possible physiological treatment.[77]

Another biological area concerning spinal deformities that is ill-understood or misunderstood is the transverse plane deformity. Although cross-sectional vertebral asymmetry has been reported, descriptions have varied from the concave pedicle being depicted as longer and thinner to the other extreme of the convex pedicle being longer and thinner.[78,79] We also extensively studied the three-dimensional nature of the deformity in idiopathic scoliosis and in particular its transverse plane component in both humans and in animals.[55] We naturally found that the most asymmetrical vertebra was at the curve apex where the pedicle on the convex side was short and stout and that on the concave side was long and slender (▶ Fig. 3.20). As, however, one goes above and below the apical area, the transverse plane geometry changes—first becoming neutral before becoming the opposite in the compensatory kyphoses that balance the central lordotic area.[31] In these regions the pedicle on the convex side was long and slender and that on the concave side short and stout. The same pattern of apical vertebral body deformation was seen in the rabbit as in the human and this accounts for why there had been previous conflicting reports about transverse plane geometry[78,79] when of course it just depends which vertebra in the deformity you happen to look at. Then Smith et al. carried out a novel and crucial piece of experimental work.[55] They studied transverse plane vertebral deformation longitudinally during growth with a textile dye similar to tetracycline which labels growing bone. With growth of a normal vertebra in terms of cross-section as regards around the spinal canal vertebral growth consistently progresses outward (▶ Fig. 3.21a).

However, in the scoliotic situation, growth in the spinal canal and vertebral body goes toward the curve concavity (▶ Fig. 3.21b). Thus, the transverse plane is trying to correct and not cause the deformity. This confirms that the transverse plane is therefore not an etiological factor in idiopathic scoliosis. This answers the not particularly logical question sometimes asked, "which comes first—the rotation or the lordosis?" In both the animal and human, with particularly big curves, the concave pedicle can not only be very long but very narrow and it is perfectly clear that pedicle screws no matter what diameter cannot pass down the pedicle and their fixation is almost certainly into the vertebral body itself.

Then on to the fascinating work of Dubousset[80] and Machida[81] who rekindled interest in experimental scoliosis by observations of pinealectomized chickens and rats. The pineal gland produces melatonin from tryptophan through a series of enzyme reactions and serotonin is intermediary in this pathway. Thillard first produced scoliosis in pinealectomized chickens to assess the role of melatonin and its associated compounds in scoliosis.[82] If chickens are pinealectomized shortly after they hatch, a scoliosis similar to human idiopathic scoliosis is consistently produced. However, if melatonin supplements are given after pinealectomy, a scoliosis does not develop.[81] But why does this happen? Research translated into the human situation has shown conflicting results with regard to melatonin levels in patients with idiopathic scoliosis and those in controls. Careful studies involving diurnal variation showed no differences between the two groups.[83,84] It is thought that melatonin activity may be mediated by growth hormone as the common denominator,[85] but this is by no means certain.

Looking at the biomechanics of this experimental model it is not only interesting but most informative. Even with the pinealectomized animal model it is accepted that the primary

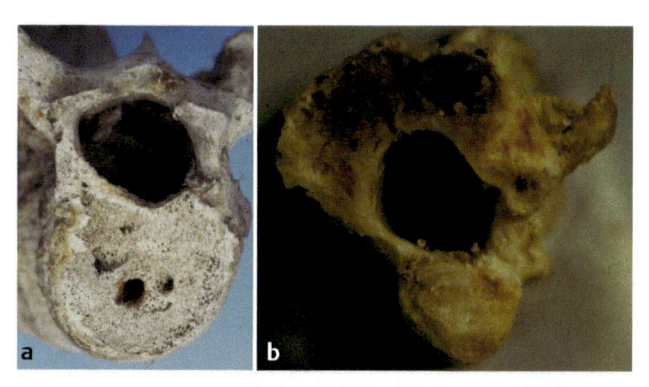

Fig. 3.20 Transverse plane asymmetry at the curve apex, with a short, stout pedicle on the convex side and a longer, thinner pedicle on the concave side. (a) Human, (b) rabbit. (Reproduced with permission from Newton P, O'Brien M, Shufflebarger H, et al. Idiopathic Scoliosis: The Harms Study Group Treatment Guide. Stuttgart/New York: Thieme; 2010: 44.)

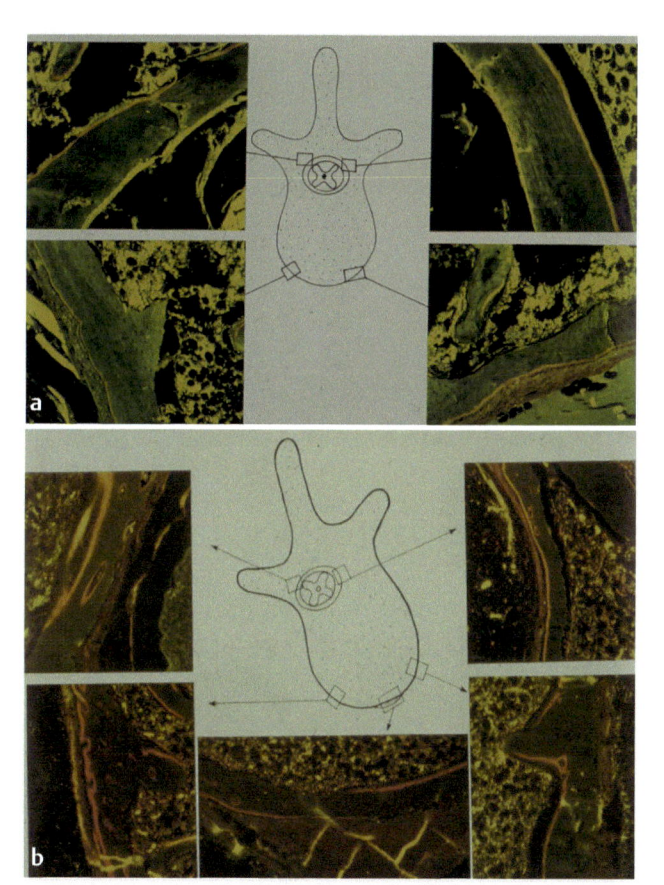

Fig. 3.21 (a) The diagram in the center shows that growth of a normal vertebra in terms of the spinal canal and the vertebral body is outward. Consequently, the orange-stained growth area in the canal above and the vertebral body below is facing outward. (b) With the apical scoliotic vertebra, the spinal canal and the vertebral body grow toward the concavity, as the orange-stained growth zones indicate. Thus, the transverse plane is therefore not an etiological factor in idiopathic scoliosis. (Reproduced with permission from Newton P, O'Brien M, Shufflebarger H, et al. Idiopathic Scoliosis: The Harms Study Group Treatment Guide. Stuttgart/New York: Thieme; 2010: 44–45.)

abnormality is a lordosis[85] which subsequently buckles to produce the typical three-dimensional lordoscoliotic deformity,[12] as stated and confirmed by Machida.[85] This does not occur spontaneously in quadrupeds while chickens are bipedal. Consequently, Dubousset and Machida went on to investigate the effects of pinealectomy in rats.[86] If they were initially rendered bipedal and then pinealectomized they developed a scoliosis comparable to that in chickens whereas the spine remained straight in rats that underwent a sham operation after being rendered bipedal (▶ Fig. 3.22). Meanwhile, quadrupedal rats when pinealectomized did not develop a spinal deformity.

Furthermore, a scoliosis was much more easily produced when the tails of bipedal rats were removed, allowing them to have an even more upright posture (they couldn't sit back on their tails). The sagittal profiles of these rats showed that the pinealectomized quadrupedal rat had a physiological thoracic lordosis whereas a thoracic hyperlordosis was produced in both the sham operated and pinealectomized bipedal rats. In other words, the effect of being bipedal was to exaggerate the existing thoracic lordosis but no buckling occurs to produce a lordoscoliosis unless the bipedal rat was pinealectomized suggesting that the hyperlordosis rendered

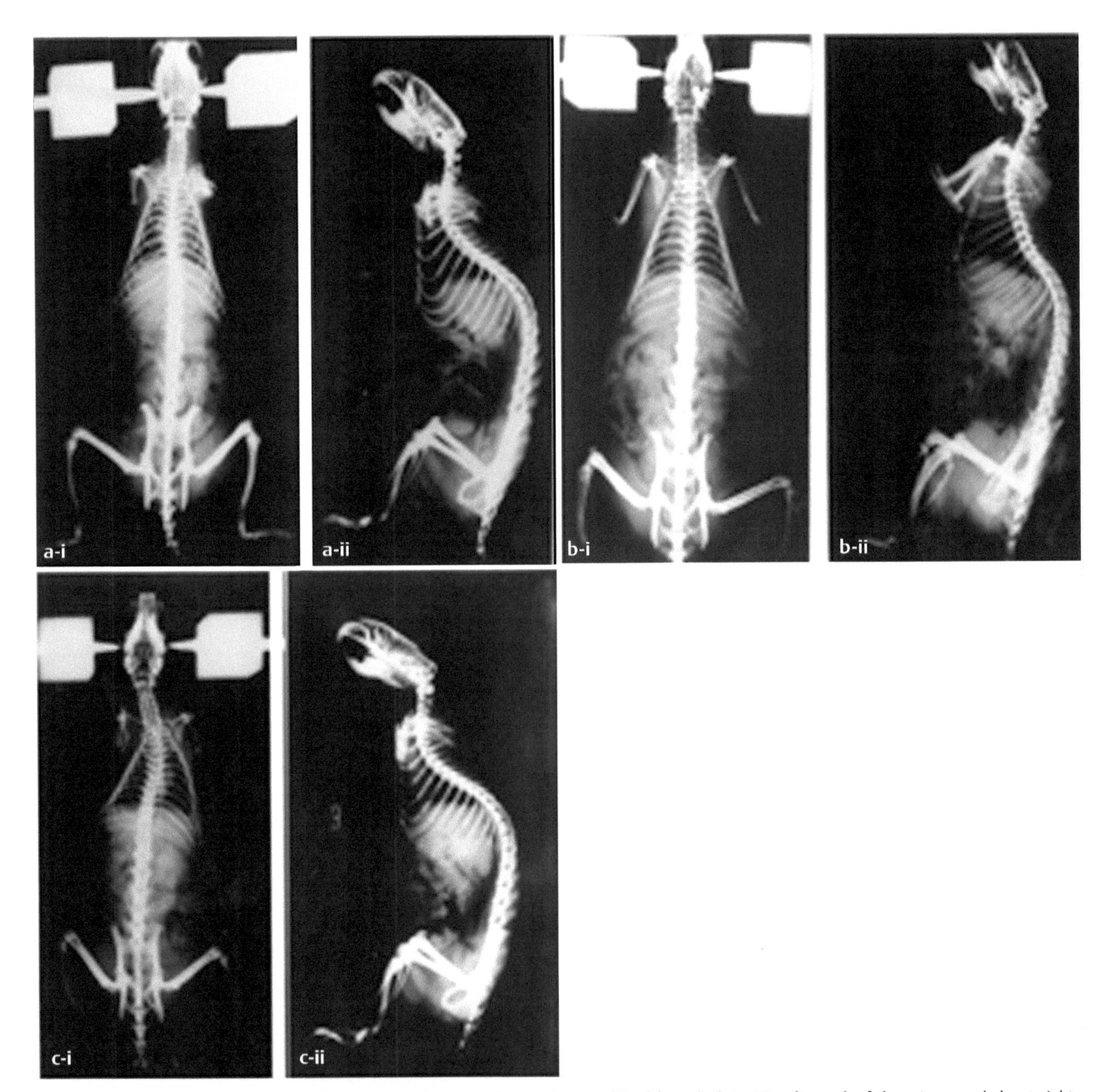

Fig. 3.22 Pinealectomy in the rat. **(a)** Sham non-pinealectomized operation on a bipedal rat. **(a-i)** An AP radiograph of the spine revealed a straight spine. **(a-ii)** A lateral view revealed a thoracic hyperlordosis of −43 degrees between C2 and T7. **(b)** Pinealectomized quadrupedal rat. **(b-i)** An AP radiograph of the spine revealed a straight spine. **(b-ii)** A lateral view revealed a physiological thoracic lordosis of −15 degrees between C2 and T7. **(c)** Pinealectomized bipedal rat. **(c-i)** An AP radiograph of the spine revealed thoracic scoliosis of 29 degrees. **(c-ii)** A lateral view revealed thoracic hyperlordosis of −48 degrees between C2 and T7. (Reproduced with permission from Newton P, O'Brien M, Shufflebarger H, et al. Idiopathic Scoliosis: The Harms Study Group Treatment Guide. Stuttgart/New York: Thieme; 2010: 47.)

The Etiology of Spinal Deformities

by the upright posture was destabilized by pinealectomy to produce the scoliosis.

Going back to the lordoscoliosis produced by Somerville[14] and the Leeds Group[54–57] we couldn't make it buckle unless the lordosis was rendered asymmetrical by producing a few degrees of concomitant scoliosis (biplanar asymmetry). Perhaps a pinealectomy would have done the same. In the bipedal chickens and rats that developed scoliosis there was no preferentiality in its developing either on the right or left side. There doesn't seem to be any other explanation for the effect of the pinealectomy performed on rats because the rats were of much the same weight at the end of the experiment and were not constitutionally disadvantaged, unlike the rabbit in ▶ Fig. 3.18.

So the clinical, epidemiological, biomechanical, and experimental evidence very nicely comes together to provide a unified etiological cause of structural scoliosis—an abnormality in the sagittal plane in the form of a primary lordosis producing scoliosis with rotation secondarily. You don't have to look anywhere else etiologically. You've got Adams, Somerville, Roaf, Dubousset, and Machida on your side, not to mention three decades of work by the Leeds Group!

3.4 What Pathogenesis Tells Us about Treatment

3.4.1 Surgical Treatment of Spinal Deformities

Essential Strategy

Based upon what we have now learned about the development of spinal deformities, and in particular idiopathic scoliosis, only now can we figure out the necessary steps that we have to take to reverse the shape alterations during their development so as (1) to make the spine as straight and acceptable as possible and (2) to prevent recurrence of the deformity with growth so that the corrected position is maintained until maturity. First of all, we shall have to go back to first principles. Our mechanical engineers' beam or column only fails in one of two ways: angular collapse or beam buckling (▶ Fig. 3.1). Then we have to ask whether the deformity is rigid or flexible. Congenital spinal deformities and spines that have undergone previous fusion are rigid whereas idiopathic deformities are flexible, to whatever degree. Angular failure of a rigid column implies breakage so that straightening a rigid bent (deformed) column implies that fracture (osteotomy) is required.

Idiopathic scoliosis is inherently flexible because it comprises a series of linked vertebrae and so deforms by intervertebral beam buckling and therefore has the potential for segmental correction. We know that every idiopathic deformity is lordotic and that the lordosis (▶ Fig. 3.6 and ▶ Fig. 3.7) starts first[30] (▶ Fig. 3.15). As it twists out of the sagittal plane so it becomes more and more visible in the frontal plane with associated rotation (see ▶ Fig. 2.10). Thus the primary deformity is lordosis and the secondary deformities are scoliosis with rotation. The deformity is therefore three-dimensional and the strategy for correction must recognize this, addressing the lordosis as well as the scoliosis itself.

Of course when the lordosis turns into the frontal plane the spinal column must point backwards which is why pseudokyphosis is seen on a lateral X-ray of the column itself and misleads the true interpretation of the three-dimensional deformity (stop taking lateral X-rays and you won't have this problem). When you rotate an articulated cadaver spine with scoliosis and X-ray it at, say, 10-degree intervals measuring Cobb angle as you go, as we did more than 30 years ago with such a museum specimen fixed to the turntable of a record player, then the graph produced shows that the Cobb angle can vary enormously just because of the plane of projection[13] (▶ Fig. 3.23). Now you can see that the lateral X-ray is just another radiograph of the same deformity. Nowadays 3D CT or 3D MRI can do all this for you (see ▶ Fig. 2.14), confirming the presence of the essential lordosis and enabling the entire spine to be visualized from any direction. Many years ago before there was any 3D scanning and using the old BBC computer we digitized scoliosis curves by marking the same anatomical points on both PA and lateral X-rays (the bases of the pedicles and the midpoints of the upper and lower end plates). Then we were able to generate through the graphics program images of the spine in any plane (▶ Fig. 3.24).[87] You can always locate the essential lordosis (▶ Fig. 3.24c).

Now, back to treatment. With a rigid beam construct then clearly osteotomy is the only way of changing shape and is the basis of apical vertebral column resection (VCR), a refinement of the closing wedge osteotomy concepts of Roaf[77] and Leatherman.[88] Quite rightly these pioneers pointed out the dangers

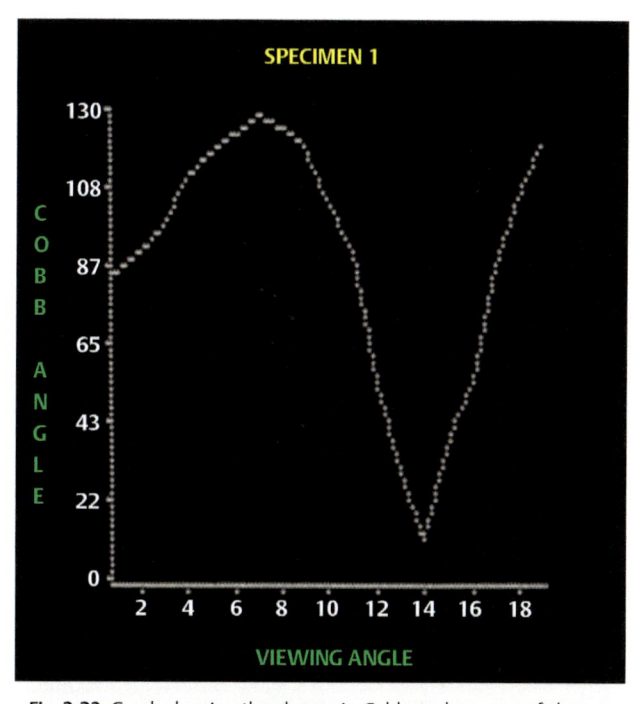

Fig. 3.23 Graph showing the change in Cobb angle as one of the museum specimens is rotated through 180 degrees. The initial Cobb angle is 78 degrees and varies in sine wave form maximizing just short of 120 degrees, dipping down to a minimum of a less than 10 degrees (where of course the apical zone is frankly lordotic) before returning to its initial Cobb angle value of 78 degrees at 180 degrees of rotation. This shows how Cobb angle can vary by more than 100 degrees just depending upon the plane of projection.

The Etiology of Spinal Deformities

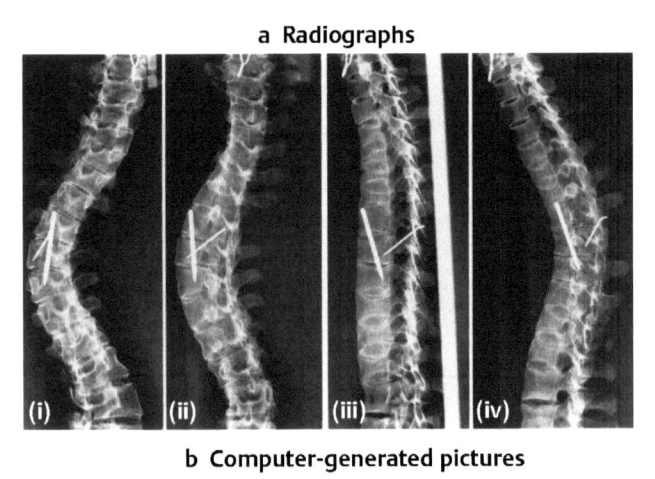

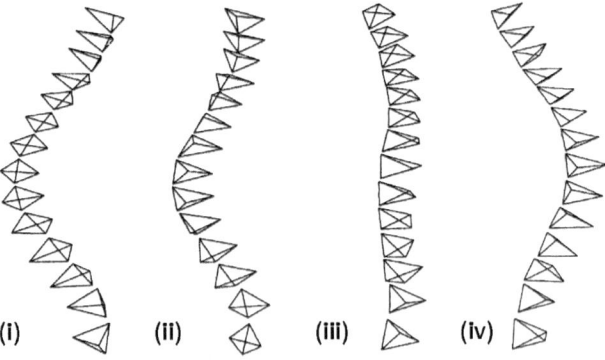

Fig. 3.24 (a) Radiographs of museum specimen showing the different appearances of the spine at selected degrees of rotation. In this case the apical vertebrae are rotated 40 degrees from the frontal plane of the patient. (i) Plan d'election true AP of the deformity (rotated 40 degrees out of the frontal plane). (ii) AP view of the patient showing the deformity with rotation in the middle. (iii) X-ray taken at 130 degrees, that is, true lateral of the curve apex and 90 degrees rotation from the true plan d'election AP (i). (iv) Lateral X-ray of the patient showing the appearance of pseudokyphosis. (b) Computer-generated spinal shape reproducing the same appearances as the X-rays.

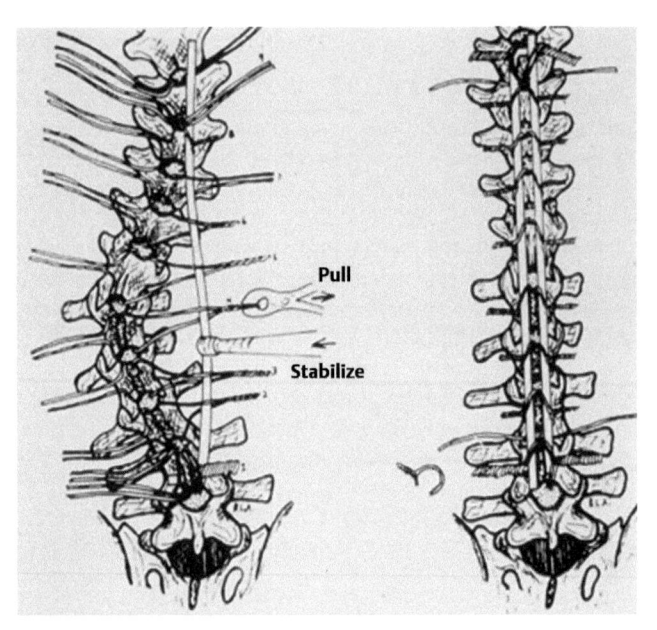

Fig. 3.25 When sublaminar wires pull a lordotic spine across to a straight rod the Cobb angle will be improved but rotation will be made worse.

and stupidity of carrying out a posterior tethering fusion on a young spine.[79] Roaf[12] stated "for many years I tried posterior spinal fusion but did not succeed in controlling the deformity. There are two reasons for this: 1) the usual area of posterior fusion for lordo-scoliosis with rotation lies in the concavity of the curve, and by acting as a tether it accentuates the inhibition of growth and even increases the deformity: and 2) the new bone of the fusion is no less plastic than the rest of the child's skeleton so that, if the deforming forces of disordered epiphyseal growth are strong, it tends to bend with growth." Going back to Harrington distraction principles this was to treat the whole deformity from top to bottom taking up whatever slack there was available when the deformity was maximally stretched. As correction proceeds by distraction, the apical region becomes stretched out and so is less responsive to distraction and needs more of a push or pull from the side. Hence the concept of sublaminar wiring at each level seemed attractive and initially was combined with a Harrington rod in the Harrington-Luque construct (▶ Fig. 3.25). There were two problems here confounding correctability. First, if you initially maximally distract then you make the deformity relatively stiff under tension so that the wires have difficulty drawing the apex across to the midline. Second, the pull of the wires is sideways (▶ Fig. 3.25), thus behind the axis of spinal column rotation for a lordosis, and so if the wires could be tightened then the apical rotation was increased not reduced.

However, the idiopathic scoliosis deformity, being a series of linkages, gives the opportunity for segmental correction, improving the rotational malalignment between each pair of vertebrae and so the Leeds procedure was devised to counter these problems and specifically address the lordosis at the curve apex. Although a Harrington distraction rod and sublaminar wires were used as in a Harrington-Luque procedure the surgical technique was quite different.[3,89,90] First of all the Harrington rod was bent into kyphosis maintained in position using square ended hooks (▶ Fig. 3.26) and secondly the rod was not distracted until the end of the procedure so as to allow maximum flexibility for the sublaminar wires to work with. Now with a kyphotic rod the concave sublaminar wires were pulling backward rather than sideways thus elevating the depressed concavity and untwisting the apex of the deformity (▶ Fig. 3.26d and ▶ Fig. 3.26e). This was fine for relatively low Cobb angle, high flexibility curves and so for these a single posterior procedure would suffice. Furthermore, with the modal age for surgery for late-onset idiopathic scoliosis of about 14 years there wasn't much time left until maturity and so, with the dangerous lordosis converted into kyphosis, the driving force for further deformation had been corrected in any event. The problem with the original Harrington procedure was that not only could it not correct the apical region satisfactorily (▶ Fig. 1.2) but the underlying lordosis persisted and so there was a tendency for further deformation to occur with subsequent growth. Indeed, Moe, in his presidential address,[91] stated quite clearly that the optimal result from Harrington instrumentation was that the curve measured the same at the end of treatment as it did at the beginning. In other

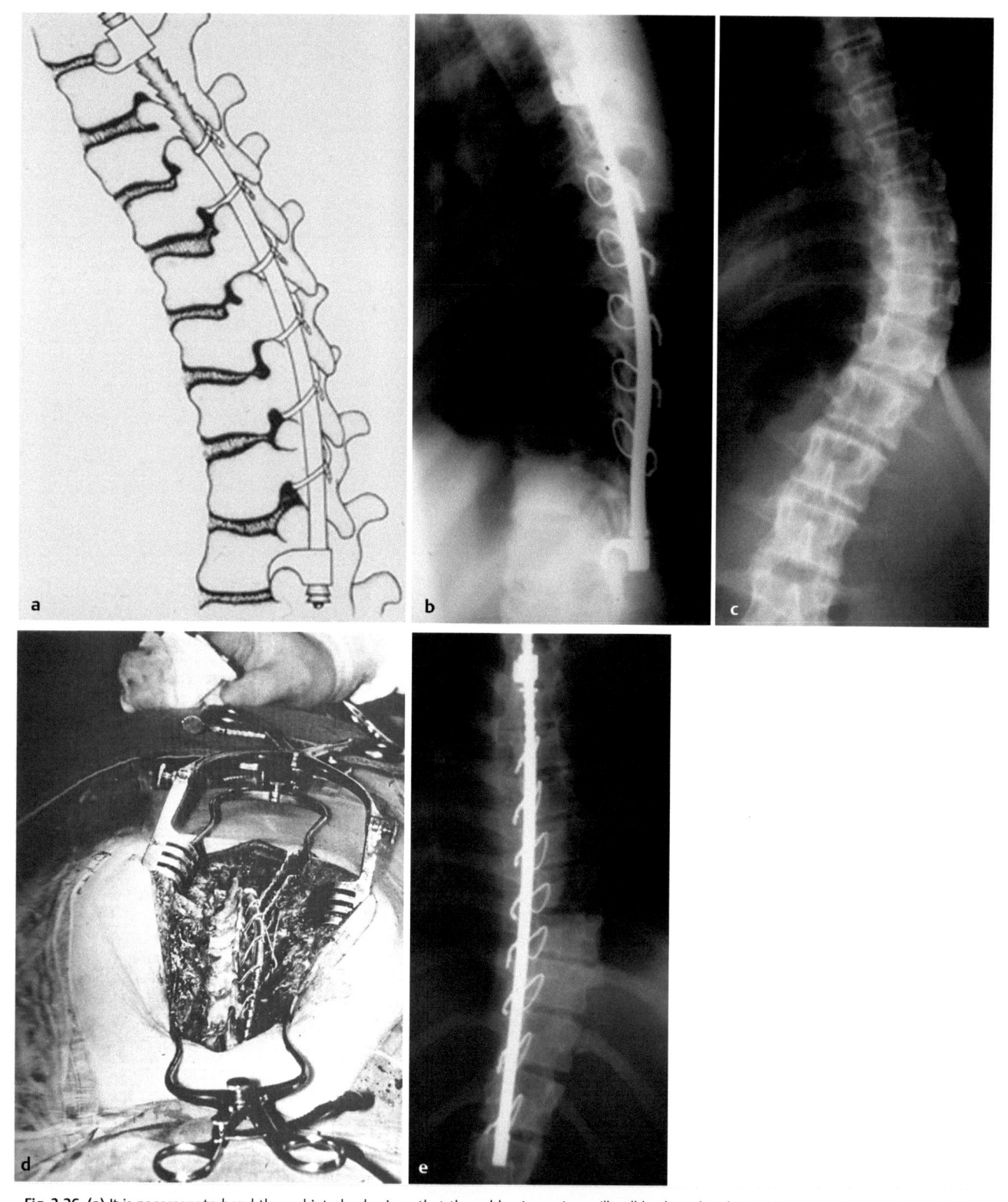

Fig. 3.26 (a) It is necessary to bend the rod into kyphosis so that the sublaminar wires will pull backward and not sideways and hence de-rotate the spine. (b) Lateral radiograph showing that this has been done. Note the diameter of the wire loops are of the same size indicating that there is bone-to-rod contact throughout confirming that the spine itself has been pulled backward and re-kyphosed. (c) PA radiograph of a right thoracic curve before surgery showing a lateral curvature with rotation and marked rib asymmetry. (d) Intraoperative photograph showing that the concave side of the back of the spine is being pulled backward and the spine is being truly untwisted. (e) PA radiograph after surgery showing the de-rotated spine with perfect rib symmetry.

The Etiology of Spinal Deformities

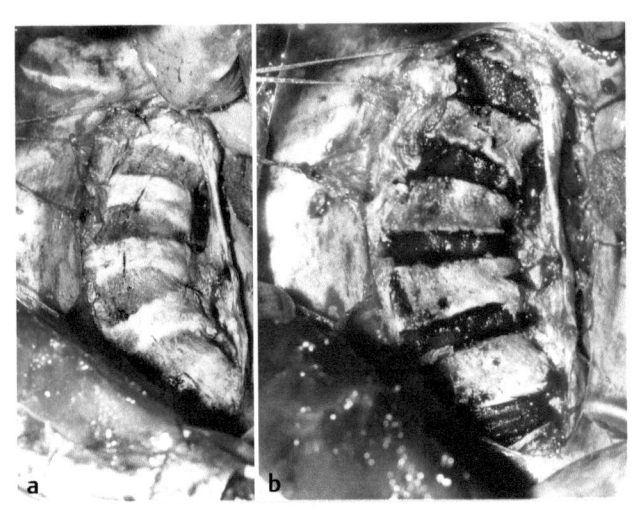

Fig. 3.27 (a) Intraoperative picture of five intervertebral disks exposed anteriorly subperiosteally. (b) Intraoperative photograph of the same set of disks after total diskectomy with gel foam in the gaps.

words, young healthy teenagers were going through this procedure for no obvious benefit and the possibility of distraction paralysis.

So what should be done with bigger Cobb angles and, in particular, younger patients? Although the modal age for surgery for late-onset idiopathic scoliosis (LOIS) is about 14, that leaves plenty of patients of a much younger age and some, hangovers from EOIS, of a particularly young age. The Leeds strategy was therefore twofold: (1) to obtain maximal correction and (2) to stop anterior growth so that recurrence of the deformity and the disastrous crankshaft phenomenon could be obviated. Growth plate ablation had already been tried with anteroconvex hemiphysiodesis but the obvious beneficial effect was negated by persistence of the biomechanical lordotic problem. Not surprisingly, the results were poor.[92] It was obvious that space had to be made available between adjacent vertebrae (adjacent asymmetric prisms) around the curve apex and this was readily achievable by anterior multiple diskectomy. Now the lordosis could be pulled back into kyphosis and untwisted so that all three planes of the three-dimensional deformity would be addressed. So what about abolishing anterior growth so that postoperative deformation would not occur? Although with bigger Cobb angles, and in particular the younger patient with a lot more growth to go, then anterior surgery was recommended as being mandatory. This was not an "anterior release" as it is now referred to after reinvention of the procedure because the front of the spine is longer than the back over the apical region in these lordoscolioses. Rather, it was a space-making procedure to allow maximum flexibility at incremental (intervertebral) level (▶ Fig. 3.27a,b). Furthermore, the reason bigger curves are stiffer is because growth has rendered the vertebrae progressively more asymmetric (▶ Fig. 3.28) and thus unstackable unless something is done about it. Now the lordosis could be pulled back into kyphosis and all three planes of the three-dimensional deformity addressed. Diskectomy means removal of all disk material back to the posterior longitudinal ligament and then using a sharp osteotome the cartilaginous endplate was detached from the contiguous surfaces of adjacent vertebrae. This then allowed the raw cancellous bone surfaces

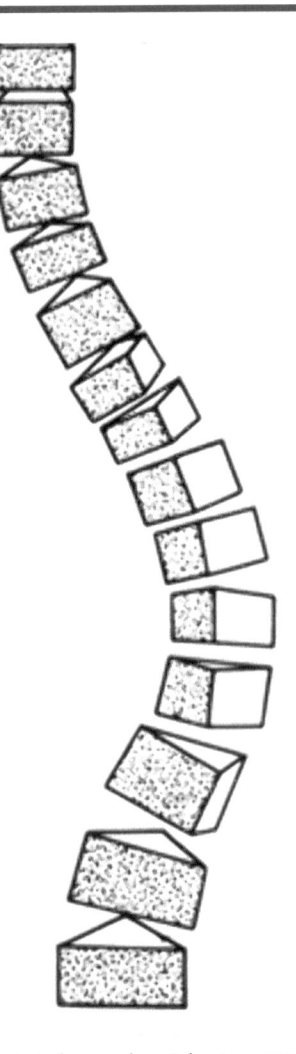

Fig. 3.28 Diagram to illustrate how each vertebra in a structural curve toward the curve apex becomes progressively more three dimensionally misshapen and thus with growth progressively more three dimensionally wedged and unstackable.

to be exposed as well as abolishing anterior vertebral growth. As each diskectomy proceeds so the disk space naturally narrows down and indeed so narrow it can become that it may require the use of a lamina spreader to obtain sufficient exposure to enable the back of the disk to be taken out. On average four to five intervertebral disks were removed in the Leeds procedure and at the end of the operation many disk spaces had closed completely and the rest did so over the next few days. An anterior interbody fusion would thereby be assured. Morselized rib bone graft was then added to any residual space after instrumentation. This was all done more than 35 years ago and the first 50 cases reported in 1987.[18] Never before had we seen such excellent corrections in three dimensions (▶ Fig. 3.29). At that time the anterior and posterior stages were separated by a week or two. More than half of the Cobb angle correction occurred between stages simply by making anterior space available and allowing the deformity to collapse into itself spontaneously. Moreover, this enabled the posterior instrumental correction to be less demanding, and thus safer.

The term "anterior release" is really not a simple matter of taking out a few disks over the apex but rather an important

The Etiology of Spinal Deformities

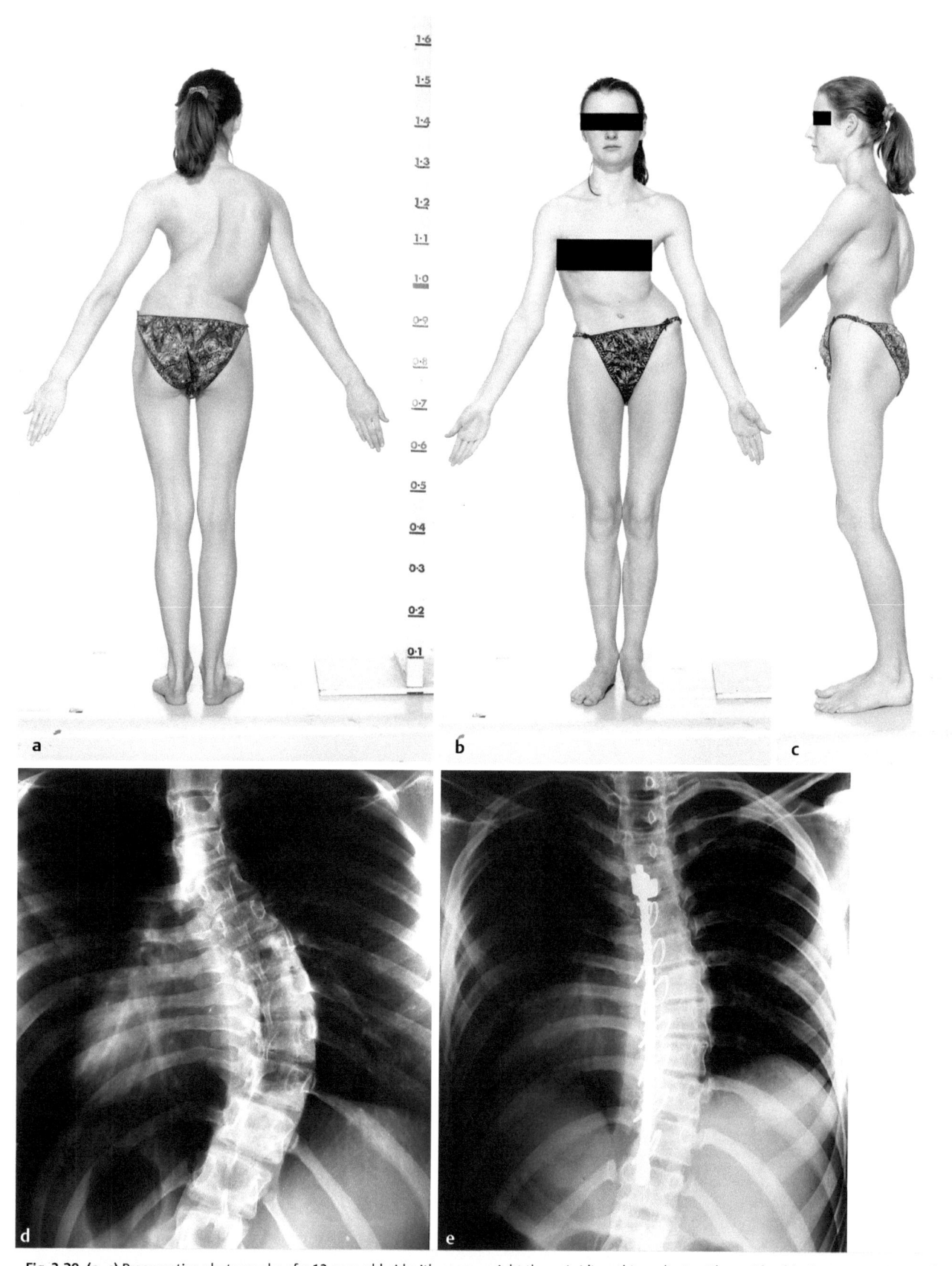

Fig. 3.29 (a–c) Preoperative photographs of a 13-year-old girl with a severe right thoracic idiopathic scoliosis with considerable decompensation and a very obvious rib hump. **(d)** PA radiograph preoperatively showing a right thoracic curve with marked rotation and rib asymmetry. **(e)** PA radiograph after surgery showing significant derotation and marked improvement in the rib asymmetry.

▶

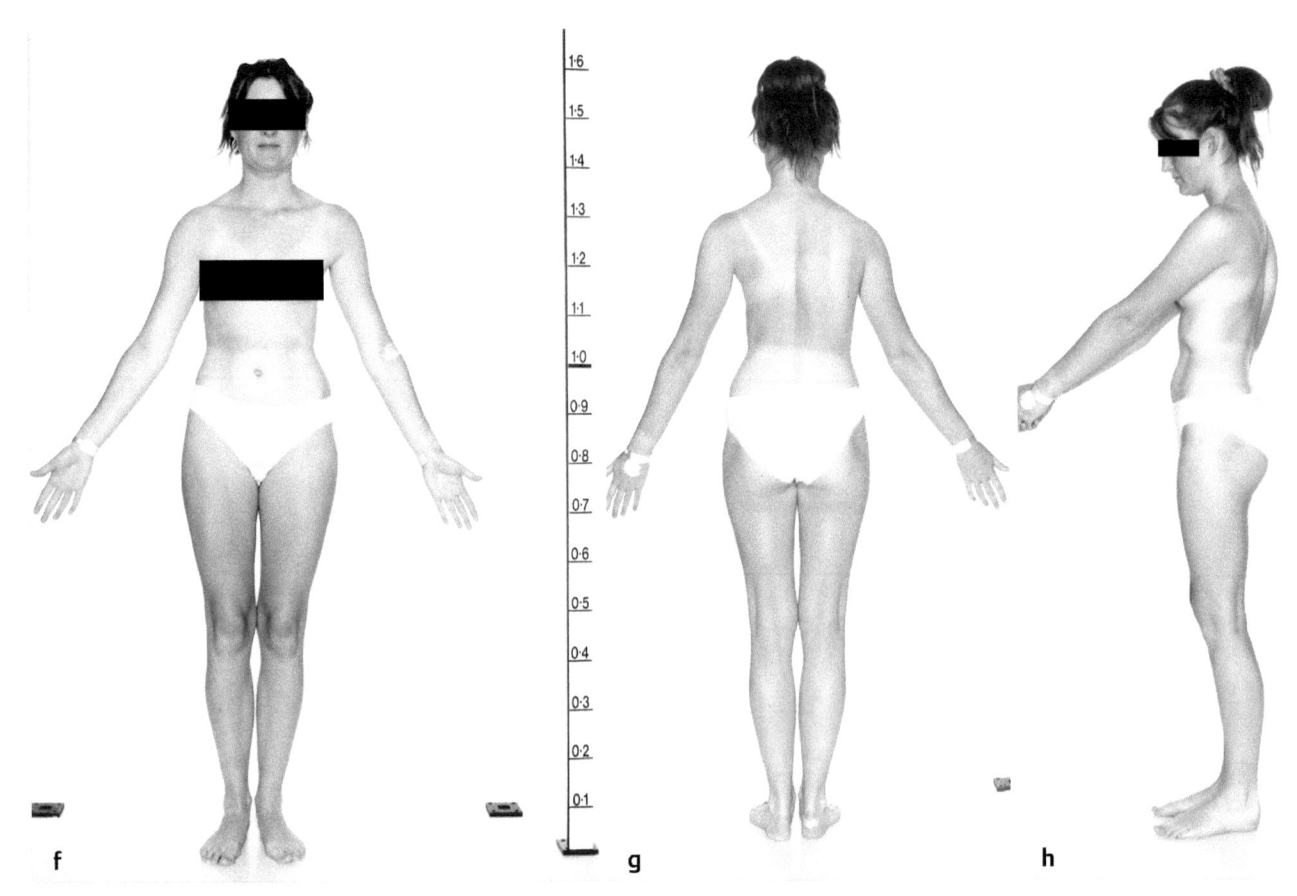

Fig. 3.29 (f–h) (*continued*) Postoperative views of the patient showing an excellent correction of the scoliosis and a perfectly balanced spine; **(f)** shows that although there has been significant improvement in the rib prominence there is still a minor residual rib hump, which there often is. This is because when the rib prominence has been present for some time—the ribs themselves deform in shape and lose their natural flexibility. This is why with ridge back or razorback deformities (usually in association with congenital deformities) costoplasty or costectomy is additionally required to obtain the most satisfactory result.[93] However the kyphosis has been re-created there has been no further increase in the rotational prominence over the 3 years since surgery.

aspect of the Leeds procedure is to abolish anterior overgrowth, so damaging with posterior fusions alone and consequently warned against by such major past authorities as Roaf and Leatherman.

To learn more about intersegmental rotation to help us in figuring out our operative strategy we carried out CT scanning on a small sample of idiopathic scoliosis patients measuring the rotational malalignment of each vertebra in the linked curve. An example is shown in ▶ Fig. 3.30 and it can be seen that there is no rotational malalignment between the two apical vertebrae. This is because in the presence of a lordosis the axis of spinal column rotation does not favor the rotational ability of the oblique orientated facet joints in the thoracic region. Where most of the intersegmental rotation occurred was well above and below the apex where the deformity is less lordotic or even kyphotic. After having fixed the top and bottom end-vertebrae with sublaminar wires it was obvious where most incremental derotation could be obtained which then dictated the sequence of wire tightening. Then and only then was additional distraction carried out, but, more often than not, the corrected position was already rigid. It is simple to translate this strategy to bilateral pedicular screw fixation tightening. Indeed hybrid constructs, a combination of pedicular metalwork with apical sublaminar wires, has a lot to be said for it biomechanically and has been tried but does not seem to be as popular as it should be, perhaps because of the various forms of wire or sling have not been as user-friendly as they might be but more probably because the idea of tackling the underlying lordotic problem and addressing the sagittal plane with surgery does not seem to have been recognized as an important part of the procedure.

Some deformities are notorious for their early onset and considerable progression potential. These would include the short sharp angular dystrophic curves of Von Recklinghausen's disease and EOIS. Of course EOIS curves that may be dealt with by posterior "growing instrumentation" must always have an anterior multiple diskectomy and removal of the growth plates otherwise anterior overgrowth will counter the potential benefits of posterior instrumentation without fusion. With Von Recklinghausen's disease there is of course a spectrum of progression potential from that of the idiopathic counterpart with relatively slow progression to the rapid progression of the maximally dystrophic curve. In our opinion all curves in Von Recklinghausen's disease should be dealt with as being dystrophic and very progressive and thus in no circumstances should an anterior first stage be missed out. There is no doubt that with modern generation transpedicular metalwork posterior correctability has been greatly enhanced with a tendency for

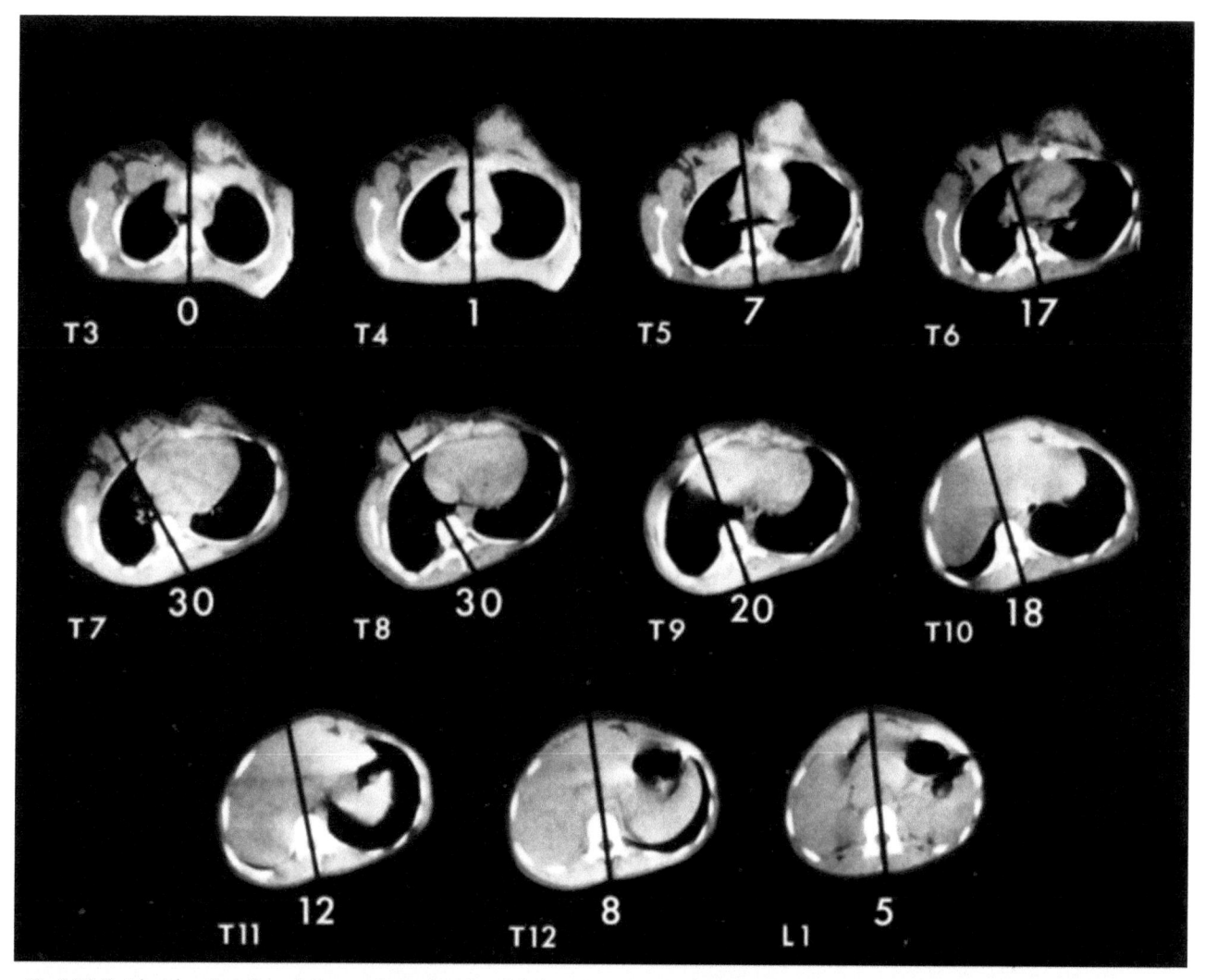

Fig. 3.30 Serial axial sections through the vertebrae of an idiopathic thoracic curve going from the neutral vertebra at the top (T3 top left) down through L1 (bottom right) which is nearly neutral. The apical vertebrae T7 and T8 are not rotated one to the other and where most of the segmental rotation occurs is above and below the apex between T5 and T6 and T6 and T7 and between T8 and T9. This is much the same picture for all idiopathic curves and it is useful to know where in the curve you want to effect significant de-rotation. Of course nowadays modern 3D CT and MRI can do this for you.

reliance on one posterior stage in these rapidly progressive curves but this should definitely be resisted.

Whereas congenital deformities requiring surgical treatment are more rigid there is more benefit to be gained from doing multiple diskectomies (two on each side of the apical VCR) so that additional correction of the deformity can be achieved above and below the apex intersegmentally. This adds very little time to the apical VCR and should be carried out before wedge resection.

Meanwhile while the Leeds Group were developing their procedure the French revolution occurred with Cotrel and Dubousset[94] introducing their two-rod system, allowing distraction and compression on the same rod. Dubousset's group, rather like our group in Leeds, has studied the three-dimensional nature of idiopathic scoliosis and has done considerable research into the subject, particularly animal work with Machida.[80] It was from this important experimental work that he and Yves Cotrel developed their unique CD instrumentation.[94] Then the derotation maneuver was carried out to try and turn the frontal plane deformity into kyphosis. This was really a form of en bloc derotation and it was subsequently shown that this technique tended to rotate the spine above and below the deformity thus reducing the beneficial effect over the deformity itself.[95] Of course the only problem with the introduction of CD instrumentation was that it was for a posterior instrumentation and took away the emphasis on preliminary anterior diskectomy and growth plate removal work. Of course Cotrel and Dubousset knew all about the lordosis but the popularity of their instrumentation led to a general persistence of posterior surgery. Ever since the time of Dwyer (▶ Fig. 1.8), and in particular Zielke (▶ Fig. 1.9), idiopathic deformities have been eminently treatable using anterior instrumentation and applying that to the front of the spine after multiple diskectomy achieved results that are as good if not better than posterior surgery alone. It was one of us (J.H.) who first applied anterior instrumentation to the thoracic spine to restore kyphosis by multiple diskectomies and thereby achieve proper three-dimensional correction, while at the same time stopping anterior overgrowth.

So it can be seen that understanding how the three-dimensional deformity develops facilitates appreciating the strategy for lasting correction of the deformity in all three planes. Structural scoliosis is not a right–left problem and dealing with it as such will never produce the optimal correction for your patient.

References

Note: References in **bold** are Key References.

[1] White AA III, Pajabi MM. Clinical biomechanics of the spine. 2nd ed. Philadelphia: Lippincott; 1990:653

[2] **Millner PA, Dickson RA. Idiopathic scoliosis: biomechanics and biology. Eur Spine J. 1996; 5(6):362–373**

[3] **Deacon P, Archer IA, Dickson RA. The anatomy of spinal deformity: a biomechanical analysis. Orthopedics. 1987; 10(6):897–903**

[4] Williams PL, Warwick R, Dyson M, Bannister LH (eds). Gray's anatomy. Edinburgh: Churchill Livingstone; 1989:321

[5] Kouwenhoven JWM, Vincken KL, Bartels LW, Castelein RM. Analysis of preexistent vertebral rotation in the normal spine. Spine. 2006; 31(13):1467–1472

[6] Kouwenhoven JWM, Bartels LW, Vincken KL, et al. The relation between organ anatomy and pre-existent vertebral rotation in the normal spine: magnetic resonance imaging study in humans with situs inversus totalis. Spine. 2007; 32(10):1123–1128

[7] du Peloux J, Fauchet R, Faucon B, Stagnara P. Le plan d'election pour l'examen radiologique des cypho-scolioses. Rev Chir Orthop Repar Appar Mot. 1965; 51:517–524

[8] **Deacon P, Berkin CR, Dickson RA. Combined idiopathic kyphosis and scoliosis. An analysis of the lateral spinal curvatures associated with Scheuermann's disease. J Bone Joint Surg Br. 1985; 67(2):189–192**

[9] Bernick S, Cailliet R. Vertebral end-plate changes with aging of human vertebrae. Spine. 1982; 7(2):97–102

[10] Adams W. Lectures on the pathology and treatment of lateral and other forms of curvature of the spine. Edinburgh: Churchill Livingstone; 1865

[11] **Roaf R. The basic anatomy of scoliosis. J Bone Joint Surg Br. 1966; 48(4):786–792**

[12] Roaf R. The treatment of progressive scoliosis by unilateral growth arrest. J Bone Joint Surg Br. 1963; 45(4):637–651

[13] Dickson RA, Archer IA. Surgical treatment of late-onset idiopathic thoracic scoliosis. The Leeds procedure. J Bone Joint Surg Br. 1987; 69(5):709–714

[14] Deacon P, Flood BM, Dickson RA. Idiopathic scoliosis in three dimensions. A radiographic and morphometric analysis. J Bone Joint Surg Br. 1984; 66(4):509–512

[15] **Somerville EW. Rotational lordosis; the development of single curve. J Bone Joint Surg Br. 1952; 34-B(3):421–427**

[16] **Dickson RA, Lawton JO, Archer IA, Butt WP. The pathogenesis of idiopathic scoliosis. Biplanar spinal asymmetry. J Bone Joint Surg Br. 1984; 66(1):8–15**

[17] Winter RB, Moe JH, Bradford DS, et al. Spine deformity in neurofibromatosis. A review of one hundred and two patients. J Bone Joint Surg Am. 1979; 61:677–694

[18] Lenke LG, Betz RR, Haher TR, et al. Multisurgeon assessment of surgical decision-making in adolescent idiopathic scoliosis: curve classification, operative approach, and fusion levels. Spine. 2001; 26(21):2347–2353

[19] Bushell GR, Ghosh P, Taylor TKF. Collagen defect in idiopathic scoliosis. Lancet. 1978; 2(8080):94–95

[20] Butterworth TR, Jr, James C. Electromyographic studies in idiopathic scoliosis. South Med J. 1969; 62(8):1008–1010

[21] **De Salis J, Beguiristain JL, Cañadell J. The production of experimental scoliosis by selective arterial ablation. Int Orthop. 1980; 3(4):311–315**

[22] **Langenskiold A, Michelsson JE. Experimental progressive scoliosis in the rabbit. J Bone Joint Surg Br. 1961; 43-B:116–120**

[23] Langenskiold A, Michelsson JE. The pathogenesis of experimental progressive scoliosis. Acta Orthop Scand Suppl. 1962; 59:1–26

[24] Piggott H. Experimentally produced scoliosis in animals. In: Zorab PA (ed). Proceedings of a second symposium on scoliosis: causation. Edinburgh: Churchill Livingstone; 1968:15–17

[25] Robb JE, Conner AN, Stephenson JBP. Normal electroencephalograms in idiopathic scoliosis. Acta Orthop Scand. 1986; 57(3):220–221

[26] Sahlstrand T, Petruson B. A study of labyrinthine function in patients with adolescent idiopathic scoliosis. I. An electro-nystagmographic study. Acta Orthop Scand. 1979a; 50(6 Pt 2):759–769

[27] Sahlstrend T, Petruson B. Postural effects on nystagmus response during caloric labyrinthine stimulation in patients with adolescent idiopathic scoliosis. II. An electro-nystagmographic study. Acta Orthop Scand. 1979b; 50(6 Pt 2):771–775

[28] Yarom R, More R. Myer p. Platelet and muscle abnormalities in idiopathic scoliosis. In: Warner JO, Mehta MH (eds). Proceedings of the seventh Philip Zorab symposium: scoliosis prevention. New York: Praeger; 1983: 3–22

[29] Zuk T. The role of spinal and abdominal muscles in the pathogenesis of scoliosis. J Bone Joint Surg Br. 1962; 44B:102–105

[30] **Stirling AJ, Howel D, Millner PA, Sadiq S, Sharples D, Dickson RA. Late-onset idiopathic scoliosis in children six to fourteen years old. A cross-sectional prevalence study. J Bone Joint Surg Am. 1996; 78(9):1330–1336**

[31] **Cruickshank JL, Koike M, Dickson RA. Curve patterns in idiopathic scoliosis. A clinical and radiographic study. J Bone Joint Surg Br. 1989; 71(2):259–263**

[32] Moe JH. A critical analysis of methods of fusion for scoliosis; an evaluation in two hundred and sixty-six patients. J Bone Joint Surg Am. 1958; 40-A(3):529–554, passim

[33] Willner S. A study of growth in girls with adolescent idiopathic structural scoliosis. Clin Orthop Relat Res. 1974(101):129–135

[34] Archer IA, Dickson RA. Stature and idiopathic scoliosis. A prospective study. J Bone Joint Surg Br. 1985; 67(2):185–188

[35] Willner S, Johnson B. Thoracic kyphosis and lumbar lordosis during the growth period in children. Acta Paediatr Scand. 1983; 72(6):873–878

[36] **Oxborrow N, Gopal S, Walder A, et al. A new surface topographical measure of spinal shape in scoliosis. J Bone Joint Surg Br. 1998; 80 Supp III:276–277**

[37] Willner S, Nilsson KO, Kastrup K, Bergstrand CG. Growth hormone and somatomedin A in girls with adolescent idiopathic scoliosis. Acta Paediatr Scand. 1976; 65(5):547–552

[38] Scheuermann HW. Kyphosis juvenile (Scheuermanns Krankheit). Fortschr Geb Rontgenstr. 1936; 53:1–16

[39] Bradford DS. Juvenile kyphosis. Clin Orthop Relat Res. 1977(128):45–55

[40] Bolk L. The menarche in Dutch women and its precipitated appearance in the youngest generation. Proc Acad Sci Amst Sec Sci. 1923; 26:650–663

[41] Hewitt D. Some familial correlations in height, weight and skeletal maturity. Ann Hum Genet. 1957; 22(1):26–35

[42] Tanner JM. Growth at adolescence. Oxford: Blackwell Scientific; 1962

[43] Cowell HR, Hall JN, MacEwen GD. Genetic aspects of idiopathic scoliosis. A Nicholas Andry Award essay, 1970. Clin Orthop Relat Res. 1972; 86(86):121–131

[44] De George FV, Fisher RL. Idiopathic scoliosis: genetic and environmental aspects. J Med Genet. 1967; 4(4):251–257

[45] Drummond DS, Rogala EJ. Growth and maturation of adolescents with idiopathic scoliosis. Spine. 1980; 5(6):507–511

[46] Duval-Beaupère G. Pathogenic relationship between scoliosis and growth. In: Zorab PA (ed). Scoliosis and growth: proceedings of a third symposium. Edinburgh: Churchill Livingstone;1971 : 58–64

[47] **Howell FR, Mahood JK, Dickson RA. Growth beyond skeletal maturity. Spine. 1992; 17(4):437–440**

[48] Riseborough EJ, Wynne-Davies R. A genetic survey of idiopathic scoliosis in Boston, Massachusetts. J Bone Joint Surg Am. 1973; 55(5):974–982

[49] Delmas A. Types rachidiens de statique corporelle. Rev Morphol Physiol Hum. 1951; 2:26–32

[50] Mardia KV, Dryden IL, Hurn MA, Li Q, Millner PA, Dickson RA. Familial spinal shape. J Appl Stat. 1994; 21:623–642

[51] Winter RB, Moe JH. The results of spinal arthrodesis for congenital spinal deformity in patients younger than five years old. J Bone Joint Surg Am. 1982; 64(3):419–432

[52] Dubousset J, Herring JA, Shufflebarger H. The crankshaft phenomenon. J Pediatr Orthop. 1989; 9(5):541–550

[53] Leatherman KD, Dickson RA. Two-stage corrective surgery for congenital deformities of the spine. J Bone Joint Surg Br. 1979; 61-B(3):324–328

[54] **Smith RM, Dickson RA. Experimental structural scoliosis. J Bone Joint Surg Br. 1987; 69(4):576–581**

[55] **Smith RM, Pool RD, Butt WP, Dickson RA. The transverse plane deformity of structural scoliosis. Spine. 1991; 16(9):1126–1129**

[56] Smith RM, Hamlin GW, Dickson RA. Respiratory deficiency in experimental idiopathic scoliosis. Spine. 1991; 16(1):94–99

[57] Lawton JO, Dickson RA. The experimental basis of idiopathic scoliosis. Clin Orthop Relat Res. 1986(210):9–17

[58] Bisgard JD. Experimental thoracogenic scoliosis. J Thorac Surg. 1934; 4:435–442

[59] Bisgard JD, Musselman MM. Scoliosis; its experimental production and growth correction: growth and fusion of vertebral bodies. Surg Gynecol Obstet. 1940; 70:1029–1036

[60] Bobechko WP. Spinal pacemakers and scoliosis. J Bone Joint Surg Br. 1973; 55B:232–233

[61] Engel D. Experiments on progductino of spinal deformities by radium. Am J Roentgenol. 1939; 42:217–234

[62] Miles M. Vertebral changes following experimentally produced muscle imbalance; preliminary report. Arch Phys Med Rehabil. 1947; 28(5):284–289

[63] Nachlas IW, Borden JN. Experimental scoliosis; the role of the epiphysis. Surg Gynecol Obstet. 1950; 90(6):672–680

[64] Ottander HG. Experimenal progressive scoliosis in a pig. Acta Orthop Scand. 1963; 33:91–98

[65] Robin GC, Stein H. Experimental scoliosis in primates. Failure of a technique. J Bone Joint Surg Br. 1975; 57(2):142–145

[66] Schwartzmann JR, Miles M. Experimental production of scoliosis in rats and mice. J Bone Joint Surg. 1945; 27:59–69

[67] Duraiswami PK. Experimental causation of congenital skeletal defects and its significance in orthopaedic surgery. J Bone Joint Surg Br. 1952; 34-B(4):646–698

[68] Ingalls TH, Curley FJ. Principles governing the genesis of congenital malformations induced in mice by hypoxia. N Engl J Med. 1957; 257(23):1121–1127

[69] Yamamoto H. Experimental scoliosis in rachitic bipedal rats. Tokushima J Exp Med. 1966; 13(1-)(2):1–34

[70] Ponseti IV. Skeletal lesions produced by aminonitriles. Clin Orthop. 1957; 9(9):131–144

[71] Alexander MA, Bunch WH, Ebbesson SOE. Can experimental dorsal rhizotomy produce scoliosis? J Bone Joint Surg Am. 1972; 54(7):1509–1513

[72] Liszka O. Spinal cord mechanisms leading to scoliosis in animal experiments. Acta Med Pol. 1961; 2:45–63

[73] MacEwen GD. Experimental scoliosis. In: Zorab PA (ed). Proceedings of a second symposium on scoliosis: causation. Edinburgh: Livingstone; 1968:18–20

[74] Pincott JR, Davies JS, Taffs LF. Scoliosis caused by section of dorsal spinal nerve roots. J Bone Joint Surg Br. 1984; 66(1):27–29

[75] Robin GC. Experimental paralytic scoliosis. Isr J Med Sci. 1966; 2(2):208–211

[76] Langenskiold A, Michelsson JE. The pathogenesis of experimental progressive scoliosis. Acta Orthop Scand Suppl. 1962; 59 suppl:1–26

[77] Roaf R. Wedge resection for scoliosis. J Bone Joint Surg Br. 1955; 37-B(1):97–101

[78] Ober FR, Belwster AH. Lovett's lateral curvature of the spine and round shoulders. 5th ed. Philadelphia: P Blakestones; 1931:3

[79] Roye DP. Scoliosis. In: Keim HA (ed). The Adolescent Spine. 2nd ed. New York, NY: Springer Verlag;1982:112

[80] Dubousset J, Queneau P, Thillard MJ. Experimental scoliosis induced by pineal and diencephalic lesions in young chickens: Its relation with clinical findings. Orthop Trans. 1983; 7:7

[81] **Machida M, Dubousset J, Imamura Y, Iwaya T, Yamada T, Kimura J. An experimental study in chickens for the pathogenesis of idiopathic scoliosis. Spine. 1993; 18(12):1609–1615**

[82] Thillard MJ. Déformations de la colonne vertébrale consécutives à l'épiphysectomie chez le poussin. C R Hebd Seances Acad Sci. 1959; 248(8):1238–1240

[83] Hilibrand AS, Blakemore LC, Loder RT, et al. The role of melatonin in the pathogenesis of adolescent idiopathic scoliosis. Spine. 1996; 21(10):1140–1146

[84] Fagan AB, Kennaway DJ, Sutherland AD. Total 24-hour melatonin secretion in adolescent idiopathic scoliosis. A case-control study. Spine. 1998; 23(1):41–46

[85] **Machida M. Cause of idiopathic scoliosis. Spine. 1999; 24(24):2576–2583**

[86] **Machida M, Saito M, Dubousset J, Yamada T, Kimura J, Shibasaki K. Pathological mechanism of idiopathic scoliosis: experimental scoliosis in pinealectomized rats. Eur Spine J. 2005; 14(9):843–848**

[87] Howell FR, Dickson RA. The deformity of idiopathic scoliosis made visible by computer graphics. J Bone Joint Surg Br. 1989; 71(3):399–403

[88] Leatherman KD. The management of rigid spinal curves. Clin Orthop Relat Res. 1973; 93(93):215–224

[89] Dickson RA, Archer IA, Deacon P. The surgical management of idiopathic thoracic scoliosis. J Orthopaedic Surgical Techniques. 1985; 1:23–28

[90] Dickson RA. Idiopathic scoliosis: foundation for physiological treatment. Ann R Coll Surg Engl. 1987; 69(3):89–96

[91] Moe JH. Methods of correction and surgical techniques in scoliosis. Orthop Clin North Am. 1972; 3(1):17–48

[92] Andrew T, Piggott H. Growth arrest for progressive scoliosis. Combined anterior and posterior fusion of the convexity. J Bone Joint Surg Br. 1985; 67(2):193–197

[93] Houghton GR. Cosmetic surgery for scoliosis. In: Dickson RA, Bradford DS (eds). Management of spinal deformities. London: Butterworths International Medical Reviews; 1984:237–251

[94] Cotrel Y, Dubousset J, Guillaumat M. New universal instrumentation in spinal surgery. Clin Orthop Relat Res. 1988; 227(227):10–23

[95] Wood KB, Transfeldt EE, Ogilvie JW, Schendel MJ, Bradford DS. Rotational changes of the vertebral-pelvic axis following Cotrel-Dubousset instrumentation. Spine. 1991; 16(8) Suppl:S404–S408

Chapter 4

Idiopathic Scoliosis

4.1	Epidemiology of Late-Onset Idiopathic Scoliosis	64
4.2	Screening for Scoliosis	65
4.3	Late-Onset Idiopathic Scoliosis	68
4.4	The Adolescent with the Bigger Curve	99
4.5	Osteotomies	102
4.6	Early-Onset Idiopathic Scoliosis	106
Case Gallery		115

4 Idiopathic Scoliosis

4.1 Epidemiology of Late-Onset Idiopathic Scoliosis

4.1.1 Scoliosis in the Community

Those of us who were young orthopaedic surgeons in the 1960s and 1970s will remember their first steps into the minefield of learning about spinal deformities and of course in particular idiopathic scoliosis. Our surgical forefathers had laid down fairly strict rules based on their very narrow and hitherto unchallenged views about management and very importantly what they were based upon.[1,2] Fortunately we all helped change the situation over the years. Even then we knew that only very few small curves progressed[3] and therefore there was nothing wrong with the observation for these. If however the curve got much beyond, say, 20 degrees, then the Milwaukee brace was empirically prescribed.[1] Moe led the way by recommending that curves of 25 degrees or more should be braced and said they indeed "responded well to bracing." This then produced the epidemic of school screening programs. Meanwhile if curves did progress they weren't allowed to get more than 60 degrees because of literature mainly from Scandinavia to the effect that if the curve went much beyond that figure patients risked cardiopulmonary dysfunction which, if severely progressive, could jeopardize life as well as quality thereof[4-7] (▶ Table 4.1).

Thus, the notion about bracing was to try and prevent curves that had progressed beyond 25 degrees from getting up to or beyond 60 degrees. So these were the rules and they were applied quite rigidly. If surgery was recommended, then in the pre-Harrington era localizer casts were applied under traction to obtain the best correction and then a window was cut out in the back of the cast through which spinal fusion was performed. The cast was then worn for at least 3 if not 6 months! With the advent of Harrington instrumentation[8] this mitigated all the previous fuss (traction, casts, windows, etc.) before carrying out spinal fusion. This was the "Harrington revolution." Although it was known that not all curves of 25 degrees or more progressed[3] (four-fifths do not), pioneers of brace treatment dictated that bracing should be worn for up to 23 hours a day because: (1) faith in brace treatment was unquestionable and (2) allowing progression to 60 degrees or more would possibly endanger their patients' lives. That was the perceived wisdom of the day and was effectively unchallengable.[9,10] If death or potential heart failure might be the outcome then, not surprisingly, both providers and recipients of health care happily endorsed this treatment program.

If there really was such a serious outcome and patients presented de novo clinically with curves of 30 or 40 degrees then it seemed quite reasonable to identify less severe curves in the community. This was the basis for the introduction of school screening programs, primarily for health reasons but fortunately, as an aside, we began to learn something about prevalence rates and progression potential of the condition of idiopathic scoliosis. At the beginning of school screening these epidemiological matters were relegated for what seemed perfectly reasonable health concerns.[11-14] Belief in bracing was so strong that it would have been quite unethical to conduct a controlled trial. Quite frankly the dictators of the time simply would not have condoned such a thing. However, over the past few decades, these rules have been challenged to the point where it is difficult to believe that we carried on with these beliefs for as long as we did. Yet there was clear evidence in the literature to go against the notion that healthy young adolescents with a bendy back could die of cardiopulmonary dysfunction.

Back in the 1960s there were several publications about the long-term follow-up of patients with untreated scoliosis. In Sweden, Nachemson[4] and Nilssonne and Lundgren[5] and in America, Collis and Ponsetti[6] reported on long-term prognosis. Nilssonne and Lundgren traced 102 patients with curve magnitudes greatly in excess of that which is normally associated with late-onset idiopathic scoliosis (LOIS) and reported that almost two-thirds of deaths were attributed to cardiopulmonary disease and that they had been disadvantaged in other ways throughout life: 76% were unmarried, 90% had back symptoms, 30% were on a disability pension, and 17% were disabled. The same can be said for Nachemson's study reporting severe cardiac and pulmonary disease and deaths.[4] Then Collis and Ponsetti reported that two-thirds of patients with thoracic curves greater than 60 degrees had diminished vital capacity.[6] Bengtsson then looked in detail at psychological and psychiatric considerations in untreated scoliosis and found much higher rates of divorce, lower marriage rates, and higher suicide rates.[7] If at the age of, say, 10 or 11, you have a curve magnitude of 130 degrees or so, and these sort of curve magnitudes in these ages typified these investigations, then the only conclusion that can be drawn is that these cases were of early-onset idiopathic scoliosis (EOIS) (or indeed congenital) and not those of late onset. Meanwhile personal experience of patients with LOIS clearly demonstrated that pulmonary function is not abnormal even if curve magnitude is well in excess of 60 degrees; the need to routinely assess cardiopulmonary function before surgery finding invariable normality in our late-onset cases. In Oxford in 1970s we wanted to give up routine cardiopulmonary testing preoperatively for teenagers about to undergo scoliosis surgery. This was regarded as being too drastic a move. Where were these so-called cardiopulmonary compromised 30 and 40 year olds? They were supposed to be filling intensive care units but of course they weren't. They were out enjoying life! Then, more recently, Pehrsson et al reported another long-term study of mortality recognizing that organic health problems of idiopathic scoliosis belonged to a much younger age of onset whereas no patient with adolescent onset scoliosis died from respiratory failure.[15]

Why then this marked discrepancy? The answer was really evident and had already been described in detail in the 1965

Table 4.1 Treatment of idiopathic scoliosis, 1970s style

Under 25 degrees	Observe
25–60 degrees	Brace
60 degrees plus	Surgery

Philip Zorab Meeting in London by the distinguished pulmonary pathologist Lynn Reid.[16] Her observations were then published in more detail in 1971.[17] She carried out postmortem examinations on children who had perished from cardiopulmonary compromise at the Brompton Hospital in London. She found very hypoplastic lungs resembling those that occur in infants with congenital diaphragmatic hernia in which the abdominal contents severely compress lung space. It was these infantile "malignant" idiopathic progressive curves (as they were called at that time) that were the main problem in producing severe cardiopulmonary compromise and fatality. Davies and Reid showed that pulmonary alveolar reduplication occurred in the first 2 or 3 years of life and certainly ended by the age of 8[17] (see ▶ Fig. 2.26). Very significant thoracic deformities can therefore cramp the developing lungs preventing further reduplication. Then Margaret Branthwaite who was a consultant chest physician at the Brompton Hospital at that time, later a distinguished barrister, published her findings about cardiorespiratory consequences of untreated idiopathic scoliosis.[18] She found that curves that started before the age of 5 years, and generally in infancy, had the bad cardiopulmonary reputation whereas curves that started beyond the age of 5 had no such cardiorespiratory concerns in the future.

As a result of being aware of these important findings it was perfectly obvious to us in Leeds why there were such bad reports about idiopathic scoliosis in the 1960s—simply because age of onset was not being considered. It was early-onset very progressive scoliosis (idiopathic or congenital) that had the bad reputation for organic health while LOIS had no such health consequences. So we thought it very important to regard idiopathic scoliosis as being either EOIS (before the age of 5) or LOIS (after the age of 5)[19] (▶ Fig. 2.25) and therefore we should reclassify accordingly. Notwithstanding, screening for scoliosis in adolescents was still championed well into 1970s, 1980s, and even 1990s. The process seemed unstoppable despite the strong retrospective evidence base against it.

What about bracing? We shall look at the efficacy (or rather lack of efficacy) later, but there is no evidence in favor of this practice now and there never was. However, screening for scoliosis did produce a valuable by-product of trying to learn more about the natural history although we do not know much more today than we knew 20 years ago. That might be because of the diminishing school screening programs but although the loss is to epidemiology the gain is that hordes of quite normal children no longer go through this harmful and unethical process.

4.2 Screening for Scoliosis
4.2.1 Definitions and Criteria

If you are going to go screening there are certain niceties to be observed. You cannot just go swanning into Marks and Spencer on a Saturday morning and start measuring blood pressure! For decades there have been strict criteria for screening. "Screening is the presumptive identification of an unrecognised disease or defect through the application of tests, examinations or other procedures that can be applied rapidly."[20] The World Health Organization (WHO) has defined several criteria that should be met before informing an unwitting individual that he or she has a problem and there are 10 of them[21] (▶ Table 4.2).

Table 4.2 WHO criteria for screening

1. The condition sought should be an important health problem for the individual and community.
2. There should be an accepted treatment or useful intervention for patients with the disease.
3. The natural history of the disease should be adequately understood.
4. There should be a latent or early symptomatic stage.
5. There should be a suitable and acceptable screening test or examination.
6. Facilities for diagnosis and treatment should be available.
7. There should be an agreed policy on whom to treat as patients.
8. Treatment started at an early stage should be of more benefit than treatment started later.
9. The cost should be economically balanced in relation to possible expenditure on medical care as a whole.
10. Case finding should be a continuing process and not a once-and-for-all project.

As regards scoliosis there are a number of prerequisites and so let's pick out a few from the WHO's list. First, the condition should be an important health problem for the individual and community. Certainly that was thought to be the case in the late 1960s and early 1970s when it spread through the scoliosis community that children might die from untreated idiopathic scoliosis. We have known all about hypoplastic infantile idiopathic lungs for decades but we knew that far too long before screening faded out. Second, there should be an accepted or useful intervention for patients with the disease. School screening detected droves of children with minor curves, less than the Scoliosis Research Society's definition of scoliosis which should be a curve of 11 degrees plus with concordant rotation (vertebral bodies turning into the curve convexity).[2] Neither is there any accepted treatment for these very small curves nor do such individuals need treatment. They are not cases of scoliosis and are better termed "schooliosis" (irrelevant curves detected in schools).

There should be a latent to early symptomatic stage of the disease and of course for LOIS there are no symptoms other than deformity. Then there should be a suitable and sensitive screening test for examination, both forward bending tests (▶ Fig. 4.1) and scoliometer readings[22] leading to far too many curves detected that are too small to be called scoliosis. In Leeds we have used the Quantec Surface Shape Measurement system (▶ Fig. 4.2) for a lot of our epidemiological and natural history work, and while this records more than 250,000 data points on surface shape in a fraction of a second it does not tell you how deformed an individual is on, say, a 0 to 100 scale basis.[23] Moving on to age criteria, the rules say that treatment at an early stage should be of more benefit than treatment started later but unfortunately we have no adequate early stage or conservative treatment.

Then while the question of costs may not be important for fully privately funded health services, it is very important, for example, in the UK where health service costs are most definitely finite. Screening for scoliosis would then compete economically with, for instance, cervical cancer screening and would fail dismally.

Children harvested then had the deformity corroborated on clinical examination and many then underwent X-ray examination of the spine. That you had scoliosis (whatever that was to the child and family) was then permanently imprinted on your

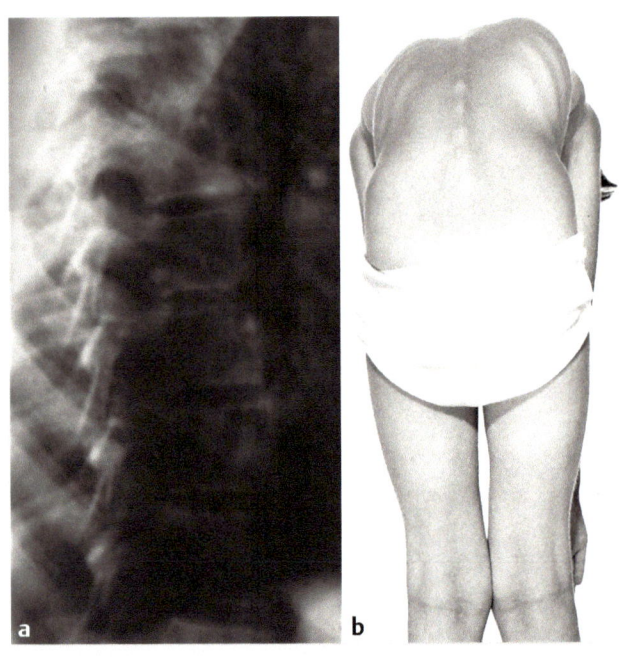

Fig. 4.1 The forward-bend test. (a) A true lateral radiograph showing the essential lordosis. (b) On forward bending this lordosis is compressed and the spine therefore buckles, enhancing the rib hump (see ▶ Fig. 3.9). (Reproduced with permission from Newton P, O'Brien M, Shufflebarger H, et al. Idiopathic Scoliosis: The Harms Study Group Treatment Guide. Stuttgart/New York: Thieme; 2010: 53.)

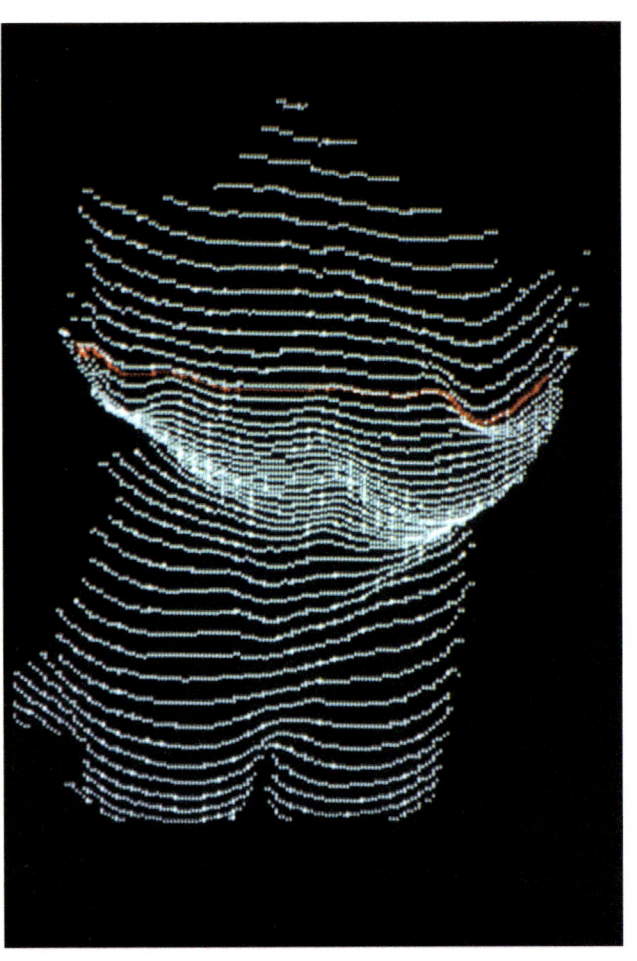

Fig. 4.2 A patient with a right thoracic idiopathic scoliosis whose surface shape has been registered by the Quantec system.

medical records, rather like a criminal record. Even chiropractors were getting in on the act. R.A.D. well remembers John Hall in Boston telling him in the late 1970s in a rather facetious manner that he spent more time telling young children and parents that they didn't have scoliosis than actually treating those that did (as a result of these nonsensical screening programs). Mercifully the U.S. Preventive Services Taskforce eventually recommended eliminating school screening for scoliosis.[24] (Hopefully it has gone for good and we shall never see its like again.)

4.2.2 Natural History

Although nearly all epidemiology surveys have involved female schoolchildren between the ages of 10 and 14, the recent MRC study in Leeds of 16,000 schoolchildren of both genders chose an age group from 6 to 14 so as to encompass all the years of LOIS,[25] the 10-year-olds reaching maturity by the end of follow-up. All of 2.2% of girls aged 12 to 14 years had idiopathic scoliosis, a curve of 11 degrees or more with concordant rotation (▶ Table 4.3). With increasing curve magnitude, thoracic curves and females became greatly over-represented with 70% of curves in excess of 15 degrees (▶ Table 4.4 and ▶ Table 4.5).

Comparing the results of the Oxford study[26] with those of the Leeds study almost 20 years later, it would appear that LOIS is perhaps pursuing a more benign course with the passage of time (2.5% of teenage girls in Oxford versus 2.2% in Leeds).

Then we know that bigger curves do tend to progress more than smaller curves and this would accord with Euler's laws of flexible columns as well as common sense (e.g., the Leaning Tower of Pisa—the more it leans the more it will carry on doing so). In addition, some useful information about other curve patterns is helpful. Right-sided thoracic curves and left-sided lumbar curves are more likely to progress, as is well known, but why? The answer lies in the transverse plane geometry of the thoracic and lumbar vertebrae. Thoracic vertebrae are asymmetric to the right in the transverse plane thus favoring a right thoracic scoliosis (due to the constant pressure of the descending thoracic aorta[27,28]) (▶ Fig. 3.2 and ▶ Fig. 3.3) but there is also an inbuilt coronal plane deformity in "normal children" with curvatures in the right and left directions being equally represented for small curves (< 10 degrees). If therefore the preexisting normal coronal plane deformity is to the left it will counter the adverse effect of right-sided transverse plane asymmetry with the two effectively canceling each other out. If, however, there is a preexisting right-sided coronal plane deformity, then right-sided transverse plane asymmetry may give momentum to a preexisting thoracic lordosis. Just in case you're wondering, the inbuilt transverse plane deformity is in the opposite direction in situs inversus[29] (see ▶ Fig. 3.3), which more than adequately confirms the Leeds theory about curve directions.[30,31]

A lot of natural history information comes from screening programs although nearly all harvested are very small curves.

Table 4.3 Overall prevalence rates for the curve sizes according to age group

Group	Age group (years)	No. of patients	Prevalence	Prevalence in girls (%)	Prevalence in boys (%)
Idiopathic scoliosis	6–8	4	0.1	0.1	0.1
	9–11	16	0.3	0.4	0.1
	12–14	56	1.2	2.2	0.3

Table 4.4 Distribution of curve sizes according to site in curves of 6 degrees or more

Apex	Size of curve		
	6–10 degrees No. (%)	11–15 degrees No. (%)	>15 degrees No. (%)
Thoracic	37 (40)	24 (51)	20 (69)
Thoracolumbar	28 (30)	17 (36)	8 (28)
Lumbar	28 (30)	6 (13)	1 (3)
Total	93	47	29

Table 4.5 Prevalence of adolescent idiopathic scoliosis

Cobb angle	Female:Male	Prevalence (%)
>10°	1.4–2:1	2.3
>20°	5.1:1	0.3–0.5
>30°	10:1	0.1–0.3
>40°	–	<0.1

Source: Reproduced with permission from Weinstein SL. Adolescent idiopathic scoliosis: Prevalence and natural history. In Weinstein SL (ed) The Pediatric Spine. Principles and Practice. 1994. Copyright © by Lippincott-Raven.

Of 134 patients detected by Brooks only 5% increased and 22% decreased.[11] Rogala detected 603 and only 7% progressed, with 2% progression in those less than 10 degrees and 10% progression in those that were greater. A total of 52 immature patients whose curves were between 20 and 30 degrees progressed.[14] In 1984 Lonstein, a key figure in the epidemiology of idiopathic scoliosis, published a very important natural history paper.[32] A total of 727 patients with LOIS curves measuring from 5 to 29 degrees were reviewed having been followed either to the end of skeletal growth or curve progression: 23% progressed while 11% showed improvement in the curve of 5 degrees or more. Risser 0 and curves of less than 15 degrees favored improvement while curve progression was related to bigger curve magnitudes, a more advanced Risser sign, and greater chronological age. Double curves progressed more than single (27% versus 18%) and single thoracic curves were the most progressive.

Much emphasis was placed on the Risser sign (see ▶ Fig. 2.23) and indeed the Risser sign is very widely used in the clinical management of patients with LOIS.[33] He noted on posteroanterior (PA) X-rays of the pelvis that the iliac apophysis appeared laterally and anteriorly (capping) and with continued growth it developed posteriorly in its excursion of ossification across the iliac crest to dip down to contact the ilium medially at its junction near the sacrum (completion). Meanwhile closure of the line between the apophysis and the ilium was of no growth significance but might take a further 2 or 3 years. The average time of completion of excursion of the iliac apophysis to its medial and posterior attachment was about a year although there was considerable variation. The average chronological age when the iliac apophysis excursion was completed was 14 years in girls and 16 years in boys although in girls it could vary from 10 to 18. Spinal growth is slow in the period from 5 to 10 years of age and curve progression was about 4 to 5 degrees a year while in the pre-adolescent phase of 10 to 15 years the average annual curve increase was 10 degrees.

Weinstein, a key figure in so much that we know about the behavior of idiopathic scoliosis, and Ponseti published about curve progression after maturity in patients with LOIS.[3] They followed 102 patients with 133 curves for an average of more than 40 years. These were evaluated as regards progression by X-rays at maturity and then at follow-up although some had intervening radiographs. More than two-thirds of curves progressed after skeletal maturity while curves of less than 30 degrees tended not to progress regardless of curve pattern. Important prognostic factors for thoracic curves were Cobb angle, apical vertebral rotation, and the RVAD of Mehta[34]; while in the lumbar spine additional factors, such as the relation of the fifth lumbar vertebra to the intercristal line and translatory shifts, were important for progression (translatory shifts are where with, say, lumbar curves, L3 appears to be displaced laterally to L4). It should be noted however that skeletal maturity was regarded as either Risser 4 (iliac apophysis completely ossified) or 5 (iliac apophysis fused to the ilium). Of course the vertebral end plates do not fuse until up to the middle of the third decade[35] and this prompted the Leeds Scoliosis Study Group to measure in an epidemiological survey sitting height for several years after Risser maturity and found that teenagers grew beyond Risser maturity by an average of 2 cm.[36] It was therefore felt that starting at Risser maturity, possibly 10 years before spinal maturity, may not be the best starting point for analysis of curve progression in adult life.

This unrecognized gap between pelvic maturity and spinal maturity led to publications to the effect that pregnancy was bad for curve progression.[37-39] Nachemson even went to the length of suggesting the avoidance of pregnancy in such women in their 20s, particularly in those who have been brace treated.[40]

Notwithstanding there were several of Weinstein's cases where there was an interim film beyond which there was still significant curve progression.[3] Curves that measured between 50 and 75 degrees at Risser maturity, particularly thoracic curves, progressed the most. Some of the examples in his paper were quite striking although it was not possible to tell whether this was due to coincidental disk degeneration.

More recently Weinstein summarized the state of knowledge of natural history in a review article with more than 250 references and this should be obligatory reading for all scoliosis surgeons.[41] There are easy-to-remember tables about prevalence, probability of progression, and progression factors (e.g., ▶ Table 4.6). For curves of more than 10 degrees the prevalence rate is 2 to 3% with a quite even female to male ratio which the Leeds Scoliosis Study Group confirmed.[25] With increasing curve magnitude to curves of more than 30 degrees the female to male ratio is now 10:1 and the prevalence rate 1-3:1,000. ▶ Table 4.6 is interesting as it shows the probability of progression changes with curve magnitude and age.

The matter of back pain in relationship to scoliosis has challenged scoliosis surgeons ever since surgery was introduced. We all assumed without any statistical analysis that long Harrington fusions to L4/L5 produced back pain making us take the metalwork out and carry out extension osteotomies in several cases although whether this altered the natural history was certainly unclear. It made sense to pay attention to sagittal curves and to restore lumbar lordosis but was flattening of the normal sagittal profile the reason for the pain or was it over-stressing the available joints below? Nowadays by paying attention to sagittal curvatures with modern instrumentation we hope the problem of long-term low back pain will be very much less but we certainly aren't in a position to say so at the moment. In any event we have an annual incidence of back pain in the general population varying from about 60 to 80%. We all know this and if more specifics are required then you only have to consult Weinstein's 1999 Natural History paper for the exact references.[41] Incidentally, incidence and prevalence are not interchangeable but are quite different. They are both rates—incidence rate being the rate of new cases and prevalence rate being the number of existing cases. It is generally accepted that the problem of back pain in scoliosis patients is no greater than in the general population.[42] However, a quarter of scoliosis patients had reported to their doctor with back pain mainly those with lower curves and lumbar curves with translatory shifts. In this Iowa long-term series whereas at Risser maturity only 2% of patients had evidence of osteoarthritis, at age 40 at follow-up all of 38% of patients had radiographic evidence of degenerative joint disease of the spine and at 50 at follow-up in all of 91%. Again this is very difficult to separate from the natural history in the general population bearing in mind that the great majority of scoliosis patients are female who do have "the gene" for primary generalized osteoarthritis of which significant facet joint arthropathy in the lumbar spine is an important part. Furthermore, we have to look at comparable aged nonscoliotic females to assess the prevalence of degenerative changes in the lumbar spine to form a proper comparison group. One would also have to look at those who have been treated surgically and those who have not. The evidence would suggest that with the use of long straight Harrington rods decades ago it was a problem but whether it is now or will be in the future with modern instrumentation and recognition of the importance of sagittal shape one simply does not know (see later under *Specific Curve Patterns*).

4.3 Late-Onset Idiopathic Scoliosis

4.3.1 Clinical Presentation and Evaluation

It is important to look at LOIS in some detail because this condition is the "bread and butter" of scoliosis surgeons worldwide in terms of occupying their clinical time. More than 90% of cases of scoliosis we see are of the LOIS variety. Furthermore, the treatment methods for LOIS are the cornerstone of treatment for scoliosis of many other diagnostic categories. Whereas 40 years ago, and indeed for the next 10 or 15 years thereafter many patients presented because they had been noted to have some asymmetry of the torso on school screening, the only mode of presentation now and for the last at least 20 years has been because of concern by patient or family about body shape. Presentation is quite different from, say, an underdeveloped 11-year-old girl to a relatively mature 14-year-old. For the 10 or 11 year old, it is more often the parents who see a shape abnormality and they are very concerned about their daughter whereas it is the 14-year-old more mature girl that herself is very worried about the fact that she is not of normal shape like her friends. The common denominator however is that the spine is buckling during adolescent growth and they want to know why this has happened, what does the future have in store, and if there is any satisfactory treatment. Compared to 30 to 40 years ago, we now have good sound answers to these very important questions.

The history is almost universal, namely that the last time we saw our daughter or she saw her shape herself in the mirror her

Table 4.6 Probability of progression with magnitude of curve at initial detection versus age

Curve magnitude at detection (*)	Age at detection		
	10–12 yr	13–15 yr	16 yr
<19	25%	10%	0%
20–29	60	40	10
30–59	90	70	30
>60	100	90	70

*Values are percentages.
Source: Reproduced with permission from Nachemson A, Lonstein J, Weinstein S. Report of the Scoliosis Research Society Prevalence and Natural History Committee 1982. Presented at the Scoliosis Research Society Meeting, Denver.

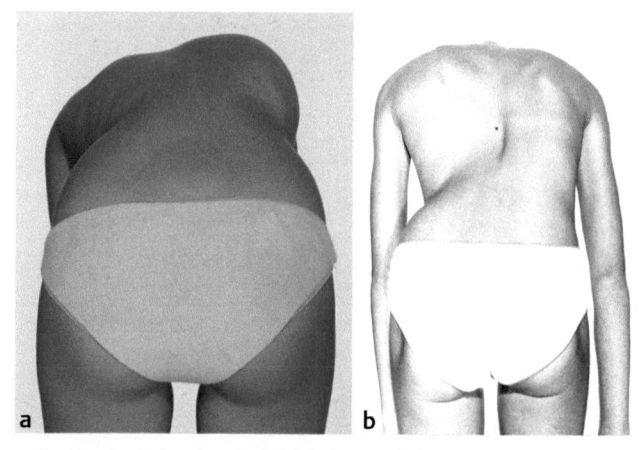

Fig. 4.3 The deformity of LOIS. **(a)** The unsightly rib hump of a thoracic curve. **(b)** The ugly waist asymmetry of a lumbar curve.

back was normal but now it has become unsightly, with usually either a rib or loin prominence (▶ Fig. 4.3). With a thoracic curve there may be concern that one developing breast is bigger or smaller than the other. With a thoracic curve the whole torso is twisted (plagiothorax) so that with a right thoracic curve then the left breast may seem larger than the right. It has even been suggested ludicrously that this may be indicative of the cause of idiopathic thoracic scoliosis with the underlying ribs having hypervascularity and so asymmetric rib length is secondarily produced.[43] This spurious hypothesis even predicated rib length surgery for LOIS. One might ask how this correlates with idiopathic scoliosis in boys not to mention infants! With a thoracolumbar or lumbar curve there is often marked waist asymmetry and this may be a presenting feature. Indeed, girls may find the ugly waist just as concerning as the rib hump. Then asymmetric shoulder height is also common with the right shoulder being higher for a right thoracic curve while a higher left shoulder may indicate the characteristic signe d'epaule[44] of a double thoracic curve (▶ Fig. 2.17). Decompensated patients also present with a significant list of the torso (▶ Fig. 2.19). Whatever feature of body disfigurement is the presenting symptom it is a matter of deformity only and the family can be reassured that there are no organic health consequences.

On further questioning the child is absolutely normal with no associated problems. That is certainly the case in the vast majority of LOIS patients. There are however a number of red flags to watch out for. Back pain should not be a problem in children to begin with, let alone those with a scoliosis, and is a red flag for primary health care and accident and emergency doctors. For the scoliosis patient this is particularly important. Pain, particularly if present at night, would indicate a pathological basis for the scoliosis and mandates further examination and imaging. The main suspects are a spinal cord tumor or syrinx (▶ Fig. 2.38) or a bony tumor such as an osteoblastoma or osteoid osteoma. These must be excluded by MRI or skeletal scintigraphy and CT. More often than not plain X-rays will localize the lesion. For example, with an osteoid osteoma/osteoblastoma there is enlargement of the pars/transverse process junction (▶ Fig. 4.4) while with an intradural tumour or syrinx there may well be widening of the interpedicular distance at

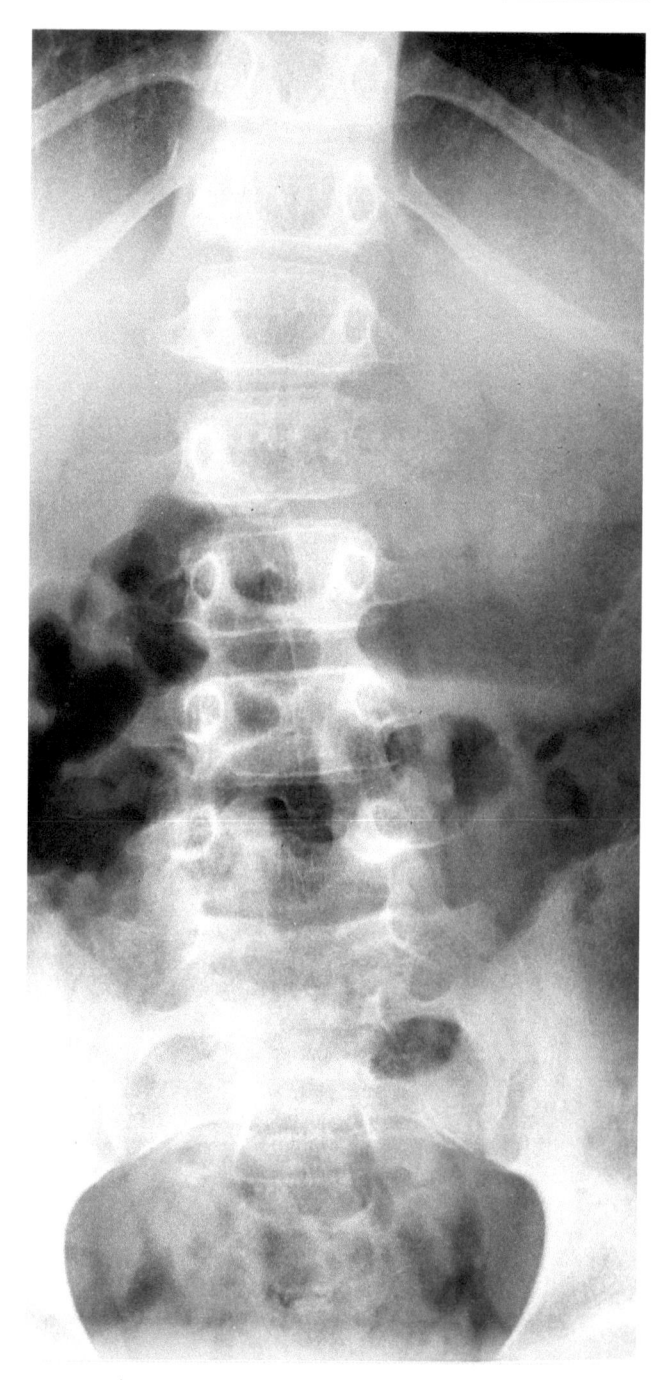

Fig. 4.4 Plain film appearances of an osteoblastoma with enlargement of the right L2 pedicle/transverse process junction and no clear pedicle ("winking owl" sign).

the site of the lesion. MRI is definitive in the diagnosis of spinal cord tumors and syrinxes while CT scanning and isotope scanning are strongly positive for bone lesions. For individuals with these lesions, on examination the curve is more often very stiff whereas with LOIS they remain very flexible until curve size is considerable. The most important neurological abnormality for intradural lesions is absence or asymmetry of the abdominal reflexes whereas no neurological abnormalities would be expected with bone lesions. With osteoid osteomas the often late diagnosed cause of night pain can lead to psychological or behavioral problems during adolescence and it is remarkable how curative for these nonorganic problems, as well as pain, surgical removal is. The scoliosis in association with these bone tumors is never great, generally not exceeding 20 or 30 degrees. Curve regression after removal is the rule and these curves never become autonomous in their own right unless the process of posterior excision tethers the back of the spine.

Because the typical idiopathic-type scoliosis deformity is also present in other diagnostic categories it is important to observe the musculoskeletal system in its totality. A very tall slim child should be checked for arachnodactyly, a high arched palate, and joint laxity for Marfan syndrome, whereas some café-au-lait spots and, in particular, axillary freckling would demand considerable further investigation as regards neurofibromatosis type 1 (NF1). Collagen diseases and neurofibromatosis very often present with an idiopathic-type scoliosis as the first clinical feature. It is only those with the severe dystrophic bone change that have the short sharp angular curve with lots of rotation diagnostic of NF1. Meanwhile a high stepping gait would indicate a peripheral neuropathy whereas a wide-based unsteady gait would suggest Friedreich's ataxia. It is very important for the scoliosis surgeon not to divorce themselves from the rest of the musculoskeletal system and so in this book we cover the general orthopaedic principles of these various conditions in which a scoliosis might also be an important clinical feature because it is often the spine surgeon to whom these patients first present.

Other than for the above nonidiopathic conditions that might present or masquerade as idiopathic scoliosis, far too many investigations are performed and, importantly, far too many X-rays are carried out unnecessarily, dangerous in particular to the developing thyroid and breasts.[45,46] The only reason for radiographing the spine of the typical idiopathic case at first visit is to make sure that it is idiopathic and does not belong to another category, such as, to exclude a congenital anomaly of the spine. One full length PA radiograph of the patient erect and one lateral with a reference grid is quite sufficient for this initial consultation (▶ Fig. 4.5). These views are principally to exclude a congenital spinal anomaly and not to register the deformity which can be clearly seen on examination of the patient. The lateral X-ray is commonly misinterpreted as showing a kyphosis when of course all these deformities are lordoscolioses (see Chapter 3). A PA X-ray of the left hand and wrist to measure bone age is useful to titrate these appearances with chronological age so as to more accurately measure maturation status and growth velocity.[47]

Registering Cobb angles on the initial film is important to guide the understanding of natural history but measuring Cobb angles on an annual basis is quite unnecessary and should indeed be an inadmissible radiation hazard. What matters is not what the X-ray tells you but what the patient and family tell you about the deformity itself. First of all, reassurance is the most important thing so that the family can understand that there is no disease present, that the spine is perfectly normal except that it has decided to buckle with growth, that this condition is very common affecting more than 2% of normal growing girls, and that it produces no organic ill-health consequences whatever. Then the family should be taken through what the future may hold. There is then only one question to be

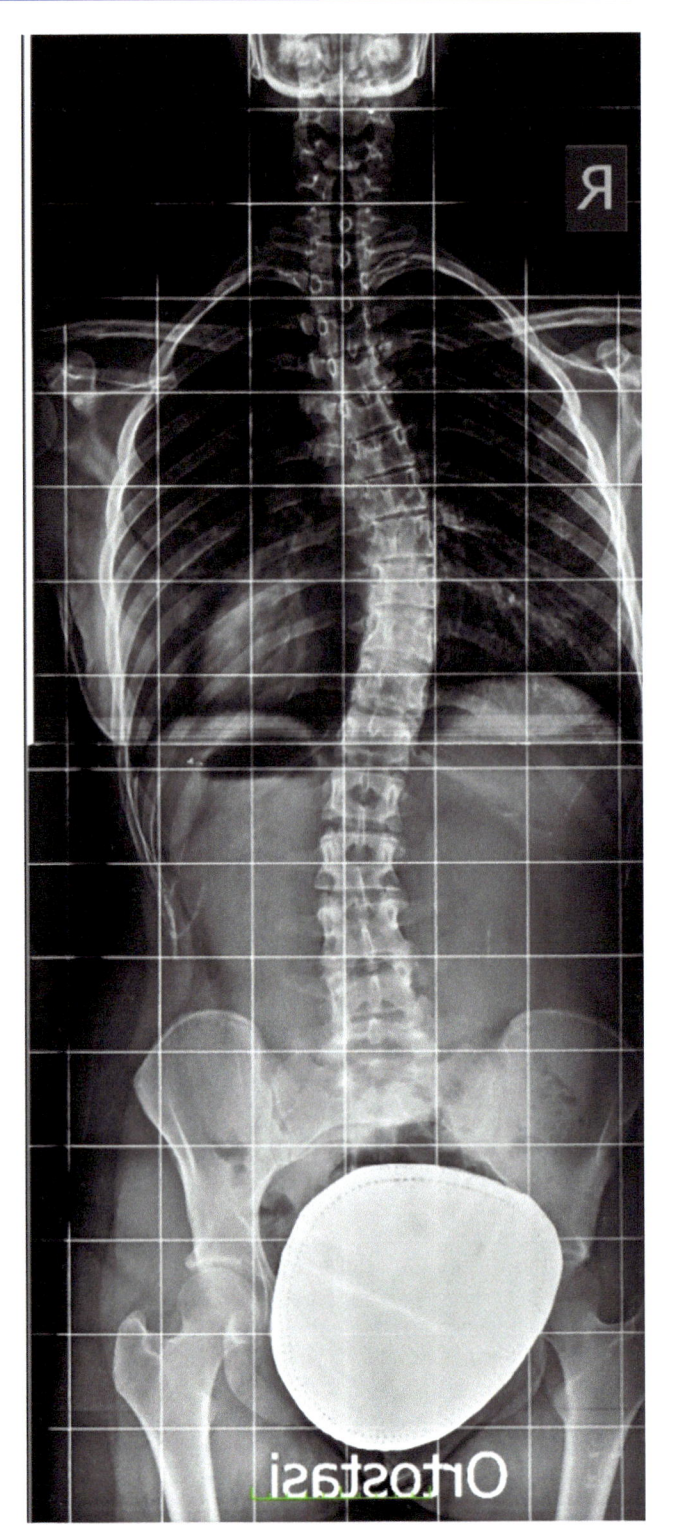

Fig. 4.5 Erect PA X-ray spine (whole) with grid.

asked: is the deformity acceptable or not? Acceptability must mean that the patient and family are quite happy with the deformity as it is now, provided it doesn't worsen significantly. Unfortunately, we have no way of preventing progression nonoperatively. Unacceptability means that the patient and the family are not satisfied with the deformity to the point where they will undergo surgical correction to improve/correct the situation.

Nowadays with modern instrumentation systems not only is correction a real possibility it is very much what surgeons and their patients expect. Of course full correction of the deformity does not necessarily mean a Cobb angle of zero degrees. The reason the initial X-ray looks so bad at 30 degrees or so is that the spine, fairly deep inside the torso, has to buckle appreciably from the midline before it alters surface shape and so the essential principle of surgical correction is to put it back to where it was before it impinged on the surface of the body.

The surgeon has no role at all to decide whether the deformity is acceptable or not, that is for the patient and family to decide. What the surgeon must do is to provide all the information necessary to the family so that they can make this often difficult decision in a proper risks and rewards equation. It is quite inappropriate for the surgeon to look at the X-rays, and, tell the patient the deformity measures 45 degrees and that surgery is necessary.[48] It is for the family and patient to decide upon surgery regardless of Cobb angle and if they have gone through this very important risks and rewards equation with the surgeon then the only decision that they can make is the right one. Fortunately, nowadays rewards greatly outweigh risks—the latter being minimal. Families do often come nowadays with some knowledge about scoliosis from the Internet and the sensible way forward is to provide them with knowledge that is really essential to their case and then afterward deal with any questions that might arise from their Internet experience.

If the deformity is considered acceptable it is very unfortunate that we do not have a method of treatment that will maintain acceptability. It was thought in the days of Milwaukee and Boston bracing that these contraptions might alter natural history favorably but unfortunately that has not proved to be so. In that situation observation is the only way forward and that should not be radiographically measuring Cobb angle, say, every 6 months or yearly, but should be by inspection of the patient and, most importantly, listening to how the patient and family regard the deformity and how intrusive it is in their way of life. At the end of the visit standing height can be measured using a calibrated stadiometer and the reading recorded on standard centile charts,[49] kept in the records.

It is quite unnecessary to take any more spine X-rays on the first visit and indeed for evermore unless the patient's deformity becomes unacceptable when of course, as we shall see, there are important images to take before surgery that help operative planning. For idiopathic patients, flexibility is a function of curve size and the bigger the curve gets the less flexible it will be simply because the component parts have become more and more three-dimensionally deformed with growth. There is no point in looking at it radiologically before the decision for surgery when it is perfectly self-evident on clinical inspection.

The first visit is extremely important and the patient and family should not be overdosed with information about scoliosis that is not particularly germane at this point in time. An early introduction to scoliosis can well be supplemented by further important information at the second and subsequent visits. Normality, with the exception of the spinal deformity, is the name of the game and should be stressed repeatedly as consultations continue.

It is commonly asked what the cause of this condition is and this is something that can be discussed more and more as the consultations progress. At the first consultation it should be impressed that this is not a simple right–left growing problem or wearing school bags on one shoulder rather than the other, but a front–back problem with the spine growing more quickly at the front than the back. This is abundantly clear when they look at their child's back and see that overall it is very flat sideways on, more so than others of their age. Then to produce a deformity the spine simply has to buckle with growth and that is perhaps all they need to know about the etiology of this problem. With a 14-year-old more mature girl there may already be considerable psychosocial distress and it is often very helpful to have a few words with the girl in the presence of the nurse but without the rest of the family, indeed many such girls request this.

One of the research fellows in the Leeds Scoliosis Study Group, Dr. Fiona Smith, an honors psychology graduate doing her PhD, looked at degree of deformity in girls with idiopathic scoliosis in relation to psychosocial distress using validated psychological questionnaires to tease out and measure their problems.[50] One of the parameters she measured was body mass index (BMI) and for those with severe deformities eating disorders and a low BMI were common. The normal prevalence rate of eating disorders in adolescent schoolchildren is of the order of 2 or 3% but this was 10 times higher, 20 to 30%, in those with severe idiopathic scoliosis. In the worst cases there was frank osteoporosis just when peak bone mass in females should be achieved. Occasionally one finds a patient so distressed as to be grossly underweight and almost emaciated (▶ Fig. 4.6). Such individuals may need hyperalimentation before they can be deemed fit enough to undergo surgical intervention. We are therefore not relegating this condition of idiopathic scoliosis as simply a matter of cosmetic deformity but rather there is very much more to having a deformity than perhaps meets the eye. It is of course the amount of psychosocial distress that drives the patient with the deformity toward surgery and as this condition is a matter of appearance and deformity only then that is all that matters. Patients nowadays tend to present with deformities of between 20 and 30 degrees and so at initial presentation it is unusual for the deformity to be unacceptable although acceptability might be a 50-degree curve in one more stoical patient and family and a 35-degree curve may be unacceptable in another. It is important not to suddenly stick up the X-ray on the viewing box as many patients and families express shock and guilt that they could have allowed the deformity to become so apparently large. They should therefore be forewarned that the appearance on X-ray grossly exaggerates the surface shape deformity lest you frighten the life out of them. It is obsession with X-rays and Cobb angles that drives scoliosis surgeons to unnecessarily take radiographs on every visit which only upsets them. Reassurance is the name of the game.

4.3.2 Classification

New classifications seem to be irresistible; however, of course, there is nothing wrong with the original SRS classification[2] (▶ Table 4.7). We don't really see any need to produce new

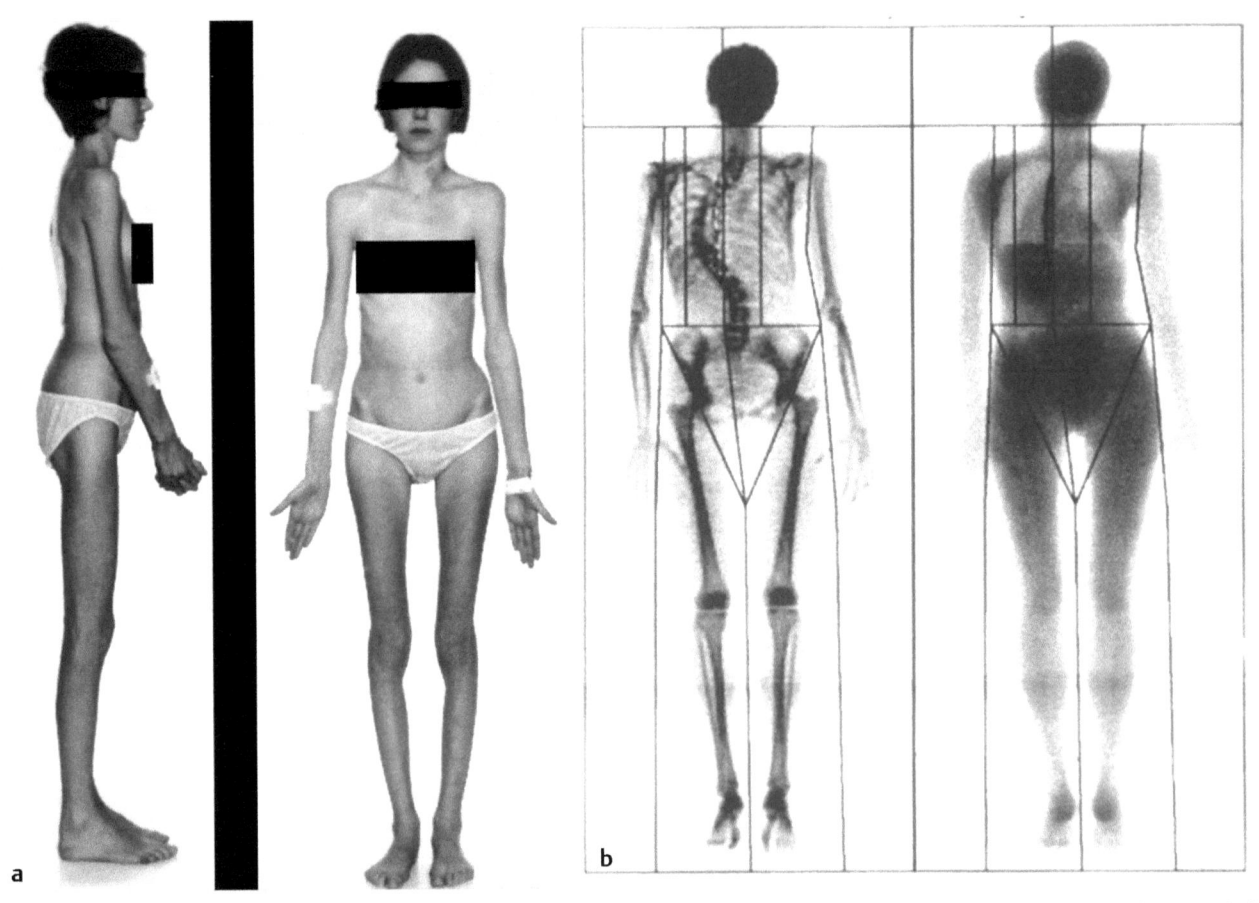

Fig. 4.6 (a) This 15-year-old girl had severe anorexia and was severely undernourished and had amenorrhea. (b) DEXA scanning revealed a T score (−2) on the border between osteopenia and osteoporosis.

Table 4.7 The original SRS classification

- Single structural curves
  - Thoracic
  - Thoracolumbar
  - Lumbar
- Double structural curves
  - Double thoracic
  - Thoracic and thoracolumbar
  - Thoracic and lumbar
- Triple structural curves

Table 4.8 The King classification

Type 1	Double structural right thoracic and left thoracolumbar or lumbar curves with the lower curve bigger than the thoracic curve.
Type 2	Double right thoracic and left thoracolumbar and lumbar curves of equal magnitude or the thoracic curve being bigger.
Type 3	A single thoracic curve.
Type 4	Unbalanced thoracic curves with significant decompensation to the side of the convexity of the curve.
Type 5	Double thoracic major curves with a main right thoracic curve and above that a left upper thoracic curve.

classifications if they are limited in their applicability or indeed validity. The King classification[51] (▶ Table 4.8) is to do with posterior surgery for thoracic curves only while the Lenke classification (▶ Table 4.9) is to do with posterior surgery for all curve patterns[52] although there are problems with the perception of kyphosis.

We shall see later how the introduction of anterior spinal surgery for idiopathic scoliosis has affected selection of fusion levels.

Before anterior surgery came in the generally perceived wisdom with posterior spinal surgery was to fuse all vertebrae in the structural curve. A look at any PA radiograph of a thoracic curve would indicate that the first neutral (unrotated) vertebra may be one or even two above and below the upper and lower end vertebrae, respectively (▶ Fig. 2.7). Therefore, quite obviously, a fusion from end vertebra to end vertebra will be too short leaving out two or three vertebrae in the structural curve that are not incorporated in the fusion. Not surprisingly this was a fundamental reason why curves could progress after operation until the end of growth, quite simply because the whole curve hadn't been fused. In addition, this could lead to imbalance and decompensation. In the old days we said that too short a fusion could lead to "adding on"—that is, the curve size as measured by Cobb angle could progress above or below the

Table 4.9 The Lenke classification

Type 1	Main thoracic
Type 2	Double thoracic
Type 3	Double thoracic and thoracolumbar/lumbar where both curves are of much the same size
Type 4	Triple major—double thoracic curve with a structural thoracolumbar or lumbar curve below
Type 5	Single thoracolumbar or lumbar curve
Type 6	Double structural curve—main thoracic and thoracolumbar or lumbar curve below where the main thoracic curve is less and may be nonstructural

central fused area. With early-onset curves too short a posterior fusion was said to lead to the crankshaft phenomenon[53] of further deformation which indeed was perfectly obvious all along without introducing the phrase crankshaft phenomenon if you don't curtail anterior spinal growth at the same time. In the past if you wanted to do posterior surgery for a double curve with long instrumentation down to the mid or lower lumbar spine then these fusion levels, neutral to neutral, more often than not led to a long stiff spine, flat in the sagittal plane obliterating the lumbar lordosis, and adding low back pain to the problem for which subsequent surgery in the nature of lumbar extension osteotomy was often required to try and relieve symptoms.

The whole idea of the King classification[51] came from the great John Moe himself, the founder of the world famous Twin-Cities Scoliosis Center, and he figured that these long posterior flattening fusions were not good practice and therefore introduced the concept of selective fusion[54,55] whereby the thoracic curve could be instrumented and fused sparing the lower spine to allow continued lumbar spine mobility and hopefully to reduce postoperative back pain. The original paper is quite wordy but in essence led to an alteration in the recommended posterior fusion levels based on full radiographic analysis (standing, supine, bending, etc.).[51] That's why you don't need those sets of X-rays until you've decided on surgery. Of course we were all doing selective thoracic fusions anyway based upon curve size and side-bending correction clinically as well as radiologically.

In days gone by Harrington himself always insisted that the lower end of his posterior fusion should be "in the stable zone of Harrington."[56] If vertical parallel lines are drawn through the lumbosacral facets then the vertebral bodies that remained within these lines are in the stable zone. The authors of the King paper[51] felt as the study progressed that a more accurate determination could be gained by a single vertical line drawn through the center of the sacrum perpendicular to the iliac crests which they called the center sacral line (CSL). This important line has persisted to the present day although now is referred to as the center sacral vertical line (CSVL). The vertebra that is bisected or almost bisected by this line is determined and is recorded as being the so-called stable vertebra (▶ Fig. 4.7).

Then one of the most important criteria was the degree of flexibility on side bending and they introduced the concept of

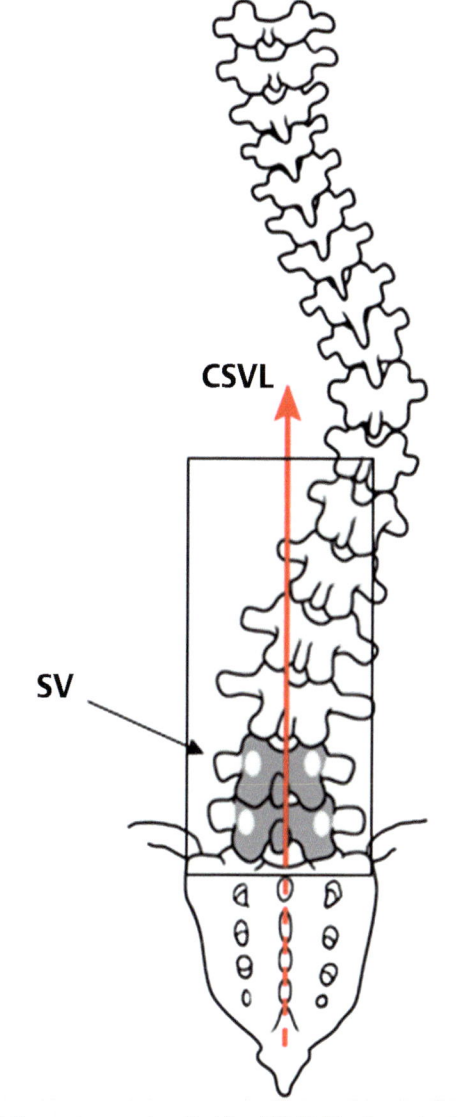

Fig. 4.7 The center sacral vertical line (CSVL). The figure has been modified to include the stable vertebra (SV) and Harrington's stable zone (shaded area). (From the Spinal Deformity Study Group Radiographic Measurement Manual, page 47, published by Medronic, Inc., 2004)

the flexibility index. If the percentage correction of the thoracic curve was then subtracted from the percentage correction of the thoracolumbar or lumbar curve, this was designated as the flexibility index. They then produced the King classification of different curve types based upon this, as shown in ▶ Table 4.8, for posterior thoracic scoliosis surgery only.

Type 1 curves were double structural right thoracic left thoracolumbar or lumbar curves with the lower curve bigger than the thoracic curve and the thoracic curve more flexible. Not surprisingly these did not do well with a selective thoracic fusion so had to be fused all the way down to the bottom of the lumbar curve. However, they do very well with an anterior selective instrumentation of the lower curve.

Type 2 curves were double structural curves where the thoracic and lumbar curves were of equal magnitude, or the thoracic curve was bigger, and most of these can be treated by selective thoracic fusion. This is based upon the premise that the greater flexibility of the lumbar curve would allow the spine below to restack, or indeed improve in response to upper curve correction.

Type 3 were thoracic curves that were subdivided according to the basic pattern of the thoracic and compensatory curves. In essence, a type 3 curve was a straightforward single thoracic curve which of course could be dealt with by a selective fusion.

Type 4 curves were unbalanced thoracic curves listing way to the side of the convexity of the curve and for this a longer posterior fusion was required.

Type 5 curves were what we used to term Moe double thoracic majors,[55] whereby the thoracic curve to the right has to be treated with metalwork going up to the cervicothoracic region on the right side, or beyond, to maintain shoulder symmetry.

That really was the prescribed treatment for idiopathic thoracic curves going back to the early 1980s. However, without being unnecessarily critical it really didn't seem to add anything to our knowledge if one persisted with posterior Harrington instrumentation but it did categorize what we were doing in a simple and memorable way. For instance, type 3 is a straightforward single right thoracic curve, say no more. Then again for type 1 curves one obviously cannot leave out the bigger lumbar curve. Then for type 4 curves treated posteriorly we have always known that we have to go down to the lower lumbar spine and for type 5 Moe double thoracic majors we have always known that we have to go up to the cervicothoracic junction or above to treat what is called the signe d'épaule.[44] We always thought this phrase was coined by Pierre Stagnara but Jean Dubousset (personal communication) reassures us that the sign was taught to him by Pierre Queneau, although it may have originally emanated from Pierre Stagnara.

Notwithstanding, the King classification was a review of a huge number of patients (more than 400) from the major center at the time. We rather liked this classification although it was how thoracic curves were always approached from the back. We could also see clearly the important role of anterior surgery.

The next most important determinant of fusion levels was contained in the paper describing the Lenke classification (▶ Table 4.9) in 2001 which is in common use today.[52] Again it focuses on posterior surgery only. It also tries to incorporate the sagittal profile using the lateral radiograph of the patient which of course is not valid as explained in Chapter 2 (▶ Fig. 2.10). With a three-dimensional deformity each vertebra occupies a different position in space as regards inclination and rotation and therefore there is no one plane in which the whole deformity can be visualized.[57-61] Stagnara's plan d'election views are with reference to the curve apex but they are only true planar views of the apical area[62] (the apical body and probably one or two above and below). They are obviously better than AP and lateral radiographs of the patient but it simply isn't in any way meaningful to try and register the sagittal profile with lateral views of the patient—so why take them? Let alone then use strange terms like hypokyphosis and hyperkyphosis when they're all lordotic! One of us (J.H.) didn't like the sagittal modifiers for the above reasons and the other (R.A.D.), having spent most of his career showing that kyphosis doesn't exist with idiopathic scoliosis, could not have faith in a system devised by a group most of whom didn't appear to appreciate the real three-dimensional deformity of structural scoliosis.

These Lenke curve patterns, as shown in ▶ Table 4.9, are the same established curve patterns going back to the days of Goldstein and Waugh.[2] The curves themselves do not change, just the classifications! The lumbar modifier for type 1 main thoracic curves is thought to be useful to help to decide if the thoracolumbar or lumbar curve is likely to be structural or not (▶ Fig. 4.8). Of course these are not really structural curves but

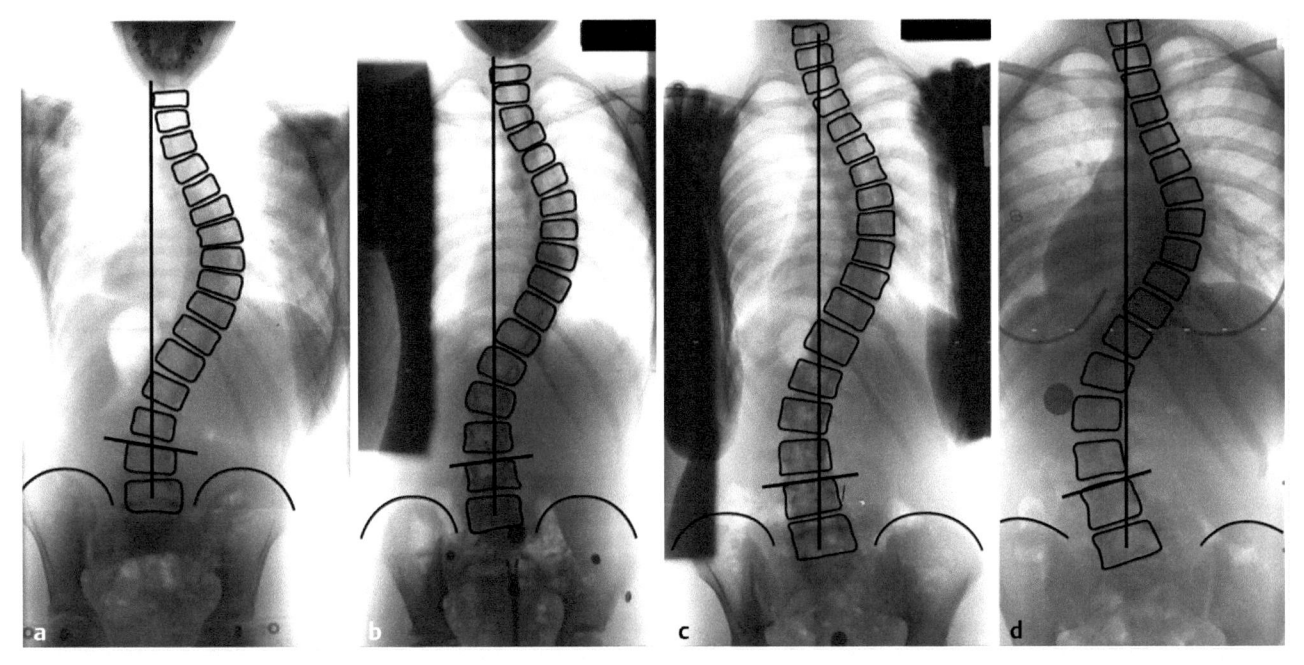

Fig. 4.8 Radiographic PA images with outlined vertebral bodies, CSVL, and L4 tilt for **(a)** a Lenke type 1AR curve (L4 tilts to the right); **(b)** a Lenke type 1 AL curve (L4 tilts to the left); **(c)** a Lenke type 1B curve; and **(d)** a Lenke type 1C curve. (Reproduced with permission from Newton P, O'Brien M, Shufflebarger H, et al. Idiopathic Scoliosis: The Harms Study Group Treatment Guide. Stuttgart/New York: Thieme; 2010: 202.)

represent what is happening below the main thoracic curve—either the lumbar spine is straight (A), or there is a small left lumbar curve (B), or the lumbar curve is a bit bigger (C). The CSVL is the same as the CSL of King based upon Harrington. If this line runs up the middle of the lumbar spine then it is a lumbar modifier A, if it still lies within the lumbar spine it is a B and if it is on the concave side of the lumbar spine it is a C. Therefore, initially for diagnostic registration of curve pattern you have 1 to 6 then for type 1 curves you add on A, B, or C according to the lumbar spine. Then you add on the thoracic sagittal profile measured from T5 to T12 as being N for normal (10 to 40 degrees, – (hypo) less than 10 degrees, and then +(hyper) if it is more than 40 degrees. Therefore, a 1AN is a main thoracic curve with a straight thoracolumbar spine below and a lateral X-ray of the patient showing a sagittal profile of 10 to 40 degrees. Incidentally T5 cannot be easily identified on a lateral because of shoulder overlap. Furthermore, thoracic kyphosis changes during adolescence (▶ Fig. 3.11) so there isn't a normal thoracic kyphosis as a basic reference. God knows what the true intraobserver error is let alone the interobserver error, never mind what they tell you,[52] but do scoliosis surgeons want to be so regimented and more importantly do they find such a busy classification (invalid in part) really helpful? For instance, a type 1AN is a simple single thoracic curve, why say anything else? The lumbar curve is purely compensatory and doesn't need a lumbar modifier. Type 1B is always going to have a sufficiently mobile lumbar spine below while a 1C has always had a lumbar curve below that needs its mobility checked out.

While this thoracic sagittal profile assessment is spurious based on the lateral view of the patient and invalid as regards this classification it is still worth thinking again about what this pseudokyphosis really means.[58–61] As the primary lordosis rotates out of the sagittal plane so of course it is less well seen on the lateral view of the patient which shows a progressively greater amount of pseudokyphosis. Thus what this pseudokyphosis really registers is the amount by which the lordosis has rotated. Therefore, if, in Lenke language, the sagittal modifier is + (i.e., the pseudokyphosis has got bigger than 40 degrees), then this means that this particular curvature is big and has a lot of rotation. This is particularly well seen in scolioses in dystrophic neurofibromatosis. With a lot of structural skeletal problems, including dystrophic spinal bone producing a very sharp angular scoliosis, the lateral view of the patient may register a pseudokyphosis of 50 degrees or more. This led to the recommendation that if there was 50 degrees of kyphosis on the lateral view then this warranted anterior surgery, as well as posterior surgery.[63] It was not of course kyphosis at all but a scoliosis with a lot of rotation particularly at the apex and clearly these very big deformities manifestly cannot be managed by posterior surgery only so the call to add an anterior stage while being entirely correct was based on a misunderstanding of what the lateral X-ray of the patient really shows. In simple terms you cannot specify a particular angle but if the pseudokyphosis is particularly big or the patient very young then watch out for the need to do an anterior procedure as well, if not before.

Then going on to pseudokyphoses of less than 10 degrees, these are particularly well seen in double-structural curves, thoracic, and thoracolumbar or lumbar, where the whole spine is lordotic throughout (▶ Fig. 2.21) and that is all that minus in the thoracic sagittal modifier really means. This is where the expression junctional kyphosis between two curves is again spurious. If this junctional vertebra lies between two structural lordoscolioses then the junctional vertebra cannot be kyphotic (▶ Fig. 2.22) but it may look as if it is on the lateral view of the patient[64] because the junctional area is less lordotic than the curves above and below.

For a classification to be useful it has to be straightforward and readily applicable and because the lateral view of the patient doesn't mean anything then it is better to leave out the sagittal modifier altogether and then the Lenke classification can have some use (for posterior surgery only), but then it isn't much different from King.

In any case, it does not really matter which classification you use because they are all trying to describe the same original curve patterns.[2] ▶ Table 4.7 is the original SRS classification slightly amended and highly recommended. It is more important to understand what, say, pseudokyphosis really means. In addition, the Lenke classification addresses posterior surgery only whereas many of these curves can be treated anteriorly with a much shorter fusion and just as good a result, if not better. For instance, all Lenke type 6 have a major structural curve in the thoracolumbar or lumbar region eminently, and we would say only, treatable anteriorly. There has been a marked trend in recent years, probably because of these classifications, to go with posterior surgery only—or the trend to do posterior surgery only has generated these classifications—and as a result anterior surgery seems to be less frequently carried out although it has been shown to be superior than equivalent posterior surgery.[65,66] We have enormous anterior experience being disciples of Leatherman and Zielke, and we feel it right and proper to guide learning scoliosis surgeons through the front of the spine as well rather than just the back.

4.3.3 Treatment

Nonoperative Treatment

Going back to our simple treatment philosophy we have asked the patient and family if they find the deformity acceptable as it is and if they do so then ideally we want a nonoperative treatment modality that can do just that—namely, prevent progression and maintain acceptability.

It would be marvellous if we had a bracing or casting system that really was effective. Unfortunately, there is no evidence of such nor does it seem possible to conceive of an effective orthosis (see Chapter 3). The great problem is the Hueter-Volkmann law because as soon as the lordosis buckles out of the sagittal plane, the vertebrae, particularly around the apical region, become progressively more three-dimensionally deformed and thus progressively more unstackable in a straight position (▶ Fig. 4.9). The best way of seeing this in one's mind is to consider blocks of Lego that progressively become more deformed and less rectangular as one proceeds through the curve to the apex. It might be possible to consider some form of corrective treatment if the blocks of Lego remained rectangular but when deformed three-dimensionally they can only be restacked in the original deformed scoliotic position (▶ Fig. 4.9), unless space is made available between adjacent vertebral bodies or the end plates are refashioned perpendicular (▶ Fig. 3.9). This is only necessary around the apical region (4 or 5 vertebrae) where three-dimensional deformation is maximal (the

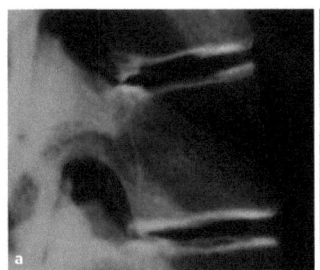

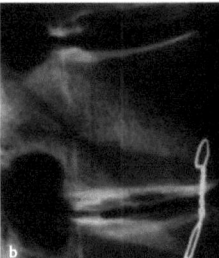

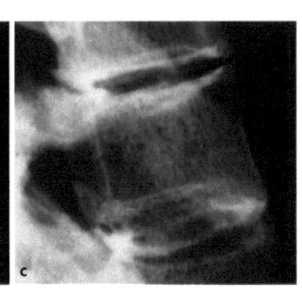

Fig. 4.9 Progressive asymmetrical wedging with growth. True lateral X-ray films of the apical vertebrae of different size curves. **(a)** Curve of 20 degrees with reasonable sagittal shape. **(b)** Curve of 40 degrees, showing that the back and inferior surfaces of the vertebral body are ellipsoid. **(c)** Curve of 80 degrees, showing marked asymmetrical 3D vertebral wedging. These vertebrae will not stack straight unless something is done about it. (Reproduced with permission from Newton P, O'Brien M, Shufflebarger H, et al. Idiopathic Scoliosis: The Harms Study Group Treatment Guide. Stuttgart/New York: Thieme; 2010: 95.)

Leeds procedure)[67–69] (see surgical treatment section). What orthosis on this earth, or in any other galaxy, could possibly redress that progressive growth deformity and imbalance? Not surprisingly side-bending radiographs show progressively less flexibility as Cobb angle increases. There is no added fibrosis or tightness or whatever to produce lack of flexibility, rather it is simply a question of unstackability, and if it wasn't then it wouldn't be idiopathic scoliosis!

By contrast an idiopathic spinal deformity without significant vertebral deformation, at least in three dimensions, is the opposite of idiopathic scoliosis, namely Scheuermann's thoracic hyperkyphosis.[59] This progresses in the sagittal plane because it is always behind the axis of spinal column rotation and, being under tension, will not buckle.[70] Certainly as Scheuermann's disease progresses the vertebrae become more wedged with anterior compression but not in three dimensions. Not surprisingly therefore when an extension orthosis is prescribed or extension casting the deformity is correctable over time provided there is sufficient growth remaining.[71,72] After about, say, 60 degrees, the deformity of Scheuermann's disease is less responsive to extension bracing or casting and there may not be enough growth left. This is where surgical treatment may be required, only of course if the patient finds the deformity unacceptable and nothing to do with any X-ray measurements suggested by the surgeon. As hyperkyphosis needs extension then lordoscoliosis needs flexion and that of course is precisely what causes it to buckle further[19] (▶ Fig. 4.1). The condition of LOIS is therefore not readily treatable externally although one hears through the grapevine that yet another brace trial is being considered,[73] surely not.

Of course for a prospective controlled trial to have any substance then there should already be very good evidence that the treatment works and, not surprisingly, such evidence is conspicuous by its absence; two retrospective trials[74,75] did not show any benefit for brace treatment while a prospective nonrandomized study had far too many progressive thoracic curves in the nontreatment group,[76,77] thus favoring brace treatment.

Since the time of Hippocrates there have been innumerable contraptions applied to scoliosis patients with no effect whatsoever.[78] Even the diligent work of Cotrel and his colleagues in Berck-Plage with adolescent girls wandering about the town with their elongation derotation flexion (EDF) casts trying to stand and walk upright balancing a book on their heads had no beneficial effect on curbing the progression of their deformities.[79]

What happened in idiopathic scoliosis was that the Milwaukee brace was empirically prescribed. It is difficult to understand why this should happen because the Milwaukee brace was specifically designed to prop up the spine with a poliomyelitis scoliosis after surgery and had nothing at all to do with idiopathic scoliosis let alone as a preventative measure.[80] It was primarily designed to distract the spine and not surprisingly with the initial mandibular counter-distraction piece significant dental problems arose.[81] Then this was exchanged for a choker round the neck to actively maintain the patient upright. It was felt in the initial phases of treatment that the lumbar spine should be flattened by the orthosis which seemed to provide an improvement in Cobb angle when brace wearing. Of course this is easily understandable because with the lumbar spine effectively flexed this caused active hyperextension of the thoracic spine above and led to movement of the thoracic lordosis toward the midline.[19] However, the improvement in the thoracic spine Cobb angle was only about half of that which would be achieved by natural daily side bending and if the brace was worn for the prescribed 23 hours a day then the spine was never able to achieve its maximum side bending position with ordinary activities of daily living that would happen with any normal adolescent with their sporting and other physical activities. However, the proponents dictated that it must be worn for curves beyond, say, 25 degrees without any objective data to support their insistence.

Evidence-based medicine has been "in" for many years now. It means "the integration of individual clinical expertise with the best available external evidence from systematic research, particularly concerning the scientific principles governing treatment."[82] It is not possible to identify any criteria by which the nonoperative treatment of LOIS adheres to the principles of evidence-based medicine. Not only was the orthosis used for treating LOIS devised for a completely different type of scoliosis under entirely different circumstances but the early experience with this orthosis was reported at a time when it was not conventional to apply statistical methods or any other rigorous analytical approach to the problem. This is what we have done, this is what has happened, and because we are the senior scoliologists of the day, you'd better do the same. Dissent or challenge did not seem to be the most prudent route to a successful career in spinal surgery! In the 1970s there were various retrospective reports with poor numbers followed up, usually less than half, suggesting benefit from brace wearing.[9,10,83] However even these papers did highlight their problem: "there have been no published data with regard to long-term end results comparable to the available follow-up studies of untreated patients."[9] Another commented "the role of the Milwaukee brace in the treatment of idiopathic scoliosis is still unclear" …

"what then is the proper role of the Milwaukee brace in scoliosis treatment ... further follow-up must be obtained in these patients."[9]

Then some common sense came into the situation and in 1984 the Gothenburg Group carried out a retrospective comparison of 144 braced patients versus 111 untreated, both groups with a mean deformity of less than 30 degrees. There was no statistical benefit for the braced patients.[74]

Caroline Goldberg then assessed the efficacy of the Boston brace and, like Gothenburg, no difference was reported between the braced and unbraced controls. She quite rightly stated "this raises very seriously the question of whether bracing can be considered an effective way of altering the natural history of late-onset idiopathic scoliosis."[75] Notwithstanding, bracers continued unabated. In 1994 the Minneapolis Group published their results of more than 1,000 patients treated with a brace between 1954 and 1979.[83] The braced patients were compared with 727 patients who were not braced but just followed up. Failure was defined as an increase in Cobb angle of at least 5 degrees or surgical intervention. The results would suggest that failure rates were lower in the braced group although of course no statistical evidence was produced. Despite the fact that it had been previously stated that "the role of the Milwaukee brace in the treatment of idiopathic scoliosis is still unclear,"[10] academic criticism was not well tolerated[84] and it was further stated "in the 1980s, a negative attitude about bracing existed, it was so extreme that Professor Robert Dickson of Leeds, England, stated that 'there was no place at all for brace treatment.'"[19] It is always advisable before you go into print to make sure that what you are quoting is correct. R.A.D. never stated that there was no place at all for brace treatment, rather he chose his words more precisely: "set against the background of natural history there is no evidence that Milwaukee brace treatment alters the course of scoliosis"—a quite different statement. Noonan and Weinstein expressed concern about the large number of patients being excluded from the Minneapolis study and that only 28% of the study questionnaires had been completed.[85] Then the Puerto Rico Group suggested better results from bracing but there were far more thoracic curves in the untreated group compared to the treated group—thoracic curves well known to have a greater progression potential.[86] They also talked about the patients fully complying with treatment whereas Houghton in Oxford with hidden compliance meters showed that adolescent children in Oxford only wore the brace 10% of the prescribed time.[87] RAD's great friend, the late Greg Houghton's (he was knocked off his bicycle by a drunk driver and suffered severe and fatal head injuries) results have been challenged at international meetings but R.A.D. knew this study from his alma mater and it was impeccable.

Not surprisingly with so many vested interests and so many stake holders a prospective randomized controlled trial was recommended. Those carrying out this trial quite rightly stated as regards previous reports "none of these studies met the stringent criteria for scientific evidence that must be used to prove the effectiveness of treatment." They added "a well-designed study must include a large cohort of similar patients with similar patterns and sizes of deformity and that they should be randomized to different treatment methods and followed until at least skeletal maturity."[76] Not surprisingly randomization was impossible because bracers wouldn't stop bracing and nonbracers wouldn't start. Notwithstanding and for very good reasons, a nonrandomized study was carried out of 286 patients comprising 129 observed patients, 111 braced patients, and, for whatever reason, 46 electrically stimulated although this latter treatment method had been discarded years earlier. Perhaps they thought that the electrically stimulated group might form another control group. The results are shown in ▶ Table 4.10 and it can be seen that failure (6 degrees or more of progression) occurred most in the electrically stimulated and least in the braced group. A 6-degree threshold might be statistically significant but can a change in Cobb angle of 6 degrees really be regarded as clinically significant?

The next article in the *Journal of Bone and Joint Surgery* concerned the proportions of thoracic and thoracolumbar curves in these groups as is shown in ▶ Table 4.11. Dangerous thoracic curves[32] were much less prevalent in the braced group than the observed group while the electrical group had many more thoracic curves.[77] You simply couldn't stack the odds better! The only conclusion that can be drawn from this trial was that no benefit could be attributed to bracing for scoliosis. Or alternatively that the differences between the three groups actually was measuring not failure but the difference in the proportions of significantly progressive thoracic curves among the three groups. Indeed, at this point, Stuart Weinstein and R.A.D. surveyed the world literature on bracing for idiopathic scoliosis and we found no evidence base for brace wearing.[88]

Bracers apparently cannot be subdued and another trial is planned.[73] Prospective trials are designed to follow on from good retrospective or other data that suggest that treatment is beneficial. The prospective trial then looks at different categories of patients, such as, 20 to 30 degrees, 30 to 40 degrees, thoracic vs. lumbar, to see in which way the treatment is beneficial and not to assess whether it is beneficial in the first place. There is, therefore, on strict research principles, no evidence to support any further trials on the nonoperative treatment for idiopathic scoliosis. A silver bullet might however be required.

Bracers have published some papers beyond the Nachemson trial paper suggesting again that bracing might be beneficial. Katz et al in 2010 published a study of 126 patients with curves between 25 and 45 degrees who were braced with a heat

Table 4.10 Results of the trial between braced, observed, and electrical stimulation

	Brace	Observed	Electrical
No. of subjects	111	129	46
Failed	40	56	29
Percent failure	36%	52%	63%

Note: Failure = 6 degrees of progression.

Table 4.11 Percentages of thoracic and thoracolumbar curves in the braced, observed, and electrical stimulation groups

	Brace	Observed	Electrical
Thoracic	68	81	89
Thoracolumbar	32	19	11

sensor measuring the exact number of hours of brace wear.[89] A total of 100 patients completed the study and were managed with a Boston brace; 82% of patients who wore the brace for more than 12 hours had a successful outcome (less than 6 degrees of progression). For those who wore the brace 7 to 12 hours the success rate was 61% and for those who wore it less than 7 hours, 31%. Again, like other studies, the main endpoint criterion was a Risser scale of 4 or 5, although they did measure height at the same time. In patients who were Risser 0 or 1 with curves of more than 35 degrees there was only a barely significant difference between brace wear times ($p=0.05$). Of course what happens a year or two or three after the cessation of brace treatment, bearing in mind that the spine is still growing, is uncertain. However, once again one can question the significance of 6 degrees of progression, or indeed of 6 degrees of improvement.[89]

In 2011 Negrini et al in Italy published an extraordinary paper about brace treatment for individuals whose curves were in excess of 45 degrees and who had steadfastly refused surgery.[48] First, a one-off operation to make a straight spine nowadays is a very safe and reliable procedure. Whether or not that was a properly and fully discussed option for them is unclear but in any event they declined surgery and were "treated" with a brace. There were 28 subjects whose age at the start of treatment was 14.2 years on average and whose Cobb angle measured on average almost 50 degrees (49.4 degrees), range 45 to 58 degrees. Reported compliance was allegedly 94%! Six patients (21%) finished with a curve of between 30 and 35 degrees and 12 patients (45%) finished up between 36 degrees and 40 degrees. Improvements were found in 71% of patients overall. Their alleged improvements were an average of 8 degrees for thoracic curves and 16 degrees for lumbar curves. One finds these figures unbelievable simply because with curves of more than 45 degrees at the age of more than 14 years then the apical three-dimensionally wedged vertebrae can simply not be corrected by any form of external orthosis.

While we were writing this last section on bracing it has now become quite clear that another trial has been set up and indeed is under way.[90] This paper was published to describe the design and development of the brace trial, referred to acronymously as BrAIST (Bracing in Adolescent Idiopathic Scoliosis Trial). We were interested to read that one of us (R.A.D.) was part of the brace protocol development committee. A Cobb angle of 50 degrees was regarded as being the surgical threshold and the question that the trial was primarily addressed to was "do braces lower the risk of curve progression to a surgical threshold in patients with adolescent idiopathic scoliosis relative to watchful waiting alone?" The endpoint was either skeletal maturity or the surgical threshold. There seem to be two main problems here one of which was the surgical threshold of 50 degrees Cobb angle and the other the taking of lateral X-rays evaluating them as showing either kyphosis or lordosis when of course all idiopathic scolioses are lordotic. Indeed they are lordotic to begin with before the spinal column turns out of the sagittal plane to become more and more visible in the frontal plane as the scoliosis with rotation. In this regard lateral X-rays are meaningless. While 10 to 40 degrees might be a reasonable range of normality for kyphosis on a lateral X-ray of normal children, such appearances of kyphosis are spurious in the presence of idiopathic scoliosis and are better described as "pseudokyphoses" (see Chapter 3 for more detail). Then the Cobb angle of 50 degrees has not as far as we know been validated as a threshold for surgery. Rather it is the patient and family finding the deformity unacceptable, regardless of Cobb angle, which is the essential driver for surgical treatment. There are lots more criticisms one can level at this trial design but there is one good thing about it; namely, the lead investigator is Stuart Weinstein. It is a pity the reference list does not include any of the publications from the Leeds Group. They did not, for instance, include the publication by Weinstein and Dickson on "Bracing and Screening – Yes or No."[87]

We do hope the proposed trial[90] is carried out properly with rigorous separation and stratification for the important variables such as curve pattern and compliance. It certainly should be with Stuart Weinstein at the helm and then it might lead to some definitive results. Although it is difficult to conceive why an external orthosis should work in this progressive three-dimensional deformity, we do not want to know about preventing a few degrees of progression. What we do want to know is that if the brace does work then what are the real benefits so that we can take these to our patient population in a risks and rewards equation. With excellent results with modern instrumentation and surgery being an ever more safe procedure it is going to take some persuasion for a teenager to wear a brace for a longish time each day for years without a goal at the end.

Surgical Treatment

In guiding the patient and family as regards surgical treatment it is important to understand that the only criterion that has to be fulfilled for surgery to proceed is that the deformity has become unacceptable to the patient to the point where they are prepared to undergo surgery in an attempt to restore acceptability. If they have reached general skeletal maturity, usually about 15 years of age in girls, then the deformity should not substantially progress although we have already seen that the vertebral epiphyses do not fuse until the early 20 s.[35] Some degree of progression may therefore occur up until this age but usually not of any great clinical significance. Therefore, if the deformity is still acceptable at the age of 15 it probably will continue to be so and can of course still be observed serially until the early 20 s to make sure that unacceptability is not reached in the interim. The idea that it will progress a degree or so throughout the rest of life is a possibility although quite why is uncertain.[41] A few degrees, say 10 degrees at most, may occur in terms of progression up until the early 20 s when the spine finally stops growing[35] but there is no evidence to support the notion that any further progression is due to pregnancy.[37,38]

If of course unacceptability has been achieved by the age of 15 then that is the essential indication for surgical intervention and it is extraordinary to see that when acceptability has been restored by surgical intervention how they rejoin their happy and healthy peers, a real sensation of achievement for both patient and surgeon.

Once surgery has been decided upon, only now do we restart taking X-rays. Hitherto we have taken only one diagnostic PA X-ray and one lateral, or should have done, when we first saw the patient. Until unacceptability is reached there is absolutely no need to take any further X-rays. Why should we? The lateral is generally misunderstood and we don't want or need to see radiographic progression when it can be seen by the patient who is the chief and only determinant of whether the deformity is acceptable or not. Far too many X-rays are taken of these growing children, usually girls, and this practice must be stopped. The only requirement to take further X-rays of the spine is when unacceptability has been reached and surgery is being planned, other than harmless X-rays of the left hand and wrist for bone age as and when necessary.

4.3.4 Radiological Evaluation

The surgeon should already know the curve pattern from the initial PA X-ray as well as visual clinical inspection. The flexibility of the curve should also be known by clinical examination and so these preoperative films are important for precision in choosing the length of the curve and for deciding overall surgical strategy. It is standard to take PA and lateral standing X-rays against a grid (▶ Fig. 4.5). The following statement might be contentious but if the lateral X-ray is only for adding +, N, or − to so-called kyphosis then why should a lateral X-ray be taken at all?

Of course it has been traditional in orthopaedic surgery to take AP and lateral X-rays so that we have information about the problem in two planes at rectangles. This is clearly very important for fractures, tumors, and many other pathologies but it is less useful for looking at deformities. The main reason for taking X-rays in the typical idiopathic case is to make sure there isn't some form of subtle congenital anomaly producing or contributing to the deformity and in this regard lateral films are certainly beneficial to pick up for example minor degrees of failure of segmentation which may induce a nearby idiopathic-type lordoscoliosis.

As regards assessing the spinal deformity itself the lateral view in particular has been confusing showing the spurious appearance of kyphosis when all these idiopathic deformities are lordoscolioses. If you do however know the importance of lordosis in the three-dimensional deformity of idiopathic scoliosis, then the lateral X-ray can give you lots of useful information. For relatively small Cobb angles the lateral X-ray does show a flat thoracic spine and you may still see the original lordosis over the T7, 8, 9, and 10 levels. This is because with smaller curves the lordosis has not rotated much from the sagittal plane but as it does so and with bigger Cobb angles then the more it moves away from the sagittal plane into the frontal plane the more it will wrongly register a thoracic kyphosis. The bigger the pseudokyphosis, the bigger the scoliosis and the bigger the amount of rotation. Not only does this mean a worse progression potential in terms of prognosis but also that the more the need is for anterior surgery to shorten the front of the spine and make space available for the deformed vertebrae to collapse into. This is particularly well seen with the short sharp angular curves of dystrophic von Recklinghausen's disease where rotation is excessive. However, do not take a lateral X-ray and assign it (−, N, +) to fit into the Lenke classification because that is misleading and means that you have not understood the contents of Chapter 3.

Maximum lateral bending films to right and left can then be taken and these should be with maximum patient effort plus a pull from the arms of a radiographer or resident or over the fulcrum of a cylindrical bolster at the curve apex. Interpretation of maximum side bending films is not straightforward. If you select the end-vertebrae on the PA erect film then sometimes with a flexible curve the side bending film will register a Cobb angle of 0 degrees or even a negative one. However, what this is doing is really testing the flexibility of the upper and lower compensatory curves and not of the apical region (▶ Fig. 4.10). An alternative strategy would be to take the maximum side bending film and select the end-vertebrae on this film and compare it with the same end-vertebrae on the PA erect film. Then what you are really looking at is the degree of flexibility over the stiffer apical region, which is much more important than the overall flexibility of the curve from end-vertebra to end-vertebra on the erect film. Supine maximum traction films are also commonly taken but if such views are not going to be acted upon then don't take them. We quite like these stretch films as they can provide additional information when the flexibility on side-bending films is not clear. If you are concerned about pedicular size over the apical region, then a PA Stagnara plan d'election view can be taken to see the pedicles en face.[62] You might well be surprised how small your target is!

As MRI is so available and safe, this should be performed preoperatively just to make sure there is not some hidden problem in the neuraxis such as a syrinx, bearing in mind the high rate of neurological complications with scoliosis correction in the presence of a syrinx.[91] Huebert and MacKinnons' two cases developed paraplegia following Harrington instrumentation and subsequently died. This publication was of course more than 40 years ago when distraction was the essential force vector and a more recent publication from Auckland New Zealand was much less concerning.[92] They looked at 13 patients with thoracic curves who had undergone neurosurgical decompression for a syrinx. The degree of so-called thoracic kyphosis was much greater than comparable patients with uncomplicated idiopathic thoracic curves. Curve correction was almost 50% and no unfavorable neurological problems arose—all patients undergoing spinal cord monitoring and wake-up tests. Interestingly syrinx decompression did not lead to an improvement in the degree of scoliosis. Of course the difference between

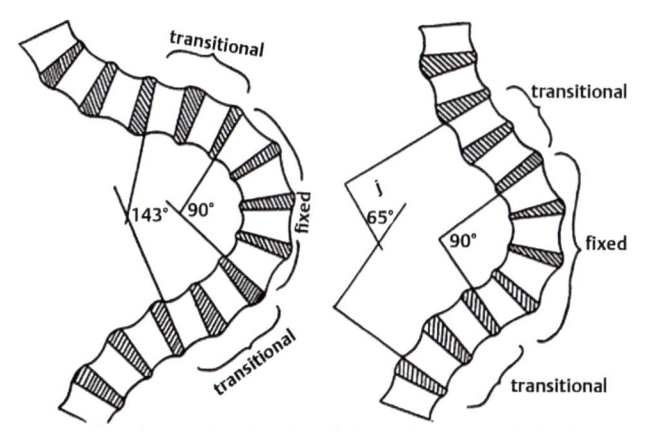

Fig. 4.10 This diagram is taken from Roaf's 1955 paper on wedge resection. It demonstrates the spurious correction of Cobb angle that can be obtained by in Roaf's case a Risser corrective jacket which could just as well be a lateral bending film or a maximum traction stretch film. **(a)** Curve with a Cobb angle of 143 degrees. **(b)** The "corrected" position where the Cobb angle now measures 65 degrees. Of course the fixed apical region doesn't change at all. (Reproduced with permission and copyright © of the British Editorial Society of Bone and Joint Surgery, Roaf R. Wedge Resection for Scoliosis. J Bone Joint Surg (Br) 1955;1:97–101.)

Huebert and MacKinnon's two cases and the New Zealand ones is that the former were undetected syrinxes whereas in the New Zealand cases the syrinx was decompressed before surgical treatment, presumably the critical factor. You might wish to ask a neurosurgical colleague to have a look at the images if the syrinx is unusually sizeable. You will almost certainly get the answer back that the syrinx does not demand neurosurgical action in its own right. But that is not the question. The question is "if I possibly distract the spinal cord or otherwise change its shape could I cause neurological problems?" If the syrinx is sizeable (we know of no particular dimensions) then it would be advisable to avoid a scoliosis lengthening procedure and thus to adopt an anterior approach with preliminary disk removal. In the presence of a syrinx paralysis is an unacceptable risk without apical shortening.

It is traditional to measure the Cobb angle using a protractor[93] (▶ Fig. 2.8) or Cobbometer[94] (▶ Fig. 2.9) in the clinic. Now there are tools on the Picture Archiving and Communications System (PACS) system to draw the lines and measure it for you. Again using the PACS system a vertical plumb line can be dropped from the spinous process of the vertebra prominens downward to check spinal balance. Spinal balance can also be assessed using a plumb line clinically, but also by looking at the size of the compensatory

curves which should be equal for a single structural curve[95] (▶ Fig. 2.18).

It is important to measure apical rotation which may vary several degrees for a given Cobb angle. The first reliable measure of vertebral rotation introduced was that of Nash and Moe[96] (▶ Fig. 2.12). This is still the best method of measuring apical rotation and, like Cobb angle, can be used in the clinic. Now new three-dimensional CT and MRI techniques have been developed that are not such a radiation hazard although they are supine images (▶ Fig. 2.14).

Then a radiograph of the left hand and wrist should be taken to check on maturity status unless one taken on a previous occasion has already shown skeletal maturity. Measuring Risser sign[33] is not really appropriate because maturity of the pelvis is not the same as maturity of the spine which may occur in girls 5 years or more later when the vertebral epiphyses themselves fuse.[35] However, the Risser sign is in such common usage and of course it does have value in gauging where patients are as they approach maturity (▶ Fig. 2.23). Clearly, as you move onward from fusion of the pelvis, growth diminishes appreciably but notwithstanding growth still does occur and while that may be of no importance at all to a straight spine it may be very important indeed for a deformed one.

4.3.5 Specific Curve Patterns

Surgical treatment differs in terms of the six curve patterns in our amended original classification (▶ Table 4.7) and the six described by Lenke (▶ Table 4.9).[52,97] Both anterior and posterior approaches are appropriate for most of these curve types. It is crucially important to select the right fusion levels so as to obtain and maintain the optimal correction and preserve spinal balance. Strategies additional to simple anterior or posterior instrumentation are required for rigid late-onset idiopathic cases which would be big very stiff curves, with less than 20% peri-apical correction on bending films if you want to try to put a figure on it.[98] These latter cases are complex ones that, more often than not, may require osteotomies.

Meanwhile there are a number of important decisions that need to be made relating to surgical treatment.[99] Which if any minor curves need to be included in the fusion? What vertebral levels should be included in the fusion? What is the best approach? Is an anterior "release" indicated? Selecting the lowest instrumented vertebra (LIV) particularly with posterior instrumentation is crucial (▶ Fig. 4.8).

Recently the concept of selective versus nonselective surgery for adolescent idiopathic scoliosis has come more into focus although it really has always been a problem and a challenge to us. Although this concept is attributable to Moe[56] it really has always been in the minds of all scoliosis surgeons because, as Sucato says, "the goals of surgical treatment in late-onset idiopathic scoliosis are to prevent progression of the curve and to correct the spinal deformity while maintaining overall coronal and sagittal balance. These goals should be achieved with fusion of as few spine motion segments as possible."[100] Selective posterior fusion really applies only to thoracic curves. Whether or not a selective thoracic fusion is carried out depends upon assessment of the flexibility of the lower curve so that the mobility and health of the lumbar spine can, if possible, be preserved. For thoracic and thoracolumbar/lumbar double patterns (Lenke 3 curves) selective fusion is often all that is required but that is nothing new and has been challenging scoliosis surgeons ever since Harrington introduced his instrumentation.[56] If the lower curve straightens out or restacks in balance below the expected thoracic curve correction then selective fusion is the treatment of choice.

There are a number of controversial matters to be taken into consideration in deciding site and length of fusion as well as balance and the question of future pain and degeneration. It would seem obvious that if you just do a selective fusion leaving the lumbar spine free then the lower spine would have more movement to compensate for the fusion higher up. Indeed that seems to almost be the perceived wisdom about selective fusion until you start looking at the matter in detail as Engsberg et al did when they looked at 30 patients with adolescent idiopathic scoliosis undergoing instrumented fusion assessed objectively by videography with reflective surface markers.[101] Whereas range of motion was obviously reduced in the fused regions of the spine it was also reduced in the unfused regions and the lack of compensatory increase in motion at unfused regions contradicted the current theory addressing the need for early postoperative range of motion therapy to facilitate motion in unfused segments. Meanwhile Cochrane worked with Alf Nachemson in Gothenburg and demonstrated that with the old fashioned Harrington instrumentation if the lower hook went down to L4 or 5 then retrolisthesis was locally produced along with significant low back pain as well as degenerative facet joint changes and disk space narrowing in 11% of patients.[102] Certainly there would appear to be mechanical problems and pain at the bottom of a long Harrington fusion but the question of degenerative changes is quite unclear as there is a natural trend for degenerative disk disease to be located at L4/5 and L5/S1 and a natural trend for primary facet joint osteoarthritis to occur at L3/4 and L4/5. A lot more work needs to be done to sort out who really is going to be disadvantaged by way of degeneration caused or accelerated by scoliosis surgery. Furthermore, degenerative disk disease is quite different from degenerative posterior facet joint primary osteoarthritis. The pathologies are different and the processes are different, with degenerative disk disease tending to affect a younger age group than degenerative posterior facet joint osteoarthritis—the latter occurs much more commonly in older individuals and females who more often have the gene and also of course progressive idiopathic scoliosis.

The term adjacent segment degeneration is used to describe radiographic changes seen at levels adjacent to a previous spinal fusion procedure but do not necessarily correlate with any clinical findings.[103] The term adjacent segment disease refers to those who have new clinical symptoms that do correspond with new radiographic changes adjacent to a previous spinal fusion. This matter of adjacent segment problems seems to have attracted more than considerable attention in recent years to the point where there is perhaps a general notion amongst spinal surgeons that both adjacent segment degeneration and disease do pose considerable problems. But where is the evidence?

Two earlier reports indicate that 25% of patients undergoing anterior cervical fusion for degenerative disease or cervical myelopathy over the postoperative 5 to 9 years went on to develop adjacent segment degeneration with an average prevalence rate of 2 to 3%.[104,105] Herkowitz[106] studied 44 patients randomized to either anterior cervical diskectomy and fusion or posterior foraminotomy without fusion and treated for cervical radiculopathy. More patients undergoing posterior foraminotomy without fusion developed adjacent level degeneration but there was no correlation with symptoms. Bohlman[107] reviewed more than 100 patients undergoing anterior diskectomy and fusion for radiculopathy finding that 9% went on to develop adjacent segment disease requiring additional surgery while Gore[105] described 14% of their patients requiring additional surgery for adjacent segment disease. The annual incidence of adjacent segment disease requiring surgery appeared to be between 1.5% and 4%. Lunsford[108] reported on more than 300 patients undergoing anterior cervical diskectomy some without fusion and found an annual incidence of adjacent segment disease of about 2.5% with no difference between those who were fused or not. Henderson[109] found an average annual incidence of about 3% in those undergoing posterior foraminotomy without fusion. These clinical observations suggest that anterior surgery with fusion and posterior surgery without lead to similar rates of adjacent segment disease. Hilibrand[110] reported on more than 400 anterior cervical decompression and fusion procedures for radiculopathy and/or myelopathy and looked for the development of any new neurological symptoms referable to adjacent levels calculating a Kaplan-Meier survivorship analysis. There was an overall annual incidence of approximately 3% developing adjacent segment disease but the Kaplan-Meier survivorship analysis suggested a much higher likelihood up to 25% at 10 years. Risk factors included neurological problems from adjacent levels at the time of initial surgery as well as surgery performed next to C5/6 or C6/7, the levels by far the most common for the development of natural degenerative disease anyway. Interestingly anterior fusions at more than one level significantly lowered the rate of adjacent segment disease. The conclusions of all this were that adjacent segment disease was a common problem that may reflect the natural history of the underlying cervical spondylosis and that fusion per se may not be the culprit originally thought.

In the lumbar spine Lehmann[111] and Luk[112] demonstrated instability at the segment above lumbar or lumbosacral fusions, with no correlation with the patient's symptoms. Penta[113] compared the natural history of lumbar segments in fused and nonfused patients and interestingly found no difference in the rates of adjacent segment degeneration with a third in both groups developing degenerative changes at the level above the fusion. Again increasing length of fusion did not appear to increase the extent of adjacent segment degeneration. Rahm[114] found that a third developed adjacent segment degeneration and did have worse clinical results but interestingly the development of a pseudarthrosis appeared to be a protective factor against the development of adjacent segment degeneration. Whitecloud[115] found it much more difficult to obtain a solid fusion when operating the level adjacent to a previously operated level with an 80% pseudarthrosis rate. Etebar[116] found a 14% rate of symptomatic adjacent degenerative disease while Ghiselli[117] found that only 1 of their 32 patients developed symptoms following a lumbosacral fusion. Interestingly Throckmorton[118] looked at patients whose surgery was adjacent to a degenerated disk or a normal disk and found the worse clinical outcomes occurred with normal adjacent disks. Ghiselli[119] looked at more than 200 patients with lumbar fusions and found that 37% would be expected to require additional surgery for adjacent segment disease, with highest incidences in floating lumbar fusions.

Based on the present scientific literature it is still not clear whether these radiographic and clinical findings are the result of the spinal fusion within the iatrogenic production of a rigid motion segment or whether they represent the progression of the natural history of the underlying degenerative disease. It would be therefore very unwise to blame previous surgery for the "adjacent segment degeneration and disease" and in particular additional fusion which, if anything, seems to have a protective effect. The very name "adjacent segment degeneration" implies that there is a tacit belief in trouble adjacent to an operated area and it is that belief that is so infectious amongst spinal surgeons that carrying out adjacent level fusions is endemic while there is no evidence base to support blaming the previous surgery over and above the natural and constitutional process of degeneration.

If there is no way of confirming that a degenerative motion segment is symptomatic and thus the source of pain, then spinal fusion or whatever has no particular target to aim at. It can hardly therefore be the raison d'être for concern about adjacent level disease when there is no way of knowing whether the incriminated level is the real source of symptomatic concern. It certainly makes the concept of reducing movement but not abolishing it (e.g., ligament support or disk replacement) as being beneficial as naively fanciful at best. Orthopaedic associations around the world made the problem of back pain a key issue for the "millennium" and this is well articulated by Nachemson.[120,121] Diagnosing low back pain is verging on the impossible with one level disk degeneration, spondylosis, mild scoliosis, or low grade spondylolisthesis all being shown to have no predictive value as they are as common in people with pain as in people without pain. The radiologists Roland and van Tulder have already told us to stop using unproven labels.[122] The ability to diagnose facet syndrome has been disproven in several randomized trials and degenerative disk disease, isolated disk resorption, and segmental instability have all been

Table 4.12 Recommended insertions for radiology reports on spinal radiographs

Slight degeneration	Almost half of patients with this finding on radiography do not have back pain, so this finding may not be related to the patient's pain
Advanced disk degeneration	Roughly 40% of patients with this finding do not have back pain, so this finding may be unrelated
Spondylosis	Roughly half of patients with this finding do not have back pain, so this finding may be unrelated
Spondylolisthesis	Roughly half of patients with this finding do not have back pain, so this finding may be unrelated
Spina bifida	Almost half of patients with this finding do not have back pain, so this finding may be unrelated
Transitional vertebrae	Almost half of patients with this finding do not have back pain, so this finding may be unrelated
Scheuermann's disease	More than 40% of patients with this finding do not have back pain, so this finding may be unrelated

Source: Reproduced with permission from Roland M, van Tulder M. Should radiologists change the way they report plain radiography of the spine? Viewpoint, Lancet 1998;352:229–230.

Table 4.14 Yellow flags

- Poor health beliefs
- Never pain free
- Fear of activity/movement
- Previous long disabling back pain attacks
- Frequent emergency treatment of back pain
- Whole body part numbness
- Whole extremity giving way

described as "waste baskets"[120] (▶ Table 4.12). Diagnosing these can lead some patients into a sick role behavior.

The worst culprits in all this surgical treatment of low back pain are the spine surgeons ourselves. Indeed, one of RAD's old mentors, Alf Nachemson, with whom he did a fellowship in 1974, was never backward in coming forward and entitled one of his last papers "Failed back surgery syndrome is syndrome of failed back surgeons"[123]—a paper that all back surgeons should read and particularly opinionated ones. He described our shortcomings (▶ Table 4.13) and concluded by saying that the overwhelming evidence of our failures explains the poor results of revision surgery for failed back surgery syndrome. Of course we need to pay attention to not only red flags but also yellow flags[123] (▶ Table 4.14), rid ourselves of matters that have no evidence base, and give up for good the idea that for the chronic back pain patient at the end of the line there is always a man/woman with a white coat and a scalpel in their pocket ready to do a spinal fusion. Ciol[124] found that in the United States 20% of patients over 65 who had undergone lumbar spine operations had one or more reoperations within 4 years and others have found higher rates.[125] Nachemson stated, not wholly with tongue in cheek, that at a number of meetings held in 1998 in the United States, the UK, and Sweden, orthopaedic surgeons were questioned on whether they would send a chronic low back patient to a fusion procedure and also if they would undergo the procedure themselves. ▶ Table 4.15 shows the results which speak for themselves about spinal surgeons having serious delusions of adequacy!

Table 4.13 Failed back surgery syndrome

In the absence of any scientifically admissible evidence of efficacy or efficiency for revision back surgery, the syndrome of failed back surgery is described by the following combination of back surgeons' shortcomings:
- Lack of scientific basis for proper surgical indications in patients with low back and/or leg pain, with the exception of surgery for severe nerve root pain due to a disk hernia.
- Avoidance of attempts to provide evidence of efficacy by scientifically admissible studies.
- Too easily influenced by the marketing forces of instrument manufacturers and/or well-spoken colleagues with a new method.
- Uncritical reading of published uncontrolled case series of various surgical procedures for patients with chronic low back pain.
- Disregard for the predictive value of the psychosocial factors.

The overwhelming evidence of our failures explains the poor results of revision surgery for failed back surgery syndrome.

Table 4.15 "Would you send a chronic, idiopathic low back patient to fusion surgery?": Orthopaedic surgeons' response in Mentometer polls, 1998

Country	Yes (%)	Would undergo fusion themselves (%)
United States	45	10
Great Britain	35	5
Sweden	30	7

Table 4.16 Back pain in AIS

Clinical findings	Scoliotic patients* (%) 40-yr follow-up ($n=161$)	Scoliotic Patients† (%) 50-yr follow-up ($n=106$)	Controls* (%) ($n=100$)
Never have pain	20	13	14
Rare pain (one to five times in life)	19	13	25
Occasional pain (few days per year)	24	33	36
Frequent pain (few days per month)	20	22	19
Daily pain	17	19	6

*Data adapted from Weinstein SL, Zavala DC, Ponseti IV. Idiopathic scoliosis: Long-term follow-up and prognosis in untreated patients. J Bone Joint Surg (Am) 1981;53:702–712.
†Adapted from Weinstein SL, Dolan LA, Spratt KF, Peterson K, Spoonamore M. Natural History of Adolescent Idiopathic Scoliosis: Back Pain at 50 years. Presented at the annual meeting of the Scoliosis Research Society, September 1998; New York, NY.

Anyway, this textbook is not about back pain (thank goodness) but is about the treatment of spinal deformities and so be reassured by Weinstein[41] that "the incidence of back pain in patients with scoliosis is comparable to the incidence of back pain in the general population." In the Iowa long-term follow-up study of 161 living patients with LOIS, 80% reported some backache and there were more, 86% in the control group of 100 with no deformity. ▶ Table 4.16 summarizes the position perfectly.

Idiopathic Scoliosis

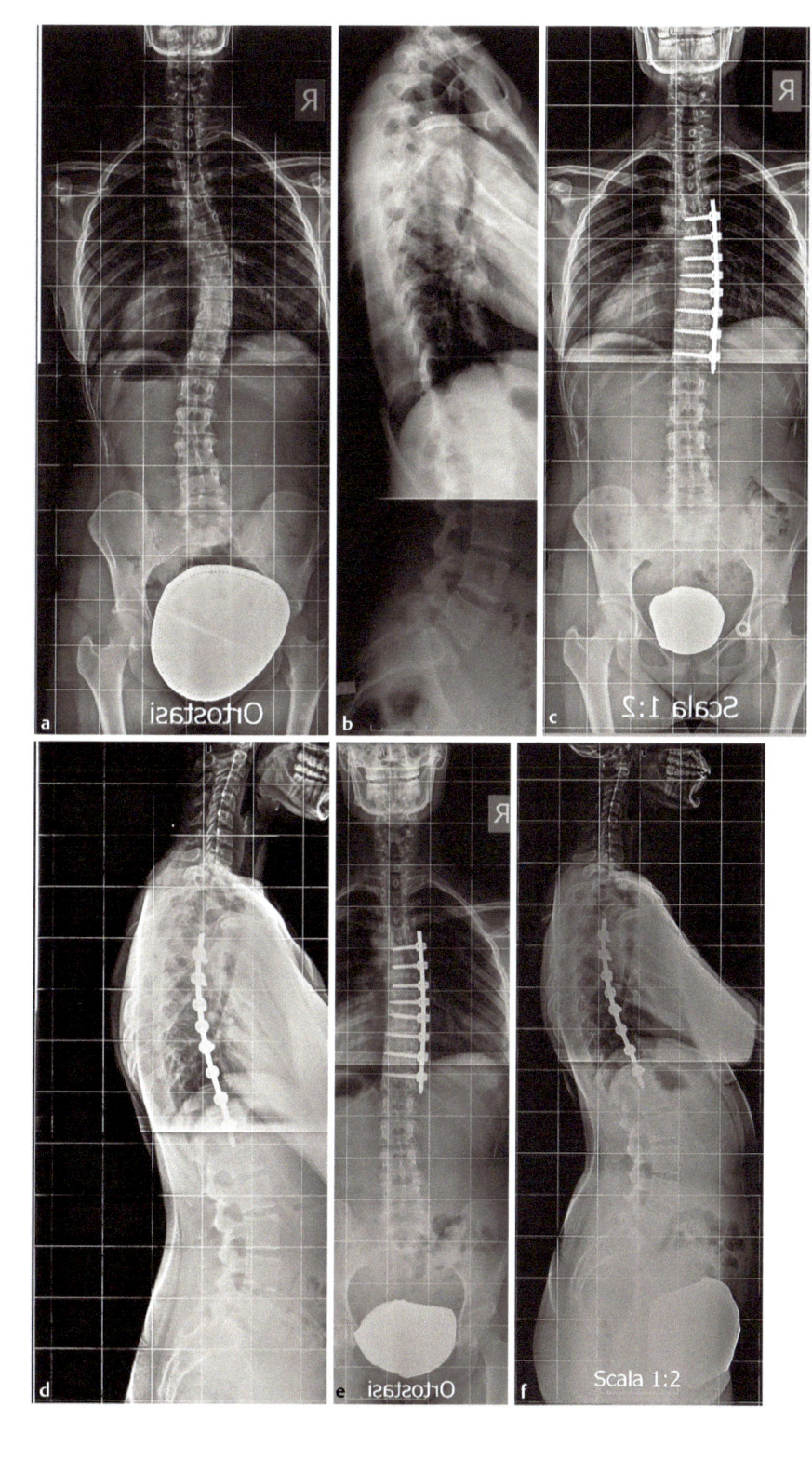

Fig. 4.11 Anterior only—thoracic curves. **(a)** PA radiograph of a Lenke 1AL right thoracic curve. **(b)** Lateral radiograph showing the typical thoracic flat back. **(c)** PA radiograph after anterior instrumentation showing an excellent correction going no lower than T12. **(d)** Lateral radiograph showing restoration of a natural thoracic kyphosis. **(e,f)** PA and lateral radiographs at follow-up 2 years later showing a solid anterior fusion with maintenance of the corrected position. A perfect result from one procedure and a very happy girl.

Single Curves

Thoracic Curves (Lenke 1, King 3)[125]

Anterior Only

You shouldn't have forgotten by now that all idiopathic curves are lordotic including thoracic ones and so a crucial part of the correction strategy is to restore thoracic kyphosis (Chapter 3). This can be carried out anteriorly (▶ Fig. 4.11 and ▶ Fig. 4.12) or posteriorly (▶ Fig. 4.13, ▶ Fig. 4.14, and ▶ Fig. 4.15). Thoracic curves tend to be stiffer than curves lower down because of the attached chest wall and because disk height is less. Of course if the curve is not too big and remains nice and flexible then it is easy to obtain correction by instrumentation only. However, for bigger curves that do not adequately correct on side-bending then something else needs to be done first to render the curve

Idiopathic Scoliosis

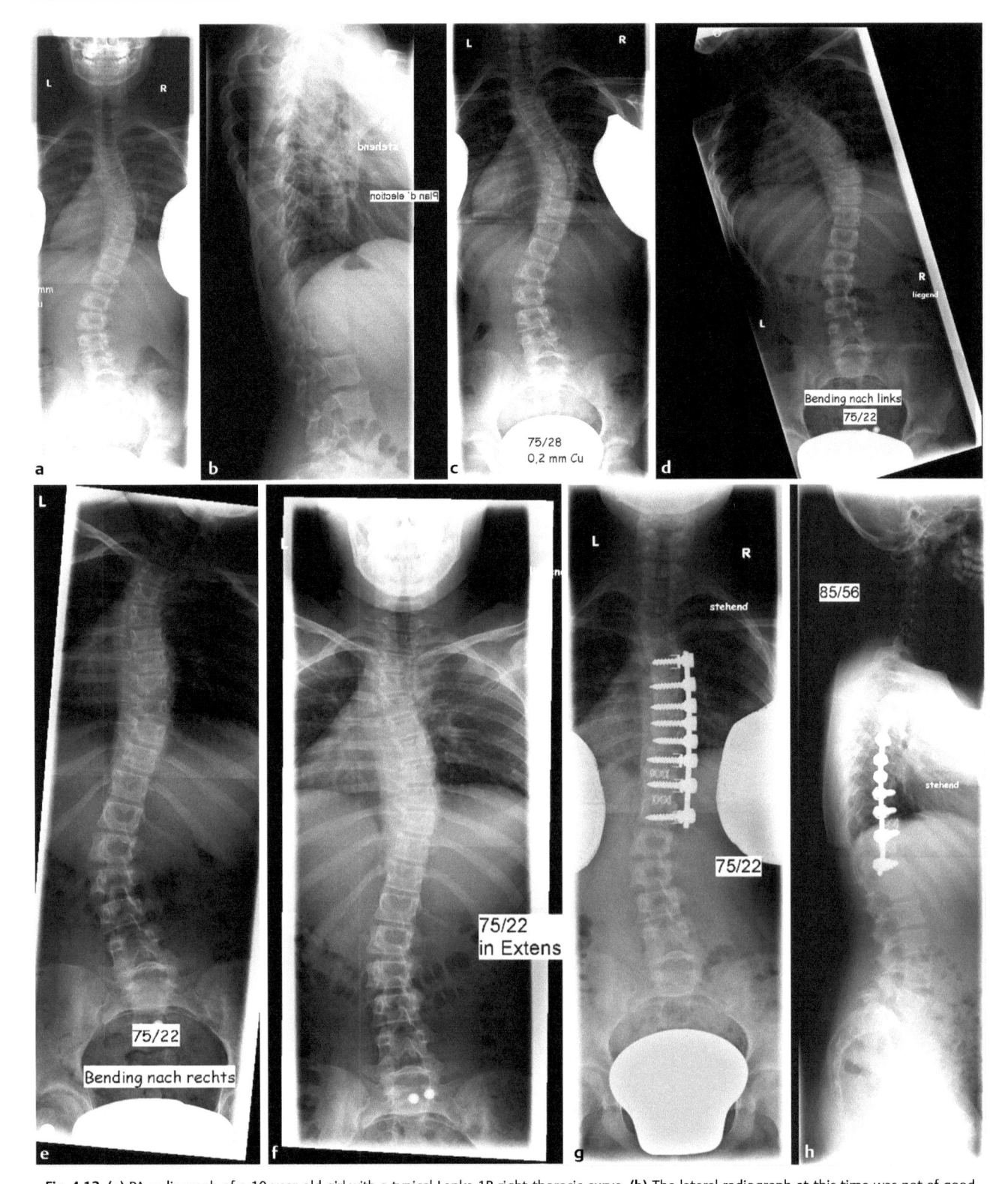

Fig. 4.12 (a) PA radiograph of a 10-year-old girl with a typical Lenke 1B right thoracic curve. (b) The lateral radiograph at this time was not of good enough quality for reproduction in the text. However, this figure is a plan d'election lateral X-ray showing the essential apical lordosis. (c) Two years later before the adolescent growth spurt the curve has progressed significantly. (d) Side bending to the left showing that the lumbar spine is nicely mobile. (e) Side bending to the right showing that the thoracic curve is more mobile than one might expect. (f) PA stretch film showing correction of the whole spine into a nice lazy-S configuration. (g) PA radiograph after surgery showing a nice correction. (h) Lateral radiograph postoperatively showing a rather flat thoracic spine.

Idiopathic Scoliosis

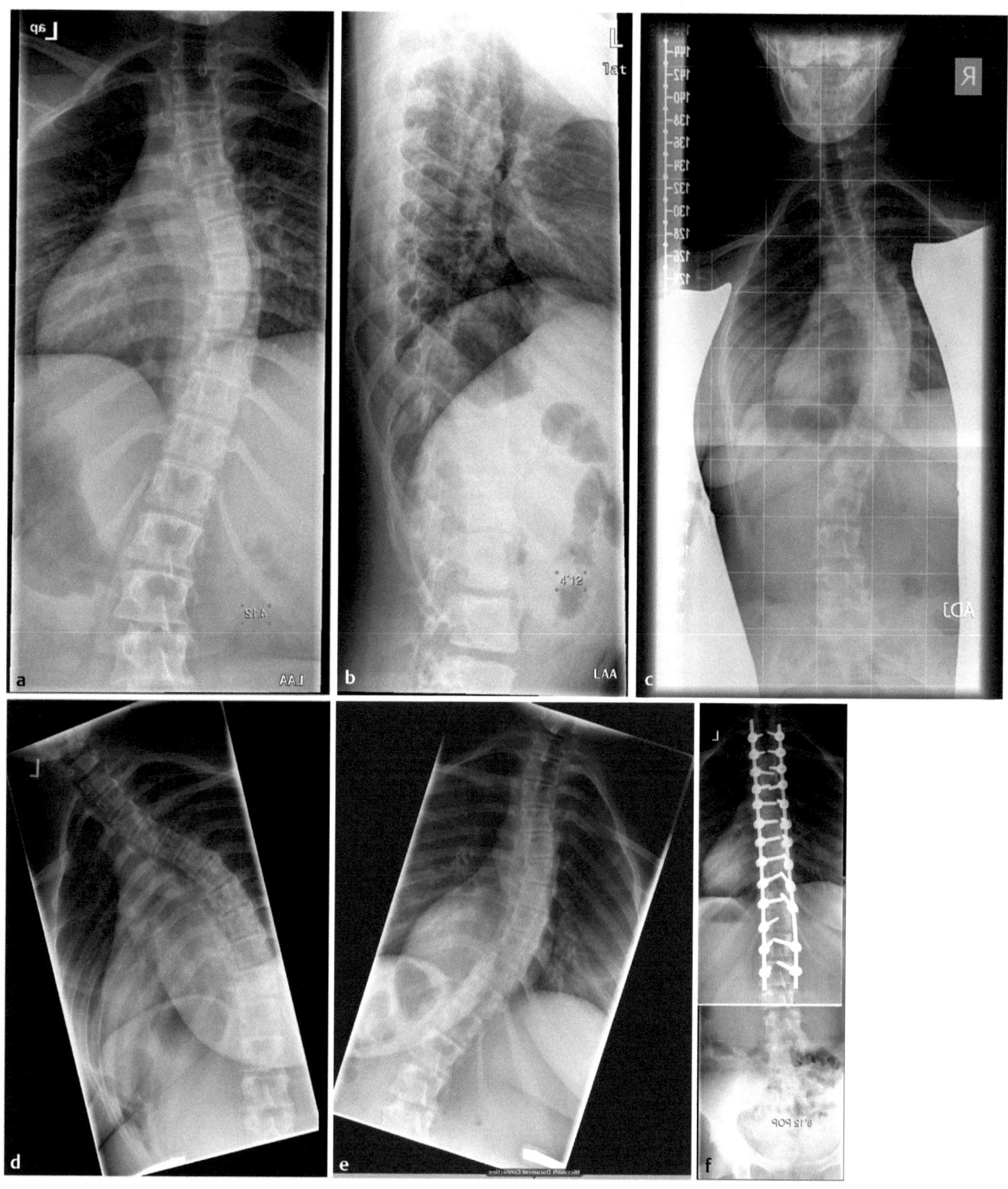

Fig. 4.13 Posterior only. **(a)** PA radiograph showing a Lenke 1A right thoracic scoliosis. **(b)** Lateral radiograph again showing the characteristic flat back with a visible apical thoracic lordosis. **(c)** PA radiograph 2 months later showing quite rapid progression synchronous with a significant adolescent growth spurt. **(d)** Side-bending film to the left showing that the lumbar spine nicely stacks up straight but the upper thoracic curve is not so flexible. **(e)** Side-bending film to the right showing moderate flexibility of the main thoracic curve. **(f)** PA radiograph after posterior instrumentation down to L2. The original intention was to treat this curve anteriorly but we were concerned about lack of flexibility of the upper thoracic curve on side bending and so posterior instrumentation was chosen going up to T2.

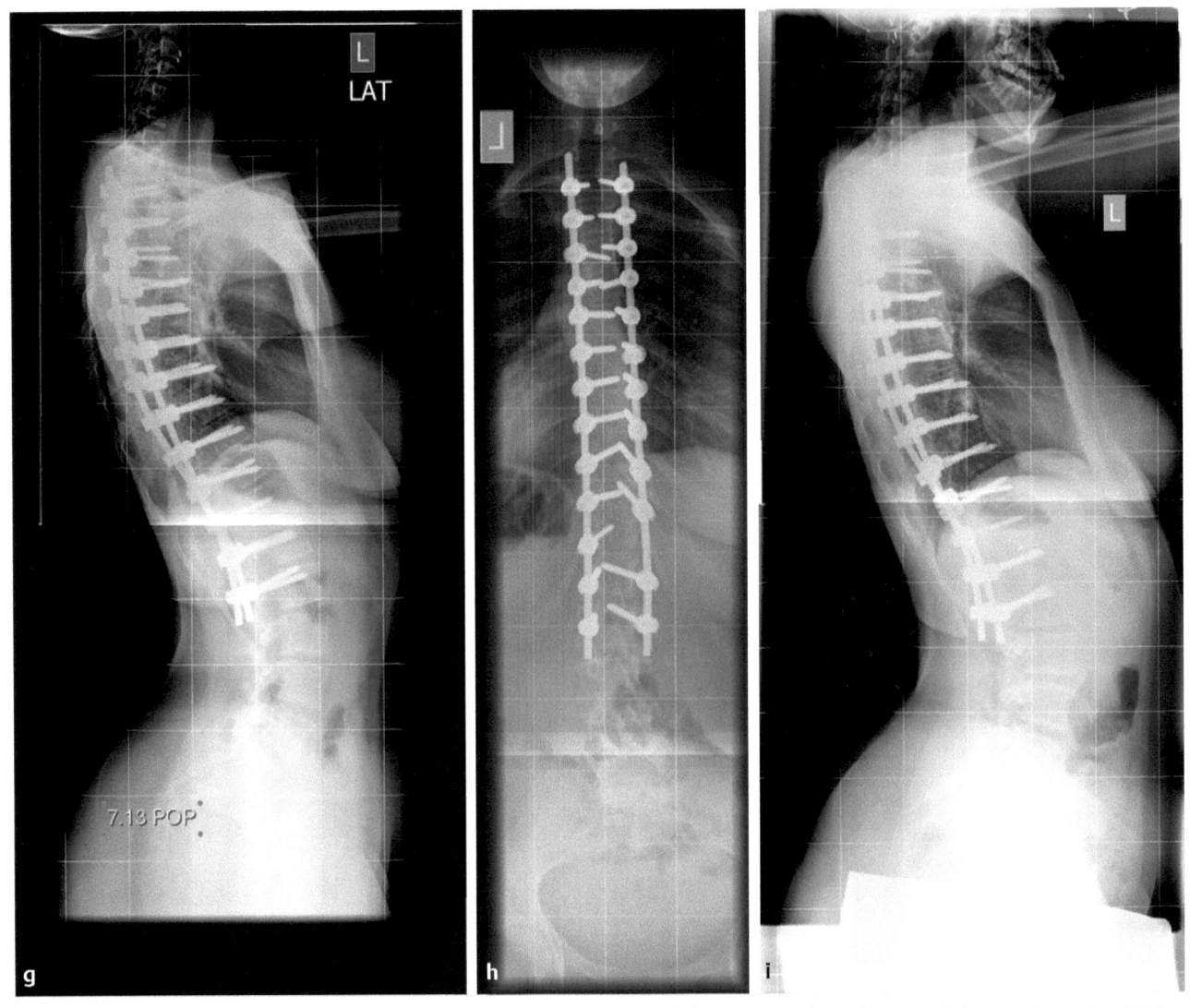

Fig. 4.13 (g) (*continued*) Lateral radiograph showing an improvement in sagittal profile but not as good as with anterior diskectomy (see ▶ Fig. 4.13d). **(h)** PA radiograph at follow-up 2 years later showing maintenance of the original corrected position. **(i)** Lateral radiograph showing better sagittal curvatures.

flexible enough to be taken up by instrumentation although one more often sees these big stiff curves perhaps unwisely being dragged into place by single posterior transpedicular instrumentation only. As a general rule if the thoracic curve does not correct by at least 50% then consideration should be given to a preliminary anterior multiple diskectomy if posterior instrumentation is your decision.[125] This so-called anterior release is the fundamental part of the Leeds procedure originally described all of 30 years ago and for precisely this reason for making curves flexible enough to be taken up by instrumentation (▶ Table 4.17).[67–69] At that time it may have appeared somewhat aggressive to be going into the chest with someone who only had idiopathic scoliosis. Of course then it was generally perceived that adolescent idiopathic scoliosis did cause irreversible chest dysfunction but we knew the Brompton experience of the difference between EOIS and LOIS[16–19] and we soon published our first few cases to show that a thoracotomy was in no way dangerous or detrimental to our patients.[68] There never is a problem with doing a thoracotomy for thoracic scoliosis and we have done hundreds and the results of subsequent instrumentation have been spectacularly good. The main purpose of the procedure was to provide space for the deformity to collapse into (now reinvented and called an anterior release) and therefore to correct spontaneously as postoperative X-rays clearly indicated with more than half of the ultimate correction being achieved before the metalwork was put in. And so we have never regretted carrying out an anterior multiple diskectomy. Four or five disks, however, are quite sufficient for the adolescent with a stiffer thoracic curve (▶ Fig. 3.27) so that a posterior second stage, if chosen, can effect an excellent correction (▶ Fig. 4.16). Looking at the lateral radiographs it can be seen how a nice physiological kyphosis is naturally restored after anterior multiple diskectomy with shortening of the front of the spine and this of course forms the other essential part of the Leeds procedure. Pari-passu with that naturally comes some correction in the frontal plane as well. It does seem rather excessive and traumatic to have done all the necessary preparatory flexibility work anteriorly to have another anaesthetic and

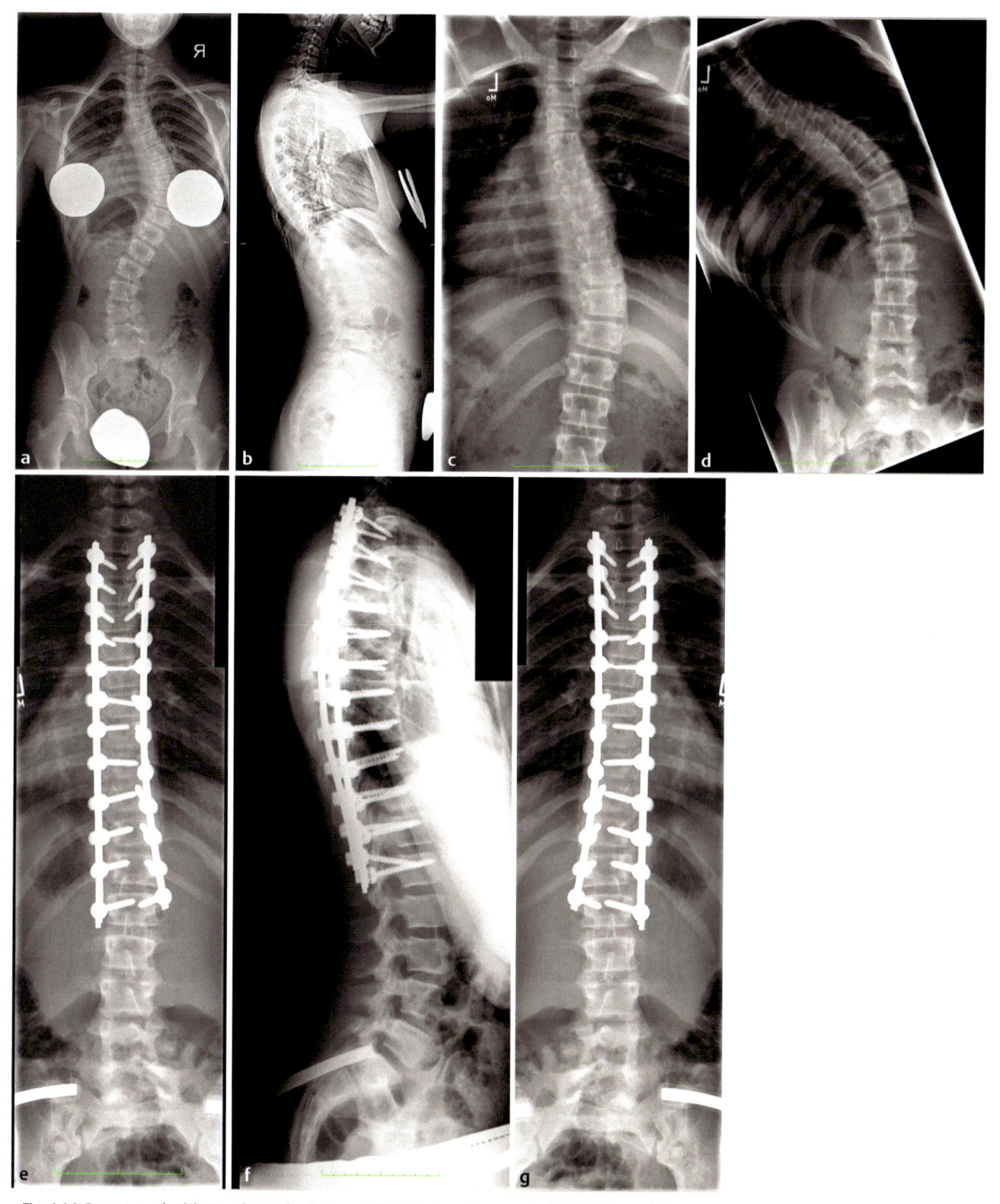

Fig. 4.14 Posterior only. (a) PA radiograph of a type 1AL right thoracic curve. Both the upper and lower compensatory curves are a bit rotated. (b) Lateral radiograph showing a flat thoracic spine. (c) PA stretch film showing a good correction of the thoracic spine and maintenance of shoulder balance. (d) Lateral bending film to the left showing that the lumbar curve stacks nicely below but the upper thoracic curve doesn't straighten. (e) PA radiograph after selective posterior thoracic fusion. (f) Lateral radiograph postoperatively showing a nice sagittal profile. (g) PA radiograph 2 years postoperatively showing maintenance of a very nice looking spine. (In many cases the follow-up is of only 1 or 2 years and this is because they were tertiary referral cases to our centers and of course returned whence they came. However, a solid fusion and a maintained correction is a reasonable illustrative endpoint).

Idiopathic Scoliosis

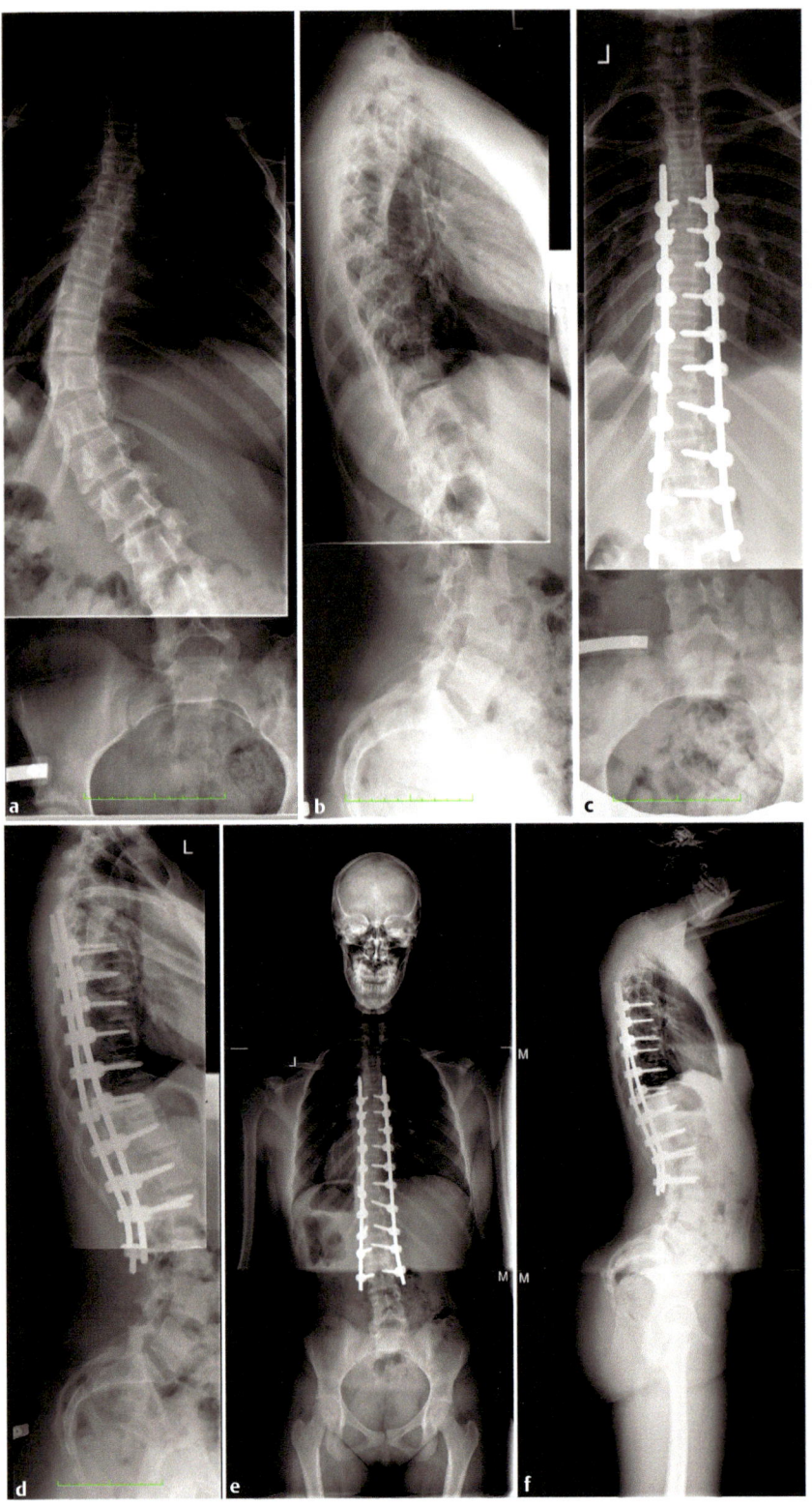

Fig. 4.15 Posterior only. (a) PA radiograph of a lowish left thoracic curve badly decompensated. (b) Lateral radiograph showing a very flat lateral profile. (c) PA radiograph after posterior instrumentation down to L3. (d) Lateral radiograph showing a rather flat thoracic profile with a natural lumbar lordosis. You cannot reliably obtain a natural thoracic kyphosis without anterior multiple diskectomy. (e,f) PA and lateral radiographs at 2-year follow-up showing maintenance of a good correction.

Table 4.17 Results in the first 50 patients with late-onset idiopathic scoliosis treated by the Leeds procedure

	Cobb angle <60° (42 patients)			Cobb angle 60–90° (8 patients)*		
	Before operation	At follow-up	Correction (%)	Before operation	At follow-up	Correction (%)
Mean Cobb angle	54°	18°	66	77°	27°	65
Mean apical rotation	31°	15°	51	54°	27°	50

*Two-stage procedure (see text).

Idiopathic Scoliosis

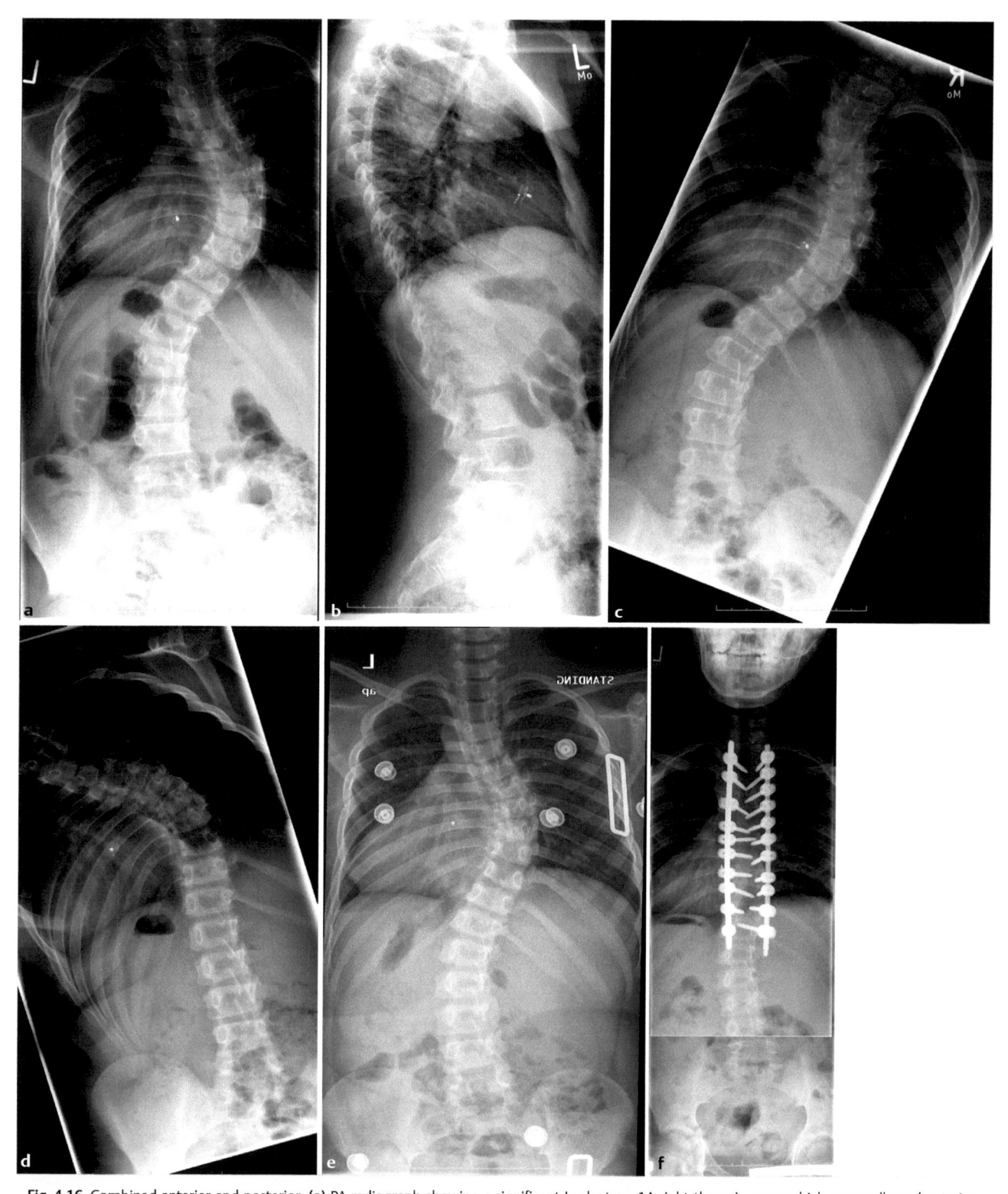

Fig. 4.16 Combined anterior and posterior. **(a)** PA radiograph showing a significant Lenke type 1A right thoracic curve which may well need anterior multiple diskectomy but the shoulders are just level indicating that posterior instrumentation is necessary to maintain level shoulders. **(b)** Lateral radiograph showing the typical flat back appearance. **(c)** Side bending to the right showing no significant improvement in the thoracic curve. **(d)** Side bending to the left showing that the lumbar spine stacks very nicely below so that a selective thoracic fusion would be preferable. **(e)** PA radiograph after anterior multiple diskectomy. **(f)** PA radiograph after posterior selective instrumentation showing an excellent correction and the value of anterior release.

▶

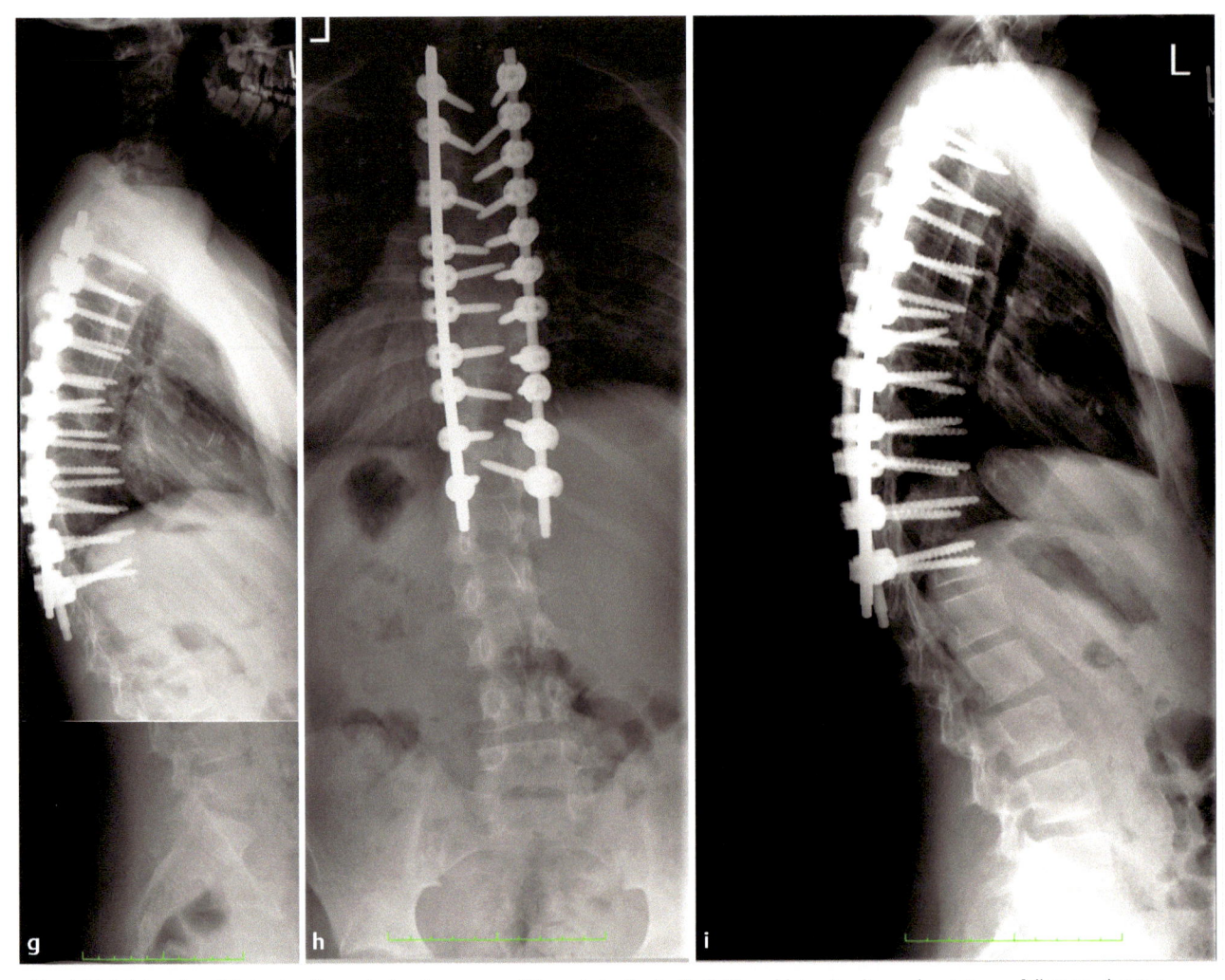

Fig. 4.16 (g) (*continued*) Lateral radiograph showing a normal thoracic kyphosis. **(h, i)** PA and lateral radiographs at 1-year follow-up showing maintenance of the corrected position.

big operation from the back when the front of the spine is asking for instrumentation then and there (▶ Fig. 4.11).

Before anterior multiple diskectomy (anterior release) became so popular we only operated from the back—tried to release the spine by cutting out facets and rib heads (posterior release) in an effort to gain some flexibility but of course we were really on the wrong side of the spine. However, for the really big stiff thoracic curves when posterior instrumentation is going to follow anterior diskectomy rib head resection can still be a useful adjunct to gain that little bit extra for the patient (▶ Fig. 4.17).

For posterior instrumentation the upper instrumented vertebra (UIV) varies according to clinical shoulder balance and this can be readily visualized both clinically and radiologically (▶ Fig. 4.18). If there is concern about the shoulders not being level and the deformity verging on a Lenke 2 with a signe d'épaule then posterior second stage instrumentation is necessary to allow higher fixation on the convex side to keep the shoulders in balance (▶ Fig. 4.13). For a single right thoracic curve, the right shoulder should be higher than the left and so the UIV should be T3 or T4, with level shoulders the UIV should be T2 or 3 but with left shoulder elevation, the signe

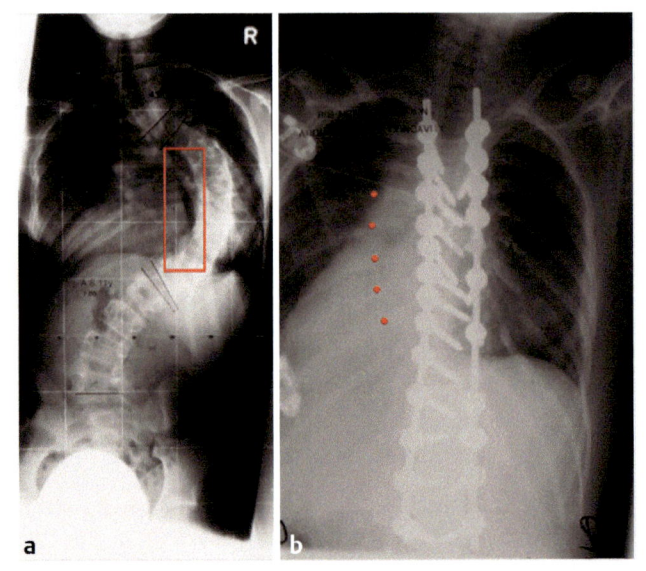

Fig. 4.17 Combined anterior and posterior. **(a)** PA radiograph of a right thoracic curve in excess of 100-degree magnitude. **(b)** PA radiograph after anterior multiple diskectomy and second stage posterior instrumentation after rib head resection showing an excellent correction.

Idiopathic Scoliosis

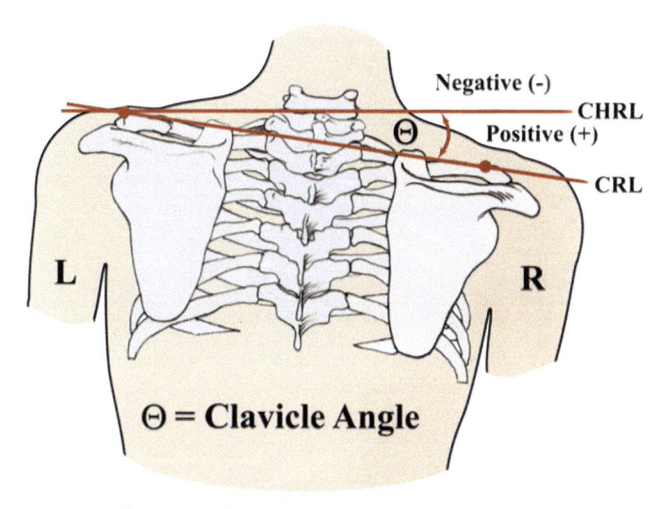

Fig. 4.18 Illustration of the clavicle angle. (From the Spinal Deformity Study Group Radiographic Measurement Manual, page 56, published by Medtronic, Inc, 2004.) CHRL, clavicle horizontal reference line; CRL, clavicle reference line.)

d'épaule (▶ Fig. 2.17). This has become a double thoracic (Lenke 2, King 5) and instrumentation may need to go even higher to maintain shoulder equality (which you can see on the operating table). You certainly cannot carry out fixation of these sorts of curves solely from an anterior approach because you have to be able to get high enough up toward the neck or actually into it.

In deciding the level of the lowest instrumented vertebra (LIV) it is important to look where the CSVL contacts the lumbar spine (▶ Fig. 4.7). For Lenke types 1A and 1B it is obvious just looking at the PA plain films but for type 1C with the lumbar spine well to the left the choice is not quite so easy. In days gone by we simply looked at the degree of flexibility of the lumbar curve and if flexible (became straight or virtually so on side-bending) then we only treated the thoracic curve, now known now as a selective fusion (▶ Fig. 4.11, ▶ Fig. 4.13, and ▶ Fig. 4.14). If not so flexible then we had to go down to L4 or possibly L3 as the LIV. To assist in this matter Lenke suggests looking at the Cobb angles for the thoracic and lumbar curves as well as the apical vertebral rotation and translation and if their ratios are less than 1.2 then a selective fusion is a possible option.[126] This is very important because we want to avoid "adding on" for both deformity and balance. Of course selective thoracic fusion is also embraced by anterior instrumentation for thoracic curves (▶ Fig. 4.11).

When the front of the spine is exposed it is best to divide the periosteum down the front longitudinally with release incisions transversely at top and bottom so that there are two nice osteoblastic periosteal curtains to close over the front of the spine at the end of the anterior stage. Stagnara suggests a layer of bone with the periosteum, his osteoperiosteal flap, to increase fusion.[127] It will be observed that the intervertebral disks look much wider than they really are because of attachment of the annulus to the vertebral bodies on each side of the disk by way of Sharpey's fibers (▶ Fig. 3.27a). Once they are reflected upward and downward using a periosteal elevator then the disk itself is exposed and the anterior annulus from side to side is excised sharply. The nucleus is then removed using rongeurs.

Then with a 1-cm osteotome the natural interface between the bony and cartilaginous plates can be exploited right down to the back of the disk and the growth plate can then be broken off from the underlying posterior annulus and removed. Then using the 1-cm osteotome turned obliquely one of its corners can be used to separate off the posterior annulus from the posterior ligament above and below so that the entire disk can be removed. It is generally not necessary to remove the posterior longitudinal ligament because anatomically we are now right back to the compression side of the deformity and the presence of the ligament will not prevent correction (▶ Fig. 3.29).

As disk excision proceeds the disk space naturally closes down so it may be necessary to use a lamina spreader to keep the disk open to remove the posterior annulus. This nicely demonstrates how the front of the spine is too long and naturally wants to shorten with diskectomy. At this point if it is noted that the apical vertebrae are markedly lordotic then the osteotome can be used to trim the end plates into a rectangular or slightly kyphotic configuration. It is important to have bone wax at the ready in case a major tributary of the basivertebral vein is encountered. Then each interspace is filled with gel foam and the spine is ready for instrumentation or closure by joining together the periosteal curtains. The endpoint will be when the two contiguous vertebral surfaces are in juxtaposition so that the ultimate result will be an anterior interbody fusion but if there is a gap then bone graft/cage is used to fill the space. There is no requirement for iliac crest bone graft, when the excised rib can be used as bone graft material. However, if there is only a small gap between the bony end plates then inserting bone graft material should be avoided as within a short period of time there is further correction of the lordosis and so any small residual gaps close completely.

Thoracolumbar/Lumbar Curves (Lenke 5)

For posterior surgery instrumentation levels should include all convex disks within the curve but it really is sacrilege to deal with these lower single curves posteriorly when there is every advantage of doing so anteriorly with a short segment, four or five vertebral level construct (▶ Fig. 4.19 and ▶ Fig. 4.20). It is easier, quicker, and far less traumatic than doing an unnecessarily long posterior fusion in amongst all the highly vascular paraspinal muscles (there are no muscles attached to the front of the whole thoracolumbar spine—the diaphragm is lashed to the side of the spine at waist level and psoas originates from the side of the lumbar spine). The maximum lateral bending toward the curve convexity is the key to levels and the stretch film helps. The first disk space that opens out against the curve above and below determines the levels of anterior instrumentation which is always significantly less than carrying out the same procedure posteriorly.

▶ Fig. 4.19 is a typical Lenke 5 right thoracolumbar curve. The stretch film shows clearly that the disk space between 3 and 4 opens up. The lateral bend to the right suggests that L3 and L4 are parallel. L4 was chosen as the LIV but the PA postoperatively shows a very nice straight spine. The instrumentation could probably have been one level shorter below with just as good result.

However, the appearance on side-bending doesn't always give you the right answer (▶ Fig. 4.20). This is a mild right lumbar curve which on side bending clearly opens up at L3/4 (the

Idiopathic Scoliosis

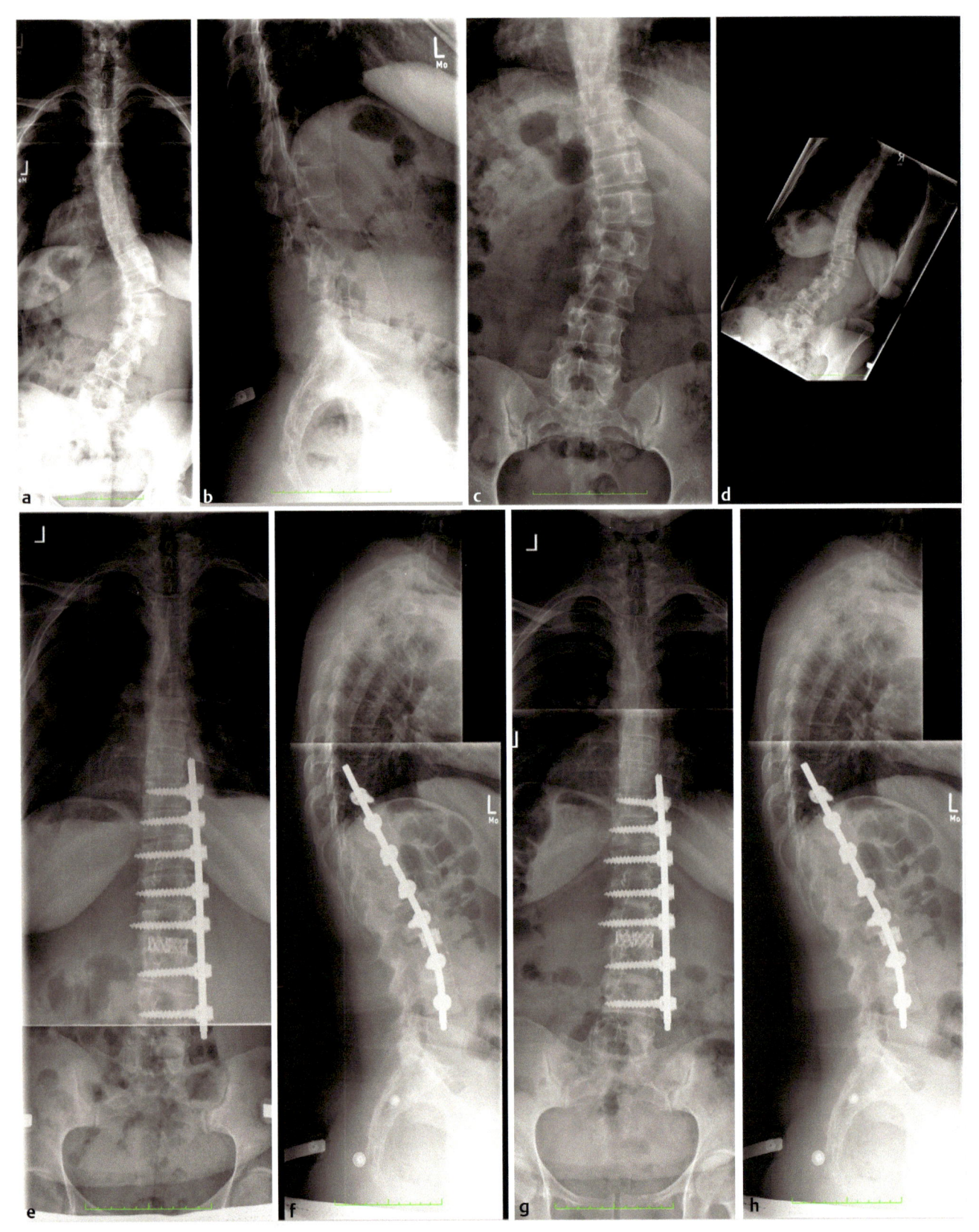

Fig. 4.19 Thoracolumbar/lumbar curves; anterior only. **(a)** PA view of this Lenke 5 right thoracolumbar curve. **(b)** Lateral radiograph showing the pseudokyphosis of a significantly rotated lordoscoliosis. **(c)** PA stretch film shows that the L3/4 disk space opens up. **(d)** The lateral bend to the right shows that L3 and 4 appear to be parallel. The L4 is chosen as the LIV. The construct might be one lower than necessary. **(e)** PA radiograph after anterior instrumentation and an excellent correction. **(f)** Lateral radiograph showing restoration of a natural lumbar lordosis. **(g,h)** PA and lateral views at 1-year follow-up.

Idiopathic Scoliosis

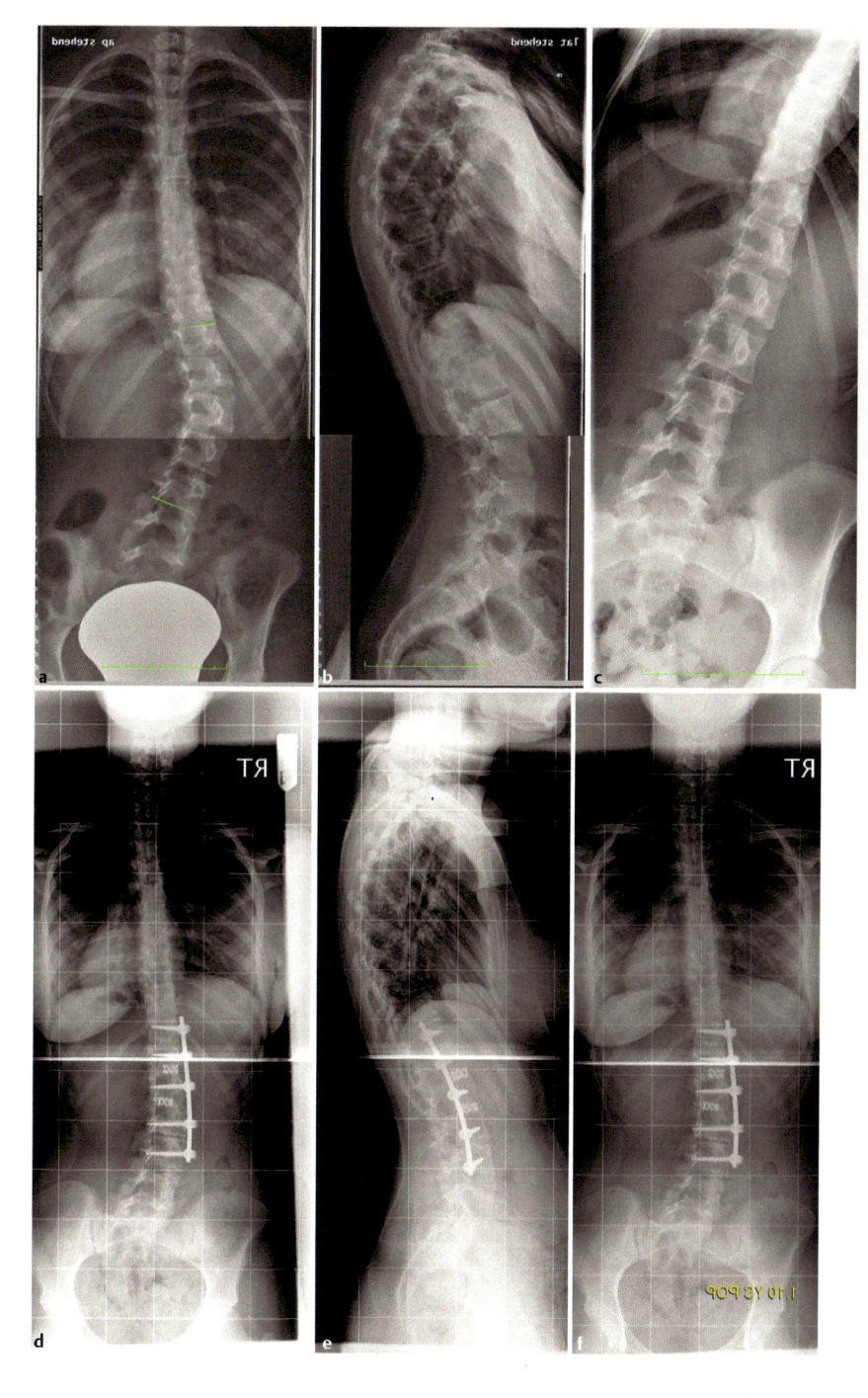

Fig. 4.20 Anterior only. **(a)** PA radiograph of a Lenke 5 right lumbar curve. It looks as though there are six lumbar vertebrae and the bottom one sacralized and so the one above we can call L5. **(b)** Lateral radiograph showing that there is a lumbar lordosis because the amount of apical rotation is not too much and so the spine points less backward. **(c)** Lateral bending radiograph to the right showing that 3/4 opens up below and so L3 should be the LIV while above T11/12 are parallel. Sacralization of L5 is well shown here particularly on the right side. **(d)** PA radiograph after anterior instrumentation down to L4 and above at T12. **(e)** Lateral radiograph showing a natural postoperative lumbar lordosis. **(f)** PA radiograph at follow-up 2 years later showing that we should have gone one lower but the clinical result was excellent with a very happy patient.

L5 vertebra is clearly sacralized and what appears to be L1 does have a rudimentary rib on the left side). However even instrumenting down to L4 does leave an obliquity below so lower fixation would have been better. In general, it is better to be one level too low than one level short because of the possibility of adding on. However, this is not always the case—particularly with the more mature patient.

Double Curves

What was initially referred to us as a Lenke 5 single thoracolumbar curve (▶ Fig. 4.21) is clearly a Lenke 6 double curve with a thoracic curve above which is not rotated but cannot really be called nonstructural. (Remember: a structural curve is defined as a lateral curvature with rotation.) A bending film to the right shows moderate flexibility but not complete and so some degree of right thoracic curve could be a residual problem. The stretch film shows better flexibility than the side-bending film. We went on to carry out anterior instrumentation of the thoracolumbar curve from T10 to L2 with a nicely balanced gentle lazy S configuration. The lateral view shows a very nice sagittal profile. All in all, the spine is in perfect balance and the deformity is not visible, at least to the patient who is very happy and after all that is the ultimate result.

Taking out the disks totally right back to the posterior ligament is essential because it is the back 10% of the disk that

Idiopathic Scoliosis

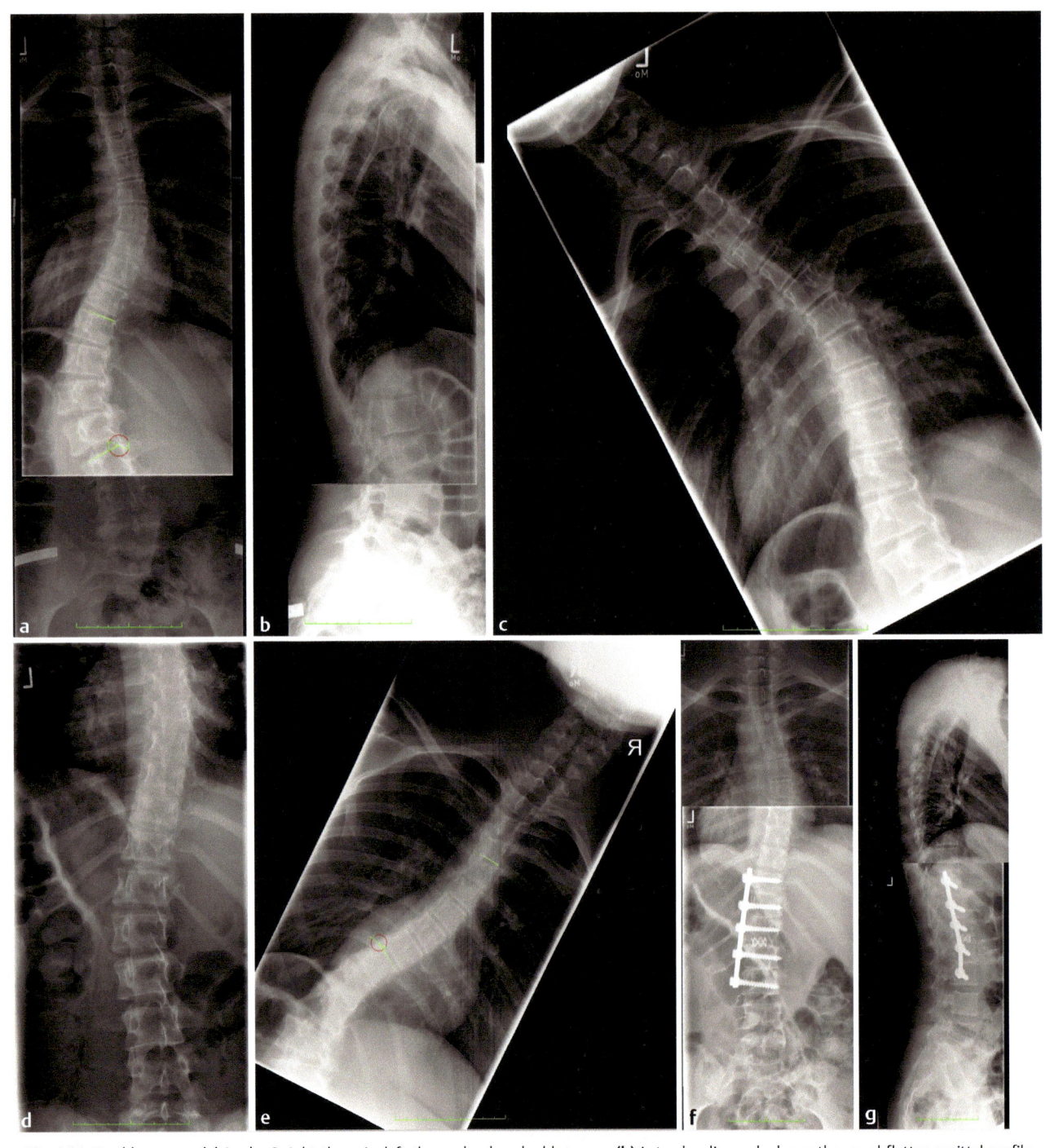

Fig. 4.21 Double curves. **(a)** Lenke 6 right thoracic, left thoracolumbar double curve. **(b)** Lateral radiograph shows the usual flatter sagittal profile throughout. **(c)** Side-bending film to the left shows good correction of the coronal plane component of the lower curve but no change in rotation. **(d)** The stretch film shows good correction of both curves. **(e)** Side-bending film to the right shows a residual thoracic scoliosis but again with no significant rotation. **(f)** PA radiograph after anterior short segment instrumentation showing a nicely balanced well corrected spine. In this case anterior instrumentation was by far the best option. **(g)** Lateral radiograph showing a very nice lateral profile.

requires removal. Indeed, so corrective is anterior instrumentation that you have to be careful not to over-correct. By putting the transverse screws in eccentrically (more anteriorly in the middle) derotation occurs and the lumbar lordosis is better safe-guarded. You shouldn't need to put bone graft or a cage anteriorly in the empty disk space; there should be bone to bone contact with only any spaces left needing filled but a cage/graft must be used if there isn't bone to bone end plate contact.

Double Thoracic Curves (Lenke 2)

Lenke 2 curves come in all shapes and sizes and ▶ Fig. 4.22 is one of the worst we have come across. The PA radiograph shows a right thoracic curve in excess of 90 degrees and above that a big upper thoracic curve and obvious signe d'épaule. The lateral X-ray shows a big pseudokyphosis indicating there is about 90 degrees of rotation of the major curve so that the front

Idiopathic Scoliosis

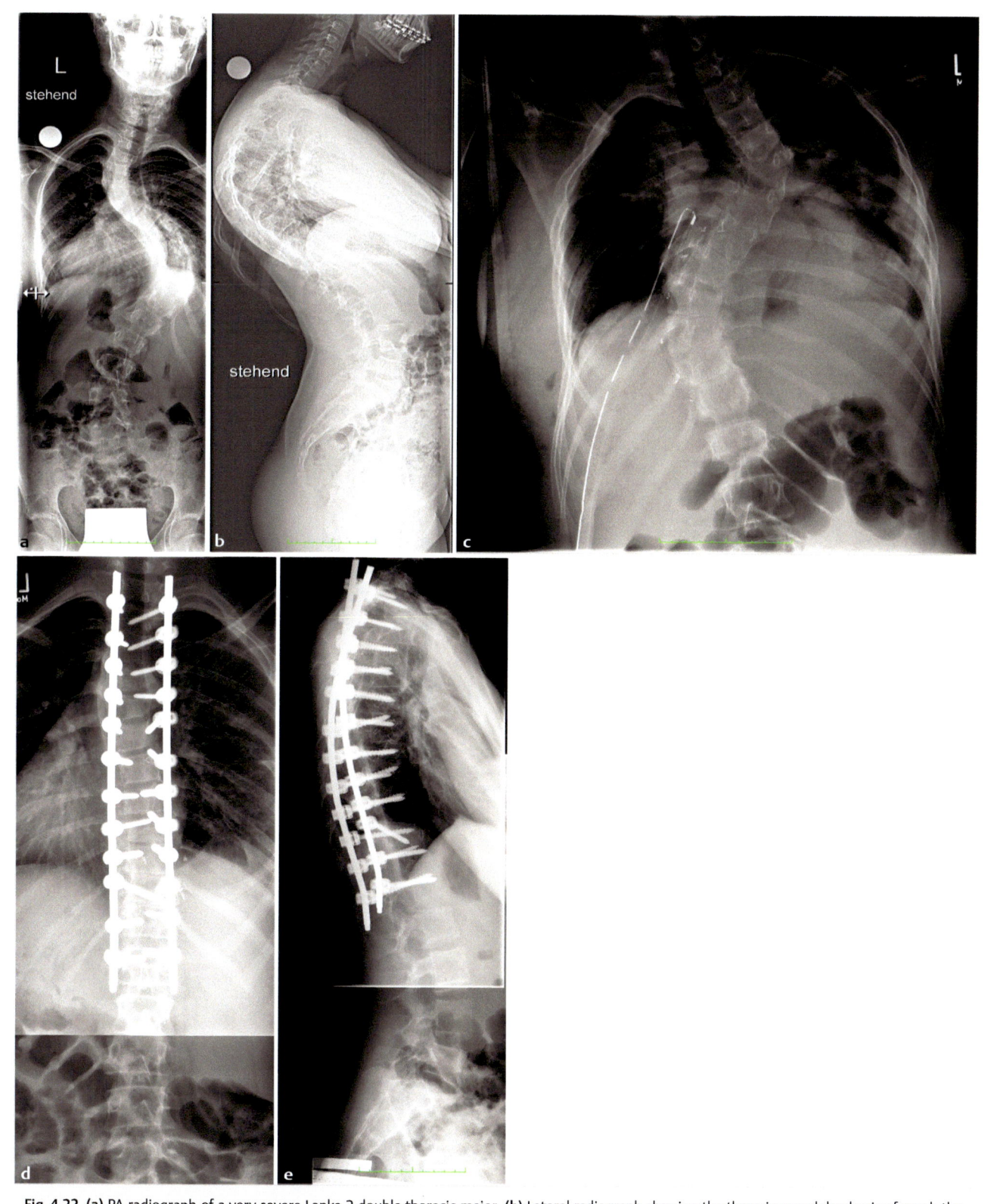

Fig. 4.22 (a) PA radiograph of a very severe Lenke 2 double thoracic major. (b) Lateral radiograph showing the thoracic pseudokyphosis of much the same magnitude as the Cobb angle of the PA view because of the excessive amount of rotation. (c) PA radiograph after anterior multiple diskectomy showing the considerable flexibility achieved. (d) PA radiograph after the second stage posterior instrumentation down to L1 and sparing most of the lumbar spine and showing a virtually straight spine above. A really excellent result and a very happy patient. (e) Lateral radiograph showing a normal thoracic kyphosis.

Idiopathic Scoliosis

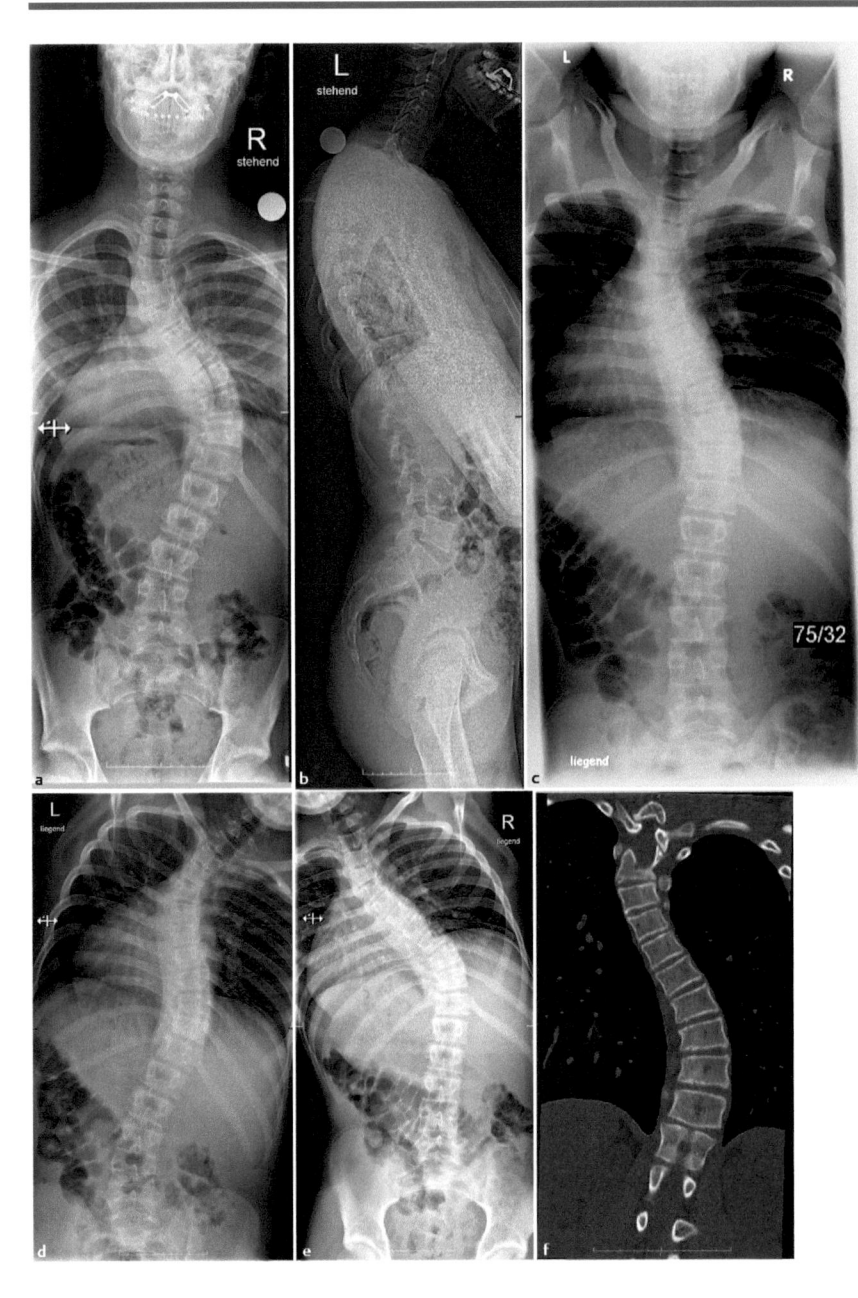

Fig. 4.23 (a) PA radiograph showing a right thoracic curve with a slight signe d'épaule high left shoulder. (b) Lateral radiograph showing the usual long flat back. (c) Stretch film showing good correction of the main thoracic curve but less so of the upper curve. (d) Bending to the right shows some mobility in the major thoracic curve. (e) Bending to the left does not show as much mobility in the upper thoracic curve as we would like. (f) PA CT showing that there is a significant signe d'épaule with a high left shoulder and a rather tight upper thoracic curve.

of the spine (not the back of the spine) points backward with a similar sort of lateral Cobb angle as the PA one. After multiple anterior diskectomy as a first stage there is incredibly good improvement in the Cobb angle and significant derotation; PA radiograph after posterior instrumentation up to T2 leaves a well corrected deformity and equal shoulders. It simply is not possible to achieve this sort of correction without an anterior multiple diskectomy.

▶ Fig. 4.23 was referred as a Lenke type 1 right thoracic curve but the PA film shows the left shoulder is higher clearly making this a Lenke 2 double thoracic. The lateral film clearly shows the typical long, flat-backed deformity along with a clear thoracic lordosis. The stretch film shows some flexibility in the major thoracic curve but not much in the upper curve. Bending films show that neither curve improves very much and the PA CT view does suggest rigidity in the upper curve. The lateral CT shows perfectly the lordosis in the main thoracic curve. The postoperative PA view after posterior instrumentation to T2 still shows a somewhat higher left shoulder. The LIV is L3 leaving three mobile joints below in this very active athletic boy. The lateral view postoperatively shows a natural spinal contour. One year after surgery the shoulders are well balanced. The boy however was delighted with his appearance.

Double Thoracic and Thoracolumbar/Lumbar Curves (Lenke 3 and 6)

Type 3: Double Thoracic and Thoracolumbar Curve

There really are three important subdivisions here with the thoracic curve being the major one, both being equal (Lenke 3) and the thoracolumbar or lumbar curve being major (Lenke 6).

If the thoracic curve is the major one these were traditionally dealt with by posterior instrumentation of both curves with the UIV the same for single thoracic curves and the LIV having to be chosen carefully, generally down to L3 or 4, to the level where the next disk opens up on maximum side bending (▶ Fig. 4.24).

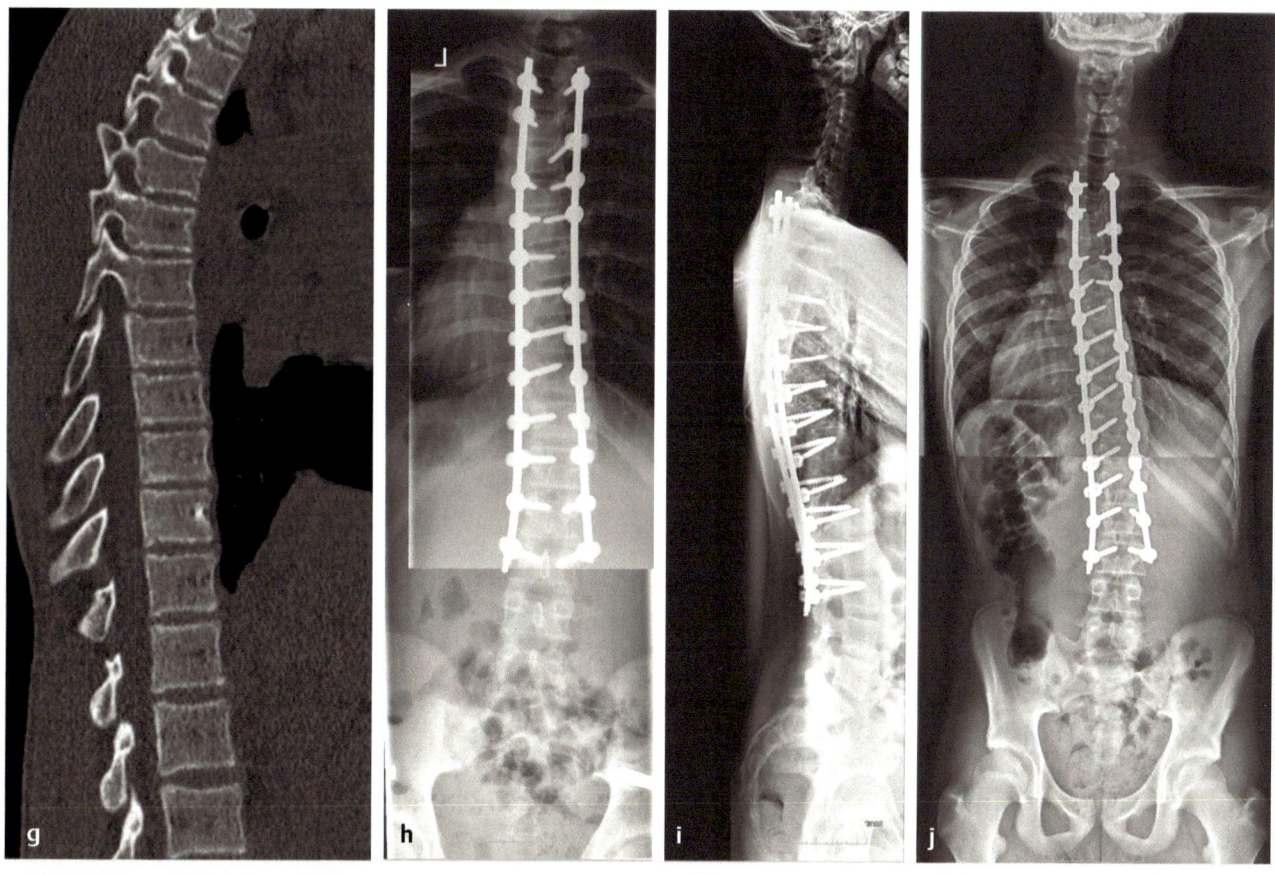

Fig. 4.23 (*continued*) **(g)** Lateral CT showing the apical lordosis. **(h)** PA radiograph after posterior instrumentation from T2 to L2 resulting in excellent correction of the major curve, but the left shoulder is still a little high. **(i)** Lateral radiograph showing restoration of the natural thoracic lateral profile. **(j)** PA radiograph 1 year later showing better shoulder balance.

Again it is important to take side bending views to the left to see how flexible the lower curve is and again don't forget the patient. Look at the lower curve when the patient maximally bends to the left to see what the clinical appearance is likely to be. Then it is possible to decide whether selective fusion of the upper curve is possible or not and if so anterior or posterior instrumentation and fusion are both possibilities. In these situations, anterior thoracic instrumentation is by far the best option and should provide a nicely balanced and corrected deformity. The health of the lumbar spine is obviously safeguarded.

Then if the curves are both major curves of relatively equal size and if the thoracic curve is particularly stiff (Lenke 3) then a long posterior instrumentation and fusion is required down to L3 or L4 after anterior thoracic diskectomy (▶ Fig. 4.25).

If the lower curve is the major one, then this is ideal territory for short segment anterior instrumentation and fusion which will lead to a good correction of the lower curve leaving a nice well balanced well corrected situation (▶ Fig. 4.26).

Triple Curves (Lenke 4)

These are Lenke 2 double thoracic majors with a lumbar curve below.

The choice of UIV and LIV is very much what we have already seen in the previous types. The UIV will be usually T2 or 3 and the LIV L3 or 4.

Although it may be said that anterior instrumentation and fusion is particularly for Lenke type 1, 5, and 6 curves it can also be used for other types provided the flexibility of the other curve is adequate. Thus for determining levels of fixation and flexibility maximum side-bending views are essential, plus a look at the patient please. If you choose to deal with the upper curve only then there is clear evidence of superior results over posterior surgery if you do so.[55,65,66]

Of course the tendency toward an anterior or posterior instrumentation in idiopathic scoliosis is very much to do with the sort of experience and training that scoliosis surgeons have gone through. The authors have had extensive experience of thousands of anterior procedures for idiopathic scoliosis and thus do tend to favor anterior procedures wherever reasonable. Less experienced scoliosis surgeons who may not have had much anterior experience would in all probability favor a posterior approach because that is what they are used to. Lack of anterior spinal experience may be because of concern about not understanding or confidence about approaches among anterior organs. Most of us who do a lot of anterior surgery have not had specific cardiothoracic training but have assisted cardiothoracic or indeed abdominal colleagues in their approaches to the spine. After a few such educational experiences it sometimes becomes apparent with the approach that "you can do it better yourself" in which case you feel confident in going solo. The approaches are simple, intrathoracic and intrapleural and intra-abdominal and extraperitoneal. Furthermore, the bigger

Idiopathic Scoliosis

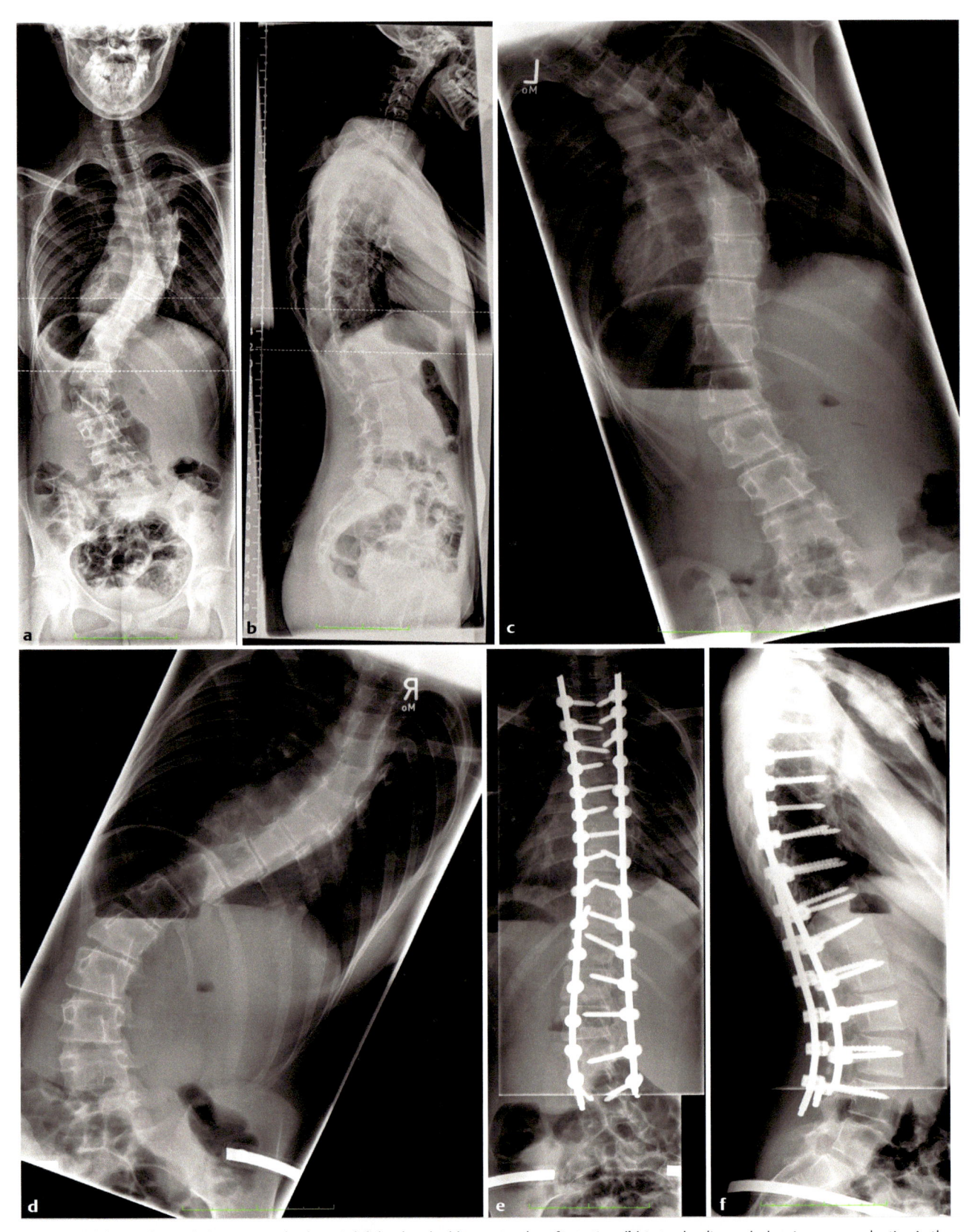

Fig. 4.24 (a) PA radiograph showing a right thoracic left lumbar double structural configuration. (b) Lateral radiograph showing some reduction in the amount of thoracic kyphosis and lumbar lordosis. (c) Lateral bending to the left showing that the lower curve has some flexibility. (d) Bending to the right shows that the upper curve is less flexible. (e) PA radiograph after posterior instrumentation down to L4 showing a nice correction. (f) Lateral radiograph showing restoration of a natural sagittal profile.

the curve the closer the spine is to the surface with the great vessels tending to fall into the curve concavity and move out of the way.

Looking therefore at the data on comparisons between open anterior spinal fusion (OASF), thoracoscopic anterior spinal fusion (TASF), and posterior instrumentation and fusion (PSF) in Peter Newton's excellent chapter in our "other" description of idiopathic scoliosis,[128] one is not surprised to know that the number of levels fused is less anteriorly than posteriorly but one is surprised that the surgical time is much the same for OASF and TASF at about 6 hours each while PSFs are just under 4 hours. Of course there were only 28 OASFs as expected, 97 PSFs and all of 63 TASFs. Not knowing surgeons' names for the TASFs nor the OASFs, we don't think either of us has taken more than 4 hours to do an anterior thoracic spinal fusion for scoliosis but perhaps it doesn't matter as long as it's done properly. Furthermore, the blood loss from an OASF being much the same as a PSF is again quite unexpected, the former generally being much less vascular. We were not surprised that OASFs produce a better correction than TASFs which didn't differ from PSFs. More results are therefore clearly required. OASFs should only take 3 or 4 hours in experienced hands and if it is transthoracic then the lung on the convex side is only deflated using a double lumen tube for not much longer than an hour of this procedure, and can of course be reinflated from time to time as necessary.

However, trying to reach a happy medium Lenke types 1, 5, and 6 can as well be treated either anteriorly or posteriorly but it is generally recommended that types 2, 3, and 4 be treated completely posteriorly although, depending upon curve size and flexibility, anterior multiple diskectomy may well be required. As David Clements rightly says "classification does not help in selecting the end vertebrae or the treatment construct."[129] He says "it is a matter that continues to be subjectively debated and we need more follow-up studies or even prospective randomized trials"—a perfectly reasonable statement.

4.4 The Adolescent with the Bigger Curve

In the late 1950s the halo was designed and fitted to the outer diploë of the skull by four screws.[130,131] This allowed a significant amount of weight, 40 kg or more, to be applied to the head end of the patient. Then when pins are inserted transversely

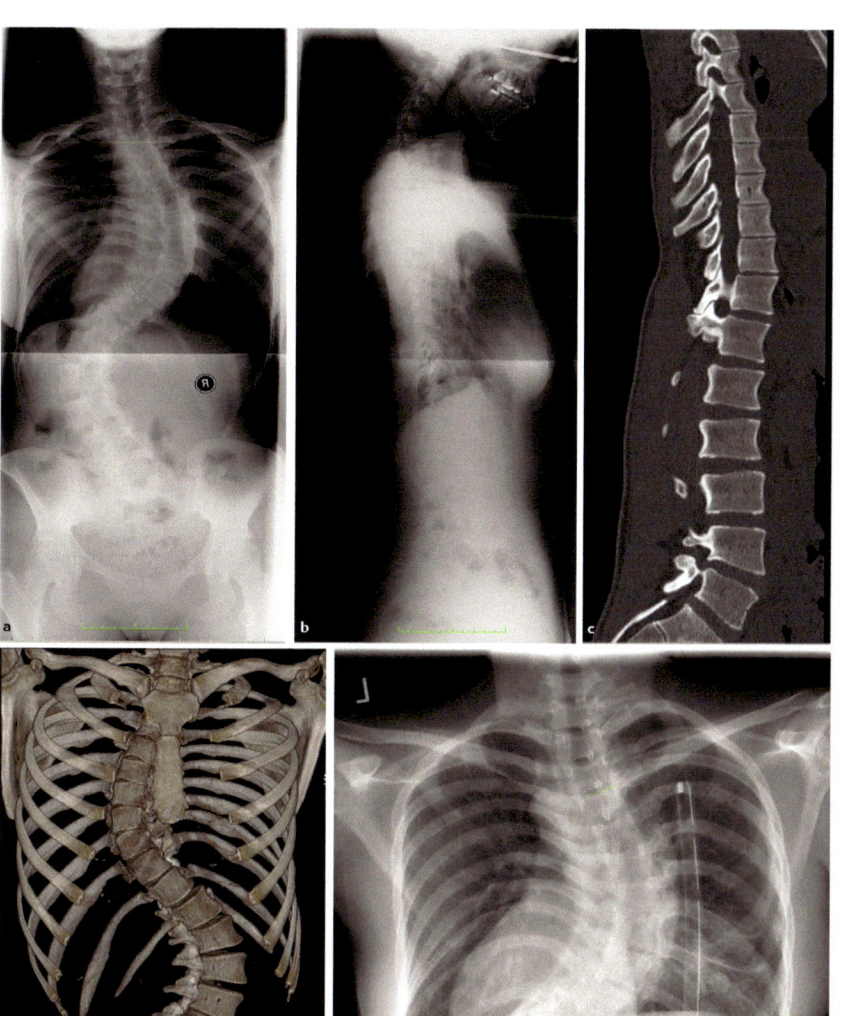

Fig. 4.25 (a) PA radiograph showing a Lenke type 3 right thoracic left lumbar double structural configuration showing big and probably relatively inflexible curves. It is typical for double structural curves to present with bigger radiological deformities because they provide much less disturbance of surface shape than single curves. This is because they rotate one way higher up and then have to stop and go the other way lower down so the amount of rotation associated with each curve is less than if either curve was present on its own. That is why double curves are much less impressive clinically than single ones of comparable magnitude. (b) Lateral profile showing an extreme flat back all the way down. (c) Lateral CT scan showing a mild thoracic lordosis with some pseudokyphosis of the lumbar spine. (d) AP 3D CT of the deformity. (e) PA radiograph after anterior multiple diskectomy of the upper curve.

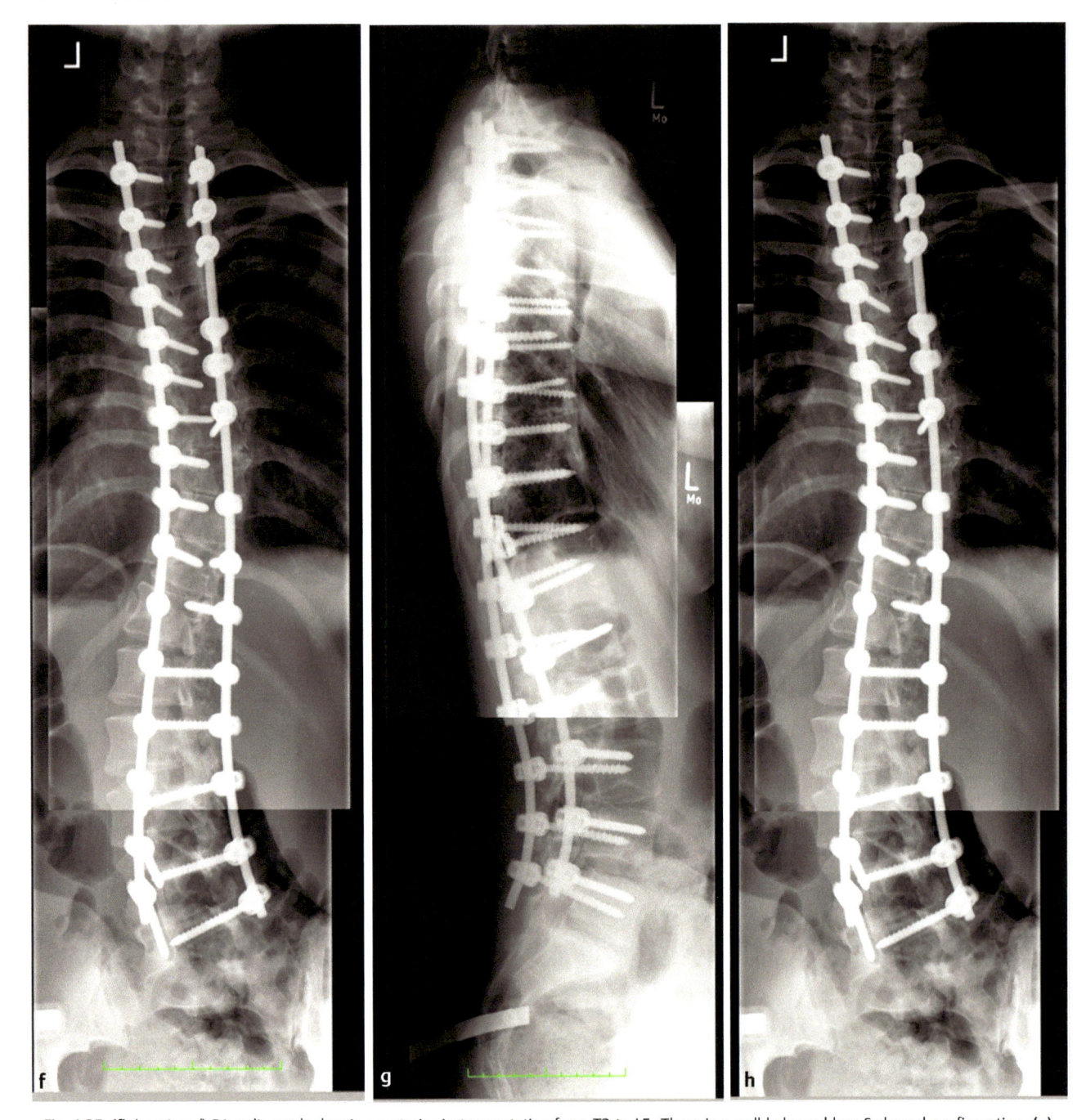

Fig. 4.25 **(f)** (*continued*) PA radiograph showing posterior instrumentation from T2 to L5. There is a well-balanced lazy S-shaped configuration. **(g)** Lateral radiograph showing a natural sagittal profile. **(h)** PA radiograph 2 years later with maintenance of the correction and good horizontalization of L4 and L5.

across the lower femurs much greater distraction forces can be produced. De Wald and Ray devised the pelvic hoop[132] whereby skeletal traction could be applied to the ambulatory patient and this was very popular in the 1960s and 1970s, particularly for polio patients in the Far East.[133] Both forms of skeletal traction require to be monitored carefully with weight being only incrementally added and should be followed by a careful neurological examination not only of the spinal cord but also the cranial nerves.[134,135] There are other complications and deep vein thrombosis and pulmonary embolus have both been reported.[136] Again in the 1960s and 1970s halo-anti-gravity traction was popular whereby the counter traction was the weight of the patient but would appear to be only rarely used these days.[137]

Traction was initially devised in the belief that with very big curves, say 80 degrees or more, then there was some mysterious tightness or stiffness factor that could be released by pulling on each end of the patient. Knowing the three-dimensional nature of the deformation of each vertebra in the curve, particularly around the apex, it is difficult to see the logic of traction. It certainly might and generally does reduce the size of the curve if the traction is continued and the weights increased. However, it is really not doing anything significant around

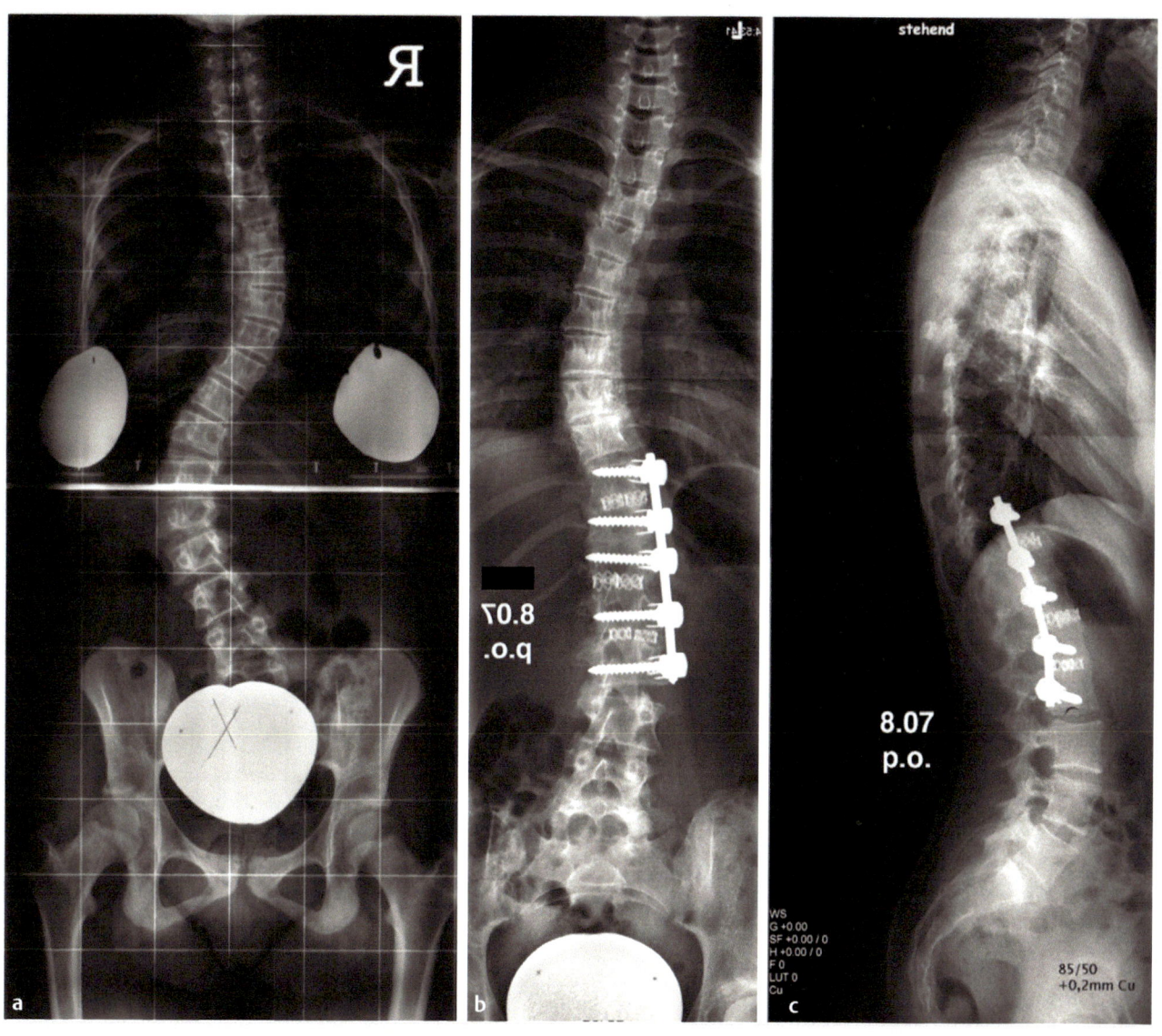

Fig. 4.26 (a) PA radiograph of a Lenke type 6 double curve pattern. (b) PA radiograph after short segment anterior instrumentation from T10 to L2 showing a very nicely balanced lazy S configuration. An excellent result with only four joints fused. (c) Lateral radiograph showing a natural sagittal profile.

the apical region rather just pulling on the compensatory curves at each end (▶ Fig. 4.10) which can be dealt with by instrumentation anyway. In any event very severe and rigid curves are more commonly encountered with congenital scoliosis or with Von Recklinghausen's disease rather than idiopathic scoliosis. The Harms Study Group (HSG) did carry out a small trial comparing 15 in the traction group and 8 controls.[138] Average curve magnitude was 97 degrees in the traction group and 93 degrees in the control group—not significantly different. Two years after surgery there was 64% correction in the traction group and 61% in the control group, again not significant either statistically and certainly not clinically. Therefore, we would not consider it to be useful to apply traction preoperatively.

4.4.1 Intraoperative Traction

This has certainly become more fashionable either using a halo or Gardner-Wells tongs. The amount of traction used is usually about a quarter to a third of the body weight if a patient is awake and obviously more if the patient is asleep and muscles relaxed. The force vector is of course longitudinal distraction which, as mentioned earlier (▶ Fig. 4.10), is in the wrong direction and will not influence the apical region merely the upper and lower compensatory curves. Furthermore, intraoperative traction with the relaxed asleep patient is potentially dangerous and if it is going to be used it mandates electrophysiological spinal cord monitoring. We have encountered a patient from elsewhere where a subtle cervical congenital anomaly was not recognized preoperatively as a potential source of cord tether and intraoperative traction rendered the patient quadriplegic. We therefore feel that intraoperative traction is contraindicated.

It is also possible to apply traction internally using a temporary rod. This rather resembles the old Harrington outrigger[8] which did exactly the same thing during the original insertion of Harrington rods. Nowadays sufficient flexibility can be achieved with soft tissue releases or even osteotomies, which would, in our experience, make traction unnecessary and outmoded. The adolescent with the bigger curve was the driver for the development of the Leeds procedure (anterior release)[67-69] so that the curve could be made more flexible and thus better able to respond to instrumentation.

4.4.2 Anterior Multiple Diskectomy

This is sometimes called anterior release, but we do not like this expression because it should mean that there is something tight on the short (posteroconcave) side of the spine. Of course the front of the spine is far too long and the whole idea of doing diskectomies is to make space at the front for the spine to collapse into itself either as a preliminary first stage to a posterior instrumentation procedure or, of course, prior to the application of anterior metalwork. Thirty years ago the Leeds Group introduced multiple diskectomy as an integral part of their Leeds procedure for bigger thoracic curves[67-69] (▶ Fig. 4.16 and ▶ Fig. 4.17). We had no idea at this stage that we could correct thoracic curves even bigger than 100 degrees. This was a preliminary procedure prior to a second stage posterior instrumentation which, at the time, was a kyphotically contoured Harrington rod with concave sublaminar wires. This instrumentation was nowhere near as powerful as modern day metalwork with multiple pedicular screws. Therefore, for curves not much more than 60 degrees we routinely did an anterior first stage and never regretted it in terms of the degree of subsequent correction obtained by the second stage posterior metalwork procedure (▶ Fig. 1.4). Of considerable interest was the fact that as soon as the patient went into recovery the routine post-thoracotomy chest X-ray demonstrated that the Cobb angle had reduced spontaneously by at least half and about 20 to 25% further correction occurred before the second stage which we routinely performed 1 or 2 weeks later. This was before it became fashionable do an anterior first stage and then turn the patient over and do the second stage all in one sitting. Thereby an opportunity to allow further spontaneous correction was denied.

Therefore, what is the place for multiple diskectomy, or anterior release, if you will, with modern multiple pedicular screw fixation systems? Luhmann et al looked at 84 patients with major thoracic curves between 70 and 100 degrees comparing preliminary anterior diskectomy with posterior spinal fusion alone.[139] If the posterior fusion used pedicular metalwork there was no significant difference in correction. Suk et al did the same sort of comparison in curves of 70 to 100 degrees and found a more than 60% correction in both groups.[140] Interestingly with pedicular systems they seem to be so strong as to avoid any crankshafting in the younger patient. Suk went on to suggest that the indication for anterior release would be curves of 110 degrees or more but it is very difficult to categorize curve size in this manner. Newton summarizes the position well when he says that "the indication for an anterior release is to some extent based on the desired result."[141]

This is precisely why the Leeds Group put safety first. If there was any doubt at all about carrying out a preliminary anterior multiple diskectomy then it was done and not just thought about and as a result we have encountered no neurological problems in hundreds of cases.

Having looked at the cases reported by Luhmann and Suk we do not understand how there seems to be no difference between carrying out a preliminary anterior diskectomy and not. Certainly the Leeds Group have been more aware of the apical lordosis for longer than any other group with the possible exception of the group led by Jean Dubousset. It isn't just a matter of a bit of hypokyphosis or a flat sagittal profile but frank lordosis in every case. Therefore, dealing with the safety side first if you are going to straighten up a significant lordoscoliosis then you are going to lengthen the apical half of the curve or so and that must be potentially dangerous neurologically with bigger curves. But also there is too much spine getting in the way and what an anterior multiple diskectomy allows is the spine to collapse into itself so it can straighten by way of shortening and importantly derotation as well (▶ Fig. 4.16). In our first few tentative cases in Leeds when we were perhaps less aggressive in our diskectomies to finish up with a curve a third of the size that you started with seemed incredible but perhaps the most important correction occurred in the transverse plane where there was 50% derotation providing a proper three-dimensional correction and not just in the frontal plane. It simply doesn't make sense that you cannot get a better correction by way of a preliminary anterior multiple diskectomy. If, as Newton says, that the indication is to some extent based on the desired result then if your desired result is a better correction of these very big curves then it goes without saying that you should do an anterior release.

Of course you also want to reshape the spine into kyphosis and that is another very good reason for doing an anterior multiple diskectomy particularly in the younger patient. The average number of disks removed by the Leeds Group was four or five. With bigger curves it may not be possible to get to more than four disks because of access. Notwithstanding that will have taken you beyond the limits of the apical lordosis anyway. To reiterate, these diskectomies are radical right back to at least the posterior longitudinal ligament and as each disk is removed the disk space promptly closes down (because it was always under tension) (▶ Fig. 1.4 and ▶ Fig. 3.27). If it doesn't then you probably have not have taken enough disk out. If you think you have gone far enough back in taking out the disk, then you haven't. Don't confuse the posterior annulus with the rather flimsy posterior longitudinal ligament which can be easily recognized after you remove the posterior annulus in the vertical direction of its fibers.

4.5 Osteotomies

For idiopathic scoliosis there really shouldn't be a need for osteotomies unless there has been a previous failed procedure such as a posterior fusion for a very young progressive curve or a lumbar flat-back syndrome because the sagittal profile hasn't been adequately addressed. Certainly, most of these cases are attributable to less than perfect surgical work. Meanwhile for congenital spinal deformities or those attributable to dystrophic neurofibromatosis then osteotomy work is more commonly required but it really should be rare for idiopathic scoliosis, even of early onset.

4.5.1 Smith-Peterson Osteotomy

Smith-Peterson osteotomies are principally for the correction of kyphotic deformities of the thoracolumbar spine as in ankylosing spondyltis.[142,143] There are much fewer "untreated" cases now than there were in the past with the greater availability of more powerful anti-inflammatory and other therapeutic agents as well as perhaps a more benign natural history. Not being able to see forward is a very distinct disability (▶ Fig. 2.40) and life tends to become a biological obstacle race. Hip hyperextension continues to allow patients to see forward until such time that the hips cannot compensate. Some patients prefer to wear prismatic glasses but spinal osteotomy is a definite option for these unfortunate individuals. With ankylosing spondylitis the whole spine is fused from front to back and therefore when the osteotomy is carried out in the lumbar region bone is taken out from the back corresponding with approximately a 40 degree angle and then the spine is fractured backward so as to make up all the leeway at the one osteotomized level.[144] The osteotomy is sited below the conus so as to obviate any spinal cord problems. Posterior bone is cut out to the anterior end of the foramen and in a chevron shape so that stability will be restored when the chevron is closed. In the old days we used to apply a Harrington compression rod to close the wedge and indeed a flexible compression system had to be used otherwise it couldn't change its radius as the wedge was closed (▶ Fig. 4.27). There certainly still is a need for a flexible rod for some of the most challenging spinal deformities rather like a Harrington compression rod so that its radius of curvature can change with the changing shape of the spine as the osteotomy is closed. Although specifically for kyphotic deformities making the osteotomy asymmetrical can assist correction in the coronal plane as well. There is a well-established complication rate, both vascular and neurological.[144,145]

Because the three-dimensional deformity of posteriorly fused idiopathic scoliosis is quite different from ankylosing spondylitis then the Smith-Peterson procedure is really not applicable but is included here for osteotomy completeness.

4.5.2 Ponte Osteotomies

Like the Smith-Peterson osteotomy this osteotomy is to allow correction in the sagittal plane.[146,147] Not surprisingly it was originally described for the correction of Scheuermann's kyphosis with correction being achieved by posterior shortening. Again each Ponte osteotomy goes as far back as the front of the foramen and includes removal of the upper and lower laminae and the entirety of the facet joint (▶ Fig. 4.28). The number of levels at which this requires to be performed characterizes the amount of correction. It is important to generously undercut the laminae so that there is no question of any interlaminar gaps being closed and thus potentially shearing the spinal cord. Geck reported on the sagittal plane correction achieved in Ponte osteotomies for Scheuermann's disease in 17 patients and noted no neurological complications but did stress that there should not be over-correction in the sagittal plane for neurological reasons.[147]

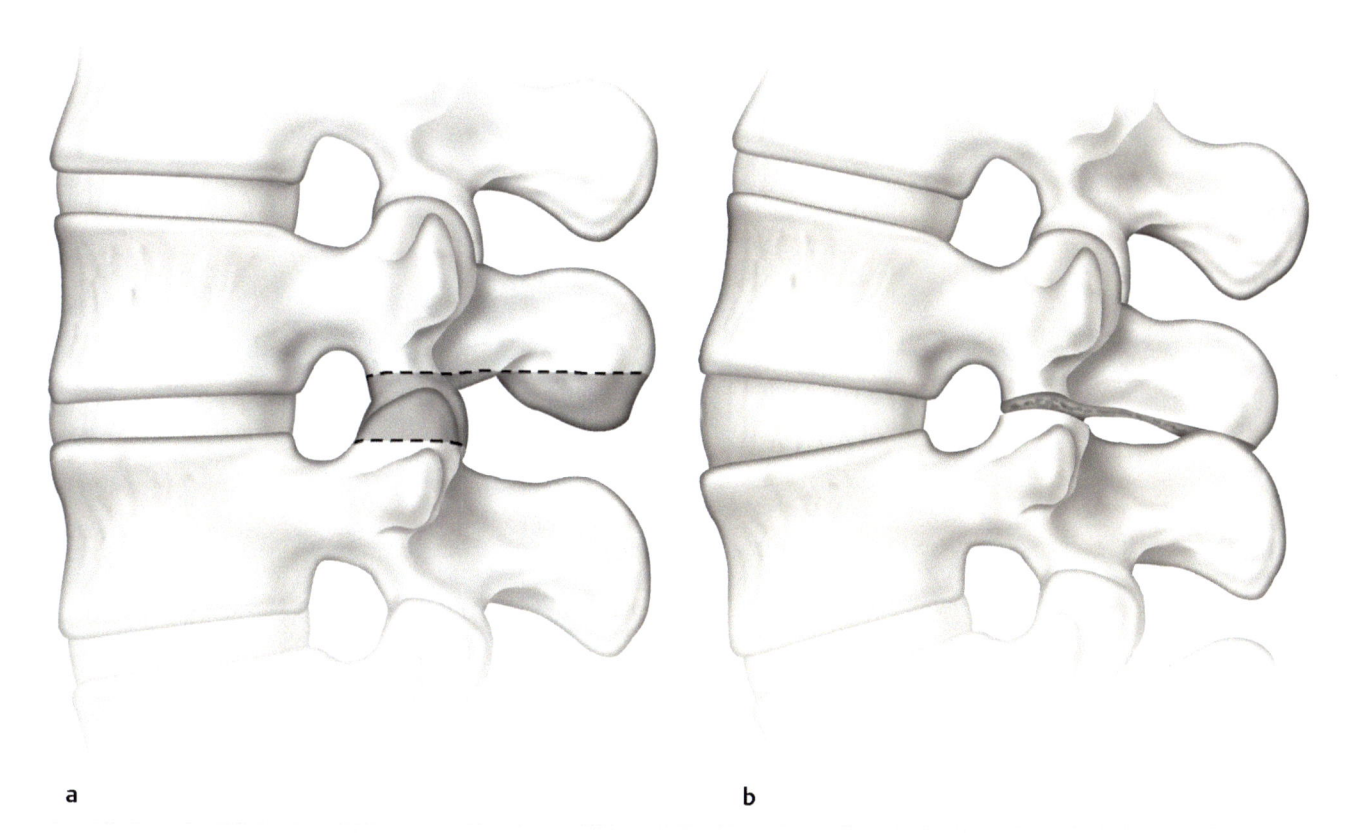

Fig. 4.27 Smith-Peterson osteotomy. (a) Lateral view of the bone to be removed (*highlighted*) for an SPO. (b) The correction expected after closure of the SPO. (Reproduced with permission from Newton P, O'Brien M, Shufflebarger H, et al. Idiopathic Scoliosis: The Harms Study Group Treatment Guide. Stuttgart/New York: Thieme; 2010: 189.)

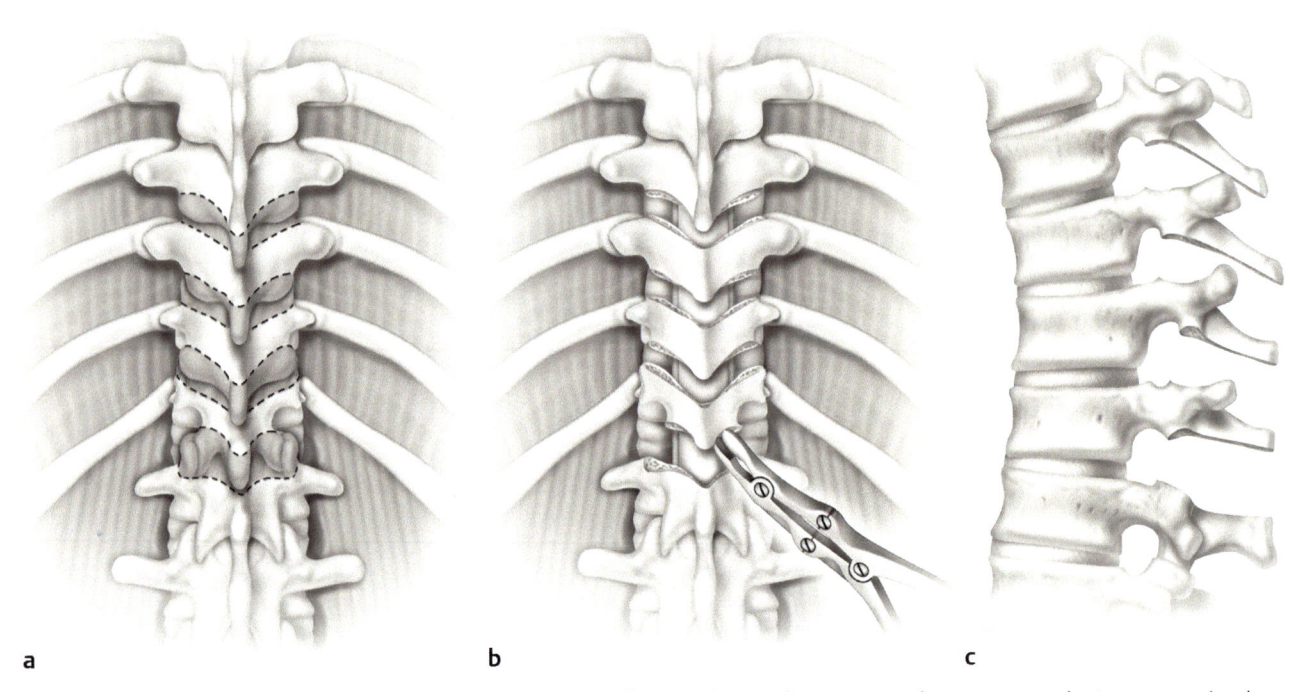

Fig. 4.28 Ponte osteotomy. (a) Outline of the structures (ligamentum flavum, inferior and superior articular processes, and spinous process) to be excised for a Ponte osteotomy. (b) Technique for a multilevel Ponte osteotomy. (c) Defects left after a multilevel Ponte osteotomy. Closure of these defects allows for shortening of the posterior column and correction of the kyphosis. (Reproduced with permission from Newton P, O'Brien M, Shufflebarger H, et al. Idiopathic Scoliosis: The Harms Study Group Treatment Guide. Stuttgart/New York: Thieme; 2010: 190–191.)

4.5.3 Pedicle Subtraction Osteotomy

This was first described by Michele and Krueger in 1949[148] but popularized by Heinig as the eggshell procedure"[149] It was originally described for pathological disease of vertebral bodies rather than deformity and again generally refers to sagittal plane correction down the pedicles to debulk the vertebral body (▶ Fig. 4.29). Of course if it is done asymmetrically then it can be of use for coronal deformity correction by fashioning the wedge resection more laterally based to the tune of about 25 to 45 degrees per level. With an extension osteotomy both pedicles are excised but with an asymmetric pedicle subtraction osteotomy only the convex pedicle is removed. This has become in recent years more popular for spinal deformity correction.[150]

After a standard posterior approach to the spine pedicle screws are inserted above and below the resection area. The posterior elements are first resected with a full laminectomy and undercutting of the laminae at adjacent levels. Then the transverse processes are removed. Then the lateral vertebral body walls at the selected resection area are exposed followed by resection of the convex pedicle only. An osteotomy is then used to create a three-dimensionally asymmetrical wedge in the vertebral body. The bone wedge is then removed and compression of the pedicle screw construct closes the osteotomy. The undercutting of the adjacent laminae is essential to avoid nerve compression. It is important to watch for posterior overhang as the wedge is closed and if so further laminar bone should be excised. For the biggest and most rigid curves apical vertebral resection is the preferred osteotomy technique.

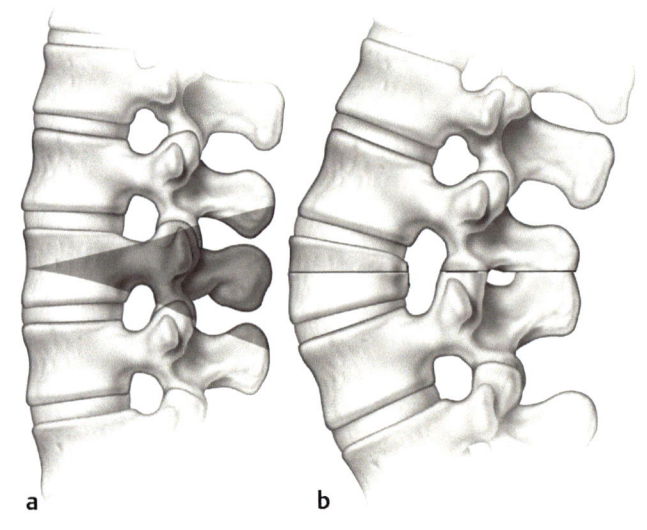

Fig. 4.29 Pedicle subtraction osteotomy. (a) Outline of a pedicle subtraction osteotomy. (b) The correction expected after closing the pedicle subtraction osteotomy. (Reproduced with permission from Newton P, O'Brien M, Shufflebarger H, et al. Idiopathic Scoliosis: The Harms Study Group Treatment Guide. Stuttgart/New York: Thieme; 2010: 192.)

4.5.4 Apical Vertebral Resection

Apical vertebral resection (AVR) can be carried out by an anteroposterior approach or a posterior-only approach. Although it is said that segmental pedicle screw instrumentation is required three levels above and three levels below to adequately stabilize the spine it should not be forgotten that there is a structural idiopathic curve here, and if it is a main thoracic (MT) curve, as usual, the whole of the structural curve requires to be instrumented and fused which may mean four above and four below or more. It would appear to be an overlooked but elementary planning principle that if a bent pipe is rigid and requires to be straightened this can only be achieved by dividing and shortening the pipe. This is made all the more biologically relevant if the hollow center of the bent pipe contains the spinal cord in which case the division must be achieved in association with shortening, or at least without lengthening. In this regard Leatherman was the real pioneer[151-154] (▶ Fig. 1.7) along with Roaf[155] (▶ Fig. 4.10). More is required to be removed from the convexity than the concavity so that straightening is effected in closing wedge fashion. In the first stage for an anterior and then posterior two-stage thoracic wedge resection procedure, there would be a standard thoracotomy and the apical bone is exposed subperiosteally. First of all the intervertebral disks are removed above and below the wedge shape of the apical vertebral body to be removed and then slivers of bone working from convex to concave side are removed with a sharp osteotome. Then, when the extradural space is exposed, up-cutting rongeurs are used to remove the final layer of bone. It is important to remove this thin layer on the concave side then work back toward the convex side. That is because half way along there is the basivertebral vein that can bleed profusely. Bone wax and layers of gel foam can then be applied to prevent bleeding while one completes excision of the convex thin layer of bone. The convex pedicle is removed back to flush with the vertebral body itself. This ends the anterior osteotomy and the gap is filled with gel foam before repair of the periosteal sleeve over it. The disks above and below should also be removed to obtain maximum correctability.

In the second stage a routine posterior approach is carried out. The whole of the structural curve is then exposed subperiosteally out to the tip of the transverse processes. Then a wedge-shaped laminectomy is carried out at the level of the anterior wedge removal and it is important to insert a metallic marker at the end of the first stage at the apex of the wedge to guide the surgeon as regards the level to be dealt with posteriorly by way of an on-table PA radiograph. The laminectomy is continued until the facet joint and pedicle on the concave side are visualized and they are then removed to complete the wedge removal. Before the final bone on the concave side is removed instrumentation is inserted on the convex side to provide stability before the convex compression rod is compressed to close the wedge. In the old Leatherman days this was the Harrington compression system but nowadays the same procedure is effected by pedicular metalwork. Once the wedge has been closed the whole of the structural curve above and below must be fused. Because this is a closing wedge osteotomy performed front and back under direct vision the integrity of the spinal cord is always visualized. This philosophy is verified by the unfortunate events that occurred during the development of anterior spinal surgery. After Royle's removal of a hemivertebra[156] others soon took up the challenge but in the early pioneering days opening wedge osteotomies were performed and accompanied by lengthening instead of shortening and therefore an unacceptably high rate of paraplegia.[157-162] One of Wiles' cases became paraplegic.[159] Hodgson in Hong Kong then carried out opening wedge osteotomies of a circumferential nature but again paraplegia was a serious and not uncommon complication.[161] Later Domisse reported four paraplegias with 68 single-stage Hodgson osteotomies.[162] Leatherman favored a two-stage approach—anterior first and then posterior—and this followed on from Von Lackum and Smith reported abandoning one-stage surgery in favor of two stages including a posterior fusion.[158] Nowadays both anterior and posterior stages can be performed at one sitting.

Posterior AVR may not produce bone-on-bone contact and thus may require a cage or bone graft material in the gap. The posterior approach is now the usual standard one and to begin with three above and three below pedicular screws are inserted (▶ Fig. 4.30). Then a wide lateral dissection is performed to allow resection of the transverse processes/concave rib and rib heads in the thoracic spine. Laminectomy then exposes the dura and this is carried out throughout the whole area to be resected. The thoracic spine nerve roots can be tied off and resected and it is very important to safeguard the great vessels anteriorly. The concave pedicle is first resected followed by the concave vertebral body and disk. Then on the concavity a rod is inserted to provide stability and prevent translation. The same is carried out on the convex side and then correction is obtained gradually through repeated shortening of the vertebral column with temporary rods. Then the convex side of the deformity is compressed and any gap between the vertebral body ends filled with cage or graft. Obviously spinal cord monitoring is required throughout as with any scoliosis operation. It is wise to put in a prophylactic chest tube as hemothoraces are not uncommon. Healthy cancellous bone does bleed in the adolescent and so any raw vertebral body end surfaces should be smeared with bone wax which should be pressed into the interstices of the ends of the vertebral bodies which considerably mitigates any subsequent postoperative bleeding.

There has now been considerable experience of this technique and Suk et al reviewed 16 patients with curves more than 80 degrees and apical flexibility of less than 25%.[163] While the correction of Cobb angles was of the order of 60 degrees, blood loss was all of 7 L. There were a number of complications but the most important one was total paralysis in one patient. Jensen reported on 23 patients with a mean correction of 78% with one transient paralysis and one death because of blood loss.[164] Why with curves of this medium magnitude did Suk do osteotomies when the safe and just as effective technique is anterior multiple diskectomies.

Letko et al reported on 16 patients half of whom had an anterior release beforehand.[165] Again mean blood loss was 7 L but mean correction was down to a virtually straight spine. There were no really worrying complications but there were a large number of hemothoraces, pleural effusions, and pneumothoraces which again would indicate the benefit of a prophylactic chest drain. However, the results can be truly spectacular (▶ Fig. 4.31).

We reported on 67 cases of two-stage wedge resection carried out in this fashion, albeit more for congenital curves rather than idiopathic ones, with no neurological complications and no fatalities.[154] R.A.D. still prefers this approach but whether done anteriorly and posteriorly or just posteriorly alone rather depends upon the surgeon's experience and choice. What matters is safety first. Paralysis or death are not acceptable complications of scoliosis surgery, least of all with idiopathic scoliosis and those carrying out AVR by posterior approach only need to be extremely skilled and very well-trained surgeons.

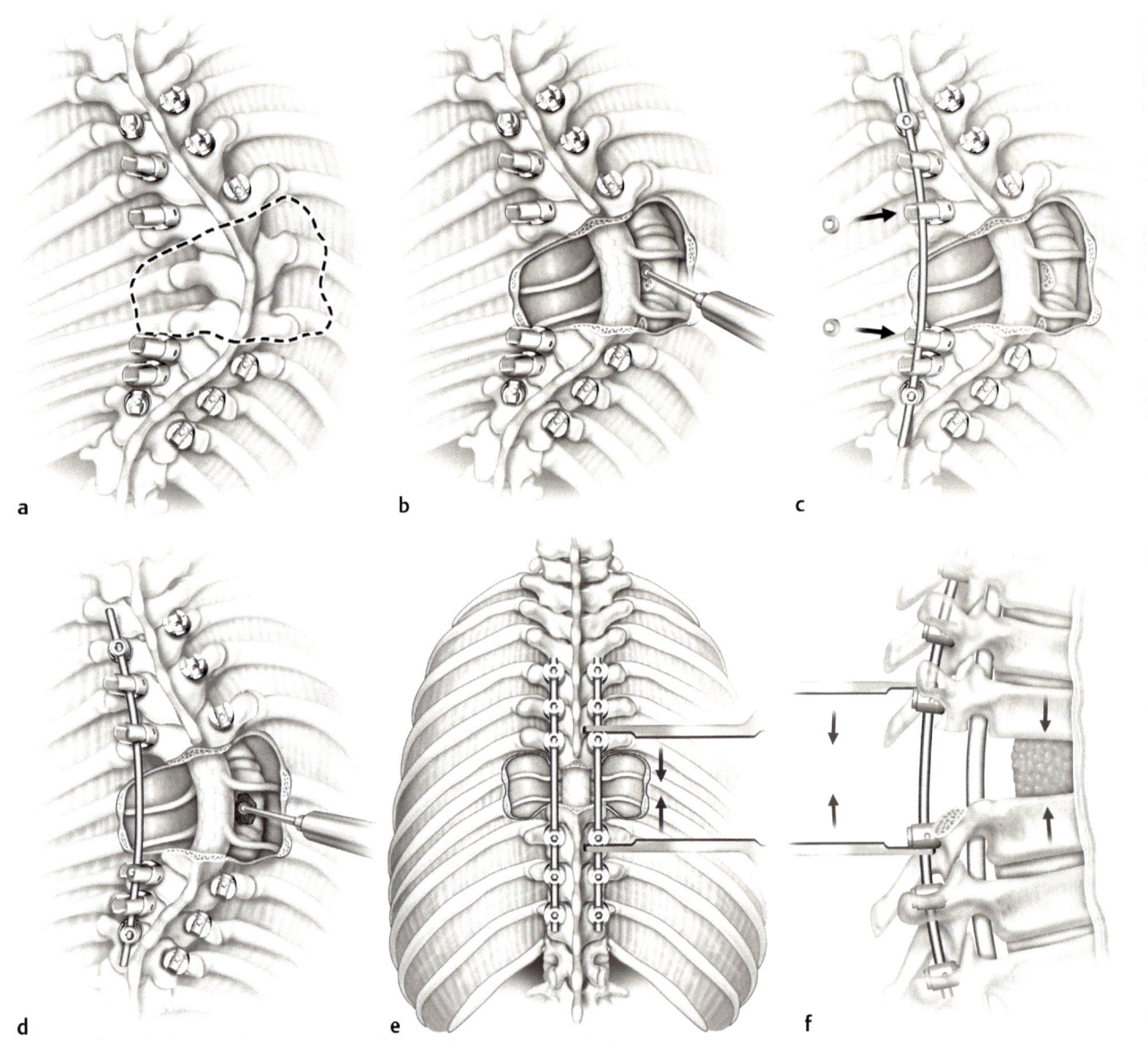

Fig. 4.30 AVR. (a) Placement of the pedicle screws (three levels above and three levels below the region of the resection) prior to the apical vertebral excision. (b) Excision of the posterior elements and concave pedicle. Wide decompression of the thecal sac and nerve roots is needed to prevent neurological injury. (c) Placement of the concave rod before excessive anterior or middle-column removal or both is needed to prevent instability and neurological injury. (d) Removal of vertebral body from the convex side. (e) Further reduction of the deformity by compression across the convex rod. (f) Incomplete closure following correction of a deformity requires the addition of anterior support (a cage or graft). Compression with the graft or cage as a fulcrum can further reduce the deformity. (Reproduced with permission from Newton P, O'Brien M, Shufflebarger H, et al. Idiopathic Scoliosis: The Harms Study Group Treatment Guide. Stuttgart/New York: Thieme; 2010: 193–197.)

4.6 Early-Onset Idiopathic Scoliosis

4.6.1 Clinical Features

This is a very interesting condition whose natural history over the last century has been a matter of almost incredulity. This is idiopathic scoliosis developing before the age of 5 years and generally within the first year or two of life.[19] This is the only form of idiopathic scoliosis that effects organic health[17,18] and does so by not allowing the pulmonary alveolar tree to properly reduplicate within the cramped environment of a severe infantile chest deformity (▶ Fig. 2.25 and ▶ Fig. 2.26). The lung on the concave side resembles the sort of hypoplastic lung seen in congenital diaphragmatic hernias when the abdominal contents occupy most of the chest.[17] This is the condition to which all the bad reports about idiopathic scoliosis in the 1960s and 1970s mainly from Sweden relate.[4-7]

It was first described in the 1920s by Harrenstein in Holland which he published in 1930.[166] He also noted that spontaneous regression could occur. Nowadays the proportion that progress would be only 5 or 10% whereas resolving cases would account for 90% or more. The extraordinary thing is that 60 years ago,

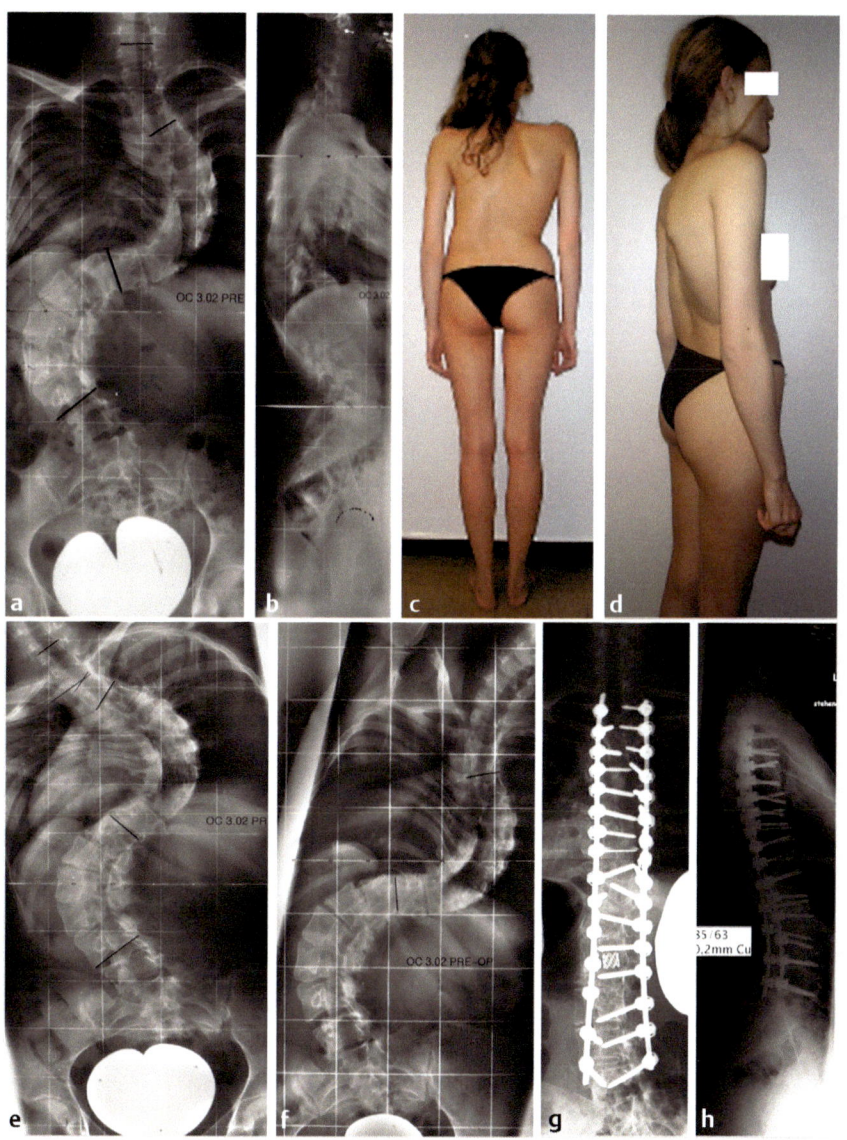

Fig. 4.31 (a,b) PA and lateral radiographs of a 21-year-old woman with a Lenke type 3CN scoliosis. The curve from T5 to T11 measures 110 degrees and the curve from T12 to L4 measures 95 degrees. (c,d) Preoperative clinical photographs of the patient. (e,f) Bending films demonstrate 12% flexibility (94 degrees) in the thoracic curve and 19% flexibility (80 degrees) in the lumbar curve. (g,h) She then underwent a staged anterior release from T4 to L1, followed by a posterior release with multiple transverse (Ponte) osteotomies, resection of periapical concave and convex rib heads, asymmetric PSOs of T8, T9, and L2, and instrumentation from T2 to L4. (Reproduced with permission from Newton P, O'Brien M, Shufflebarger H, et al. Idiopathic Scoliosis: The Harms Study Group Treatment Guide. Stuttgart/New York: Thieme; 2010: 198.)

when James in Edinburgh first looked at his cases, an estimated proportion of only 4 of his 33 cases resolved.[167] He then reviewed a further 52 cases and then all of 212 cases.[168] In the 212 there were still more progressors than resolvers although proportions were beginning to change. The Oxford Group then demonstrated that four times as many cases progressed as resolved.[169] Then over a very short period of time, by the 1960s, reports came through from London that of a further 100 cases 92 resolved and then only 5% appeared to progress.[170] This extraordinary change in natural history has hitherto been unexplained but just as the number of infantiles progressing has reduced in comparison to those resolving so has the prevalence of the condition.

McMaster, who took over the running of the Edinburgh Scoliosis Unit after James, reported in 1983 on infantile idiopathic scoliosis and how the incidence had changed over the years. Of the 672 idiopathic scoliosis patients who attended the Edinburgh clinic between 1968 and 1982, 144 had infantile scoliosis, 51 were juveniles, and 477 were adolescents (▶ Table 4.18). Between 1968 and 1971 the incidence of infantile scoliosis reduced from 41% to just 4%[171] (▶ Fig. 4.32). Meanwhile the bar chart also shows the 1967 to 1970 figures from Riseborough and Wynne Davies in Boston whose white population has a similar genetic stock showing figures not dissimilar to the much later Edinburgh figures of 1980 to 1982 (▶ Fig. 4.32), the considerable difference being thus far inexplicable. He felt that the tendency in Britain for newborn babies to be nursed prone had helped to prevent the moulding consequences of lying in an oblique decubitus position (▶ Fig. 4.33) and this was our practice in Leeds with again a marked reduction in the incidence of infantile scoliosis. Then in Britain there was a furore about the possibility of cot deaths being produced by the prone position so this was abandoned and as a consequence the incidence of infantile scoliosis has probably gone back up again somewhat. In McMaster's series 96% of patients with infantile scoliosis had a single structural curve with the great majority being thoracic, left-sided and in boys. It is interesting when we look at ▶ Table 4.18 from McMaster's 1983 paper that we see that for infantile scoliosis there is a significant majority of males while in so-called juvenile the gender ratio is about 2:1 female to male while in adolescence the gender ratio is 4:1 female to male. Why this change occurs is unknown, rather like the marked reduction in the incidence of infantile idiopathic

Idiopathic Scoliosis

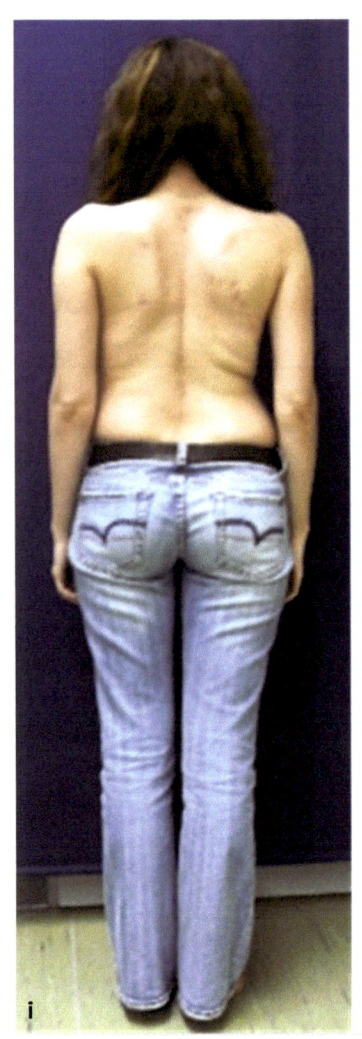

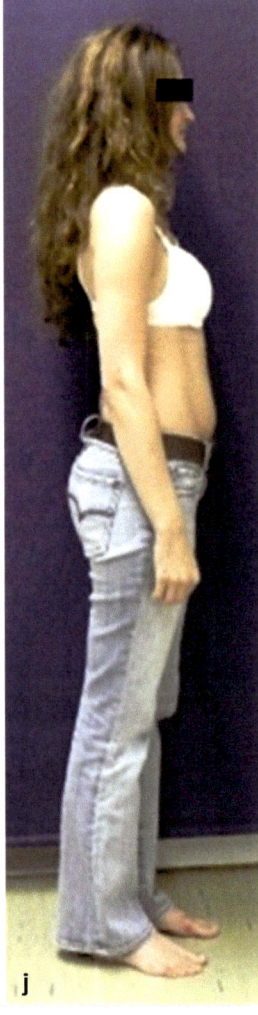

Fig. 4.31 (*continued*) **(i,j)** Postoperative clinical photographs of the patient. (Reproduced with permission from Newton P, O'Brien M, Shufflebarger H, et al. Idiopathic Scoliosis: The Harms Study Group Treatment Guide. Stuttgart/New York: Thieme; 2010: 199.)

Table 4.18 Idiopathic scoliosis patients who attended the Edinburgh clinic between 1968 and 1982

Type of idio-pathic scoliosis	No. of patients		
	Males	Females	Total
Infantile	85	59	144
Juvenile	18	33	51
Adolescent	96	381	477
Total	199	473	672

scoliosis over the years. McMaster also observed that of those who presented in the first 6 months of life more than 80% resolved and only 17% progressed whereas after the age of 1 year 70% progressed and only 30% resolved. Remembering James' three-part classification? Infants presented under the age of 3, juveniles 3 to 10, and adolescents from 10 to maturity; thus with increasing age as one goes through the juvenile period there is a move toward the more usual adolescent proportions in terms of gender ratio.

McMaster went on to review 109 consecutive patients in the juvenile idiopathic category with a mean age of 6 years and 10 months but a range from 3 years to almost 10.[172] Cobb angle at presentation for thoracic curves was of the order of 40 degrees and the gender ratio was 1:1.6 females to males in those less than 6 years old, 2.7:1 for those more than 6 years of age and so it would seem that as one progressed through the juvenile period then again the curves more resembled the adolescent variety. Curves also progressed between 1 and 3 degrees per year before the age of 10 (the relatively flat juvenile growth velocity period) and 4.5 to 11 degrees per year after the age of 10 (coming into adolescence).

We talk about juvenile idiopathic scoliosis here because, although we have a primary division of idiopathic scoliosis into early onset (before the age of 5) and late onset (after the age of 5)[19] (▶ Fig. 2.25), it is clear that only a minority of patients do present in James' juvenile period. It is also clear that the younger they are in this juvenile period the more the curves resemble James' infantile scoliosis and the older they are the more they resemble adolescent scoliosis. Of course whether these patients do have juvenile-onset scoliosis or whether they are a hangover from infancy or an early presentation of adolescent scoliosis is unclear. Growth velocity curves as produced by Tanner are very much for the average child (▶ Fig. 4.34) and the distributions around the mean are quite considerable.[173] Therefore why should an infant's growth velocity flatten out at exactly the age of 3 and why should an 8-year-old with so-called juvenile idiopathic scoliosis not have an earlier than normal growth spurt? This seems the most likely explanation for these differences.

There were two schools of thought about how the deformity was produced. Dennis Browne[174] considered intrauterine moulding as the causative agent in its production of the scoliosis and the associated deformities of plagiocephaly, plagiopelvy, and limited hip abduction; others agreed.[175–177] Meanwhile the other school of thought was introduced by Mau who thought this was due to cot positioning.[178] Postnatal pressure with a constant oblique supine position prevalent in European countries would lead to body moulding and this is why the plagiocephaly, bat ear, plagiopelvy, and limited hip abduction are all on the same side (▶ Fig. 4.33). This body moulding problem was quite clearly shown in McMaster's study of infantile idiopathic scoliosis[171] and would certainly explain why infantile scoliosis diminished in incidence so dramatically when newborn babies were nursed prone. This was confirmed by an important study on skull shape from birth onward for 6 months by Dempster from the Leeds Group who showed that plagiocephaly only developed post-natally.[179] By contrast the general method of how a baby lies in the North American continent is prone which may account for the greatly reduced prevalence rate of early onset idiopathic scoliosis in America.

In addition Wynn-Davies noted that the vast majority of her 134 cases developed the scoliosis during the first 6 months of life.[177] Mau also noted the likelihood of progression if either growth or development of the central nervous system appeared to be retarded.[178] Connor added congenital malformations such as hiatus hernia as at risk factors for progression[180] while Wynn-Davies recorded a high prevalence rate of mental

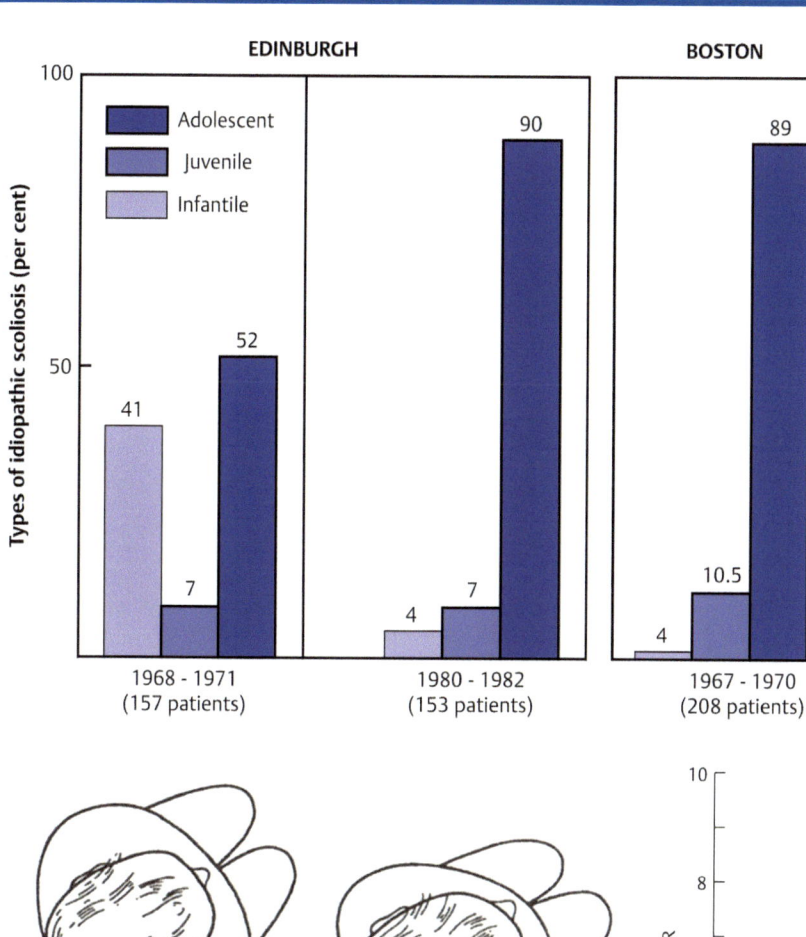

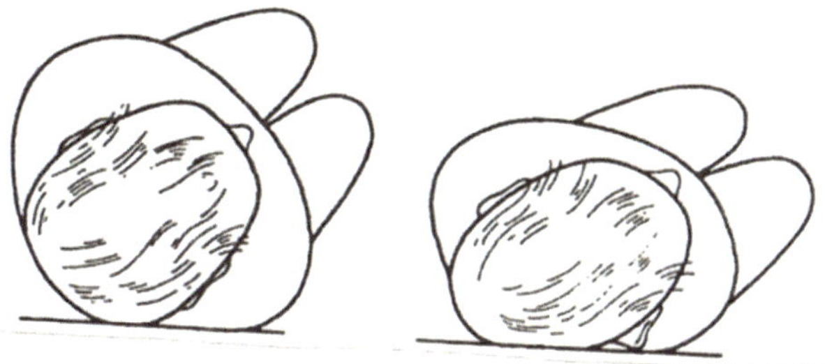

Fig. 4.32 Bar chart showing the incidence of idiopathic scoliosis in Edinburgh and Boston.

Fig. 4.33 Diagram illustrating (a) postural moulding of the skull producing left-sided plagiocephaly and (b) contralateral bat ear. Note the moulding of the thorax.

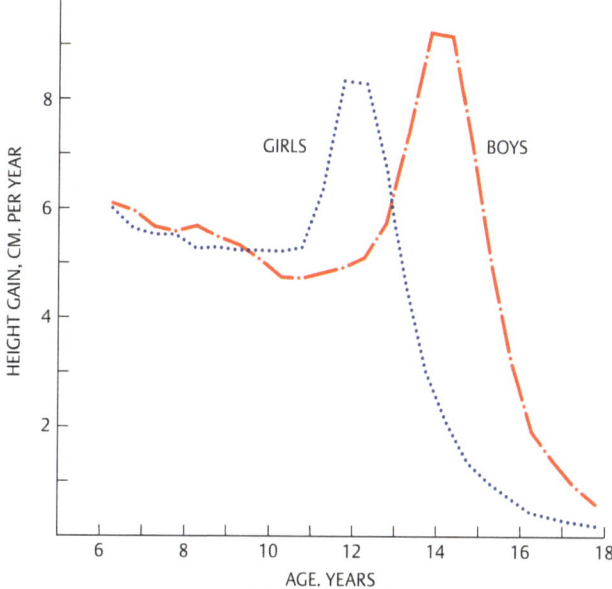

Fig. 4.34 Tanner growth velocity graph.

retardation, but only in the progressive group.[177] She also noted an increased prevalence rate of congenital heart disease, inguinal hernia, breech delivery, low birth weight, older mothers, congenital hip dislocation, and a floppy low birth weight baby. She also noted a much increased prevalence rate of scoliosis in parents and siblings of affected infants feeling that there was no genetic difference between early- and late-onset forms of idiopathic scoliosis. Males are affected more commonly than females in a ratio of 3:2, and curves can be single thoracic curves or thoracolumbar and double-structural curve patterns. With thoracic curves three-quarters are convex to the left and it has been suggested that right thoracic curves in females have a worse prognosis. While thoracic and thoracolumbar curves do tend to resolve, there is a distinctly worse prognosis for double-structural curves. Both initial curve size and amount of apical rotation are important prognostic determinants.

Mehta looked at a number of measurements on frontal radiographs to see if she could determine factors differentiating benign resolving curves from severe progressive ones.[34] A number of geometric measures were looked at but there were two that really stood out: curve size and rib vertebra angle difference (RVAD). If curve size is 30 degrees or more then this portends to a bad prognosis. This of course would not be surprising in terms of the further the leaning of the Tower of Pisa has tilted the more so it will be likely to carry on doing so (Euler's laws)—what really seemed to be important was the RVAD (▶ Fig. 2.15). On a PA radiograph a line is drawn vertically down the middle of the apical vertebra. Then on each side a line is drawn along the neck of the rib. When it meets the vertical line down the middle this angle is referred to as the rib vertebra angle (RVA). If the two are subtracted one from the other then we have the rib vertebra angle difference (RVAD). It can be readily seen on a radiograph that on the convex side the ribs droop much more downward than on the concave side but it appeared to Mehta that an RVAD of 20 degrees was the defining point above which progression could be expected. Her recommendation was that, on the initial consultation if the RVAD was 20 degrees or more, then one should wait for a period of 2 or 3 months and take an X-ray again as change can occur. Then if the curve had all the other features that signify a bad prognosis (low birth weight, floppy hypotonic baby with a very stiff curve) then immediate treatment should be started. Curve rigidity is a very important matter and if it is a very flexible curve then that should belong to the resolving variety. The best way to assess this is not by suspending the child up or down but by laying the child gently over the examiner's knee convex side downwards and letting the pelvis and the head gradually drop down. If correction does not occur then the curve is rigid and indicates a bad prognosis.

4.6.2 EDF Cast Treatment

Going back historically Cotrel and Morrell devised, as an alternative to bracing teenagers, the EDF cast[79] (▶ Fig. 4.35). Any visit to Berck-plage would see healthy teenage girls wandering around the town wearing their EDF casts and often with a book on top of their head to maintain balance. Then Mehta and Morrell applied these EDF casts to babies with progressive infantile scoliosis and noted very good results in terms of resolution particularly if the cast was applied early. The notion behind EDF casting was that when the little body jacket was applied then a derotation strap was tightened under the ribs on the convex side which then acted as paddles to try and derotate the spine. This corrected position was then maintained until the cast dried and a new cast was applied every 3 months or so to allow for the growing infant. In 1979 they reported the results of their first 21 cases.[181] The notion was that just as resolving curves became straight in the first two or three years of life then so can the infantile growth spurt help to straighten those that might progress with EDF cast management. Finally, in 2005 Min Mehta published her series of 136 infants with idiopathic scoliosis.[182] Using her clinical and geometric criteria 83% of cases followed her pattern but 17% did not and the importance here is that there are no absolutely strict criteria and of course using the RVAD of 20 degrees shows the problems of trying to categorize a continuous variable. In other words, some with a few degrees just below that figure progress and some with a few degrees above resolve. The demographics changed somewhat over the years and Mehta's recent figures were as follows—male to female gender ratio 1.1:1, 87 to 49 left to right convex curves, and an even number of single and double curves. Just as before there was a significant delay in referral to a scoliosis treatment center. The mean age at detection was 9 months but referral wasn't until 1 year and 10 months. She went on to divide these children into two groups—group 1, early referral, at 19 months with a delay of 12 months between detection and referral; and group 2, delayed referral, 12 months at detection, and all of 30 months at referral for treatment. The implications, although obvious, were borne out by the results of treatment. More than 30 years ago Alan Conner pointed out the concern about late referral[180] and it would appear that nothing has changed in the interim.[183] The only benefit that we could see as regards screening for scoliosis, and so did many others, was to raise the profile of the condition of "scoliosis" about which the public knew precisely nothing although the word sounded a bit like "sclerosis." In simple terms, if you don't get referred and treated before the age of 3 years the game is essentially over. The scoliosis was resolved in the 94 children in Group 1, but in the 42 children treated late (Group 2) correction was only partial and in some completely unsuccessful.

It is worth bearing in mind, in round figures, what infantile growth really means. When babies are born their length on average is 50 cm. In the first year of life they grow half of that (25 cm). In the second year of life they grow half of that (12.5 cm) and in the third year half of that (6 cm). That figure of 6 cm remains much the same all the way from the age of 4 to 10 when the adolescent growth spurt comes into play. Of course these figures are only approximate but they remain a very good, and memorable, guideline to growth in the early years of life. This is why Mehta recommends that treatment goes on for no more than 3 years otherwise the increased growth rate of the early years flattens out and growth acceleration cannot then be harnessed in favor of the child.[182] Then it was debatable as to what should be done once EDF casting had been stopped and many prescribed a mini-Milwaukee brace which appeared to slow down progression although of course with growth rate being only 6 cm a year until the age of 10 and therefore no increase in growth velocity this very much flattered the results of brace treatment to the point where it was probably irrelevant.

Of course the other variable in question is the curve size at the end of treatment. If the curve has completely resolved or substantially so then it can be left. But if EDF cast treatment has failed and at the age of 3 or 4 there is still a significant curve then it is very likely to progress significantly despite a flat growth velocity simply because it was much bigger and more rotated to start with. If cast treatment has therefore been seen to fail that is when surgical treatment is required. Interestingly after treatment when the spine is radiologically straight there is still a degree of plagiothorax and radiological rotation

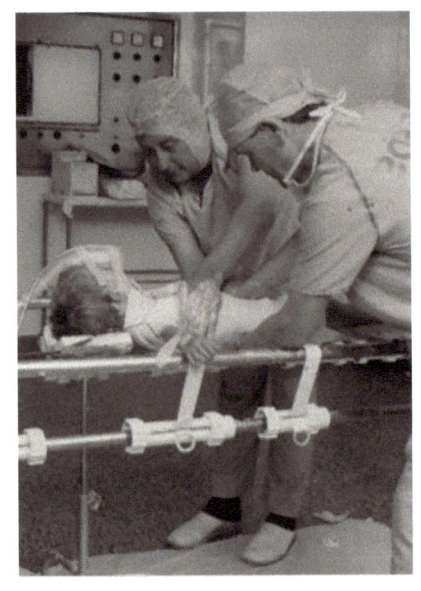

Fig. 4.35 Applying an EDF cast to an infant with progressive idiopathic scoliosis: an essential form of treatment. This treatment may need to be repeated every 2 or 3 months until the patient reaches the age of 4 years.

and this is the last component of the deformity to resolve eventually. Unfortunately it seems that fewer centers have the ability or inclination to pursue an EDF cast regime which, of course, can be curative for this potentially terrible deformity.

4.6.3 Operative Treatment

Growing Rods

Should the deformity be rapidly progressive and resist conservative treatment, although this must be tried first, surgical treatment is necessary. This is a very serious matter as it is easier to do more harm than good. But at the same time stopping progression must be the principal aim. The manner in which this is achieved is crucial. Historically this was by posterior fusion alone but this has already been shown to have significant limitations.[184,185] Cementing lordosis in bone at a young age would not at all appear sensible and would resemble doing a posteromedial fusion for club foot rather than a posteromedial release (▶ Fig. 3.16). Concern about early fusion has led surgeons back to the original thoughts of Harrington who initially performed instrumentation without fusion[186] and to distract periodically during growth by putting the rod subcutaneously so as not to raise the periosteum and thereby stimulate fusion. Having said that, raising the periosteum may not in fact be as osteogenic as generally thought[187] and so the concept was introduced of using two L rods plus sublaminar wiring but no fusion. This was referred to as the Luque trolley[188] but for early onset idiopathic scoliosis was introduced by Leatherman.[189] Again it must be remembered that the basic problem in structural scoliosis is that the front of the spine is too long and growing too fast compared to the back.[57,190] With these progressive deformities of early onset anterior spinal growth must be restrained and so for all but the unusually flexible case anterior diskectomy as a preliminary stage, combined with removal of the growth plates on each side of the disk, is an essential component of this physiological form of treatment.[67–69] Failure to appreciate this fundamental point is directly responsible for the bad results of posterior fusion in situ alone.

This approach offers enormous advantages but is still directed toward the secondary coronal plane deformity. The basic difference however between the resolving and rapidly progressive curve is that in the former growth is working for the patient while in the latter it is working against. It is therefore crucial to deal surgically with the underlying lordosis so that, the mechanics having been corrected, growth is now harnessed toward resolution of the secondary scoliotic deformity.

In the early days before dual growing rods it became fashionable to use a single Harrington rod hooked above and below into the neutral vertebrae and passed subcutaneously, distracted every 6 months to a year, or changed when the rod became too short, to try and control the coronal plane component of the deformity (▶ Fig. 4.36). However, we tried a more physiological approach using a Harrington rod bent into kyphosis and concave sublaminar wires to draw the depressed concavity back toward the rod without fusion and found that this could be very successful[69] (▶ Fig. 4.37).

Early onset malignant progressive idiopathic scoliosis deteriorates very significantly during these first 3 years of increased growth velocity and that is when these really challenging cases need to be treated. If the curve is still not too bad during years 4

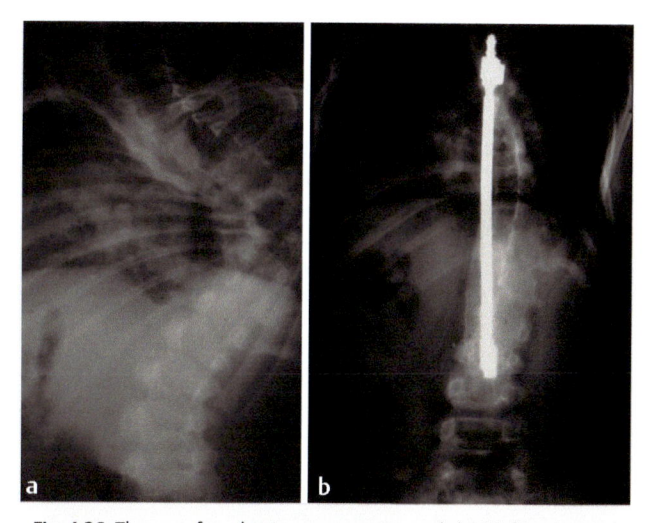

Fig. 4.36 The use of a subcutaneous growing rod. **(a)** PA film showing a 100-degree thoracic curve in a boy aged 6 years. **(b)** PA film 10 years after anterior multiple thoracic diskectomy and the insertion of a growing rod, which was lengthened or exchanged 12 times.

to 10 then probably any posterior construct without fusion will restrain further progression because this is a phase of flat childhood growth. If the curve is out of control before the age of 4 it is imperative to go anteriorly and stop the problem of significant anterior overgrowth otherwise the opportunity of really dealing with the heart of the problem is lost before the phase of flat growth velocity of 6 cm a year until the age of 10.[173] Going anteriorly at the age of 2 or 3 may seem a formidable undertaking but is mandatory for these viciously progressive curves. At thoracotomy it is extraordinary how cartilaginous the spine appears to be and, of course, it is. For the vertebral body to be half adult size at the age of 2 and not far short of full adult size at the age of 10[191] means that a lot of cartilage has to be removed on each side of the disk to get the growth plates fully out. That is all that has to be done in this first stage, stop anterior growth. The added benefit is increased flexibility and bearing in mind these very progressive early onset curves are typically very stiff then this allows posterior growing rod instrumentation to be corrective not just preventative.

In the United States the prevalence rate of EOIS is very much less than in the UK and Europe for no very obvious reason. Notwithstanding early onset scoliosis is still a problem to be treated in America and recently the multicenter Growing Spine Study Group database has been interrogated with some interesting results.[192] Names such as Akbarnia and Thompson, to mention but a couple, give this group considerable gravitas and in 2010 they published their results of 140 patients treated between 1987 and 2005 who had undergone a total of 897 growing rod procedures. In other words, the rods were lengthened or exchanged from time to time during that period. They enlarged upon the important initial contribution of Moe et al.[186] and in their 67 patients treated over 20 years there was a sustained 30% correction using their subcutaneous rod but of course there were complications to the point where some thought there was an unacceptable risk–benefit ratio.[193,194] Furthermore the 30% correction only reduced the curve from 67 degrees to a final 47 degrees which would still be well within the realms of unacceptability.

Idiopathic Scoliosis

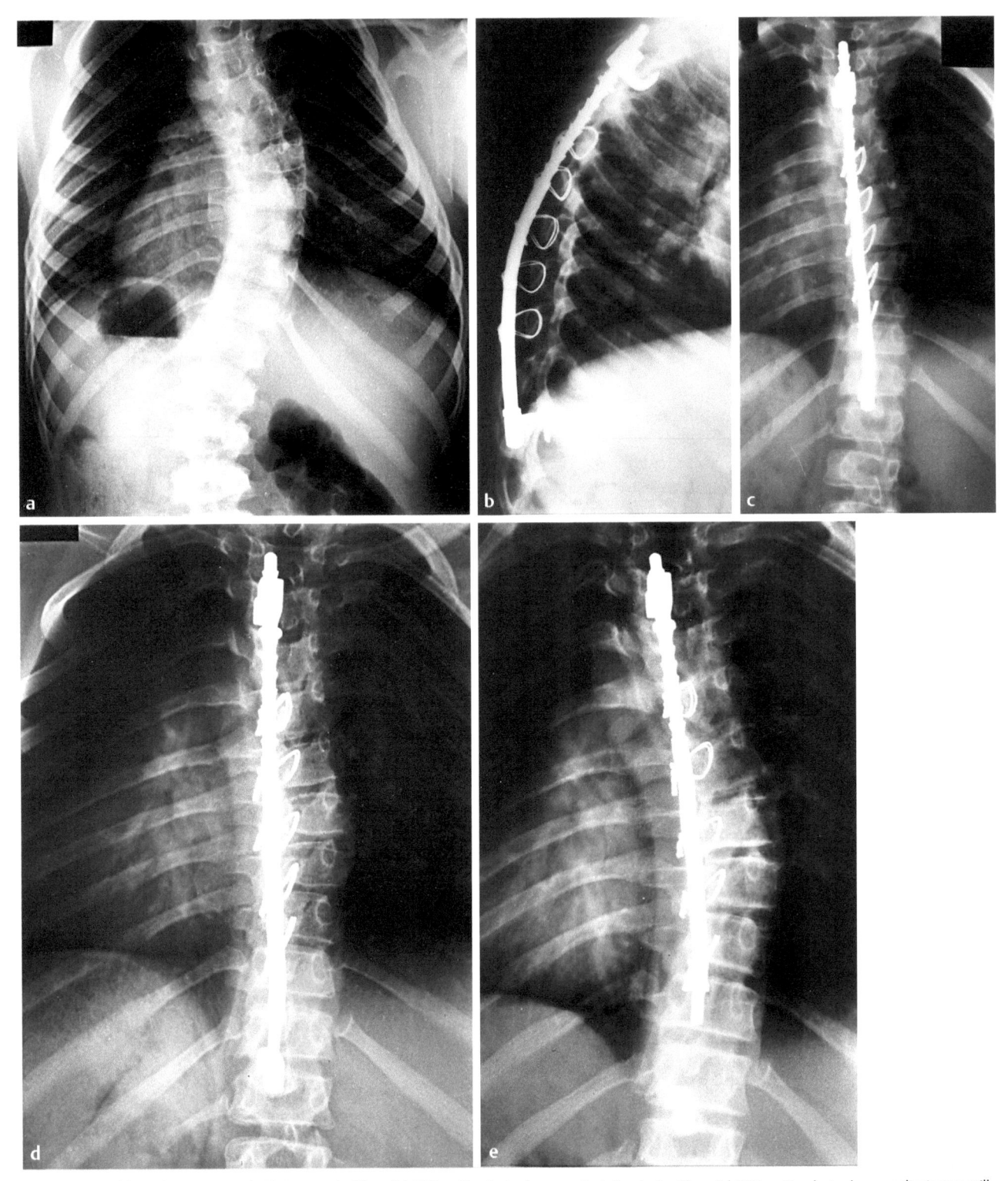

Fig. 4.37 PA films of a patient with EOIS treated with serial EDF casting but whose scoliosis treated with serial EDF casting but whose scoliosis was still progressing at the age of 5 years. (a) PA film before surgery. (b) Lateral X-ray and (c) PA X-ray: after surgery, showing that the kyphosis has been restored so as to stop subsequent buckling. (d) PA X-ray taken 3 years after surgery, showing that the lower end of the rod has come out of the lower hook, indicating growth. (e) PA film when the patient was a teenager, showing very considerable growth of the affected part of the spine, and that elevation of the periosteum for insertion of the sublaminar wires did not prevent spinal growth. At maturity, the metalwork was removed and the correction was maintained. (Reproduced with permission from Newton P, O'Brien M, Shufflebarger H, et al. Idiopathic Scoliosis: The Harms Study Group Treatment Guide. Stuttgart/New York: Thieme; 2010: 14.)

Idiopathic Scoliosis

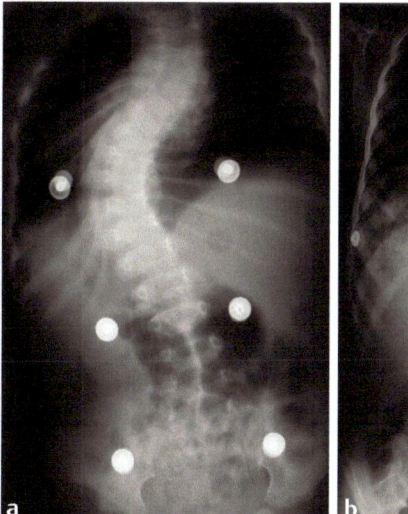

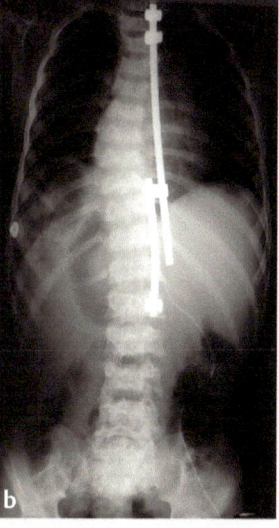

Fig. 4.38 Single rod and domino. **(a)** An 18-month old boy with early-onset scoliosis thought to be idiopathic. The patient's MRI was normal. **(b)** AP film made after insertion of a unilateral curve correction system using a crossover technique with a domino. The curve was successfully managed until the patient was 11 years of age, at which time no further correction could be obtained. The patient had broken the single rod twice, fortunately near the time of anticipated rod exchange. Conversion to a fusion was to be scheduled within the next 2 years. (Reproduced with permission from Newton P, O'Brien M, Shufflebarger H, et al. Idiopathic Scoliosis: The Harms Study Group Treatment Guide. Stuttgart/New York: Thieme; 2010: 402.)

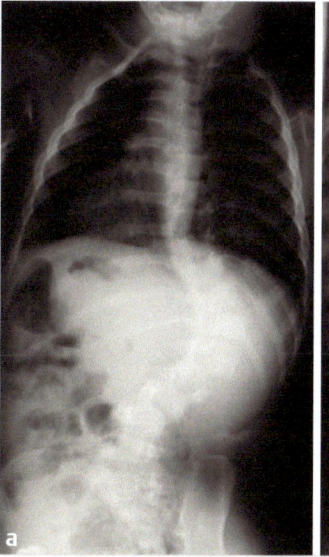

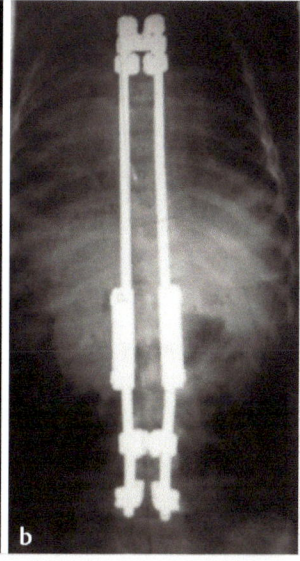

Fig. 4.39 Arkbarnia dual rod. **(a)** A 19-month old girl with idiopathic infantile scoliosis. At the age of 12 months her curve measured 21 degrees; it had progressed to 76 degrees in 7 months. **(b)** At the age of 19 months, the patient underwent dual growing rod instrumentation. Following insertion of the instrumentation, the patient's curve measured 35 degrees. (Reproduced with permission from Newton P, O'Brien M, Shufflebarger H, et al. Idiopathic Scoliosis: The Harms Study Group Treatment Guide. Stuttgart/New York: Thieme; 2010: 403–404.)

The single-rod technique is based upon that described by Blakemore et al.[195] Top and bottom hook and screw foundation sites were fused and the rod inserted either subcutaneously or submuscularly. The rod was then lengthened periodically usually about every 6 months and during the whole course of treatment a thoraco-lumbar-sacral orthosis was worn. Continued lengthening was done either by changing the rod, changing one of the segments if two overlapping rods were used, or dividing a single rod in the thoracolumbar area and applying a tandem connector (▶ Fig. 4.38).

Then Akbarnia described a modification of the growing rod technique that utilized dual rods attached to proximal and distal foundations[196] (▶ Fig. 4.39). What this meant was that the proximal and distal fixation sites were fused so that there were firm foundations top and bottom. The Leeds Group did this which then allowed fusion to occur spontaneously leaving locally some of the bone detached when making the upper and lower hook sites. Akbarnia noted better deformity correction and predicted growth maintenance during the treatment period using dual rods compared to single-rod techniques. Assorted complication rates ranged from 30 to 50% but there again that would be what would be expected using growing rods in unfused spines.[197] Complications such as rod breakage would of course be quite expected biomechanically.

Again the rods were placed subcutaneously or submuscularly and connected via a tandem connector. Then at the end of treatment (the construct couldn't be further lengthened or there had been a spontaneous fusion at least in part) the metalwork was removed and a standard posterior fusion carried out. Of the 140 patients studied by the Growing Spine Group there were only 40 idiopathic cases.[192]

When they compared the complications between single and dual growing rods, hook dislodgement and other implant problems were significantly higher in the single rod group. There were temporary spinal cord complications in four children. We always use spinal cord monitoring. On average there were six to seven surgical procedures per patient. The mean initial curve magnitude was 75 degrees and at the end of treatment 47 degrees. The mean age at the start was 6 but some were much younger and the mean duration of follow-up 5 years.

4.6.4 Other Methods of Growth Modulation

For those pre-Galilean ostriches who still believe that a structural scoliosis is a left–right problem,[43] if you experimentally reduce growth on one side then you can produce a minor nonstructural spinal deformity that is not worth further discussion except to say that for shortening rib procedures one wonders how ethical permission could ever be granted. There is also no evidence base for fiddling with the neurocentral synchondrosis.[198] As explained quite clearly in the pathogenesis chapter lordosis comes first, then rotation and not the other way round.[31]

Vertebral Body Stapling

Initial experimental work in animals promoted the use of vertebral body stapling (VBS) in the human situation.[199-202] Staples can be inserted either with a mini-thoracotomy or thoracoscopically. Either a single- or double-pronged staple can be used according to vertebral body size. Betz has done more work than anybody else as regards the use of these staples (▶ Fig. 4.40) but patients have been well beyond the infantile

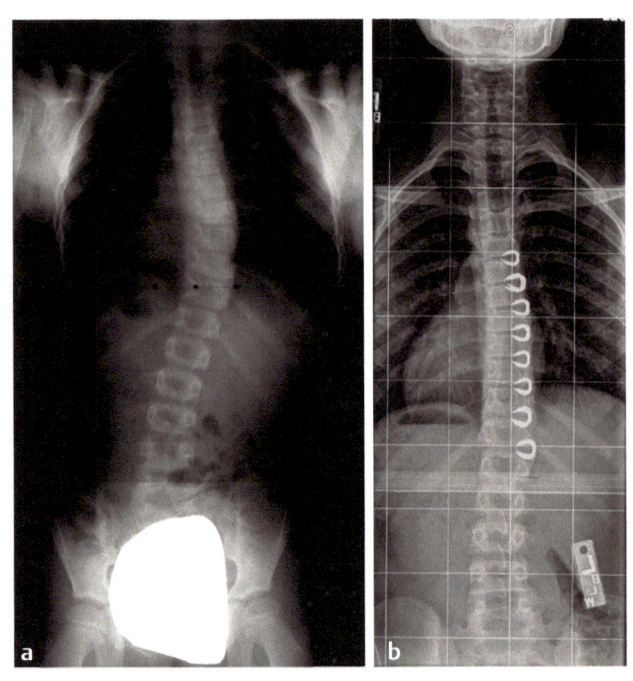

Fig. 4.40 Vertebral body stapling (VBS). **(a)** Preoperative and **(b)** postoperative PA radiographs showing the spine of a 7-year-old boy with a 30 degree right thoracic curve and 8 degrees of thoracic kyphosis. At 4 years after surgery, the thoracic curve measured 15 degrees. (Reproduced with permission from Newton P, O'Brien M, Shufflebarger H, et al. Idiopathic Scoliosis: The Harms Study Group Treatment Guide. Stuttgart/New York: Thieme; 2010: 396.)

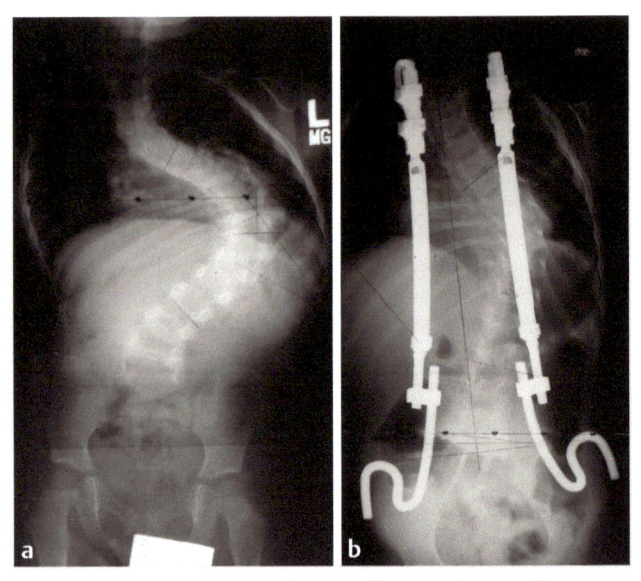

Fig. 4.41 VEPTR. **(a)** A 4-year-old girl with a 109-degree early onset scoliosis. **(b)** She was treated with a bilateral VEPTR device from T2 to the pelvis. (Reproduced with permission from Newton P, O'Brien M, Shufflebarger H, et al. Idiopathic Scoliosis: The Harms Study Group Treatment Guide. Stuttgart/New York: Thieme; 2010: 404–405.)

growth spurt when curve progression is not such a major issue. Quite rightly toward the curve apex the staples are inserted more anteriorly with the preface—that is where there is significant hypokyphosis (kyphosis less than 10 degrees), when of course every structural scoliosis is lordoscoliotic over the apical region. These staples have in the main been used for growing children with a moderate idiopathic scoliosis but notwithstanding Betz does report good results.[202,203] Initial curve size was between 20 and 45 degrees and success was considered if the curve corrected to within 10 degrees of the preoperative value. There was an 80% success rate in thoracic curves measuring less than 35 degrees. There were a number of not particularly important complications but crucially there were no instances of staple dislodgement or neurovascular injury. Best results were seen with flexible deformities, not surprisingly. This Group have inserted more than 1,400 staples and Betz doesn't recommend the use of these staples in patients younger than 8 years of age and so VBS is not really a procedure for EOIS. It has been suggested as an alternative to bracing in this sort of age group and that a controlled trial should be carried out between VBS and bracing but as we have seen, there is absolutely no evidence base whatever for bracing in idiopathic scoliosis in the first place.

Of course anteroconvex hemi-epiphysiodesis was introduced as a biological growth modulation 50 years ago.[204] Roaf knew perfectly well what the three-dimensional nature of structural scoliosis was following the important work of Adams[205] and along with Somerville[206] continued onward by the Leeds Group.[57,59,207–209] To him it was obvious that anteroconvex growth arrest was what was required for the leading edge of a progressive lordoscoliosis. It seemed entirely the logical way of dealing with this problem as opposed to those that simply wanted to cement the deformity in bone by carrying out the illogical procedure of posterior fusion for the very young spine.[184,185] Unfortunately progressive and quite rapid buckling of a progressive early onset idiopathic curve defeated Roaf's objectives because by the time the fusion could come into play biologically, the deformity had become much more progressive biomechanically.[210] Of course it wasn't just anteroconvex hemi-epiphysiodesis but posteroconvex was added as well but in spite of the unsuccessful results the procedure was repeated.[211,212]

Vertebral Expandable Prosthetic Titanium Rib

The other alternative to growing rods is the vertical expandable prosthetic titanium rib (VEPTR) technique of Campbell where the implant is attached to ribs proximally and either the spine lower down or indeed the pelvis[213] (▶ Fig. 4.41). Smith developed this device and presented his initial work in 2006 with the supposed advantage of not touching the spine and therefore not inducing an early bony fusion.[214] It certainly can produce initially good results in fairly big curves but the proximal ribs in early onset idiopathic scoliosis are not particularly substantial for load-bearing but VEPTR to the pelvis is certainly an interesting nonspinal concept. Obviously at the end of treatment instrumented spinal fusion still has to be carried out.

Refashioning of vertebral shape by wedge osteotomy is another interesting biological concept. As we have already seen, the bigger a curve is the more three-dimensionally wedged are the vertebrae particularly around the curve apex and that is what makes the curve unstackable. Refashioning vertebral shape is therefore a reasonable option and when the Leeds procedure was first introduced[67] including anterior multiple thoracic diskectomy around the curve apex, after diskectomy and growth plate removal, the apical vertebra or two or three still looked considerably asymmetrically wedged and so they were refashioned into as close to a rectangle as possible to make the spine maximally stackable again. There seems to have been a resurgence of the concept of refashioning vertebral shape more recently.[215-217] These techniques are generally addressed at the mature spine when growth has completed but of course reshaping the apical vertebrae in the growing spine is still a most useful technique.

Although nowadays even with bigger curves up to 100 degrees, modern instrumentation, particularly with a preliminary anterior multiple diskectomy, can give rise to excellent cosmetic results sometimes there is a residual rib hump that patients would like to have corrected. The concept therefore of a costoplasty was introduced in the days when rib prominences were still of considerable significance with old fashioned posterior Harrington instrumentation.[218-221] The Briard and Chopin technique of moving convex ribs putting them into the flattened concavity was certainly a preferred technique.[222] However, it is just as easy to carry out costectomy of as many ribs as are involved in the rib hump, even up to eight. The rib hump is exposed right over to almost the lateral side of the chest and then the ribs sequentially removed subperiosteally. Provided a prophylactic chest drain is introduced for a few days there are no significant pulmonary risks and no concern about paradoxical respiration. Furthermore, the rib periosteum produces new bone as well as firm fibrous tissue so that the chest wall is not reduced in strength. Do not forget that LOIS cases have no respiratory complications spontaneously and, therefore, if there is a fairly short-lived (2- or 3-month) minor reduction in pulmonary function this is of no physiological consequence whatsoever.

If the patient with EOIS with a very progressive curve somehow slips through the net and goes on untreated until the deformity measures well beyond 100 degrees at the end of growth, then complex osteotomy procedures are necessary to try and reduce disfigurement and help the patient psychosocially; but it has to be borne in mind that pulmonary function is a very important issue when going into this surgery. Anterior surgery can certainly be a problem going through the convex chest because the concave hypoplastic lung may well not be able to sustain pulmonary function while the convex lung is deflated to allow access. With skillful anesthesia anterior surgery is still possible and Leatherman's extensive experience of safe surgery testifies to that. However, nowadays posterior-only osteotomy techniques would seem to be more sensible.

Case Gallery

With so many cases for the reader to learn from, a postscript has been included after relevant chapters in the form of a case gallery where additional cases of interest have been displayed and discussed. Here are 12 more idiopathic cases to show you. Try and correctly describe the radiographs in each case, think about the surgical options, and decide how you would approach these cases; then you can compare them with what we have done. We are not always right but more often than not there are options to discuss.

Case 1: The Value of Anterior Multiple Diskectomy

See ▶ Fig. 4.42 ▶ Fig. 4.43 ▶ Fig. 4.44.

Comment

When you now come to instrument the spine you are dealing with a deformity half of its original size in both the coronal and transverse planes. Moreover, this has occurred spontaneously. It will get even better if you wait a few days before doing the posterior instrumentation stage.

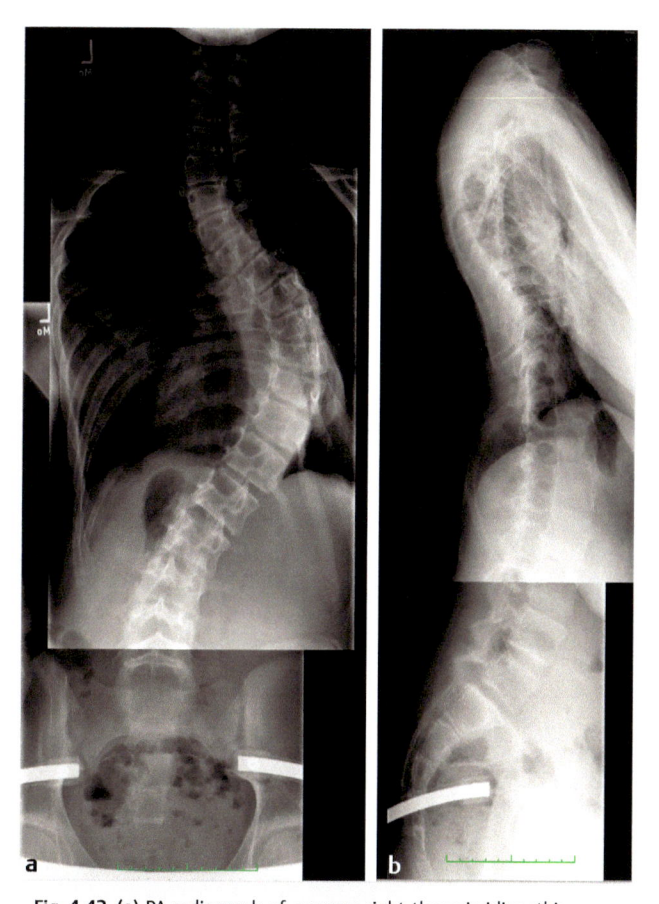

Fig. 4.42 (a) PA radiograph of a severe right thoracic idiopathic scoliosis. The Cobb angle measures in excess of 100 degrees but there is a tremendous amount of associated rotation with the deformed convex ribs overlapping the spine and producing for the patient a severe ridgeback deformity. (b) Lateral view showing the usual extreme lordosis.

Idiopathic Scoliosis

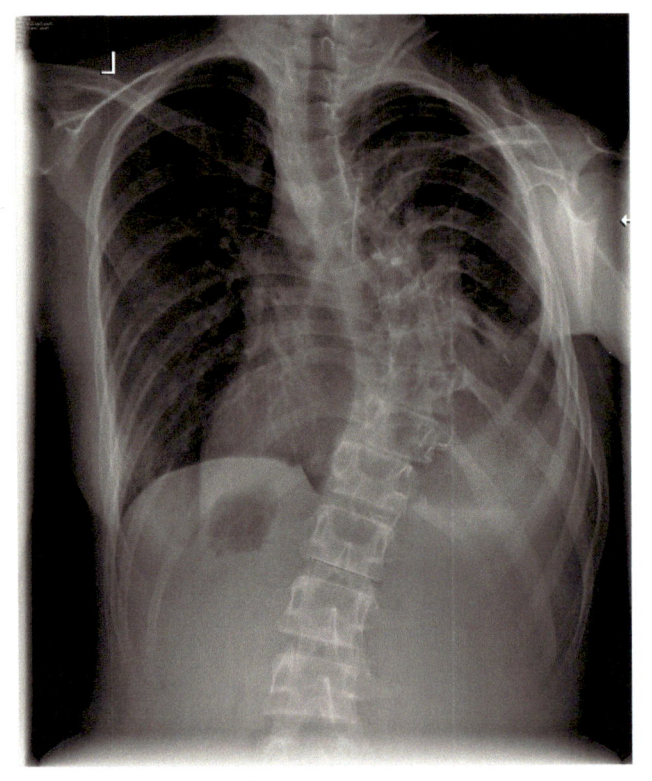

Fig. 4.43 PA radiograph after anterior multiple diskectomy showing not only has the Cobb angle reduced by at least half but the deformity has spontaneously derotated significantly.

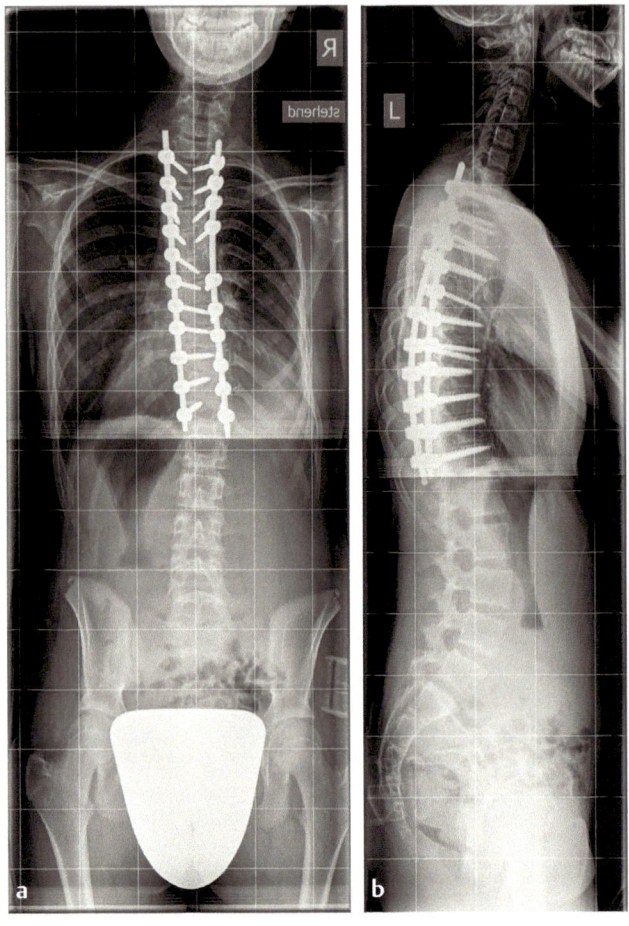

Fig. 4.44 (a,b) PA and lateral radiographs after instrumentation with a nice straight spine and a natural lateral profile.

Case 2: Anterior Instrumentation Only; Lenke 1 AR

See ▶ Fig. 4.45a-e.

Comment

Surgery has corrected the thoracic scoliosis down to a nice gentle curve but the curve carries on down to L3. L2 is neutral and so posterior instrumentation down to L2 is too short and L3 would have been better. These out of balance lumbar curves do look menacing and do need to be dealt with firmly with posterior instrumentation. Learning is a lifelong process, but in some cases doesn't need to take so long.

Idiopathic Scoliosis

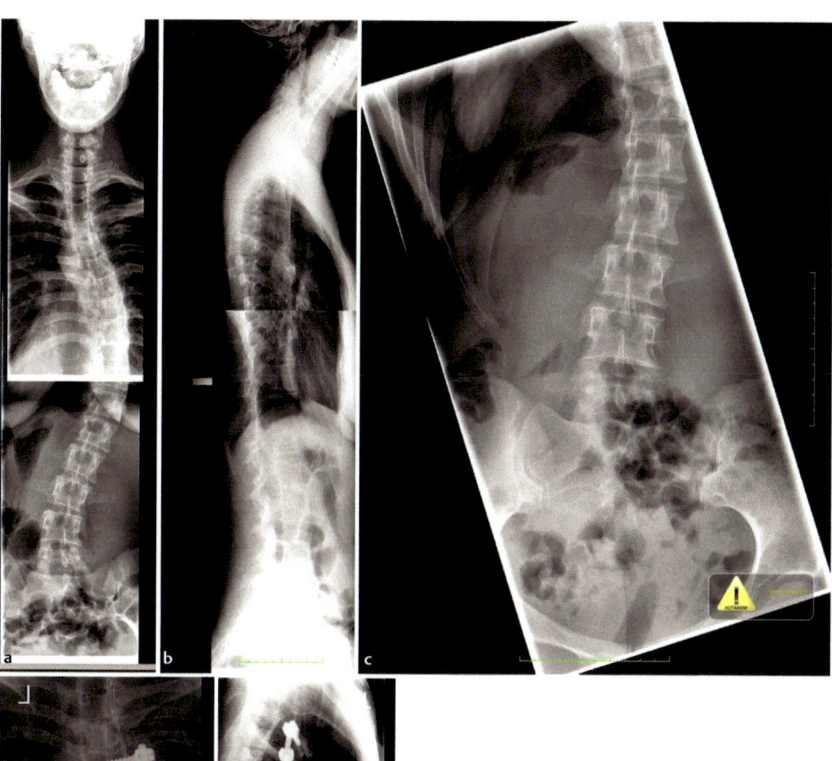

Fig. 4.45 (a) PA. This is a Lenke 1 R right thoracic curve but the lowest neutral vertebra is L2 and for posterior surgery the LIV would be L3. The lumbar compensatory curve is bigger than the thoracic compensatory curve above and she is a little out of balance. (b) Lateral X-ray showing a very flat back all the way down, indicating that the lower lumbar spine is rotated thus flattening what would be a lower lumbar lordosis. (c) Side-bending film to the left shows that the lumbar spine does straighten out in the coronal plane but the first neutral vertebra is L3 and L2 is rotated with the main thoracic curve. Do you or don't you carry out an anterior selective thoracic fusion? (d) PA radiograph after anterior thoracic instrumentation. Because the LIV was too high there is "adding-on" below. (e) Lateral X-ray showing restoration of a natural thoracic sagittal profile which you cannot achieve with posterior instrumentation only.

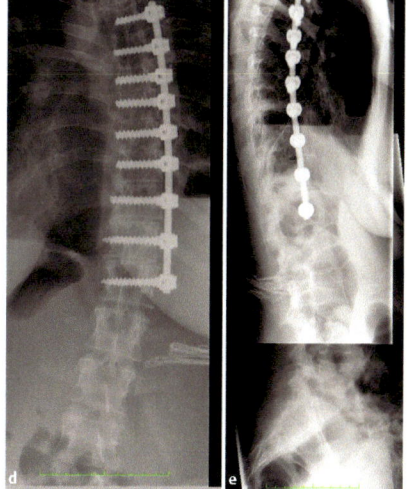

Case 3: Anterior Instrumentation Only; Lenke 1b

See ▶ Fig. 4.46a–h.

Comment

This type of thoracic curve lends itself perfectly to anterior instrumentation giving a much shorter length of instrumentation and the ability to restore the normal thoracic kyphosis. If you correct in both the coronal and sagittal planes then you must also correct rotation (the third plane) and observe the symmetry of the ribs in (d) compared to the marked asymmetry in (a). The curse of brace treatment is also well demonstrated with this case.

Case 4: Anterior Instrumentation Only; Lenke 1b

This is a decompensated right thoracic curve. See ▶ Fig. 4.47a–h.

Idiopathic Scoliosis

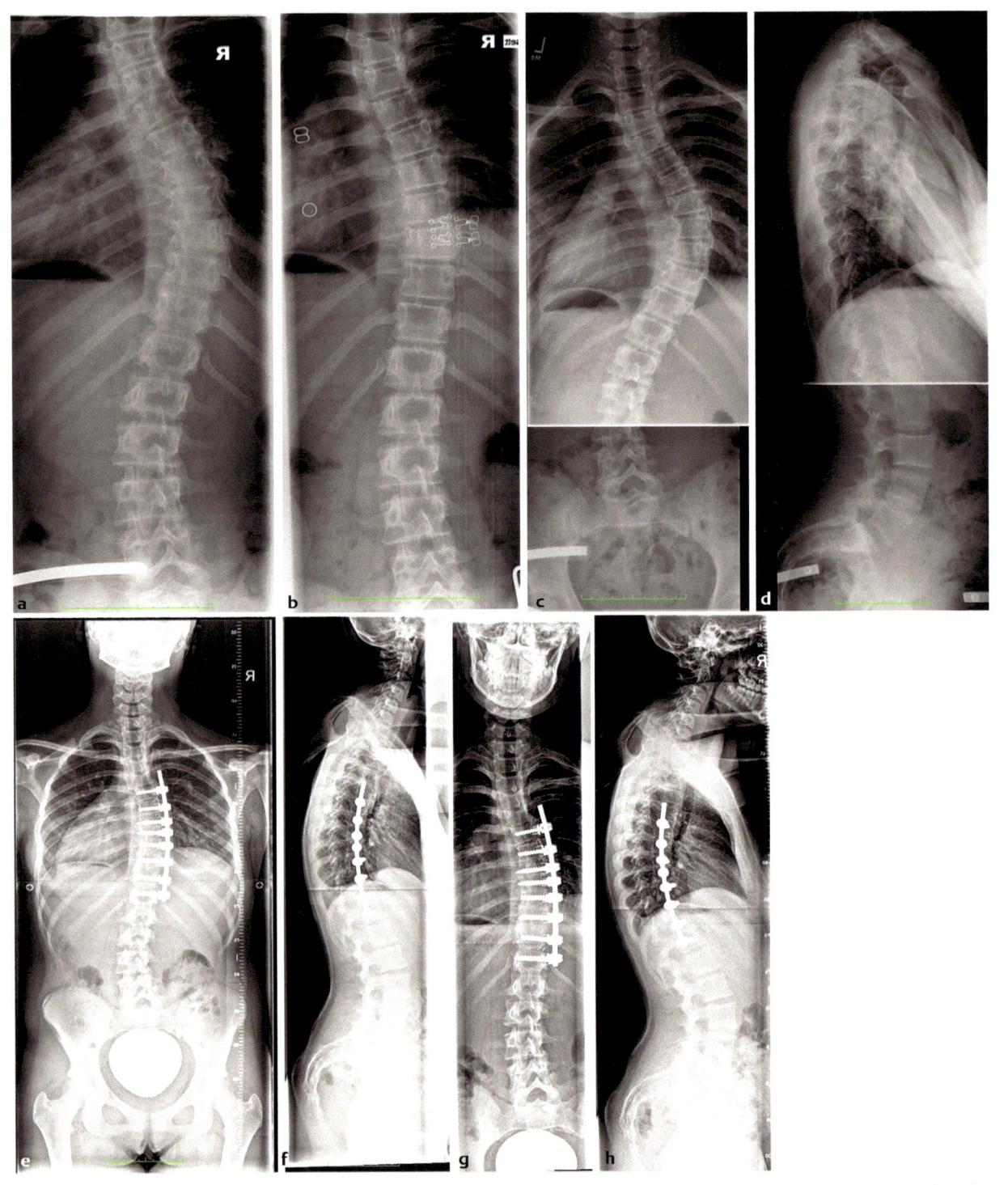

Fig. 4.46 (a) PA radiograph showing a Lenke type 1B right thoracic curve. You can see that the neutral vertebra is T12 or even T11. This is because, unlike case 1, the lumbar compensatory curve does have some structural change with rotation. Lumbar curve rotation has to turn the other way from the thoracic curve so effectively shortens the length of the thoracic curve whereas case 1 did not have such a lumbar problem. (b) This is only a moderate curve and so was initially braced. The PA radiograph shows that the curve looks better in the brace because flattening the lumbar lordosis causes thoracic hyperextension thus bringing the thoracic spine toward the midline. Of course once the brace is removed it lapses back to the original position or even worse and of course increases the lordosis. (c) PA radiograph after 18 months of brace wearing showing the futility of orthotic treatment. (d) Lateral radiograph showing that again there is flattening of the overall sagittal profile but an apical thoracic lordosis is still clearly visible. (e) PA radiograph after anterior instrumentation showing a nice correction with a well-balanced lazy-S configuration. (f) Lateral radiograph showing that a normal thoracic kyphosis has been restored. (g) PA radiograph at 2-year follow-up showing maintenance of the corrected position and (h) lateral radiograph at follow-up showing maintenance of a normal sagittal profile.

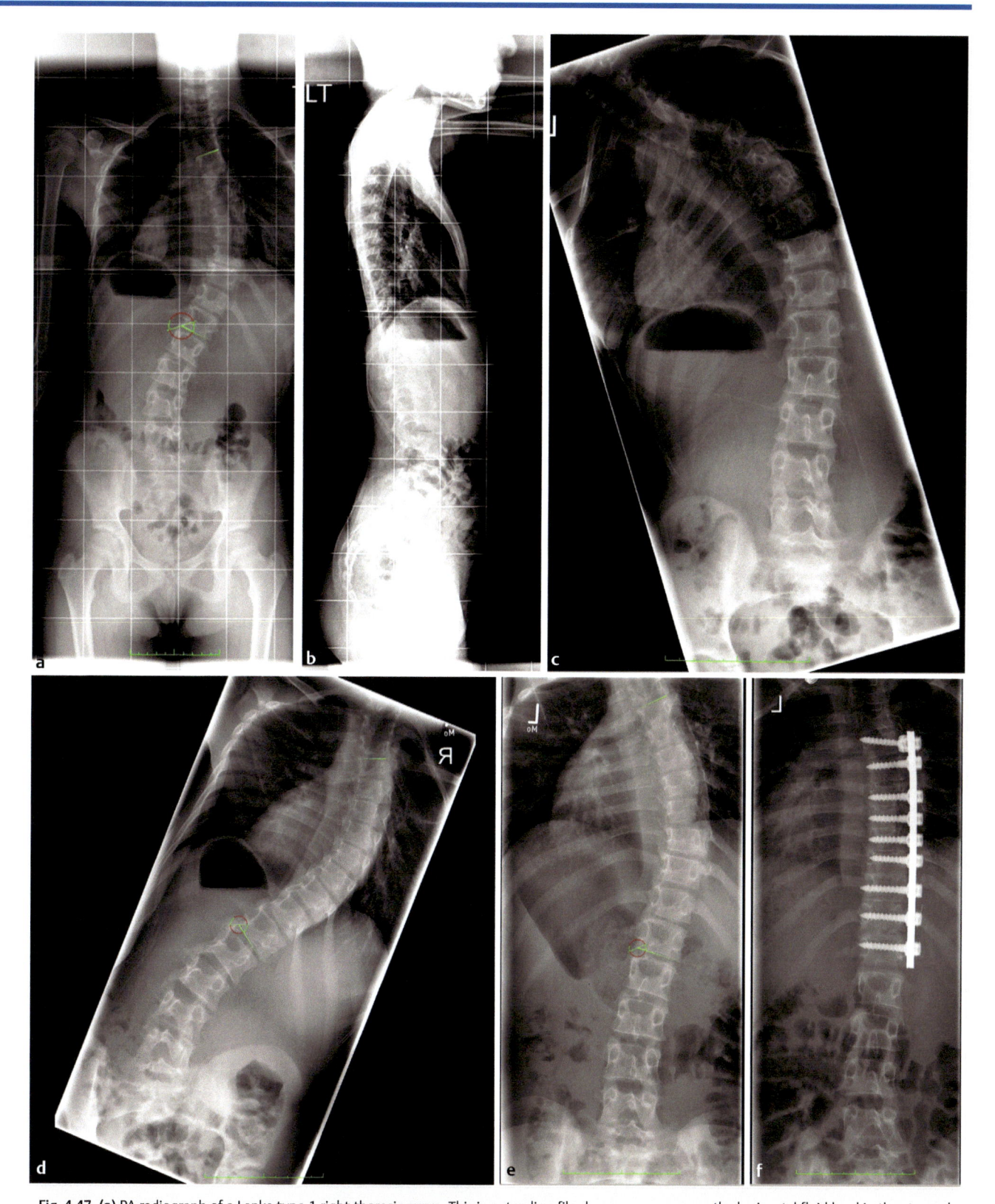

Fig. 4.47 **(a)** PA radiograph of a Lenke type 1 right thoracic curve. This is a standing film because you can see the horizontal fluid level in the stomach and note there is decompensation to the right side and, as always, this is because the lumbar compensatory curve is bigger than the upper thoracic compensatory curve (see ▶ Fig. 2.19). **(b)** Lateral radiograph showing a very long flat back with lordosis at the apex. **(c)** Side-bending film to the left showing that the lumbar spine does straighten out but no more than that. **(d)** Side-bending film to right showing that the thoracic curve is not very flexible. **(e)** PA stretch film showing better mobility of the thoracic curve. **(f)** PA radiograph postoperatively showing a nice correction.

Idiopathic Scoliosis

Comment

It was felt that there was sufficient mobility in the lumbar spine to allow an anterior selective fusion but with hindsight posterior instrumentation should have been selected down to probably L4 so that the decompensation at the time of presentation would not have recurred. These King type 4 curves always need long posterior fixation or would you accept a smidge of decompensation for a normal mobile healthy lumbar spine. Maybe you should ask the patient.

Despite reservations about axial distraction not affecting the apical region we like the PA stretch film because quite often it shows better flexibility of the thoracic curve than side bending, as in this case. Indeed, side bending may not be the best option at determining mobility of a thoracic curve in which case always do a stretch film because it can be very valuable as in this case.

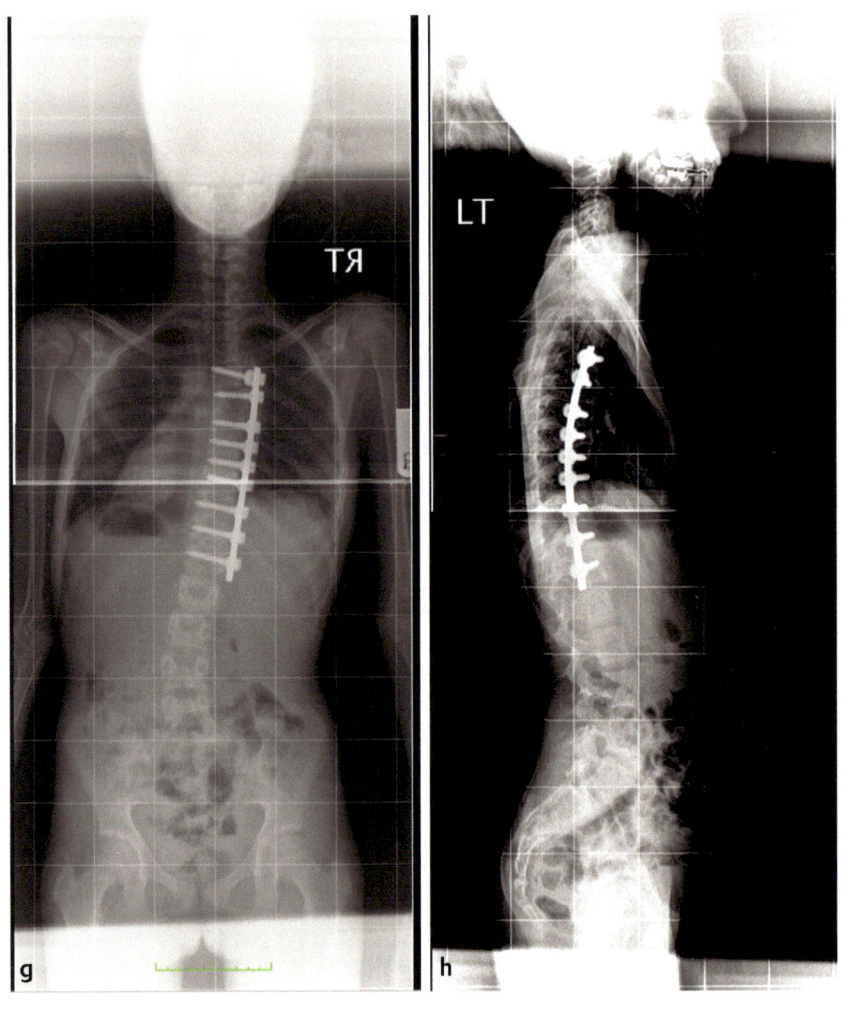

Fig. 4.47 (g,h) (*continued*) PA and lateral radiographs 2 years later showing maintenance of a very good correction.

Case 5: Posterior Instrumentation Only; King 4, Lenke 1

See ▶ Fig. 4.48a–e.

Comment

This is a perfect example of a King 4 out of balance thoracic curve which really isn't well covered by the Lenke classification. We have used stretch films from time to time and have found them of value in this kind of case to get more information as to how it might look after posterior instrumentation. These King 4 type curves must have long posterior instrumentation to get them back in balance and the PA correction is excellent in terms of curve size and balance in the frontal plane. The post-instrumentation lateral radiograph shows a flat thoracic spine and little alteration in the apical lordosis. This is the problem with posterior instrumentation only—namely, that it does not address the sagittal profile because the front of the spine isn't shortened.

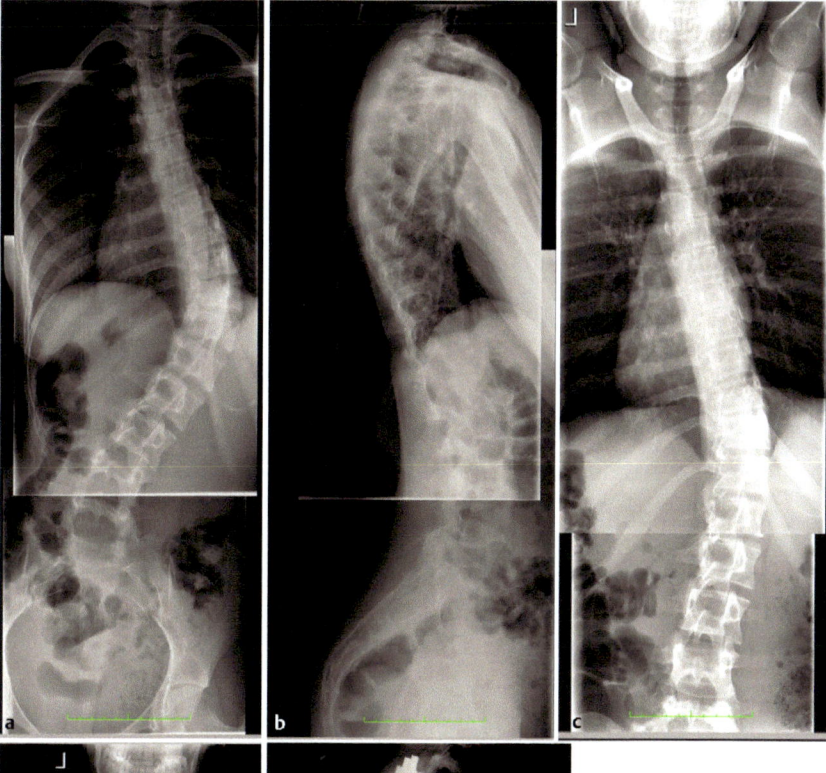

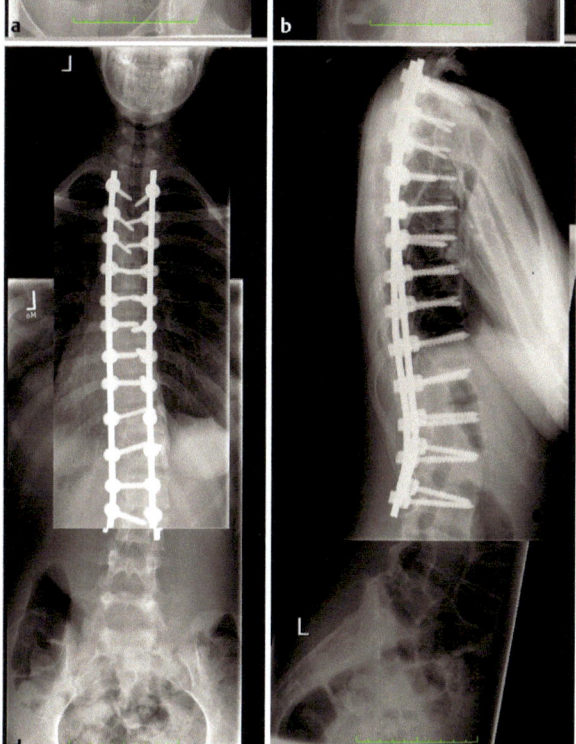

Fig. 4.48 (a) PA radiograph showing a long right thoracic curve with a low apex at T11, almost thoracolumbar. Again the lower lumbar compensatory curve is bigger than the upper thoracic compensatory curve and so the spine is out of balance. (b) Lateral radiograph showing a flat spine down to a lower lumbar lordosis. (c) PA stretch film. Although the thoracic curve corrects nicely, the spine would not be in balance if it wasn't being pulled at each end and the first neutral vertebra is at least L4 if not L5. (d) PA radiograph after posterior instrumentation down to L3 with a nice straight spine and well horizontalized L4 and L5. A very well balanced spine. (e) Lateral radiograph postoperatively showing a much flatter sagittal profile than one would like. The problem with posterior instrumentation only is that you cannot adequately influence the sagittal plane unless you do a preliminary anterior Leeds procedure (anterior release). Only then can you allow the spine to resume its normal sagittal profile and therefore help to untwist the apical region and thus address the rib hump.

Case 6: Posterior Instrumentation Only; Lenke 1c

See ▶ Fig. 4.49a–g.

Comment

The mobility of the lower curve facilitated selective thoracic fusion and this would have been a very good case for anterior thoracic instrumention thus having the benefit of optimal thoracic curve correction in both frontal and lateral planes. The end result was rather a "half way house" where the instrumentation was stopped at L3 allowing some lower lumbar mobility. Again the stretch film nicely reflects the ultimate correction.

Case 7: Combined—Anterior Diskectomy Then Posterior Instrumentation; Lenke 1AL

See ▶ Fig. 4.50a–i.

Comment

This was clearly a stiff curve to begin with and side bending confirmed that. That was fairly obvious from the initial PA film and so one might therefore question the need for a side-bending film. It is clear that anterior multiple diskectomy is required as a first stage and it achieved significant improvement in rotation which is not possible with posterior surgery only. It is also possible to re-create a natural thoracic kyphosis not achievable without an anterior first stage. We should have probably done anterior instrumentation while we were there! With a sound anterior and posterior fusion and maintenance of the original correction 2-year follow-up is quite sufficient particularly as in this case like many others the patient comes from some distance away outside Europe and so doesn't feel the need for any further follow-up.

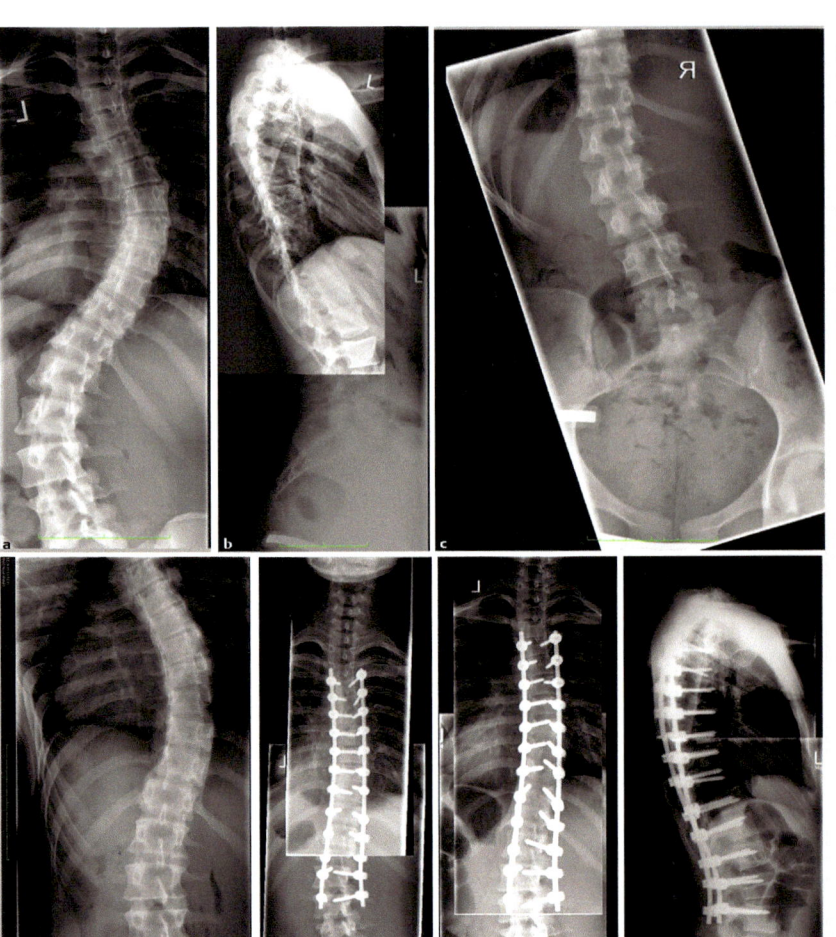

Fig. 4.49 (a) PA radiograph of a Lenke 1C right thoracic curve. (b) Lateral radiograph seeming to show a thoracic pseudokyphosis because there is a lot of rotation. Indeed, you can see the rib hump. (c) Side-bending film to the left shows a reasonably flexible lumbar curve. (d) Stretch film showing the thoracic curve is much more significant than the lumbar one. (e) PA radiograph after posterior instrumentation down to L3 saving three lower lumbar disks. (f) PA radiograph at 2-year follow-up showing maintenance of the original fixation and a well-balanced very gentle lazy-S configuration. (g) Lateral radiograph at follow-up showing a reasonable lateral profile.

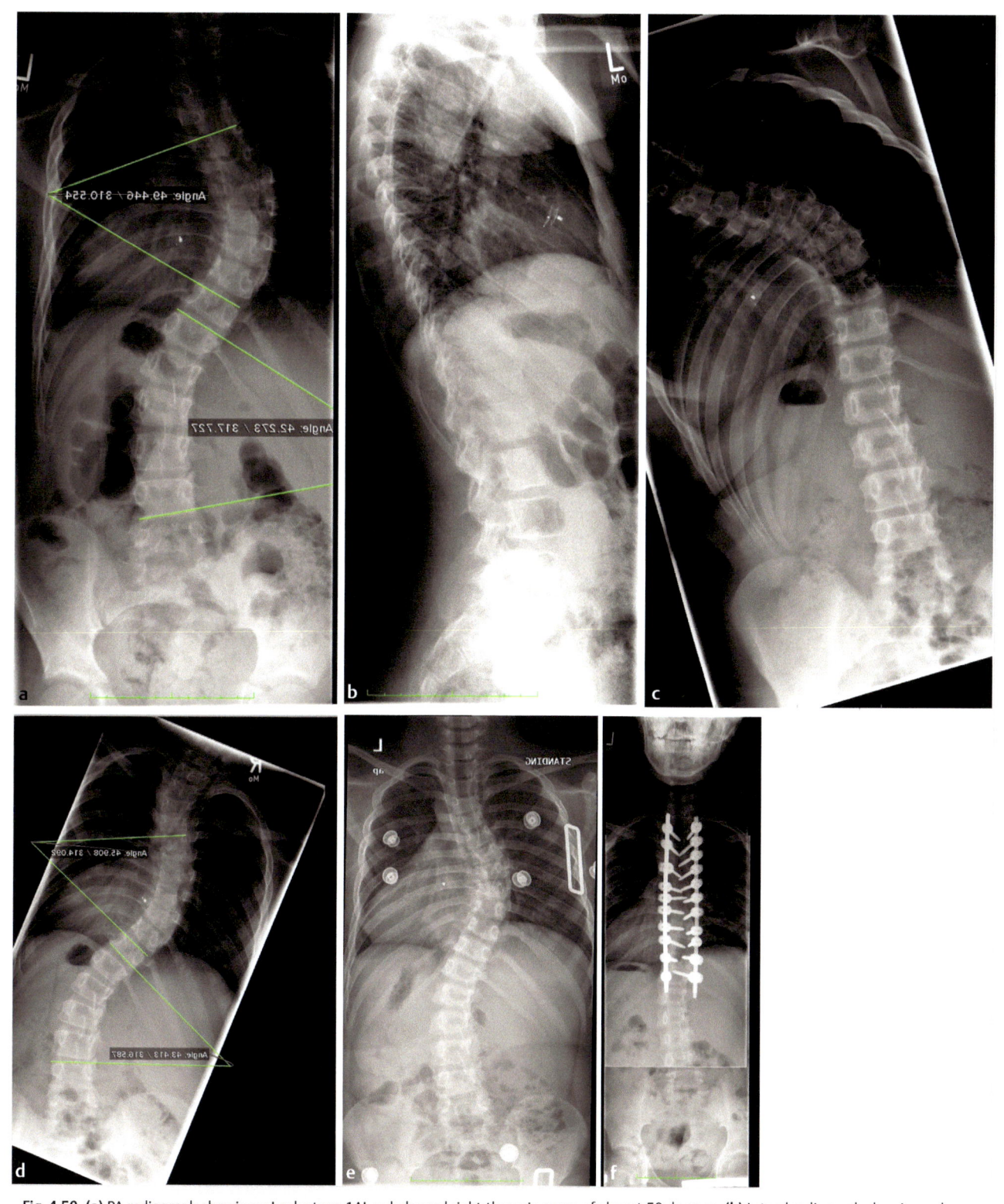

Fig. 4.50 (a) PA radiograph showing a Lenke type 1AL unbalanced right thoracic curve of almost 50 degrees. (b) Lateral radiograph showing a degree of thoracic pseudokyphosis indicating a lot of rotation. (c) Side-bending radiograph to the left showing that the lumbar spine nicely straightens below the thoracic spine. (d) Side-bending film to the right showing no significant change in the thoracic curve. (e) PA radiograph after anterior multiple diskectomy showing good initial curve correction and significant improvement in rotation (compare ribs with [a]). (f) PA radiograph after posterior selective thoracic instrumentation showing an excellent correction and a well-balanced spine.

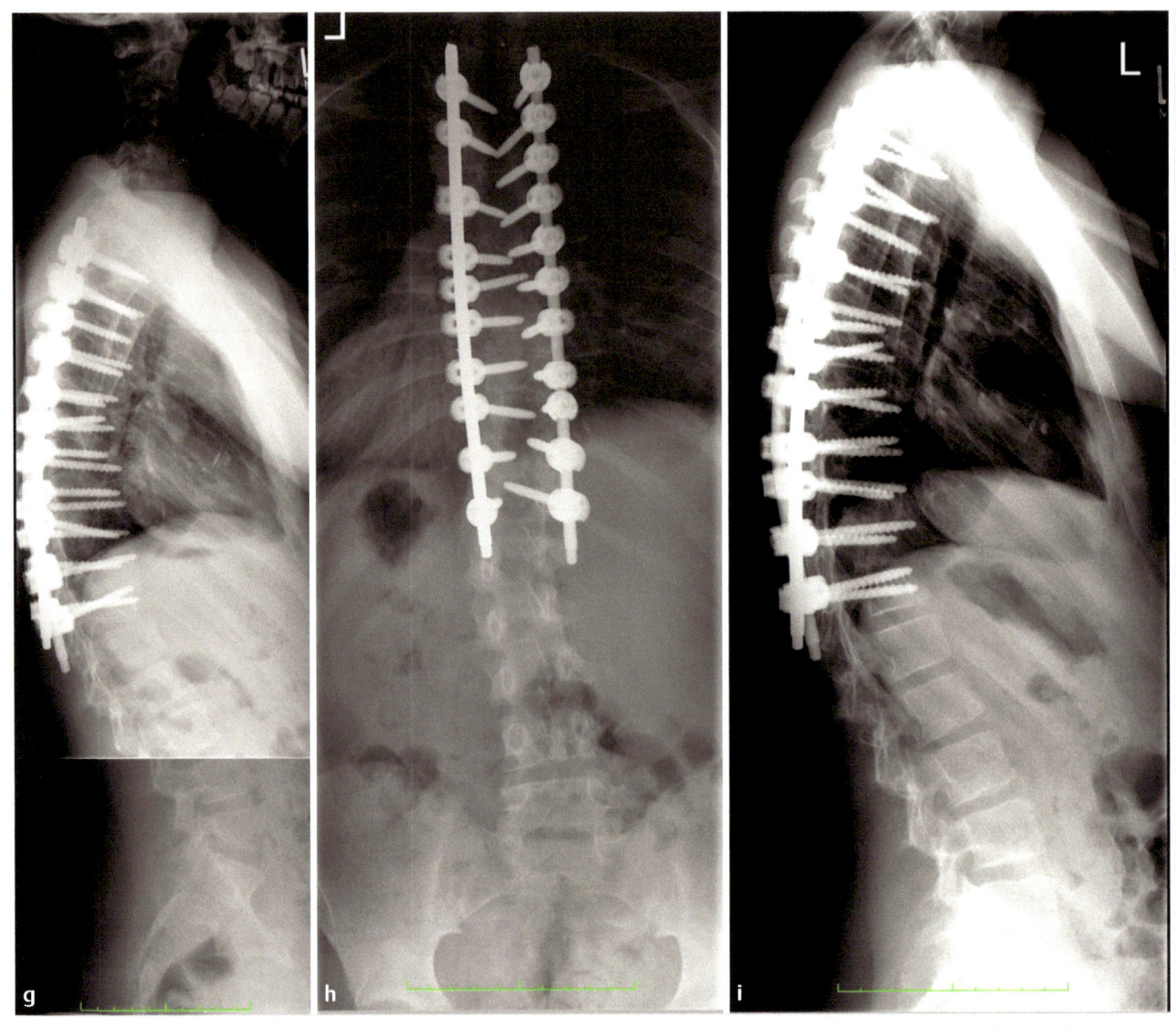

Fig. 4.50 (g) (*continued*) Lateral radiograph showing restoration of a natural thoracic kyphosis. **(h)** PA radiograph at 2-year follow-up showing maintenance of the excellent position. **(i)** Lateral radiograph at follow-up showing better development of the lumbar lordosis below the instrumentation.

Case 8: Combined—Anterior Diskectomy Then Posterior Instrumentation; Lenke 1AL

See ▶ Fig. 4.51a–h.

Comment

The initial PA film shows a significant amount of rotation with rib asymmetry as well as curve size (Cobb angle 90 degrees or so). This mandates a preliminary anterior multiple diskectomy. Note also the upper thoracic compensatory curve has undergone structural change; now the spinous processes point to the right. At this stage the shoulders are level and it will be very important to take the posterior instrumentation high enough to maintain shoulder balance. A guide to the importance of this is shown in the PA radiograph after anterior multiple diskectomy where improvement in the thoracic curve tilted the spine into a Lenke 2 thoracic double major with a signe d'epaule. It will be necessary therefore to take the instrumentation to at least T2 to improve/correct the signe d'epaule deformity. The PA post-instrumentation shows the considerable improvement in the shoulder imbalance that has occurred. Also note the almost symmetrical ribs on each side indicating that by creating kyphosis (**h**) led to significant spinal derotation which of course is what the patient with the rib hump really wants.

Idiopathic Scoliosis

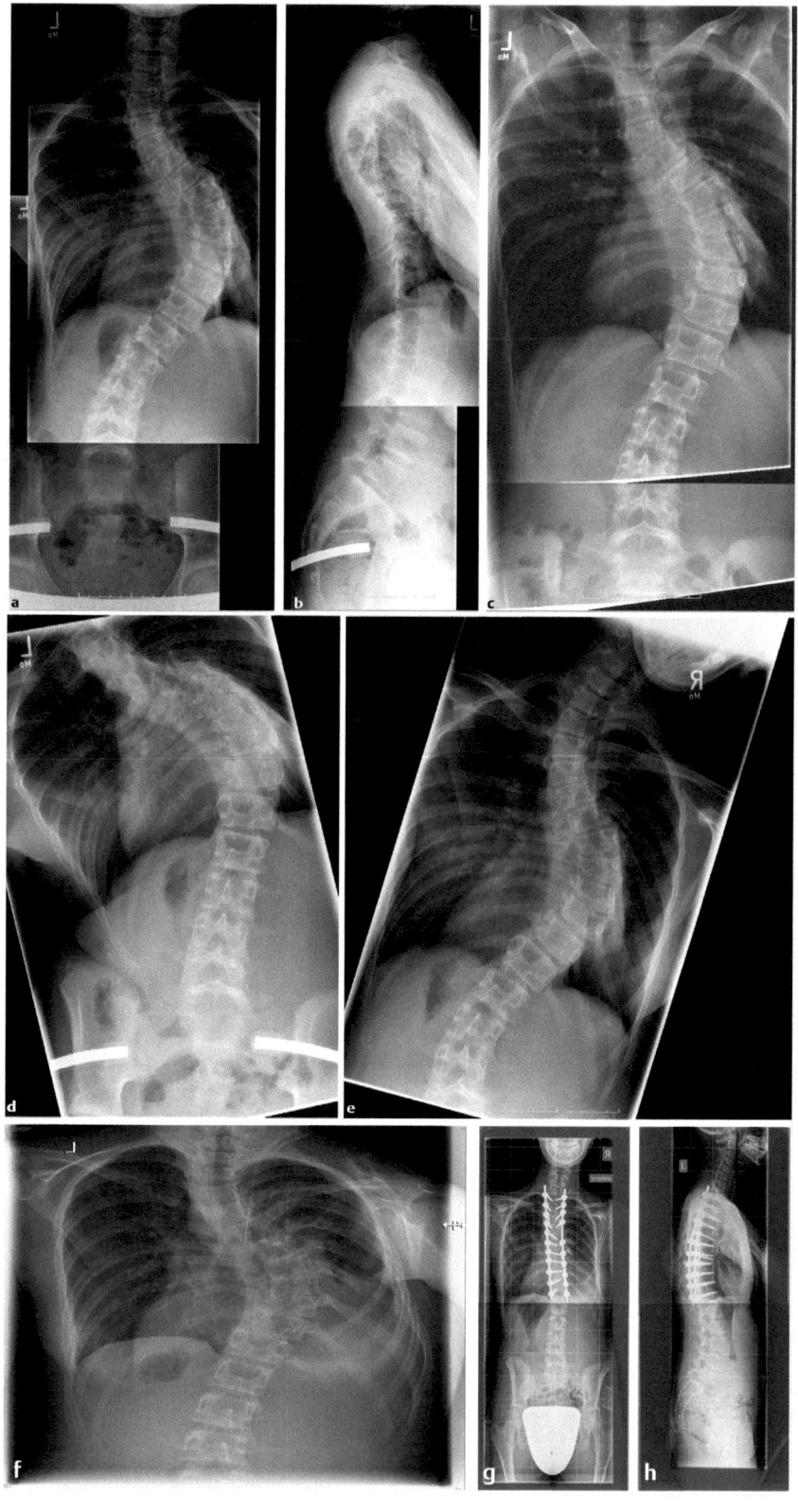

Fig. 4.51 (a) PA radiograph showing a rather low apex right thoracic scoliosis of considerable magnitude and therefore stiffness. The necks of the convex ribs overlap the spine indicating a lot of rotation. (b) Lateral radiograph showing an overall thoracolumbar lordosis. (c) PA stretch film showing only a modest improvement in the structural curve. (d) Side-bending film to the left showing good straightening of the lumbar spine below. (e) Side-bending film to the right showing no significant improvement in either the size of the right thoracic curve or the rotation. (f) PA radiograph after anterior multiple diskectomy showing improvement in both curve size, rotation, and rib overlap. Note that the disk spaces have closed down after diskectomy. (g) PA radiograph after posterior selective instrumentation showing a well-balanced spine. Importantly not only is there a great improvement in Cobb angle but also in rotation with marked restoration of rib symmetry. Comparing this radiograph with the preoperative one (a) it is difficult to see how three-dimensional improvement can occur without anterior multiple diskectomy. (h) Lateral radiograph post-instrumentation showing restoration of a natural sagittal thoracolumbar profile.

Idiopathic Scoliosis

Case 9: Thoracolumbar/Lumbar; Single Lenke 5

See ▶ Fig. 4.52a–g.

Comment

This sort of curve is begging for short segment anterior instrumentation. The lateral bend to the right shows that both L2/3 and L3/4 open up and so either L2 or L3 could have been selected as the LIV. Do you really want to do a long posterior instrumentation?

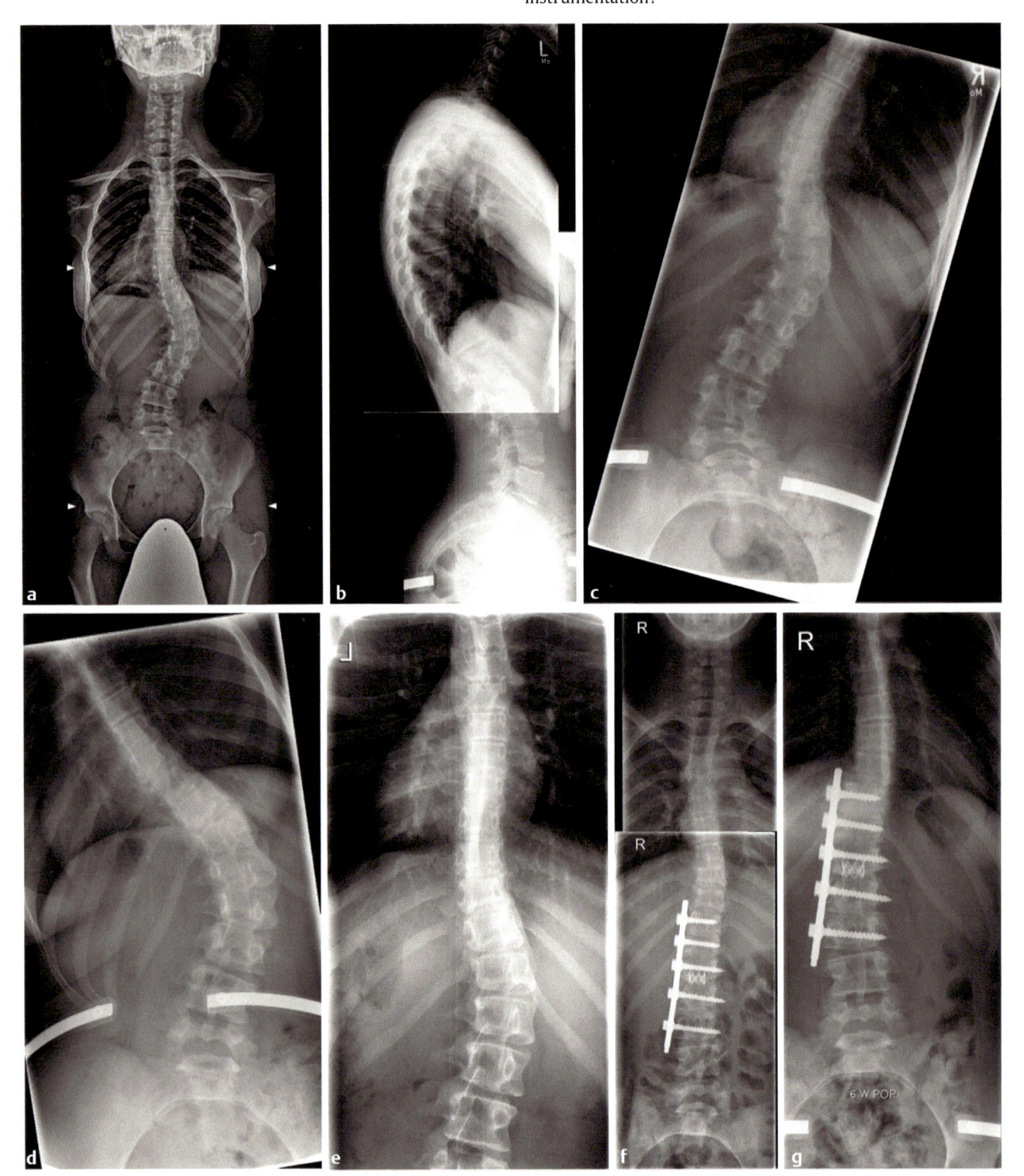

Fig. 4.52 (a) PA radiograph of a right thoracolumbar curve. (b) Lateral radiograph showing that when the thoracic spine is not involved then there is a natural thoracic kyphosis but there is of course a long lordosis from the thoracolumbar spine downward. (c) Side-bending film to the right showing reasonable flexibility and both L2/3 and L3/4 open up on the left side. There now appears to be a small left thoracic curve above. (d) Side-bending film to the left and whatever was in the thoracic spine on the side bend to the right certainly has straightened. (e) Stretch film showing good overall correction and in balance. (f) PA radiograph after anterior short segment instrumentation down to L3. There is a mild thoracic curve to the left above but the spine looks in perfect balance. (g) PA radiograph at follow-up showing a well-balanced and well corrected nice lazy-S configuration.

Case 10: Double Curves; Lenke 6

See ▶ Fig. 4.53a–h.

Comment

Although the thoracolumbar curve was flexible on side bending it wasn't mobile enough to allow anterior selective thoracic instrumentation. Consequently, the optimal result is obtained by posterior instrumentation. The thoracic curve did not show much rotation on the PA film. The side-bending film did not show a lot of flexibility. However, in the younger adolescent with, say, 2 or 3 years of growth to go, it would be well worthwhile carrying out anterior instrumentation of the thoracolumbar curve and see whether the thoracic curve above would improve with the passage of time as is often the case. That would definitely have been an option here.

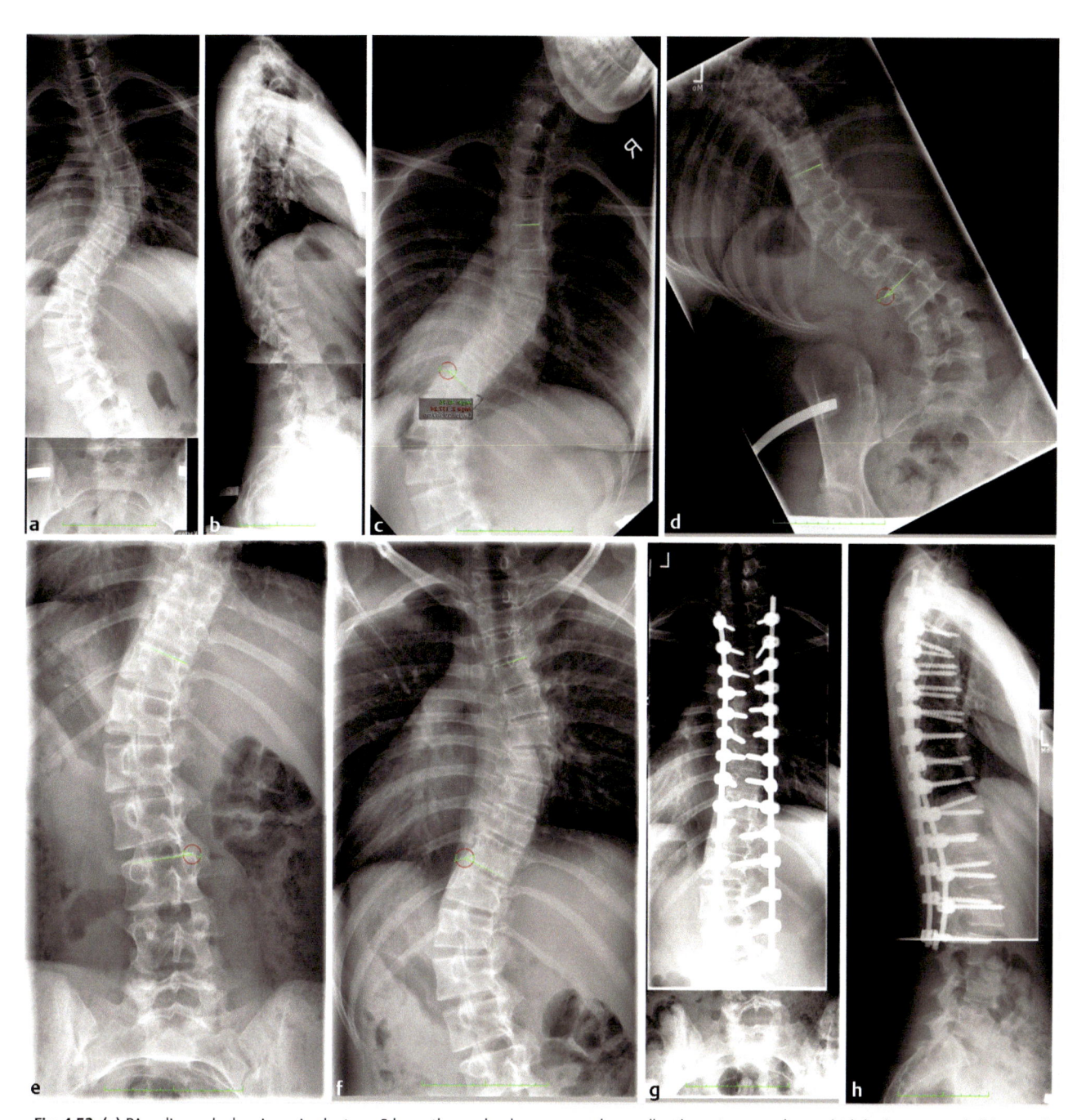

Fig. 4.53 (a) PA radiograph showing a Lenke type 6 large thoracolumbar curve and a smaller thoracic curve above which looks structural. (b) Lateral radiograph showing a flat overall profile with a bit of thoracolumbar pseudokyphosis. (c) Side-bending film to the right showing no significant improvement in the thoracic curve. (d) Side-bending film to the left showing considerable improvement in the thoracolumbar curve, perhaps more so than one would expect. (e) Stretch film from S1 up showing more flexibility in the thoracolumbar curve than to be expected. (f) Stretch film from T1 down showing more improvement in the upper thoracic curve than the side-bending view. (g) PA radiograph after posterior instrumentation from T2 to L3. (h) Lateral radiograph post-surgery showing a flat thoracic spine but reasonable lateral profile below.

Idiopathic Scoliosis

Case 11: Double Thoracic/Lumbar; Lenke 3

See ▶ Fig. 4.54a–h.

Comment

Although there seems to be good mobility of the upper thoracic curve on side bending and it was therefore hoped that the level shoulders would remain the same postoperatively at follow-up there is a slightly higher left shoulder, fortunately not unacceptable to the patient. It would have been better to have gone up higher with the instrumentation.

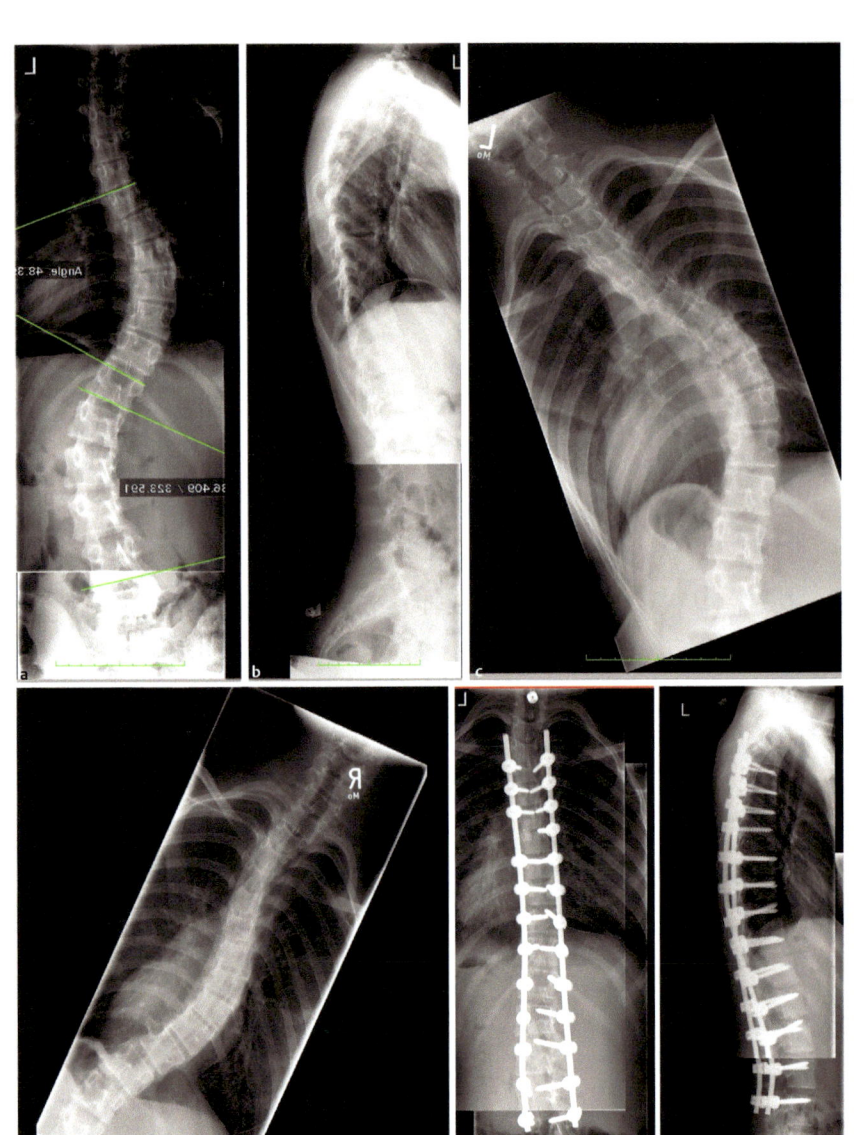

Fig. 4.54 (a) PA radiograph of a Lenke 3 right thoracic left lumbar double structural curve. (b) Lateral radiograph showing the usual very flat sagittal profile of the double curve. *Note there is no junctional kyphosis*. (c) Side-bending film to the left showing no concerns about flexibility of the high thoracic curve, note also that the lumbar curve stacks nicely vertically. (d) Side-bending film to the right showing that the thoracic curve is to a degree flexible. (e) PA radiograph after posterior instrumentation down to L4. (f) Lateral radiograph showing a better sagittal profile.

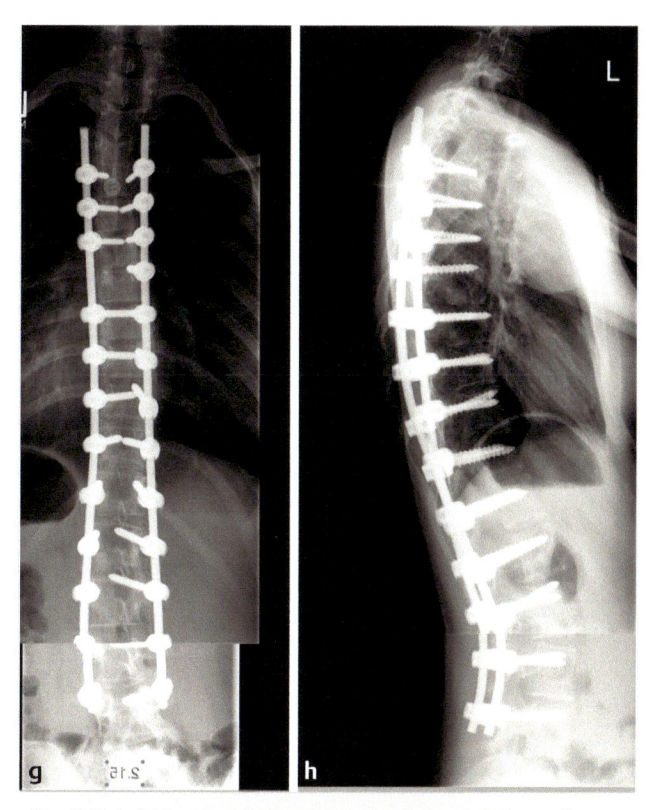

Fig. 4.54 (g,h) (*continued*) PA and lateral radiograph 2.5 years later showing maintenance of the excellent correction.

Case 12

See ▶ Fig. 4.55a–f.

Comment

One should never ignore nonidiopathic features in seemingly idiopathic cases. Pain, stiffness, and unusual curve patterns such as left thoracic are "red flags" for something potentially nasty which can indeed be a tumor or a significant intraspinal anomaly such as shown in this case. Of course a left thoracic curve pattern is not always pathological but an MRI scan is mandated to exclude that possibility or indeed confirm a problem as in this case. There are no short cuts in spinal surgery so don't be caught out.

Idiopathic Scoliosis

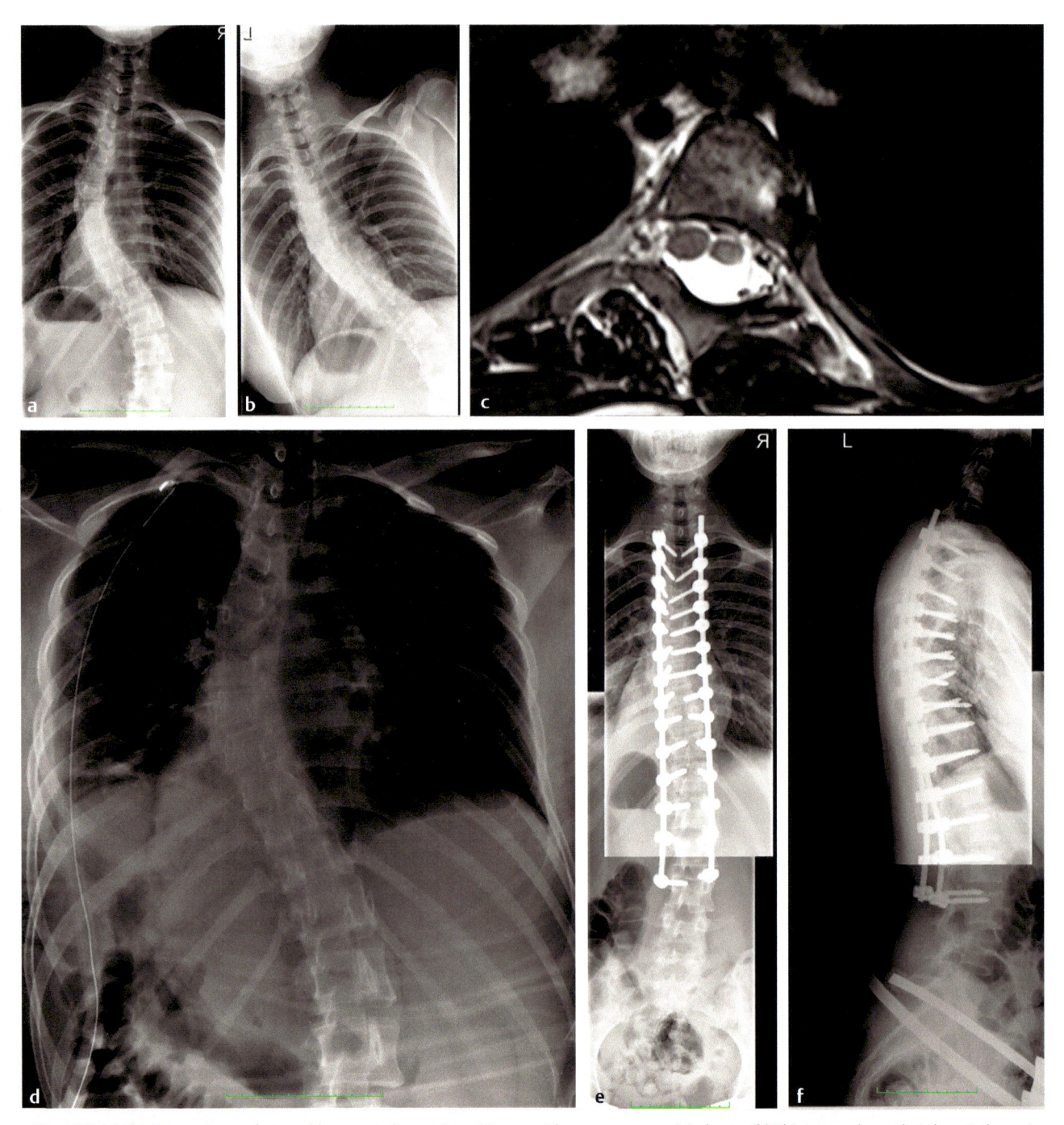

Fig. 4.55 (a) This image shows what would appear to be an idiopathic curve. There was no associated pain. (b) This image shows that there is the sort of flexibility one would expect on side bending of such a curve. Note however that the direction for this thoracic curve is convex to the left which is an unusual feature. All curves going to surgery should routinely have an MRI scan but in this seemingly idiopathic case an unusual curve direction certainly mandates a good look at the contents of the spinal canal. (c) This image shows the appearances of a typical diastematomyelia which extended from D5 to D11. There is always a danger with a tethered cord over such a length of the cord being stretched or in another way insulted if there is just posterior instrumentation and so these appearances mandated an anterior multiple discectomy first stage to allow the spine to shorten spontaneously (d). There has already been some improvement in the curve size because of shortening over the apical region. (e,f) These images are from after posterior transpedicular instrumentation with no attempt at lengthening of the deformity. There has been an excellent correction and a well balanced spine with no neurological complications.

We hope that you have enjoyed these cases and learned something from them; perhaps the most obvious point is that anterior multiple diskectomy plus growth plate removal (the Leeds procedure) produces optimal flexibility with shortening over the apical region and produces optimal correction of the scoliosis but more importantly achieves significant apical derotation. With removal of the cartilage endplates this prevents any danger of recurrence of the deformity and leads to a sound anterior interbody fusion.

References

Note: References in **bold** are Key References.

[1] Moe JH. The Milwaukee brace in the treatment of scoliosis. Clin Orthop Relat Res. 1971; 77(77):18–31

[2] Goldstein LA, Waugh TR. Classification and terminology of scoliosis. Clin Orthop Relat Res. 1973(93):10–22

[3] **Weinstein SL, Ponseti IV. Curve progression in idiopathic scoliosis. J Bone Joint Surg Am. 1983; 65(4):447–455**

[4] **Nachemson A. A long term follow-up study of non-treated scoliosis. Acta Orthop Scand. 1968; 39(4):466–476**

[5] Nilsonne U, Lundgren KD. Long-term prognosis in idiopathic scoliosis. Acta Orthop Scand. 1968; 39(4):456–465

[6] Collis DK, Ponseti IV. Long-term follow-up of patients with idiopathic scoliosis not treated surgically. J Bone Joint Surg Am. 1969; 51(3):425–445

[7] Bengtsson G, Fällström K, Jansson B, Nachemson A. A psychological and psychiatric investigation of the adjustment of female scoliosis patients. Acta Psychiatr Scand. 1974; 50(1):50–59

[8] Harrington PR. Treatment of scoliosis. Correction and internal fixation by spine instrumentation. J Bone Joint Surg Am. 1962; 44-A:591–610

[9] Mellencamp DD, Blount WP, Anderson AJ. Milwaukee brace treatment of idiopathic scoliosis: late results. Clin Orthop Relat Res. 1977(126):47–57

[10] Carr WA, Moe JH, Winter RB, Lonstein JE. Treatment of idiopathic scoliosis in the Milwaukee brace. J Bone Joint Surg Am. 1980; 62(4):599–612

[11] Brooks HL, Azen SP, Gerberg E, Brooks R, Chan L. Scoliosis: A prospective epidemiological study. J Bone Joint Surg Am. 1975; 57(7):968–972

[12] Lonstein JE. Screening for spinal deformities in Minnesota schools. Clin Orthop Relat Res. 1977(126):33–42

[13] Adair IV, Van Wijk MC, Armstrong GWD. Moiré topography in scoliosis screening. Clin Orthop Relat Res. 1977(129):165–171

[14] Rogala EJ, Drummond DS, Gurr J. Scoliosis: incidence and natural history. A prospective epidemiological study. J Bone Joint Surg Am. 1978; 60(2):173–176

[15] **Pehrsson K, Bake B, Larsson S, Nachemson A. Lung function in adult idiopathic scoliosis: a 20 year follow up. Thorax. 1991; 46(7):474–478**

[16] Reid L. Lung growth. In: Zorab PA (ed). Scoliosis and growth. Proceedings of a Third Symposium. Edinburgh: Churchill Livingstone; 1971

[17] **Davies G, Reid L. Effect of scoliosis on growth of alveoli and pulmonary arteries and on right ventricle. Arch Dis Child. 1971; 46(249):623–632**

[18] **Branthwaite MA. Cardiorespiratory consequences of unfused idiopathic scoliosis. Br J Dis Chest. 1986; 80(4):360–369**

[19] **Dickson RA. Conservative treatment for idiopathic scoliosis. J Bone Joint Surg Br. 1985; 67(2):176–181**

[20] Commission on Chronic Illness. Chronic illness in the United States, Vol I. Cambridge, MA: Harvard University Press; 1957

[21] Whitby LG. Screening for disease: Definitions and criteria. Lancet. 1974; 2(7884):819–822

[22] Bunnell WP. An objective criterion for scoliosis screening. J Bone Joint Surg Am. 1984; 66(9):1381–1387

[23] Oxborrow N, Gopal S, Walder A, et al. A new surface topographical measure of spinal shape in scoliosis. J Bone Joint Surg Br. 1998; 80 Supp III:276–277

[24] Richards BS, Vitale MG. Screening for idiopathic scoliosis in adolescents. An information statement. J Bone Joint Surg Am. 2008; 90(1):195–198

[25] **Stirling AJ, Howel D, Millner PA, Sadiq S, Sharples D, Dickson RA. Late-onset idiopathic scoliosis in children six to fourteen years old. A cross-sectional prevalence study. J Bone Joint Surg Am. 1996; 78(9):1330–1336**

[26] Dickson RA, Stamper P, Sharp A-M, Harker P. School screening for scoliosis: cohort study of clinical course. BMJ. 1980; 281(6235):265–267

[27] Inkster RG. Osteology. In: Brash JC (ed). Cunningham's textbook of anatomy. 9th ed. London: Oxford Medical; 1953:136

[28] Kouwenhoven JWM, Vincken KL, Bartels LW, Castelein RM. Analysis of pre-existent vertebral rotation in the normal spine. Spine. 2006; 31(13):1467–1472

[29] **Kouwenhoven JWM, Bartels LW, Vincken KL, et al. The relation between organ anatomy and pre-existent vertebral rotation in the normal spine: magnetic resonance imaging study in humans with situs inversus totalis. Spine. 2007; 32(10):1123–1128**

[30] **Deacon P, Archer IA, Dickson RA. Idiopathic scoliosis – biomechanics and biology. Orthopaedics. 1987; 10:897–903**

[31] **Smith RM, Pool RD, Butt WP, Dickson RA. The transverse plane deformity of structural scoliosis. Spine. 1991; 16(9):1126–1129**

[32] Lonstein JE, Carlson JM. The prediction of curve progression in untreated idiopathic scoliosis during growth. J Bone Joint Surg Am. 1984; 66(7):1061–1071

[33] Risser JC. The Iliac apophysis; an invaluable sign in the management of scoliosis. Clin Orthop. 1958; 11(11):111–119

[34] Mehta MH. The rib-vertebra angle in the early diagnosis between resolving and progressive infantile scoliosis. J Bone Joint Surg Br. 1972; 54(2):230–243

[35] **Bernick S, Cailliet R. Vertebral end-plate changes with aging of human vertebrae. Spine. 1982; 7(2):97–102**

[36] **Howell FR, Mahood JK, Dickson RA. Growth beyond skeletal maturity. Spine. 1992; 17(4):437–440**

[37] Blount WP, Mellencamp D. The effect of pregnancy on idiopathic scoliosis. J Bone Joint Surg Am. 1980; 62(7):1083–1087

[38] Berman AT, Cohen DL, Schwentker EP. The effects of pregnancy on idiopathic scoliosis. A preliminary report on eight cases and a review of the literature. Spine. 1982; 7(1):76–77

[39] Bunnell WP. The natural history of idiopathic scoliosis before skeletal maturity. Spine. 1986; 11(8):773–776

[40] Nachemson A, Cochran TP, Irstam L, Fallstrom K. Pregnancy after scoliosis treatment. Presented at SRS annual meeting, Montreal

[41] **Weinstein SL. Natural history. Spine. 1999; 24(24):2592–2600**

[42] Weinstein SL, Zavala DC, Ponseti IV. Idiopathic scoliosis: long-term follow-up and prognosis in untreated patients. J Bone Joint Surg Am. 1981; 63(5):702–712

[43] Xiong B, Sevastik JA. A physiological approach to surgical treatment of progressive early idiopathic scoliosis. Eur Spine J. 1998; 7(6):505–508

[44] Dubousset J. Signe d'epaule taught by Pierre Queneau, Personal communication via email, February 2015

[45] Ardran GM, Coates R, Dickson RA, Dixon-Brown A, Harding FM. Assessment of scoliosis in children: low dose radiographic technique. Br J Radiol. 1980; 53(626):146–147

[46] De Smet AA, Fritz SL, Asher MA. A method for minimizing the radiation exposure from scoliosis radiographs. J Bone Joint Surg Am. 1981; 63(1):156–161

[47] Tanner JM, Whitehouse RH, Takaishi M. Standards from birth to maturity for height, weight, height velocity, and weight velocity: British children, 1965. II. Arch Dis Child. 1966; 41(220):613–635

[48] Negrini S, Negrini F, Fusco C, Zaina F. Idiopathic scoliosis patients with curves more than 45 Cobb degrees refusing surgery can be effectively treated through bracing with curve improvements. Spine J. 2011; 11(5):369–380

[49] Tanner JM, Whitehouse RH. Height standard chart. Hounslow: Printwell; 1959

[50] Smith FM, Latchford G, Hall RM, Millner PA, Dickson RA. Indications of disordered eating behaviour in adolescent patients with idiopathic scoliosis. J Bone Joint Surg Br. 2002; 84(3):392–394

[51] King HA, Moe JH, Bradford DS, Winter RB. The selection of fusion levels in thoracic idiopathic scoliosis. J Bone Joint Surg Am. 1983; 65(9):1302–1313

[52] Lenke LG, Betz RR, Haher TR, et al. Multisurgeon assessment of surgical decision-making in adolescent idiopathic scoliosis: curve classification, operative approach, and fusion levels. Spine. 2001; 26(21):2347–2353

[53] Dubousset J, Herring JA, Shufflebarger H. The crankshaft phenomenon. J Pediatr Orthop. 1989; 9(5):541–550

[54] Moe JH. A critical analysis of methods of fusion for scoliosis; an evaluation in two hundred and sixty-six patients. J Bone Joint Surg Am. 1958; 40-A(3):529–554, passim

[55] Moe JH. Methods of correction and surgical techniques in scoliosis. Orthop Clin North Am. 1972; 3(1):17–48

[56] **Harrington PR. Technical details in relation to the successful use of instrumentation in scoliosis. Orthop Clin North Am. 1972; 3(1):49–67**

[57] **Dickson RA, Lawton JO, Archer IA, Butt WP. The pathogenesis of idiopathic scoliosis. Biplanar spinal asymmetry. J Bone Joint Surg Br. 1984; 66(1):8–15**

[58] **Deacon P, Flood BM, Dickson RA. Idiopathic scoliosis in three dimensions. A radiographic and morphometric analysis. J Bone Joint Surg Br. 1984; 66(4):509–512**

[59] **Deacon P, Berkin CR, Dickson RA. Combined idiopathic kyphosis and scoliosis. An analysis of the lateral spinal curvatures associated with Scheuermann's disease. J Bone Joint Surg Br. 1985; 67(2):189–192**

[60] Dickson RA. Aetiology of idiopathic spinal deformities. Arch Dis Child. 1985; 60(6):508–511

[61] Dickson RA. Scoliosis: how big are you? Orthopedics. 1987; 10(6):881–887

[62] du Peloux J, Fauchet R, Faucon B, Stagnara P. Le plan d'election pour l'examen radiologique des cypho-scolioses. Rev Chir Orthop Repar Appar Mot. 1965; 51:517–524

[63] Winter RB, Moe JH, Bradford DS, et al. Spine deformity in neurofibromatosis. A review of 102 patients. J Bone Joint Surg Am. 1979; 61:677–694

[64] Cruickshank JL, Koike M, Dickson RA. Curve patterns in idiopathic scoliosis. A clinical and radiographic study. J Bone Joint Surg Br. 1989; 71(2):259–263

[65] Newton PO, Upasami VV. Surgical treatment of the right thoracic curve pattern. In: Newton P, O'Brien M, Shufflebarger HL, Betz RR, Dickson RA, Harms J (eds). Idiopathic scoliosis. The Harms Study Group Treatment Guide. New York: Thieme; 2010:200–223

[66] Halm H, Richter A, Thomsen B, Köszegvary M, Ahrens M, Quante M. [Anterior scoliosis surgery. State of the art and a comparison with posterior techniques]. Orthopade. 2009; 38(2):131–134, 136–140, 142–145

[67] Dickson RA, Archer IA, Deacon P. The Surgical Management of Idiopathic Thoracic Scoliosis. J Orthopaedic Surgical Techniques. 1985; 1:23–28

[68] Dickson RA, Archer IA. Surgical treatment of late-onset idiopathic thoracic scoliosis. The Leeds procedure. J Bone Joint Surg Br. 1987; 69(5):709–714

[69] Dickson RA. Idiopathic scoliosis: foundation for physiological treatment. Ann R Coll Surg Engl. 1987; 69(3):89–96

[70] Millner PA, Dickson RA. Idiopathic scoliosis: biomechanics and biology. Eur Spine J. 1996; 5(6):362–373

[71] Bradford DS. Juvenile kyphosis. Clin Orthop Relat Res. 1977(128):45–55

[72] Bradford DS, Moe JH, Montalvo FJ, Winter RB. Scheuermann's kyphosis and roundback deformity. Results of Milwaukee brace treatment. J Bone Joint Surg Am. 1974; 56(4):740–758

[73] Shah SA. The case for bracing. In: Newton P, O'Brien M, Shufflebarger HL, Betz RR, Dickson RA, Harms J (eds). Idiopathic scoliosis. The Harms Study Group Treatment Guide. New York: Thieme; 2010:88

[74] Miller JAA, Nachemson AL, Schultz AB. Effectiveness of braces in mild idiopathic scoliosis. Spine. 1984; 9(6):632–635

[75] Goldberg CJ, Dowling FE, Hall JE, Emans JB. A statistical comparison between natural history of idiopathic scoliosis and brace treatment in skeletally immature adolescent girls. Spine. 1993; 18(7):902–908

[76] Nachemson AL, Peterson L-E. Effectiveness of treatment with a brace in girls who have adolescent idiopathic scoliosis. A prospective, controlled study based on data from the Brace Study of the Scoliosis Research Society. J Bone Joint Surg Am. 1995; 77(6):815–822

[77] Peterson L-E, Nachemson AL. Prediction of progression of the curve in girls who have adolescent idiopathic scoliosis of moderate severity. Logistic regression analysis based on data from The Brace Study of the Scoliosis Research Society. J Bone Joint Surg Am. 1995; 77(6):823–827

[78] Jones WHS. Hippocrates (4 vols). London: Heinemann; 1922–1931

[79] Cotrel Y, Morel G. La technique de l'EDF dans la correction des scoliosis. Rev Chir Orthop. 1964; 50:59–75

[80] Blount WP, Moe JH. The Milwaukee Brace. Baltimore: Williams & Wilkins; 1973

[81] Alexander RG. The effects on tooth position and maxillofacial vertical growth during treatment of scoliosis with the Milwaukee brace. Am J Orthod. 1966; 52(3):161–189

[82] Sackett DL, Richardson WAS, Rosenberg W, Haynes RB. Evidence-Based Medicine: How to Practice and Teach EBM. London: Churchill Livingstone; 1997

[83] Lonstein JE, Winter RB. The Milwaukee brace for the treatment of adolescent idiopathic scoliosis. A review of one thousand and twenty patients. J Bone Joint Surg Am. 1994; 76(8):1207–1221

[84] Winter RB. The pendulum has swung too far. Bracing for adolescent idiopathic scoliosis in the 1990s. Orthop Clin North Am. 1994; 25(2):195–204

[85] Noonan KJ, Weinstein SL. Letter to Editor. J Bone Joint Surg Am. 1997; 76:954–955

[86] Fernandez-Feliberti R, Flynn J, Ramirez N, Trautmann M, Alegria M. Effectiveness of TLSO bracing in the conservative treatment of idiopathic scoliosis. J Pediatr Orthop. 1995; 15(2):176–181

[87] Houghton GR, McInerney A, Tew A. Brace compliance in adolescent idiopathic scoliosis. J Bone Joint Surg Br. 1997; 69:852

[88] Dickson RA, Weinstein SL. Bracing (and screening)—yes or no? J Bone Joint Surg Br. 1999; 81(2):193–198

[89] Katz DE, Herring JA, Browne RH, Kelly DM, Birch JG. Brace wear control of curve progression in adolescent idiopathic scoliosis. J Bone Joint Surg Am. 2010; 92(6):1343–1352

[90] Weinstein SL, Dolan LA, Wright JG, Dobbs MB. Design of the bracing in adolescent idiopathic scoliosis trial (BrAIST). Spine. 2013; 38(21):1832–1841

[91] Huebert HT, MacKinnon WB. Syringomyelia and scoliosis. J Bone Joint Surg Br. 1969; 51(2):338–343

[92] Bradley LJ, Ratahi ED, Crawford HA, Barnes MJ. The outcomes of scoliosis surgery in patients with syringomyelia. Spine. 2007; 32(21):2327–2333

[93] Cobb JR. Outline for the study of scoliosis. American Academy of Orthopaedic Surgeons Instr Course Lect. 1948; 5:261–275

[94] Whittle MW, Evans M. Instrument for measuring the Cobb angle in scoliosis. Lancet. 1979; 1(8113):414

[95] Leatherman KD, Dickson RA. The Management of Spinal Deformities. Wright: London; 1988:6

[96] Nash CL, Jr, Moe JH. A study of vertebral rotation. J Bone Joint Surg Am. 1969; 51(2):223–229

[97] Lenke LG, Betz RR, Harms J. Adolescent Idiopathic Scoliosis. A new classification to determine extent of spinal arthrodesis. J Bone Joint Surg. 2001; 83A(8):1169–1181

[98] Suk SI, Kim JH, Cho KJ, Kim SS, Lee JJ, Han YT. Is anterior release necessary in severe scoliosis treated by posterior segmental pedicle screw fixation? Eur Spine J. 2007; 16(9):1359–1365

[99] Newton PO, Upasani VV. Surgical treatment of the right thoracic curve pattern. In: Newton P, O'Brien M, Shufflebarger HL, Betz RR, Dickson RA, Harms J (eds). Idiopathic scoliosis. The Harms Study Group Treatment Guide. New York: Thieme; 2010:200–223

[100] Sucato DJ. Selective versus nonselective surgery for adolescent idiopathic scoliosis. In: Newton P, O'Brien M, Shufflebarger HL, Betz RR, Dickson RA, Harms J (eds). Idiopathic Scoliosis. The Harms Study Group Treatment Guide. New York: Thieme; 2010:88–93

[101] Engsberg JR, Lenke LG, Reitenbach AK, Hollander KW, Bridwell KH, Blanke K. Prospective evaluation of trunk range of motion in adolescents with idiopathic scoliosis undergoing spinal fusion surgery. Spine. 2002; 27(12):1346–1354

[102] Cochran T, Irstam L, Nachemson A. Long-term anatomic and functional changes in patients with adolescent idiopathic scoliosis treated by Harrington rod fusion. Spine. 1983; 8(6):576–584

[103] Hilibrand AS, Robbins M. Adjacent segment degeneration and adjacent segment disease: the consequences of spinal fusion? Spine J. 2004; 4(6) Suppl:190S–194S

[104] Baba H, Furusawa N, Imura S, Kawahara N, Tsuchiya H, Tomita K. Late radiographic findings after anterior cervical fusion for spondylotic myeloradiculopathy. Spine. 1993; 18(15):2167–2173

[105] Gore DR, Sepic SB. Anterior cervical fusion for degenerated or protruded discs. A review of one hundred forty-six patients. Spine. 1984; 9(7):667–671

[106] Herkowitz HN, Kurz LT, Overholt DP. Surgical management of cervical soft disc herniation. A comparison between the anterior and posterior approach. Spine. 1990; 15(10):1026–1030

[107] Bohlman HH, Emery SE, Goodfellow DB, Jones PK. Robinson anterior cervical discectomy and arthrodesis for cervical radiculopathy. Long-term follow-up of one hundred and twenty-two patients. J Bone Joint Surg Am. 1993; 75(9):1298–1307

[108] Lunsford LD, Bissonette DJ, Jannetta PJ, Sheptak PE, Zorub DS. Anterior surgery for cervical disc disease. Part 1: Treatment of lateral cervical disc herniation in 253 cases. J Neurosurg. 1980; 53(1):1–11

[109] Henderson CM, Hennessy RG, Shuey HM, Jr, Shackelford EG. Posterior-lateral foraminotomy as an exclusive operative technique for cervical radiculopathy: a review of 846 consecutively operated cases. Neurosurgery. 1983; 13(5):504–512

[110] Hilibrand AS, Carlson GD, Palumbo MA, Jones PK, Bohlman HH. Radiculopathy and myelopathy at segments adjacent to the site of a previous anterior cervical arthrodesis. J Bone Joint Surg Am. 1999; 81(4):519–528

[111] Lehmann TR, Spratt KF, Tozzi JE, et al. Long-term follow-up of lower lumbar fusion patients. Spine. 1987; 12(2):97–104

[112] Luk KD, Lee FB, Leong JC, Hsu LC. The effect on the lumbosacral spine of long spinal fusion for idiopathic scoliosis. A minimum 10-year follow-up. Spine. 1987; 12(10):996–1000

[113] Penta M, Sandhu A, Fraser RD. Magnetic resonance imaging assessment of disc degeneration 10 years after anterior lumbar interbody fusion. Spine. 1995; 20(6):743–747

[114] Rahm MD, Hall BB. Adjacent-segment degeneration after lumbar fusion with instrumentation: a retrospective study. J Spinal Disord. 1996; 9(5):392–400

[115] Whitecloud TS, III, Davis JM, Olive PM. Operative treatment of the degenerated segment adjacent to a lumbar fusion.(comment). Spine. 1994; 19(5):531–536

[116] Etebar S, Cahill DW. Risk factors for adjacent-segment failure following lumbar fixation with rigid instrumentation for degenerative instability. J Neurosurg. 1999; 90(2) Suppl:163–169

[117] Ghiselli G, Wang JC, Hsu WK, Dawson EG. L5-S1 segment survivorship and clinical outcome analysis after L4-L5 isolated fusion. Spine. 2003; 28(12):1275–1280, discussion 1280

[118] **Throckmorton TW, Hilibrand AS, Mencio GA, Hodge A, Spengler DM. The impact of adjacent level disc degeneration on health status outcomes following lumbar fusion. Spine. 2003; 28(22):2546–2550**

[119] Ghiselli G, Wang JC, Bhatia NN, Hsu WK, Dawson EG. Adjacent segment degeneration in the lumbar spine. J Bone Joint Surg Am. 2004; 86-A(7):1497–1503

[120] Nachemson A. Back pain: delimiting the problem in the next millennium. Int J Law Psychiatry. 1999; 22(5–6):473–490

[121] Nachemson AL. Back pain in workplace: A threat to our welfare states. In: Walter D, Seide K (eds). Berufsbedingte Erkrankungen der Lendenwirbelsäule. Berlin: Springer; 1998:191–206

[122] **Roland M, van Tulder M. Should radiologists change the way they report plain radiography of the spine? Lancet. 1998; 352(9123):229–230**

[123] **Nachemson AL. Failed Back Surgery Syndrome is syndrome of failed back surgeons. Pain Clin. 1999; 11(4):271–284**

[124] Ciol MA, Deyo RA, Kreuter W, Bigos SJ. Characteristics in Medicare beneficiaries associated with reoperation after lumbar spine surgery. Spine. 1994; 19(12):1329–1334

[125] Malter AD, McNeney B, Loeser JD, Deyo RA. 5-year reoperation rates after different types of lumbar spine surgery. Spine. 1998; 23(7):814–820

[126] Lenke LG. Selection of fusion levels. In: Newton P, O'Brien M, Shufflebarger HL, Betz RR, Dickson RA, Harms J (eds). Idiopathic Scoliosis. The Harms Study Group Treatment Guide. New York: Thieme; 2010:153

[127] **Stagnara P, Gounot J, Fauchet R, et al. Les greffes antérieures par voie thoracique dans le traitement des déformations et dislocations vertébrales en cyphose et cyphoscoliose. Rev Chir Orthop Repar Appar Mot. 1974; 60:39–56**

[128] Newton PO, Upasani VV. Surgical treatment of the right thoracic curve pattern. In: Newton P, O'Brien M, Shufflebarger HL, Betz RR, Dickson RA, Harms J (eds). Idiopathic Scoliosis. The Harms Study Group Treatment Guide. New York: Thieme; 2010:214

[129] Clements DH, Pahys JM, Cahill P. Classification of adolescent idiopathic scoliosis for surgical intervention. In: Newton P, O'Brien M, Shufflebarger HL, Betz RR, Dickson RA, Harms J (eds). Idiopathic Scoliosis. The Harms Study Group Treatment Guide. New York: Thieme; 2010:104

[130] **Perry J, Nickel VL. Total cervicalspine fusion for neck paralysis. J Bone Joint Surg Am. 1959; 41-A(1):37–60**

[131] Nickel VL, Perry J, Garrett A, et al. Applications of the halo. Orthop Prosthet Appliance J. 1960; 14:31–35

[132] **DeWald RL, Ray RD. Skeletal traction for the treatment of severe scoliosis. J Bone Joint Surg Am. 1970; 52:233–238**

[133] O'Brien JP, Yau ACMC, Smith TK, Hodgson AR. Halo pelvic traction. A preliminary report on a method of external skeletal fixation for correcting deformities and maintaining fixation of the spine. J Bone Joint Surg Br. 1971; 53(2):217–229

[134] Ransford AO, Manning CWSF. Complications of halo-pelvic distraction for scoliosis. J Bone Joint Surg Br. 1975; 57(2):131–137

[135] O'Brien JP. The management of severe spinal deformities with the halo-pelvic apparatus; pitfalls and guidelines in its use. J Bone Joint Surg Br. 1977; 59:117–118

[136] Leslie IJ, Dorgan JC, Bentley G, Galloway RW. A prospective study of deep vein thrombosis of the leg in children on halo-femoral traction. J Bone Joint Surg Br. 1981; 63-B(2):168–170

[137] Stagnara P. Traction cranienne par le "Halo" de Rancho los Amigos. Rev Chir Orthop Repar Appar Mot. 1971; 57:287–300

[138] Sponseller PD, Takenaga R. The use of traction in treating large scoliotic curves in idiopathic scoliosis. In: Newton P, O'Brien M, Shufflebarger HL, Betz RR, Dickson RA, Harms J (eds). Idiopathic Scoliosis. The Harms Study Group Treatment Guide. New York: Thieme; 2010:181–184

[139] **Luhmann SJ, Lenke LG, Kim YJ, Bridwell KH, Schootman M. Thoracic adolescent idiopathic scoliosis curves between 70 degrees and 100 degrees: is anterior release necessary? Spine. 2005; 30(18):2061–2067**

[140] Suk S-I, Lee SM, Chung ER, Kim JH, Kim SS. Selective thoracic fusion with segmental pedicle screw fixation in the treatment of thoracic idiopathic scoliosis: more than 5-year follow-up. Spine. 2005; 30(14):1602–1609

[141] Newton PO, Upasani VV. Surgical treatment of the right thoracic curve pattern. In: Newton P, O'Brien M, Shufflebarger HL, Betz RR, Dickson RA, Harms J (eds). Idiopathic Scoliosis. The Harms Study Group Treatment Guide. New York: Thieme; 2010:215

[142] Smith-Petersen MN, Larson CB, Aufranc OE. Osteotomy of the spine for correction of flexion deformity in rheumatoid arthritis. Clin Orthop Relat Res. 1969; 66(66):6–9

[143] McMASTER PE. Osteotomy of the spine for correction of fixed flexion deformity. AMA Arch Surg. 1958; 76(4):603–610

[144] **McMaster MJ, Coventry MB. Spinal osteotomy in akylosing spondylitis. Technique, complications, and long-term results. Mayo Clin Proc. 1973; 48(7):476–486**

[145] Adams JC. Technique, dangers and safeguards in osteotomy of the spine. J Bone Joint Surg Br. 1952; 34-B(2):226–232

[146] **Ponte A. Posterior column shortening for Scheuermann's kyphosis: an innovative one-stage technique. In: Haher TR, ed. Surgical Techniques for the Spine. New York: Thieme Medical Publishers; 2003:107–113**

[147] Geck MJ, Macagno A, Ponte A, Shufflebarger HL. The Ponte procedure: posterior only treatment of Scheuermann's kyphosis using segmental posterior shortening and pedicle screw instrumentation. J Spinal Disord Tech. 2007; 20(8):586–593

[148] Michele AA, Krueger FJ. Surgical approach to the vertebral body. J Bone Joint Surg Am. 1949; 31A(4):873–878

[149] **Heinig CF. Eggshell procedure. In: Luque ER (ed). Segmental Spinal Instrumentation. Thorofare: Slack Inc., 1984**

[150] Yamin S, Li L, Xing W, Tianjun G, Yupeng Z. Staged surgical treatment for severe and rigid scoliosis. J Orthop Surg. 2008; 3:26

[151] Leatherman KD. Resection of vertebral bodies. J Bone Joint Surg Am. 1969; 51:206

[152] Leatherman KD. Resection of Vertebral Bodies. American College of Surgeons Fellowship Thesis

[153] **Leatherman KD. The management of rigid spinal curves. Clin Orthop Relat Res. 1973(93):215–224**

[154] **Leatherman KD, Dickson RA. Two stage corrective surgery for congenital spine deformities. J Bone Joint Surg Br. 1977; 59:497**

[155] Roaf R. Wedge resection for scoliosis. J Bone Joint Surg Br. 1955; 37-B(1):97–101

[156] Royle ND. The operative removal of an accessory vertebra. Med J Aust. 1928; 1:467–468

[157] Compere EL. Excision of hemivertebrae for correction of congenital scoliosis. J Bone Joint Surg. 1932; 14:555–562

[158] Von Lackum HL, Smith A de F. Removal of vertebral bodies in the treatment of scoliosis. Surg Gynecol Obstet. 1933; 57:250–256

[159] Wiles P. Resection of dorsal vertebrae in congenital scoliosis. J Bone Joint Surg Am. 1951; 33 A(1):151–154

[160] Herbert JJ. Osteotomie vertebrale pour cyphose congenitale. Rev Chir Orthop Repar Appar Mot. 1951; 37:506–508

[161] **Hodgson AR. Correction of fixed spinal curves. J Bone Joint Surg Am. 1965; 47:1221–1227**

[162] Dommisse GF, Enslin TB. Hodgson's circumferential osteotomy in the correction of spinal deformity. J Bone Joint Surg Br. 1970; 52B:778

[163] Suk SI, Chung ER, Kim JH, Kim SS, Lee JS, Choi WK. Posterior vertebral column resection for severe rigid scoliosis. Spine. 2005; 30(14):1682–1687

[164] Jensen R, Letko L, Melcher R, et al. Posterior resection of the apical vertebral allows excellent correction in rigid scoliosis. 12th International Meeting on Advanced Spine Techniques, Banff, Canada, July 7–9, 2005

[165] Letko K, Jensen R, Harms J. Partial or complete apical vertebral resection in the treatment of cases of moderate and severe rigid AIS. 13th International Meeting on Advanced Spine Techniques, Athens, Greece, July 12–15, 2006

[166] Harrenstein RJ. Die Skoliose bei Saueglingen und ihre Behandlung. Z Orthop Chir. 1930; 52:1–40

[167] **James JIP. Idiopathic scoliosis; the prognosis, diagnosis, and operative indications related to curve patterns and the age at onset. J Bone Joint Surg Br. 1954; 36-B(1):36–49**

[168] James JIP, Lloyd-Roberts GC, Pilcher MF. Infantile structural scoliosis. J Bone Joint Surg Br. 1959; 41-B:719–735

[169] Scott JC, Morgan TH. The natural history and prognosis of infantile idiopathic scoliosis. J Bone Joint Surg Br. 1955; 37-B(3):400–413

[170] Lloyd-Roberts GC, Pilcher MF. Structural idiopathic scoliosis in infancy: A study of the natural history of 100 patients. J Bone Joint Surg Br. 1965; 47:520–523

[171] **McMaster MJ. Infantile idiopathic scoliosis: can it be prevented? J Bone Joint Surg Br. 1983; 65(5):612–617**

[172] Robinson CM, McMaster MJ. Juvenile idiopathic scoliosis. Curve patterns and prognosis in one hundred and nine patients. J Bone Joint Surg Am. 1996; 78(8):1140–1148

[173] Tanner JN. Growth at Adolescence. Oxford: Blackwell; 1962

[174] Browne D. Congenital postural scoliosis. Proc R Soc Med. 1956; 49(7):395–398

[175] Dunn PM. Congenital postural deformities. Br Med Bull. 1976; 32(1):71–76

[176] Watson GH. Relation between side of plagiocephaly, dislocation of hip, scoliosis, bat ears, and sternomastoid tumours. Arch Dis Child. 1971; 46(246):203–210

[177] Wynne-Davies R. Infantile idiopathic scoliosis. Causative factors, particularly in the first six months of life. J Bone Joint Surg Br. 1975; 57(2):138–141

[178] Mau H. Does infantile scoliossi require treatment? J Bone Joint Surg Br. 1968; 50B:881

[179] Dempster DW, Dickson RA. The epidemiology of plagiocephaly and infantile idiopathic scoliosis. Proceedings and Reports of Universities, Colleges, Councils, Associations and Societies. British Scoliosis Society. J Bone Joint Surg Br. 1987; 69(5):851

[180] Conner AN. Developmental anomalies and prognosis in infantile idiopathic scoliosis. J Bone Joint Surg Br. 1969; 51(4):711–713

[181] Mehta MH, Morel G. The non-operative treatment of infantile idiopathic scoliosis. In: Zorab PA and Siegler D (eds). Scoliosis. Proceedings of the Sixth Symposium. London: Academic; 1979:71–84

[182] Mehta MH. Growth as a corrective force in the early treatment of progressive infantile scoliosis. J Bone Joint Surg Br. 2005; 87(9):1237–1247

[183] McMaster MJ, Macnicol MF. The management of progressive infantile idiopathic scoliosis. J Bone Joint Surg Br. 1979; 61(1):36–42

[184] Letts RM, Bobechko WP. Fusion of the scoliotic spine in young children. Clin Orthop Relat Res. 1974(101):136–145

[185] Winter RB, Moe JH. The results of spinal arthrodesis for congenital spinal deformity in patients younger than five years old. J Bone Joint Surg Am. 1982; 64(3):419–432

[186] Moe JH, Kharrat K, Winter RB, Cummine JL. Harrington instrumentation without fusion plus external orthotic support for the treatment of difficult curvature problems in young children. Clin Orthop Relat Res. 1984 (185):35–45

[187] Fisk JR, Peterson HA, Laughlin R, Lutz R. Spontaneous fusion in scoliosis after instrumentation without arthrodesis. J Pediatr Orthop. 1995; 15(2):182–186

[188] Luque ER. Segmental spinal instrumentation for correction of scoliosis. Clin Orthop Relat Res. 1982(163):192–198

[189] Leatherman KD, Dickson RA. The management of spinal deformities. London: Wright; 1988:105

[190] Dickson RA, Lawton JO, Deacon P, et al. The pathogenesis of idiopathic scoliosis. In: Philip Zorab Symposium 1983. New York: Praeger; 1985:64–79

[191] Dimeglio A. Growth in pediatric orthopaedics. J Pediatr Orthop. 2001; 21(4):549–555

[192] Bess S, Akbarnia BA, Thompson GH, et al. Complications of growing-rod treatment for early-onset scoliosis: analysis of one hundred and forty patients. J Bone Joint Surg Am. 2010; 92(15):2533–2543

[193] Acaroglu E, Yazici M, Alanay A, Surat A. Three-dimensional evolution of scoliotic curve during instrumentation without fusion in young children. J Pediatr Orthop. 2002; 22(4):492–496

[194] Mineiro J, Weinstein SL. Subcutaneous rodding for progressive spinal curvatures: early results. J Pediatr Orthop. 2002; 22(3):290–295

[195] Blakemore LC, Scoles PV, Poe-Kochert C, Thompson GH. Submuscular Isola rod with or without limited apical fusion in the management of severe spinal deformities in young children: preliminary report. Spine. 2001; 26(18):2044–2048

[196] Akbarnia BA, Marks DS, Boachie-Adjei O, Thompson AG, Asher MA. Dual growing rod technique for the treatment of progressive early-onset scoliosis: a multicenter study. Spine. 2005; 30(17) Suppl:S46–S57

[197] Akbarnia BA. Management themes in early onset scoliosis. J Bone Joint Surg Am. 2007; 89 Suppl 1:42–54

[198] Zhang H, Sucato DJ. Unilateral pedicle screw epiphysiodesis of the neurocentral synchondrosis. Production of idiopathic-like scoliosis in an immature animal model. J Bone Joint Surg Am. 2008; 90(11):2460–2469

[199] Akyuz E, Braun JT, Brown NA, Bachus KN. Static versus dynamic loading in the mechanical modulation of vertebral growth. Spine. 2006; 31(25):E952–E958

[200] Aronsson DD, Stokes IA, Rosovsky J, Spence H. Mechanical modulation of calf tail vertebral growth: implications for scoliosis progression. J Spinal Disord. 1999; 12(2):141–146

[201] Braun JT, Ogilvie JW, Akyuz E, Brodke DS, Bachus KN, Stefko RM. Experimental scoliosis in an immature goat model: a method that creates idiopathic-type deformity with minimal violation of the spinal elements along the curve. Spine. 2003; 28(19):2198–2203

[202] Betz RR, Ranade A, Samdani AF, et al. Vertebral body stapling: a fusionless treatment option for a growing child with moderate idiopathic scoliosis. Spine. 2010; 35(2):169–176

[203] Betz RR. Correction without fusion. In: Newton P, O'Brien M, Shufflebarger HL, Betz RR, Dickson RA, Harms J (eds). Idiopathic Scoliosis. The Harms Study Group Treatment Guide. New York: Thieme; 2010:392–407

[204] Roaf R. The treatment of progressive scoliosis by unilateral growth arrest. J Bone Joint Surg Br. 1963; 45(4):637–651

[205] Adams W. Lectures on the pathology and treatment of lateral and other forms of curvature of the spine. London: Churchill and Sons; 1865

[206] Somerville EW. Rotational lordosis; the development of single curve. J Bone Joint Surg Br. 1952; 34-B(3):421–427

[207] Dickson RA. Scoliosis in the community. Br Med J (Clin Res Ed). 1983; 286(6365):615–618

[208] Deacon P, Archer IA, Dickson RA. The anatomy of spinal deformity: a biomechanical analysis. Orthopedics. 1987; 10(6):897–903

[209] Smith RM, Dickson RA. Experimental structural scoliosis. J Bone Joint Surg Br. 1987; 69(4):576–581

[210] Andrew T, Piggott H. Growth arrest for progressive scoliosis. Combined anterior and posterior fusion of the convexity. J Bone Joint Surg Br. 1985; 67(2):193–197

[211] Winter RB. Convex anterior and posterior hemiarthrodesis and hemiepiphyseodesis in young children with progressive congenital scoliosis. J Pediatr Orthop. 1981; 1(4):361–366

[212] Bradford DS. Partial epiphyseal arrest and supplemental fixation for progressive correction of congenital spinal deformity. J Bone Joint Surg Am. 1982; 64(4):610–614

[213] Campbell RM, Jr, Smith MD. Thoracic insufficiency syndrome and exotic scoliosis. J Bone Joint Surg Am. 2007; 89 Suppl 1:108–122

[214] Smith JT, Smart MP, Emans JB, et al. Results of surgical experience using the VEPTR device for the treatment of thoracic insufficiency syndrome: A multicenter study. Paper presented at: 13th International Meeting on Advanced Spine Techniques, Athens, Greece, July 12–15, 2006

[215] Parent S, Labelle H, Skalli W, de Guise J. Vertebral wedging characteristic changes in scoliotic spines. Spine. 2004; 29(20):E455–E462

[216] Guille JT, Betz RR, Balsara RK, Mulcahey MJ, D'Andrea LP, Clements DH. The feasibility, safety, and utility of vertebral wedge osteotomies for the fusionless treatment of paralytic scoliosis. Spine. 2003; 28(20):S266–S274

[217] McCarthy KP, Chafetz RS, Mulcahey MJ, Frisch RF, D'Andrea LP, Betz RR. Clinical efficacy of the vertebral wedge osteotomy for the fusionless treatment of paralytic scoliosis. Spine. 2010; 35(4):403–410

[218] Manning CW, Prime FJ, Zorab PA. Partial costectomy as a cosmetic operation in scoliosis. J Bone Joint Surg Br. 1973; 55(3):521–527

[219] Laughlin TT, Mohlenbrock WC. Rib hump resection in scoliosis surgery. Orthop Trans. 1980; 4:24–25

[220] Steel HH. Convex rib resection in scoliosis. Orthop Trans. 1982; 6:25

[221] Schollner D. Steigerung der Vitalkapazität durch Rippenbuckelresektion mit der Brustkorbdehnungstechnik. Z Orthop Ihre Grenzgeb. 1966; 101:323–333

[222] Chopin D, Briard JL, Seringe R. Surgery for thoracic deformity in scoliosis. In: Zorab PA, Siegler D (eds). Scoliosis. London: Academic; 1979:161–168

Chapter 5

Scheuermann's Disease

5.1	Pathogenesis	*136*
5.2	Clinical Diagnosis	*137*
5.3	Radiological Diagnosis	*139*
5.4	Management	*141*

5 Scheuermann's Disease

Scheuermann's disease is a rigid angular kyphosis usually occurring after puberty. The apical vertebral bodies are wedge shaped in the median sagittal plane with a shorter anterior height. The prevalence rate of thoracic Scheuermann's kyphosis is of the order of 8%, not dissimilar to idiopathic scoliosis, and there is also a familial trend (▶ Fig. 5.1).[1] However, the condition is bimodal as regards site, with two-thirds of cases apical at T8, similar to idiopathic thoracic scoliosis, and the remainder at the thoracolumbar junction or upper lumbar region.[2] The clinical features of the kyphosis at these sites differ such that there is merit in considering two types: type I, apical at T8 (▶ Fig. 2.27 and ▶ Fig. 5.2a), and type II, apical lower down (▶ Fig. 5.2b), as implied by Scheuermann. Type I appears to be an idiopathic deformity and would merit being called idiopathic kyphosis. While an epidemiological survey has not been performed, boys are affected more commonly than girls.[1,2] The preponderance of females in Bradford's study of those presenting clinically suggests that girls may be more concerned about their appearance and hence present more frequently than boys, rather than having a truly higher prevalence rate.[3] In contradistinction, type II Scheuermann's kyphosis appears to be related to strenuous physical activity, affects almost solely males, and presents around maturity usually with pain rather than deformity.[1,4–8] Accordingly it is referred to as "apprentice's spine."

The most important factor governing the behavior of the deformity is the axis of spinal column rotation which, in Scheuermann's, or any other kyphosis, lies well in front of the apex, thus protecting the spine from rotation (▶ Fig. 3.4). The deformity is therefore not rotationally unstable and so remains in the median plane[9] unlike the opposite condition of idiopathic thoracic scoliosis.

5.1 Pathogenesis

In all respects type I Scheuermann's disease appears to be precisely the opposite deformity to idiopathic scoliosis in the median sagittal plane (kyphosis vs. lordosis) (▶ Fig. 5.3). This is primarily another example of median sagittal plane spinal asymmetry with anterior vertebral wedging and end plate irregularity, the reverse of idiopathic scoliosis. Both conditions show the same site of predilection at the lower two-thirds of the thoracic spine, both start from a normal spine in normal children during growth, both are familial, and both have a strong tendency to stop progressing at spinal maturity. Whatever the fundamental mechanisms in play, the final common pathway is a disturbance of growth between the front and back of the spine, the former having relatively decreased growth in Scheuermann's disease.

Scheuermann's original concept that this was an apophysitis, avascular necrosis of the cartilage ring apophysis,[10] was subsequently invalidated by the observations that the ring apophysis has nothing whatsoever to do with spinal growth, which is the responsibility of the end plate epiphysis.[11–15] Furthermore, the common radiographic finding of apophyseal irregularity is not more prevalent in patients with Scheuermann's kyphosis than straight-backed counterparts. Meanwhile Schmorl felt that the growth asymmetry between the front and back of the growth

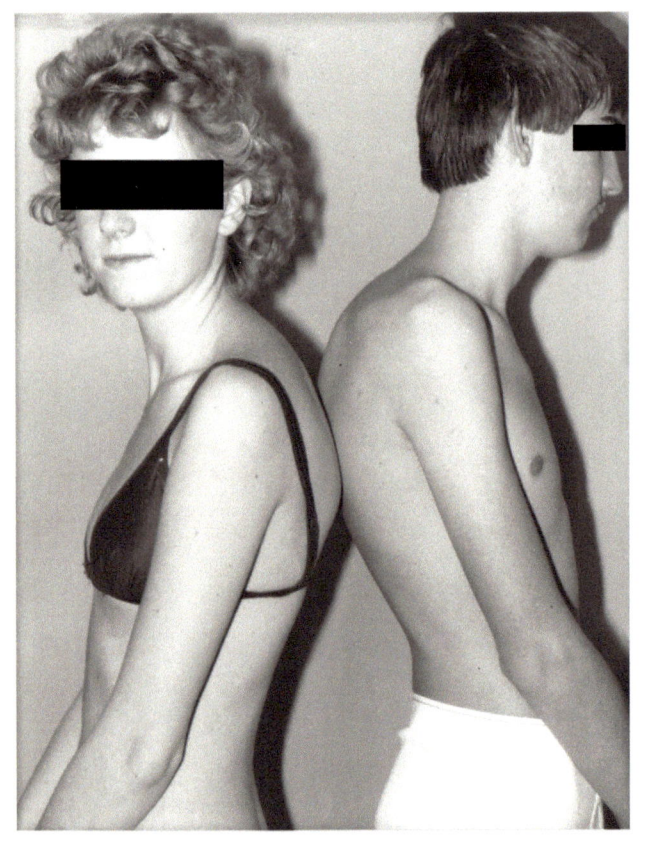

Fig. 5.1 Brother and sister standing sideways, both showing mild Scheuermann's disease. They were unhappy about being round backed (Ponte's disease).

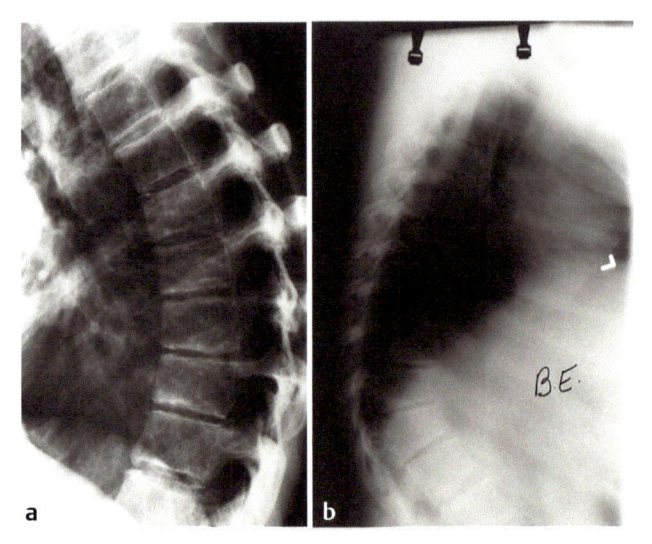

Fig. 5.2 (a) Lateral radiograph showing type I Scheuermann's disease with apical wedging of three consecutive vertebrae by 5 degrees. (b) Lateral radiograph of type II thoracolumbar Scheuermann's disease with two consecutive thoracolumbar vertebrae significantly wedged anteriorly.

plate was attributable to intravertebral protrusions of disk material more anteriorly so that anterior growth was relatively suppressed.[16] That central Schmorl's node formation is a common finding on a lateral radiograph of the normal-shaped spine does not invalidate this hypothesis and may well reflect that during the phase of spinal growth we are all vulnerable to the consequences of vertical loading, with Scheuermann's kyphosis being one severe end of the spectrum and idiopathic scoliosis the other. Indeed, in Scheuermann's kyphosis the Schmorl node formation is clearly anterior[17,18] (▶ Fig. 5.3), and in idiopathic scoliosis clearly posterior,[9] whereas in normal spines this node formation is randomly scattered and more central.[16]

There is certainly no clear evidence that Scheuermann's kyphosis is associated with any upset of endocrine balance or calcium homeostasis.[3,19] Anteroposterior (AP) views of the kyphotic region often show bilateral paravertebral shadows, suggesting that thickening of the anterior longitudinal ligament and periosteum are also associated with the end plate pathology, although very probably secondarily. Certainly at surgery on the front of a Scheuermann's kyphosis these structures do appear thickened and rather tight. The common factor among all these different pathological findings is a disturbance of end plate growth anteriorly, such that anterior vertebral body height progressively lags behind posterior around the apex of the curve. This could occur as a result of a series of repetitive minor traumatic events which may have the effect of producing a type V epiphyseal plate injury[20] with growth suppression anteriorly, while precisely the opposite would occur with idiopathic scoliosis, where the reduction in vertebral height is posterior. Histological examination of vertebral body material removed through anterior surgery shows nothing more than would be compatible with this theory.[19,21-23]

Ascani has considered that growth hormone secretion might be excessive[24] and although Murray[25] has shown normal heights in patients with Scheuermann's disease, these heights were uncoiled. Meanwhile when heights were titrated against the height measures of the normal population in Leeds heights did seem to be increased in both males and females.[26] That Scheuermann's disease might be a form of juvenile osteoporosis[19] has been disproven by the work of Gilsanz who has reported normal vertebral bone density.[27]

Very interestingly, both Willner in Sweden[28] and Oxborrow with the Leeds Group[29] have shown that the thoracic kyphosis changes markedly in shape with growth in normal children and that in both boys and girls the thoracic kyphosis flattens from around the age of 10 to 12 years (▶ Fig. 3.11) but increases again at the age of 14 when boys are growing fastest. Thus, the shape of the spine in the sagittal plane is under very subtle control and while the child goes through these changes without succumbing to a progressive deformity; the range would also include unfortunate individuals at each end, one group with an increased kyphosis and the other with a lordosis and subsequent idiopathic scoliosis (▶ Fig. 3.14 and ▶ Fig. 3.15). The latter is far more important as this group is vulnerable to the consequences of rotational progression because of the more posteriorly situated axis of spinal column rotation.[9]

Delmas[30] and Stagnara[31] have both studied the lateral profile in normal children and have observed a wide range with flat backs on the one hand and increased round backs on the other. This, like all other aspects of growth and shape, is genetically determined[32] (flat-backed children come from flat-backed families and round-backed children, from round-backed families) and therefore it is quite reasonable to expect Scheuermann's kyphosis and idiopathic scoliosis to have a similar prevalence rate and familial trend.[1] The similarity of the median plane changes in vertebral body shape in the two conditions has also been remarked upon.[33,34] However, the more obvious change in shape of the apical Scheuermann's vertebral bodies is due to this progressive deformity staying in the median plane (▶ Fig. 5.4). With idiopathic scoliosis the degree of pathological change in the median plane (the lordosis) is very much less because the instability of the lordotic configuration leads to progressive rotation away from the midline and a gradual reduction of the compression on the back of the end plate.[34] Accordingly while a severe Scheuermann's kyphosis may measure in excess of 100 degrees, the lordosis in severe idiopathic thoracic scoliosis is only of the order of 10 to 15 degrees,[35] the rest of the deformity being expressed as Cobb angle in the frontal plane (▶ Fig. 3.1 and ▶ Fig. 3.16).

5.2 Clinical Diagnosis

The clinical presentation and features of Scheuermann's kyphosis vary according to whether the deformity is type I (thoracic) or type II (thoracolumbar or lumbar). Type I (thoracic) deformities present as a result of the deformity (▶ Fig. 5.5), with relatively few patients complaining of pain. It is the appearance of the back which is the problem and this is combined with poor general posture with the shoulders drooping forward. In less severe cases it is not usually the patient who complains of the specific deformity but the parents who are aware of the bad shoulder posture. On examination while standing the angular

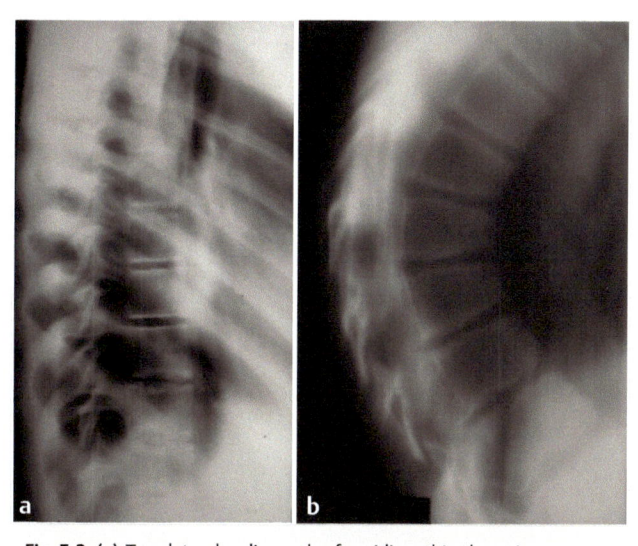

Fig. 5.3 (a) True lateral radiograph of an idiopathic thoracic curve showing more posterior Schmorl's node formation in the lower vertebrae which are lordotically shaped. (b) Lateral X-ray of a type I Scheuermann's idiopathic thoracic hyperkyphosis. The Schmorl's node formation is clearly seen anteriorly. Idiopathic thoracic scoliosis and type I Scheuermann's disease are opposite deformities in the sagittal plane. (Reproduced with permission from Newton P, O'Brien M, Shufflebarger H, et al. Idiopathic Scoliosis: The Harms Study Group Treatment Guide. Stuttgart/New York: Thieme; 2010: 36.)

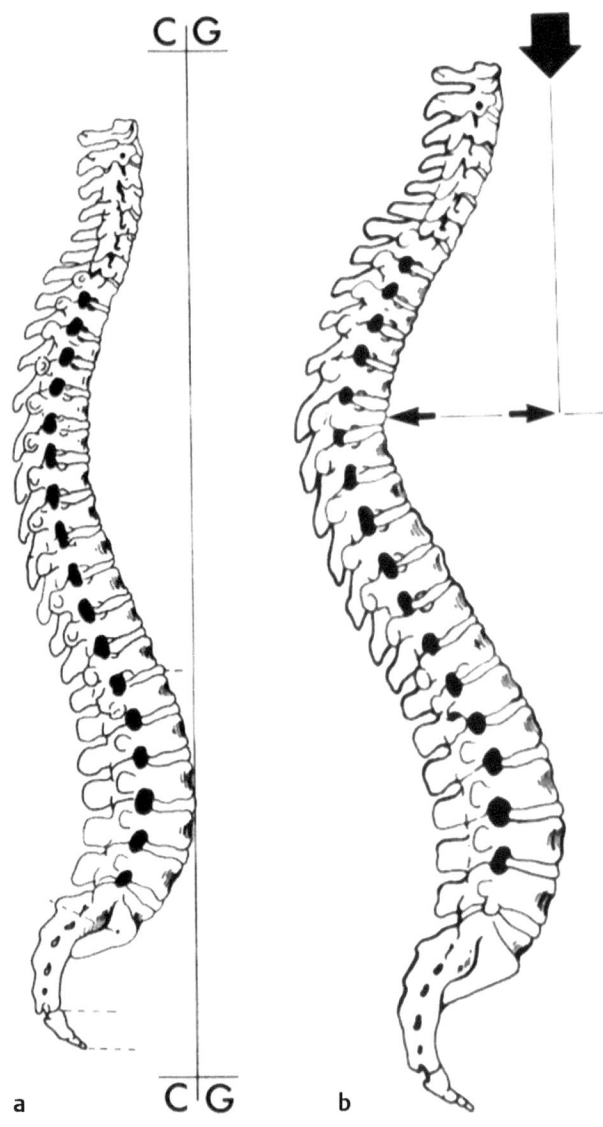

Fig. 5.4 (a) The center of gravity of the body lies just in front of the lumbar spine, and with hyperkyphosis the thoracic spine is therefore progressively behind the axis of spinal column rotation. (b) Consequently, the deformity progresses solely in the sagittal plane, with no buckling potential. (Reproduced with permission from Newton P, O'Brien M, Shufflebarger H, et al. Idiopathic Scoliosis: The Harms Study Group Treatment Guide. Stuttgart/New York: Thieme; 2010: 37.)

kyphosis is visible apical at T8/9 and is more apparent on forward spinal flexion (▶ Fig. 5.5b). In the erect position with shoulder retraction the deformity is less obvious but the kyphosis itself remains unchanged. In the prone position pressure over the apex of the kyphosis demonstrates it to be rigid, and this important clinical feature is what allowed Scheuermann himself to differentiate the condition from postural roundback deformity.[10] There is a compensatory increase in the normal lumbar lordosis. Straight-leg raising is commonly reduced by hamstring tightness which is considered to be secondary to the tilted pelvis position rather than a primary deforming mechanism as Lambrinudi postulated.[36] In all but the most severe degrees of Scheuermann's kyphosis the neurological examination is normal. However, rarely the spinal cord

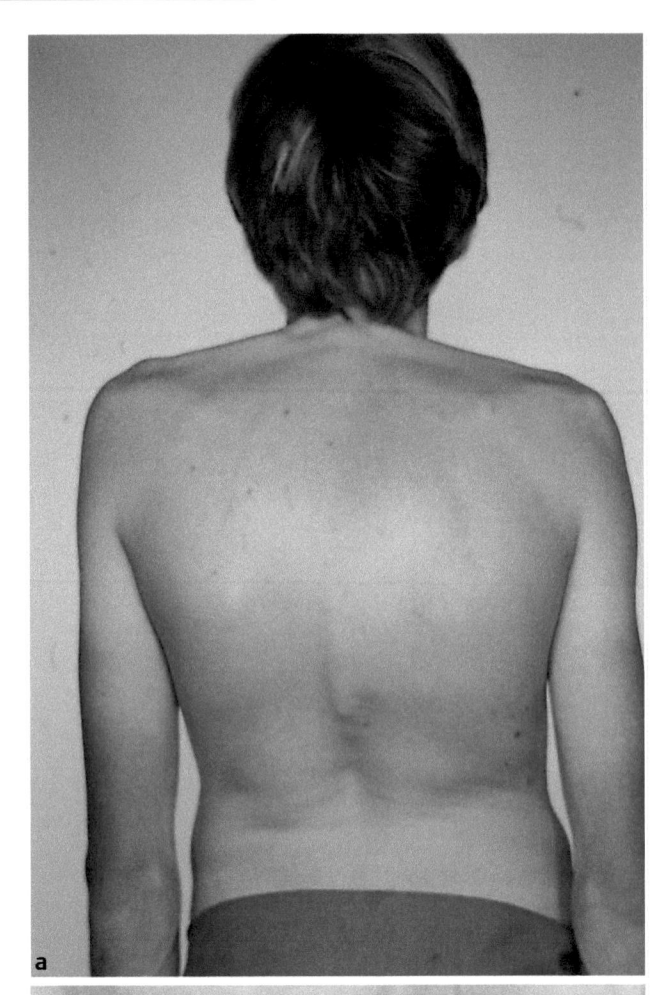

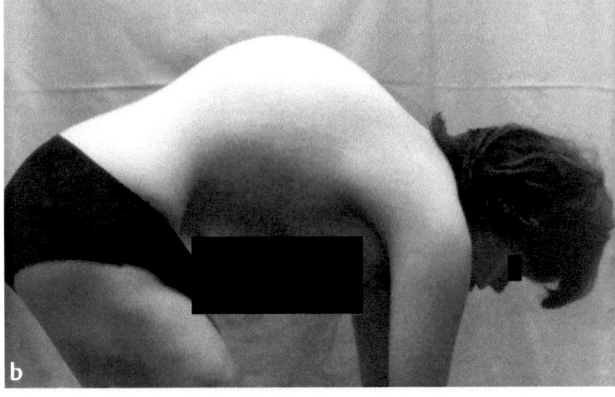

Fig. 5.5 (a) Severe angular thoracic kyphosis of type 1 Scheuermann's disease is often better seen from the back where it can also be seen that there is a mild coexistent scoliosis. (b) On forward bending the type I Scheuermann's deformity has an angular appearance over the apex.

can be bow-strung over the back of the kyphotic apex, in which case there may be objective neurological signs of impending paraplegia with clonus, hyperreflexia, and up-going plantar responses[37–39] (▶ Fig. 5.6).

Pain is an unusual presenting complaint with type I but the prevalence rate would appear to rise with the duration of the deformity,[40] and is not uncommon in the older patient. The site of the pain is generally at the apex of the deformity but can

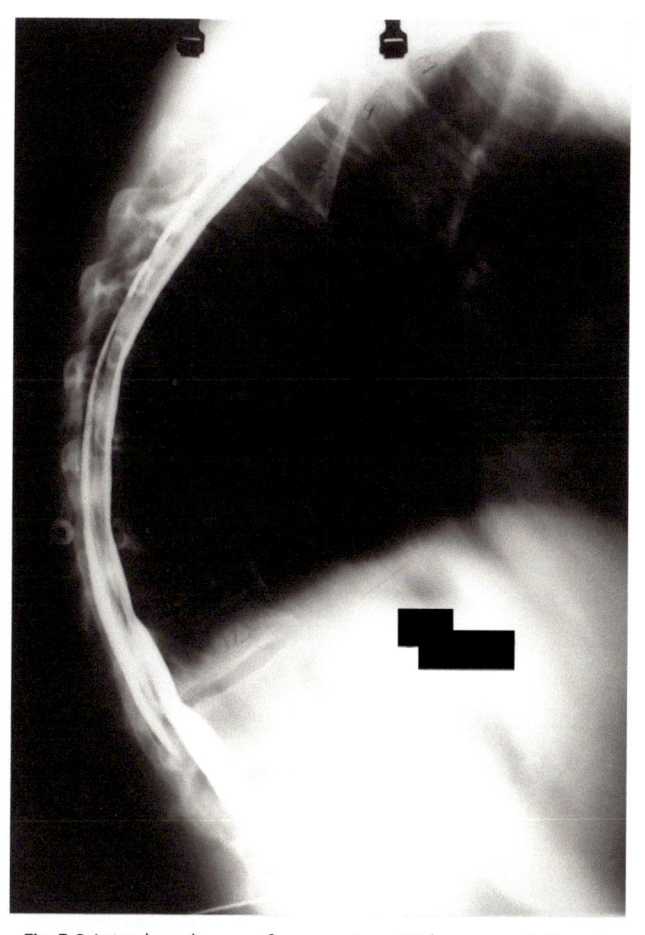

Fig. 5.6 Lateral myelogram of a severe type I Scheuermann's thoracic hyperkyphosis. There is no specific area of cord compression but the cord is thinned over several levels over the curve apex. This was sufficient to produce upper motor neurone symptoms.

spread upward and downward. It would be imagined that pain would be worse the bigger the deformity but that correlation doesn't seem to be particularly good.[24]

It was conjectured that about one-third of patients with thoracic Scheuermann's kyphosis had a mild, generally nonprogressive scoliosis.[1,41] This is not so. A careful analysis of 50 cases of thoracic Scheuermann's disease demonstrated that a mild lateral curvature of the spine was present in 85%.[34] In the minority this was present in the region of the kyphosis (▶ Fig. 5.5a) and was strictly an asymmetric kyphosis in the nature of a lateral curvature of the spine but with the spinous processes not rotated or rotated toward the curve convexity (discordant rotation). Where the majority of scolioses in association with Scheuermann's kyphosis occur is four or five vertebral segments below the apex of the kyphosis (▶ Fig. 2.27). This is in the region of the compensatory hyperlordosis below which has rotated to the side in precisely the same way as in the production of the idiopathic scoliotic deformity, nicely confirming the lordotic etiology of idiopathic scoliosis. We found that the average curve size was 14 degrees and the spinous processes were rotated toward the curve concavity (concordant rotation).[34] However, progression was minimized by the older age of the adolescent with Scheuermann's kyphosis and an axis of spinal rotation placed more anteriorly because of the presence of the kyphosis.

In type II (thoracolumbar or lumbar) kyphosis pain is the presenting complaint in the majority of patients.[7,8] This tends to be in association with increased physical activity, and is therefore generally relieved by rest. There is a definitely increased prevalence rate of spondylolysis and spondylolisthesis in patients with type II Scheuermann's kyphosis,[7] and the spondylolyses may indeed be multiple. It may be that symptomatic pain from these derangements is the mode of presentation in some. Because the vertebral wedging process occurs lower down the deformity is less marked, and is therefore not usually the cause of clinical presentation.

Indeed, on clinical examination mild degrees of type II Scheuermann's kyphosis are difficult to detect. On forward flexion, however, the kyphotic area becomes more obvious and does not correct by manual pressure or spinal hyperextension. An associated lateral curvature of the spine is much less common in type II Scheuermann's disease.[7]

5.3 Radiological Diagnosis

The "normal" thoracic kyphosis extends from T3 to T9 or T10 and is caused by the shape of the thoracic vertebral bodies in the median sagittal plane (▶ Fig. 5.2).[42] Disk height does not contribute to the kyphosis. Therefore, the thoracic vertebral bodies are normally wedge-shaped, having a shorter anterior than posterior height. There is a wide range of the normal thoracic kyphosis and this range is generally regarded to be between 20 and 40 degrees.[3,43] However, there have been several reports about so-called "normal" thoracic kyphosis either using empirical measurement points (e.g., T2 to T12), or using end-vertebrae, and these have been means of normal children of varying ages—27 degrees in one study,[43] 33 in another,[44] and for instance 36 degrees in another.[45] Mixing boys and girls and different ages altogether to derive a mean is not particularly clever because as Willner and Oxborrow clearly showed there is considerable change in thoracic kyphosis with growth[28,29] (▶ Fig. 3.12). This is really important in the pathogenesis of both idiopathic scoliosis and Scheuermann's disease because when girls go through their peak adolescent growth velocity their thoracic kyphosis is at a minimum and if they overgrow then they can easily develop a lordosis. However, boys don't mature until of the order of 3 years later when they are regaining a maximum thoracic kyphosis and of course if they overgrow then they are liable to develop Scheuermann's disease. This accounts for the marked gender discrepancy with idiopathic scoliosis being much more prevalent in females and Scheuermann's disease being much more prevalent in males.[31,42,44,45] Sorensen felt that an overall thoracic kyphosis of more than 40 degrees should be one radiographic index of the presence of Scheuermann's disease,[1] but this is clearly much less important than the shape of the apical vertebral bodies themselves. Furthermore, measurements of the overall thoracic kyphosis also include the compensatory lordoses above and below which have the effect of masking what is going on in the middle. Therefore, wedging of the apical three vertebrae by 5 degrees or more each is the best diagnostic guide (▶ Fig. 5.2).[1] In addition, vertebral wedging is the only constant radiological finding. Such end plate irregularity and Schmorl node formation

Scheuermann's Disease

as is present is situated anteriorly (▶ Fig. 5.3). However, the minimum of three consecutive apical vertebrae wedged by 5 degrees or more as the essential criterion seldom appears to be adhered to. Ponte's phenomenal series of more than 3,000 cases of so-called Scheuermann's disease[46] was only based upon the apical vertebra alone being wedged. While this might be better called Ponte's disease, it certainly is not Scheuermann's disease.

Interestingly, Knutson observed that appositional growth of the apical vertebral bodies in Scheuermann's kyphosis occurs only anteriorly, such that any Schmorl's node tends to move relatively toward the middle of the vertebrae in the median plane with time.[17] He also pointed out that there is an increased sagittal dimension of the vertebral bodies in Scheuermann's kyphosis. Persistence of the anterior vascular groove in the thoracic vertebral bodies is an index of general immaturity but has been suggested as a means by which anterior collapse could occur.[47] As the phase of spinal maturity approaches so any Schmorl's node formation or end plate irregularity tends to heal.

AP views of the thoracic spine in Scheuermann's kyphosis reveal the associated lateral spine deformity in 85% of patients, with an apex four or five segments below the kyphosis (▶ Fig. 2.27).[34] Oblique or lateral projections of the lumbar spine reveal a defect in the pars interarticularis in one-third of type II cases,[7] and AP and lateral projections of the lumbar spine show an increased lumbar lordosis in type I cases with a tendency toward early so-called degenerative change. Similar projections of the Scheuermann's kyphosis with increasing age also show changes with anterior bone spurring, the deformity occasionally progressing to apparent bony union anteriorly (▶ Fig. 5.7).[1,2,40] One has to be very careful to suggest that these appearances truly represent degenerative change.[40] What in fact is being seen are anterior bony spurs which have been erroneously called either osteophytes or syndesmophytes. Osteophytes are projections of new bone around effete hyaline cartilage cells in osteoarthritis while syndesmophytes are bony spurs projecting from the margins of syndesmoses. It should be remembered that intervertebral body joints are neither synovial joints nor syndesmoses (bone-fibrocartilage-bone). Intervertebral body joints are symphyses (bone-hyaline cartilage [cartilaginous end plate]–fibrocartilage [intervertebral disk]-hyaline cartilage-bone)[48] (▶ Fig. 5.8). However, what occurs with intervertebral joints on the concave side are marginal spurs of new bone formation simply because they are under compression as per Wolf's law (see Chapter 3). Such appearances should not be

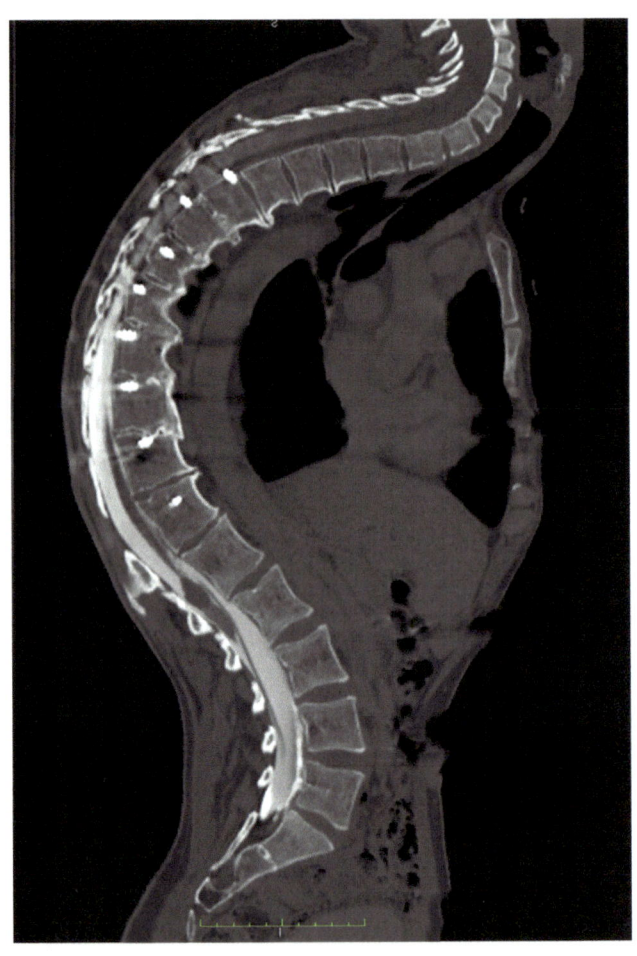

Fig. 5.7 Lateral CT scan of a patient who underwent unsuccessful posterior instrumentation for a type I Scheuermann's disease. Note the multilevel anterior spurring with possible fusion in some places.

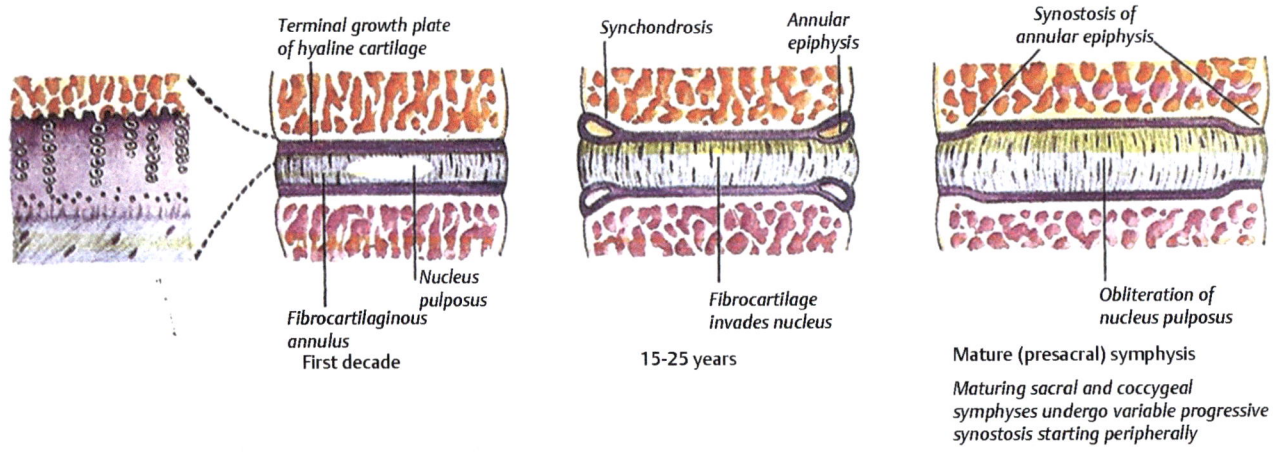

Fig. 5.8 Intervertebral body joints are symphyses – bone (vertebral body) – highline cartilage (endplate cartilage) intervertebral disk (fibrocartilage) – highline cartilage – bone. (Reproduced with permission from Gray's anatomy. Williams PL, Warwick R, Dyson M, Bannister LH (eds). Churchill Livingstone, Edinburgh 1989: Fig 4.1b.)

First decade: Terminal growth plate of hyaline cartilage, Fibrocartilaginous annulus, Nucleus pulposus

15–25 years: Synchondrosis, Annular epiphysis, Fibrocartilage invades nucleus

Mature (presacral) symphysis: Synostosis of annular epiphysis, Obliteration of nucleus pulposus. Maturing sacral and coccygeal symphyses undergo variable progressive synostosis starting peripherally

misconstrued as showing evidence of degenerative joint disease.

The characteristic three level apical vertebral wedging helps to differentiate Scheuermann's kyphosis from other forms of local kyphosis, in particular congenital kyphosis, neurofibromatosis kyphosis, the kyphosis associated with bullet-shaped vertebrae in mesenchymal disorders (see Chapter 10), and the kyphosis associated with infection and tumors.[49] However, radiologists not infrequently report a classical Scheuermann's kyphosis as osteomyelitis of the spine, particularly if the end plate irregularities are pronounced and the hypertrophied anterior soft tissues give the appearance of a paravertebral shadow. In this situation the clinical findings of an otherwise healthy child help to differentiate the two. Where the differential diagnosis is occasionally in doubt occurs when there has been a vertical loading with flexion injury to the adolescent thoracic spine. In this case the vertebral bodies are wedged and very closely resemble that of Scheuermann's disease. Perhaps the two need not be strictly differentiated apart from medicolegally, as Scheuermann's kyphosis is presumably the result of decreased growth anteriorly leading to further compression and further reduction in growth and may indeed have very minor repetitive trauma as an adjunct.

5.4 Management

Former treatment methods, which included bed rest or prolonged periods of recumbency on various frames, are both anachronistic and quite out of proportion to the nature of the underlying process, to which the term pathological is probably not semantically correct. As serious neurological complications are exceedingly rare, treatment concerns itself with body topography and the patient's, and certainly to a much lesser extent the surgeon's, view thereof. Type II (thoracolumbar or lumbar) kyphosis is not usually a problem of deformity but of pain and this can generally be alleviated by the traditional conservative measures for back pain, which include extension exercises plus hands-on physiotherapy and a supportive brace or corset for periods of severe pain.[7,8] Surgical treatment is less often required for type II kyphosis. Type I kyphosis, however, can be a major problem of deformity with potential progression during growth.

5.4.1 Conservative Treatment

Thoracic Scheuermann's kyphosis is perhaps the only spinal deformity (except early onset idiopathic scoliosis) that can be satisfactorily treated conservatively as it is a two-dimensional deformity behind the axis of spinal column rotation and therefore is not rotationally unstable and so does not buckle. Progressive change in vertebral shape producing the condition is caused by the anterior end of the growth plates being under compression, with a consequent reduction in anterior height. Accordingly, treatment that seeks to extend the kyphotic area reduces the amount of compression,[49] and a true physiological reconstitution of normal vertebral shape in the median plane is possible (▶ Fig. 5.9). Conservative treatment for Scheuermann's kyphosis works by extension.[50] An extension cast or brace that obliterates the lumbar lordosis causes thoracic hyperextension above in order to produce the desired physiological effect, whereas with idiopathic scoliosis the hyperextension so produced will bring the lordosis back toward the sagittal plane with apparent improvement of the scoliosis on X-ray. However, all that will do is to increase the underlying lordosis, the undesirability of which has already been commented upon.[51] Although the Milwaukee brace has been the mainstay of

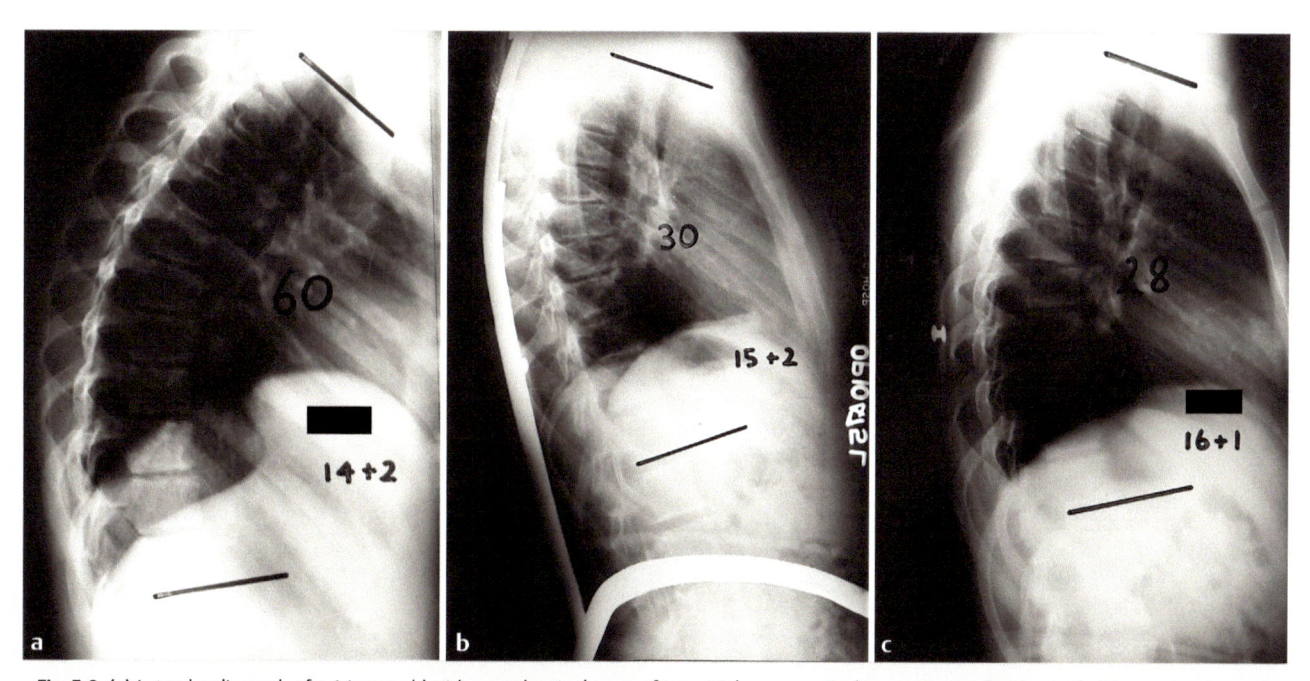

Fig. 5.9 (a) Lateral radiograph of a 14-year-old with a moderate degree of type I Scheuermann's disease. He was first treated with an extension cast. (b) Lateral radiograph in an underarm TLSO showing a correction of 50%. (c) Lateral radiograph at the age of 16 on removal of the brace a month previously. The correction has been sustained.

conservative treatment for Scheuermann's disease,[41] it is not necessary to have an orthosis with super-structure. Indeed the underarm Boston-type brace is better because of its superior powers of obliteration of the lumbar lordosis. Flexion of the spine above can be prevented by increasing the anterior height of the orthosis. We have found that wearing the brace for 12 hours at a time is quite sufficient and patients agree! According to Bradford[41] the indications for brace treatment are initial curves of less than 70 degrees with a Risser sign lower than grade 3 and minimal vertebral wedging in fewer than three vertebrae (is that really Scheuermann's disease?). However, the critical initial curve magnitude should surely be the level at which the patient finds the deformity unacceptable. Obviously the more growth to go the better the prognosis for conservative treatment. However, minimal vertebral wedging in fewer than three vertebrae will be difficult to equate with the diagnostic criteria of Sorensen[1] and Scheuermann[10] who insist that there must be at least 5 degrees of wedging over three consecutive apical vertebrae.

Bradford's rationale of getting in the end a thoracic kyphosis of 50 degrees is that if you obtain an initial correction of 50% in the brace you may then lose 20 degrees at follow-up to finish up at 50 degrees. However, that must represent an only moderate result to improve an ugly roundback by a mere 20 degrees. We have not found such a loss in brace treatment satisfies customers. Nowadays patients want a better correction than that. Stagnara and colleagues[52-55] developed the Lyons method of treatment: physiotherapy, casting, and bracing. Ponte (personal communication) treated more than 3,000 Scheuermann's patients but not all of them had the strict diagnosis of Scheuermann's disease. He used a combination of casting followed by bracing. Initial curve magnitude was just under 60 degrees and the improvement was about 40%. The best predictor of a good result was initial curve flexibility which was at least 40%. Again this would suggest that not very many of these patients had true Scheuermann's disease because the characteristic of the apical three vertebrae is that they are totally rigid.

Two factors govern the response to treatment. The younger the age of onset, the more growth can be harnessed in favor of the patient such that vertebral shape can be reconstituted. Indeed, so successful can this treatment be at this age, that the response must be carefully monitored, lest a thoracic lordosis is produced[41] which could result in a mild idiopathic scoliosis. Such young and favorable spines are unfortunately not the rule, however, as the age of onset tends to be closer to the attainment of general skeletal maturity. As the vertebral growth plates do not fuse until the 25th year on average,[11-15] there is no reason why conservative treatment cannot be prescribed for the older adolescent, although the results are generally not as satisfactory. The second factor is the degree of deformity at presentation, and clearly, the worse the situation is to start with, the less good can be the expected response. Should the patient with a sizeable deformity of the order of 70 degrees not wish to undergo the risks of surgical intervention then clearly conservative treatment should be prescribed but it may well be that several hyperextension casts are required prior to the use of bracing.[53-55] Indeed that might not be a bad idea for every patient so as to get off to the best possible start.

However, there is much about the natural history of Scheuermann's disease that is unclear. For example, the incorrect assumption that the spine stops growing at the time of the general skeletal maturity has led to cessation of bracing too soon. This is exemplified by a report of 39 cases braced for only 18 months who lost virtually all of their 30% correction over the next year and a half out of the brace.[56] Conservative treatment cannot be blamed if it was stopped too soon. Soo followed up 63 patients with Scheuermann's kyphosis for a mean of 14 years and 60% of these had radiographic evaluation.[57] There were three treatment modalities: exercise, bracing, and surgery. As would be expected the most severe curves (mean 74 degrees) had surgery, intermediate were the brace group (65 degrees), while the exercise group had a mean curvature of 58 degrees. Braced patients were younger with an average age of 12.2 years which is perhaps unusually young but does allow the adolescent growth spurt to be utilized. Exercise produced a negligible change in deformity while bracing achieved an average improvement of 13 degrees.

Meanwhile the Wilmington group looked at 22 patients with type 1 Scheuermann's kyphosis treated with the DuPont kyphosis brace and followed them until skeletal maturity.[58] The results were not good with 9 patients only showing an improvement of just 9 degrees and 7 remaining unchanged while 6 progressed by an average of 9 degrees. Optimal conservative treatment results appear to accompany an aggressive treatment regimen that starts with extension casting which is more rigid and initially corrective followed by extension bracing, and thus the two treatments are rather more complementary than alternative. Our view is that as Scheuermann's kyphosis is at least treatable nonoperatively then extension casting followed by bracing should be prescribed (▶ Fig. 5.9). The results of so doing are definitely better the earlier the age of the patient and the more flexible and less sizeable the deformity. It is certainly not worth persisting with bracing unless an early significant benefit is appreciable. Therefore, a trial of extension casting followed by bracing should first of all demonstrate a good initial improvement and that should be sustained for a year; otherwise, surgical correction should be considered. Again it is important to get away from the Cobb angle. Patients should be treated conservatively if they find the deformity unacceptable and want to avoid surgery at least to start with and a significant round-back deformity seems to be just as intrusive psychosocially as a bad rib hump in idiopathic scoliosis.

Electrospinal stimulation has been used for Scheuermann's disease.[59] However, the correction of not more than 20% indicates that, while improvement is possible because of the uncomplicated uniplanar nature of the deformity, this is at best only half as effective as cast and/or brace. More importantly, time for a better physiological correction has been wasted and we therefore consider electrical treatment contraindicated.

With the uncertain outcome of brace treatment and the more body awareness of teenagers nowadays there has been a steady reduction in the prescription of brace treatment and a reciprocal increase in the choice of surgery.

5.4.2 Surgical Treatment

Surgical treatment for Scheuermann's disease is indicated if the deformity relapses after too short a term of brace treatment for the younger adolescent with progressive kyphosis or for the mature patient with an established unacceptable kyphotic deformity. Leatherman found that better corrections were obtained with preliminary multiple anterior diskectomy or indeed apical vertebral resection. Then in a second stage two Harrington compression systems were inserted and the kyphosis was fused posterolaterally[40,60,61] (▶ Fig. 5.10). Posterior surgery alone did not consistently produce the desired effect and although kyphoses not in excess of 70 degrees fared better than bigger curves, correction was not impressive and loss of correction postoperatively was the rule rather than the exception.[40] This is not surprising as these deformities are quite rigid and it is the front of the spine that is short, contracted, and under compression while the surgical attack has been on the back. Consequently, posterior fusions on the tension side of the spine did tend to fail. Thus a little later, in the 1970s, it was felt that anterior surgery was the critical factor in obtaining a good and lasting correction and this included anterior release of the anterior ligament and periosteum followed by anterior multiple diskectomy right back to the posterior ligament plus apical body resection if necessary and then anterior apical interbody or strut grafting[61–65] (▶ Fig. 5.10). A strut of autogenous iliac crest bone was much stronger than rib or fibula graft and could be keyed in place over the apex of the kyphosis[65,66] (▶ Fig. 5.11).

In those days it was generally felt that it would be better to separate the anterior and posterior stages by a week or two. Then in the posterior second stage bilateral Harrington compression systems were inserted followed by a posterolateral fusion. Some felt that it would be advantageous if the strut graft (in this case rib) came with its own blood supply on a vascular pedicle.[67,68] In those days it was not unreasonable to consider that that might be beneficial but the chief factor governing the need for a pedicle graft anywhere is a poorly vascularized recipient area and, if there is a good healthy bed for the graft, as with the front of the spine in Scheuermann's disease, then that is not necessary but of course, particularly with post-irradiation kyphosis, any strut graft needs all the help it can get to incorporate and a free vascularized graft can be helpful. In those days it was thought to be beneficial to have interval traction between stages.[69] Although it was traditional to insert two Harrington compression systems Leatherman went on to use one distraction rod and one compression system, the former applying downward cantilever pressure on the apex of the kyphosis and the latter gathering up the slack.[70] Furthermore sublaminar wires could be added to the distraction rod to better distribute load.

Then as instrumentation techniques were progressively developed the use of Cotrel-Dubousset (CD) instrumentation became very popular not only for scoliosis but also for kyphosis[71] (▶ Fig. 5.12). Then the first CD instrumentation put in in the United States was in Louisville, Kentucky, by Jean Dubousset and Yves Cotrel a long-time friend of Dr. Leatherman himself who assisted in the procedure. Zielke popularized the idea of posterior pedicle screw fixation using his ventral derotation spondylodesis (VDS) system applied posteriorly into the body through pedicle screws following an anterior release and fusion in the first stage.[72]

For the past 10 years at least pedicle screws have become the norm for fixation of posterior instrumentation to the back of the spine. Operative results do seem to vary and some report rather poor results while those with better outcomes still do not achieve corrections anywhere near comparable to similar curve sizes in idiopathic scoliosis.

Henk Been's group in Amsterdam reported treatment of Scheuermann's disease using a combined anterior and posterior fusion.[73] There were 23 patients and in the anterior first stage the apical four to six disks were removed and then in the posterior stage either CD instrumentation or Moss-Miami was applied using double two-hook claw constructs above and pedicular screws below. The initial preoperative kyphosis was 70 degrees which was initially reduced to 40 degrees which then lapsed to 55 degrees at follow-up. They thought that the late deterioration was caused by early removal of the metalwork

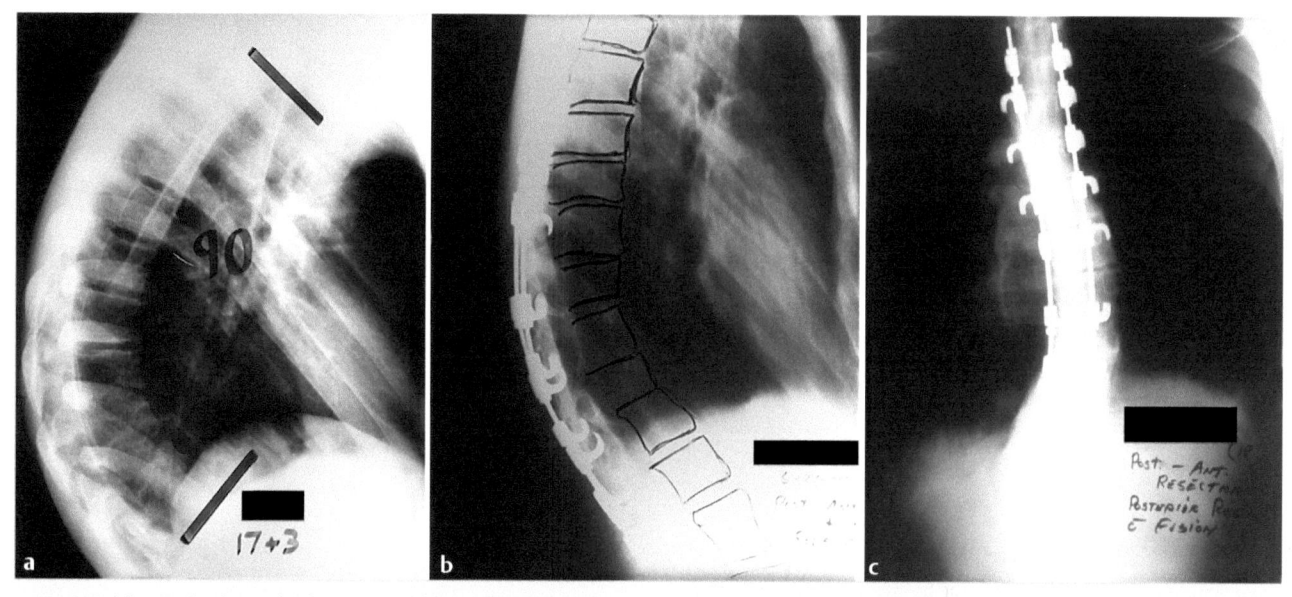

Fig. 5.10 (a) Lateral radiograph of a 17-year-old boy with a 90-degree thoracic kyphosis who found the deformity unacceptable. (b) Lateral radiograph after anterior vertebral body resection at the apex showing an excellent correction. (c) PA radiograph showing that the two compression symptoms had to be contoured over a coexistent mild degree of scoliosis.

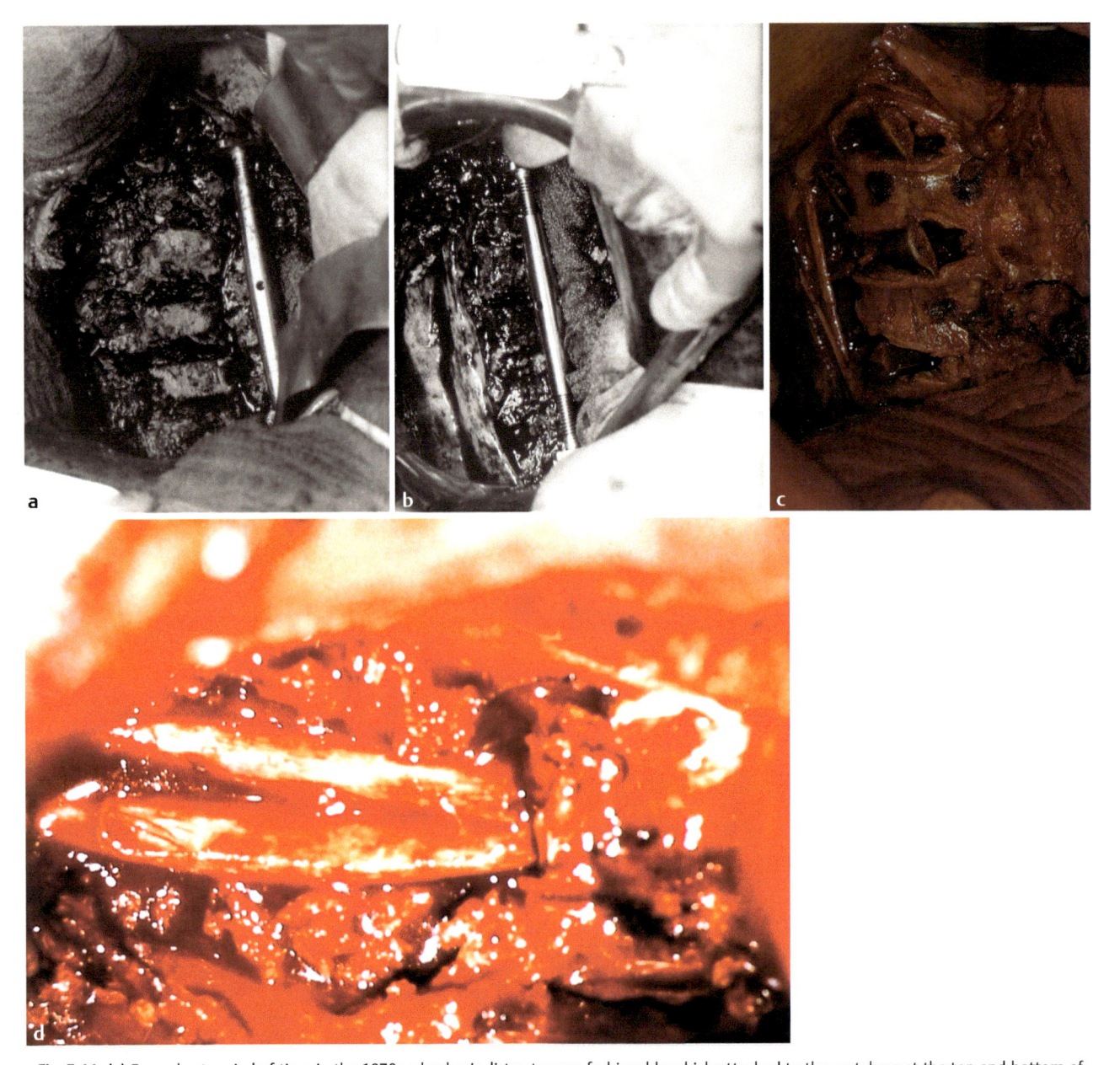

Fig. 5.11 (a) For a short period of time in the 1970s a kyphosis distractor was fashionable which attached to the vertebrae at the top and bottom of the proposed anterior graft area. (b) The body of the distractor was then rotated to extend its length and thus aid correction. This was the distractor of Gardner, similar to that of Pinto. (c) When the disk spaces were then distracted open pieces of rib could be inserted to jack open the disk space and then morselized bits of graft added to fill the rest of the interbody area. (d) Alternatively, and preferably, a strut graft could be keyed into place propping open the corrected position after removal of the distractor. Clearly only one of the struts would be under compression but the other was inserted along with cancellous bone chips to enhance a good fusion mass.

despite the fact that various radiographic measures had suggested a solid fusion.

Then Alvin Crawford's group in Cincinnati reported their experience of combined thoracoscopic anterior release with posterior spinal fusion.[74] There were 19 patients with an average age of 17 years and a follow-up of 2.7 years. They released an average of 8 disks anteriorly while 13 levels were fused posteriorly. They managed to achieve a correction from 85 degrees preoperatively to 45 degrees at follow-up which represents a very good correction. In 2006 the St. Louis group reported a comparative study between 18 patients with Scheuermann's disease who underwent posterior only thoracic pedicle screw fusions and 21 who underwent an anterior/posterior fusion.[75] The groups were reasonably well matched with an initial Cobb angle of 89 degrees in the anterior/posterior group and 84 degrees in the posterior only fusion group. However, 12 of the 18 posterior group also underwent Smith-Petersen osteotomies. The posterior only group finished up at follow-up with a kyphosis of 40 degrees while the anterior/posterior group finished up with a kyphosis of 58 degrees from which the authors concluded that an anterior release was not essential. Because in the posterior only group the majority had posterior shortening osteotomies (a very logical way of dealing with a too long back of the spine) then the results are not surprising and perhaps

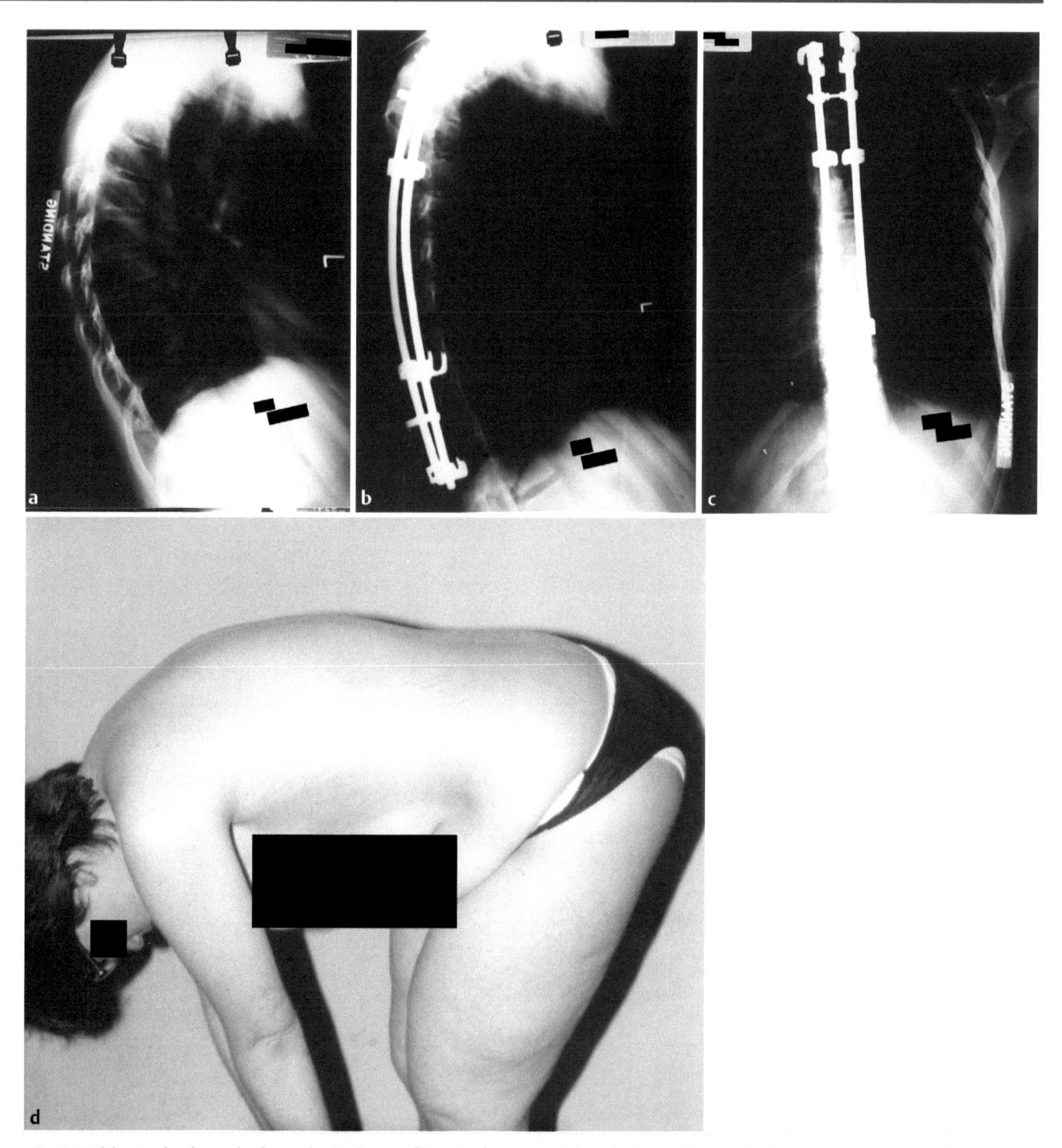

Fig. 5.12 (a) Lateral radiograph of a moderate degree of type I Scheuermann's hyperkyphosis. (b) Lateral radiograph after anterior multiple diskectomy and insertion of posterior CD instrumentation showing a good correction. (c) PA view showing the extent of the instrumentation. (d) Forward bending picture postoperatively of this patient who is depicted in ▶ Fig. 5.5.

the optimal correction would be achieved by a preliminary anterior release followed by posterior fusion incorporating osteotomies. Do not forget the front of the spine.

The Nottingham group compared autogenous rib graft versus cages for the anterior part of the management of Scheuermann's kyphosis.[76] They compared eight patients who had rib graft versus seven with cages packed with bone graft. The preoperative mean kyphosis was all of 86 degrees and there was no difference in the long-term correction down to 42 degrees at more than 5 years.

Then the Austin Texas group which included Ponte and Shufflebarger reported on 17 patients with Scheuermann's kyphosis treated with posterior thoracic pedicle screw instrumentation in association with multiple Ponte osteotomies.[77] Correction of the instrumented levels was more than 60% and the Cobb angle over the apical region was corrected to 50 degrees. This again shows the benefit of posterior bone shortening. Their comment that no patient needed an anterior approach to achieve sufficient correction or fusion is slightly oblique and certainly does not confirm that an anterior release in addition to posterior Ponte osteotomy correction would not be the ideal. They state benefits of reduced morbidity and not extending operative time with the inclusion of an anterior approach but surely the goal must be an operation for life with the best possible correction particularly bearing in mind how successful modern anaesthesia is.

Then came a report from Korea including the names of Lenke and Bridwell of a number of thoracic hyperkyphoses including 29 with Scheuermann's disease. Indeed, only one had a post-traumatic kyphosis and one a post-laminectomy kyphosis and so perhaps it would have been better for uniformity to leave out the two non-Scheuermann's patients.[78] Anyway the point of the paper was to determine principally the distal fusion level and this was confirmed to be when the sagittal stable vertebra (SSV)—the most proximal lumbar vertebral body touched by the vertical line from the posterosuperior corner of the sacrum—was included.

Then in 2010 the Scoliosis Research Society Morbidity and Mortality Committee reported on the complications of spinal fusion for Scheuermann's kyphosis.[79] There was a total of 683 procedures and pediatric and adult patients were arbitrarily divided as being equal to or below 19 years of age or older respectively; 49% of cases were posterior spinal fusions alone, 11% anterior spinal fusions alone, and 40% combined anterior and posterior procedures. Wound infection was the most common complication at 4% and the acute neurological complication rate was almost 2% including four spinal cord injuries. The mortality rate was 0.6%. Complications were significantly more common in adult patients than children. This paper is extremely important in being so comprehensive and providing such a useful database with which to discuss surgery with patients and families in a proper risks and rewards equation.

Recently the San Diego group looked at the opening of disks anteriorly in 11 patients who underwent thoracoscopic anterior release followed by posterior instrumentation and 11 who underwent posterior instrumentation only.[80] The posterior only patients also underwent Ponte osteotomies. Again the results might suggest that the optimal situation would be an anterior release followed by posterior instrumentation and fusion after multiple Ponte osteotomies. The posterior only group corrected from 83 degrees to 48 degrees while the anterior and posterior group corrected from 85 degrees to 49 degrees. Most of the correction occurred at or below the apex and they found that the addition of an anterior release didn't alter either the correction or the disk shape. Again one wonders whether thoracoscopic anterior release can really be so radical as via open thoracotomy.

We have found the best corrections follow anterior multiple diskectomy and posterior transpedicular instrumentation (▶ Fig. 5.13 and ▶ Fig. 5.14). Perhaps the most common cause for tertiary referral with type I Scheuermann's disease is instrumentation that is too short. Fusion from end to end vertebrae is quite inadequate for Scheuermann's disease which not only needs to go well beyond the upper and lower end vertebrae but should extend both upward and downward into the

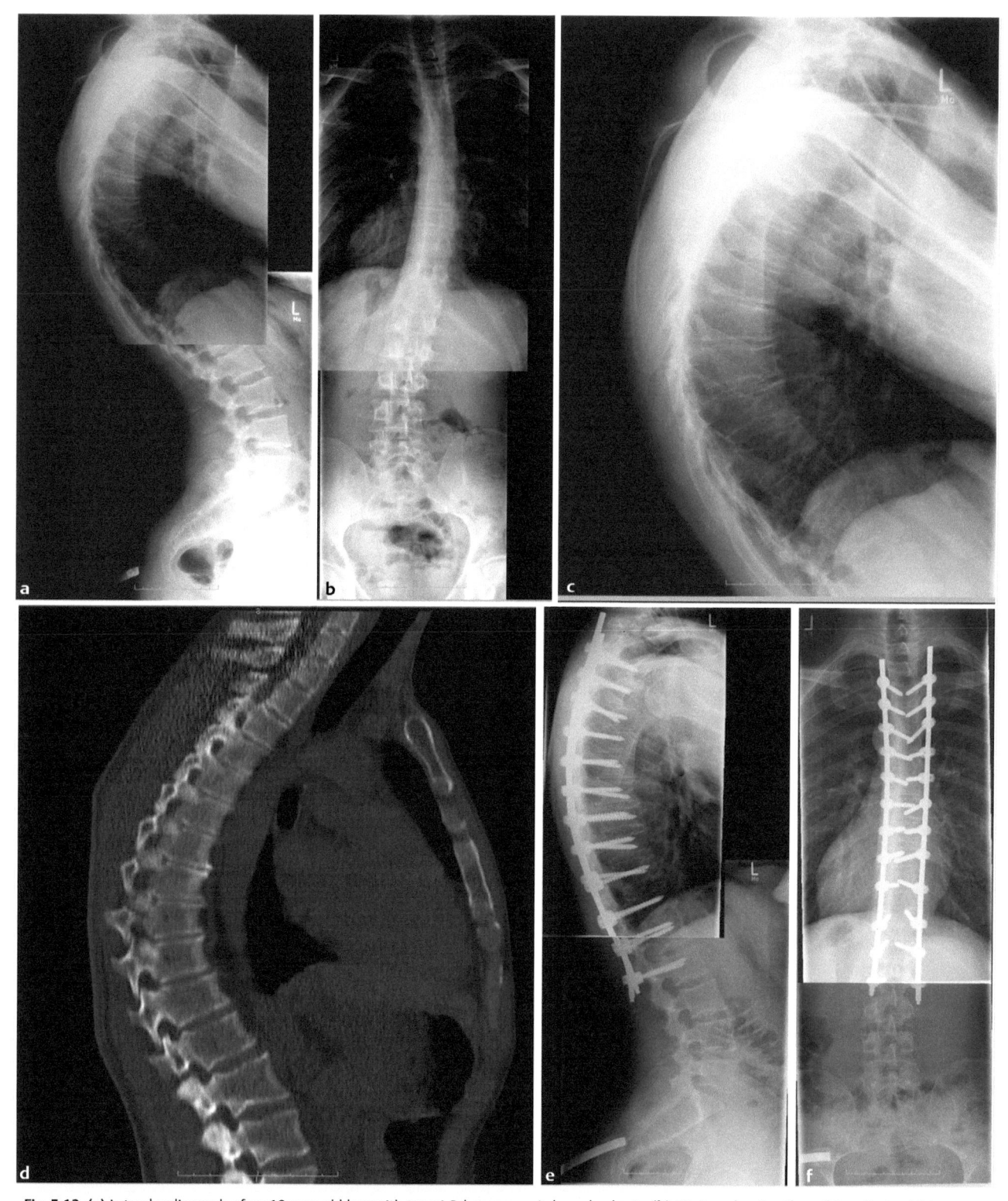

Fig. 5.13 (a) Lateral radiograph of an 18-year-old boy with type I Scheuermann's hyperkyphosis. (b) PA view showing the mild scoliosis which occurs because the kyphotic process is not exactly symmetrical in the frontal plane. (c) Lateral X-ray of the thoracic spine only showing typical features of Scheuermann's thoracic type I hyperkyphosis—significant kyphosis, elongation of vertebral bodies in the transverse plane, Schmorl node formation anteriorly, the beginnings of anterior spur formation. (d) Sagittal CT scan of the thoracic spine shows the pathoanatomy very well. (e) Lateral radiograph 2 years after posterior-only instrumentation showing an excellent correction. (f) PA radiograph showing a straight spine in the coronal plane.

Scheuermann's Disease

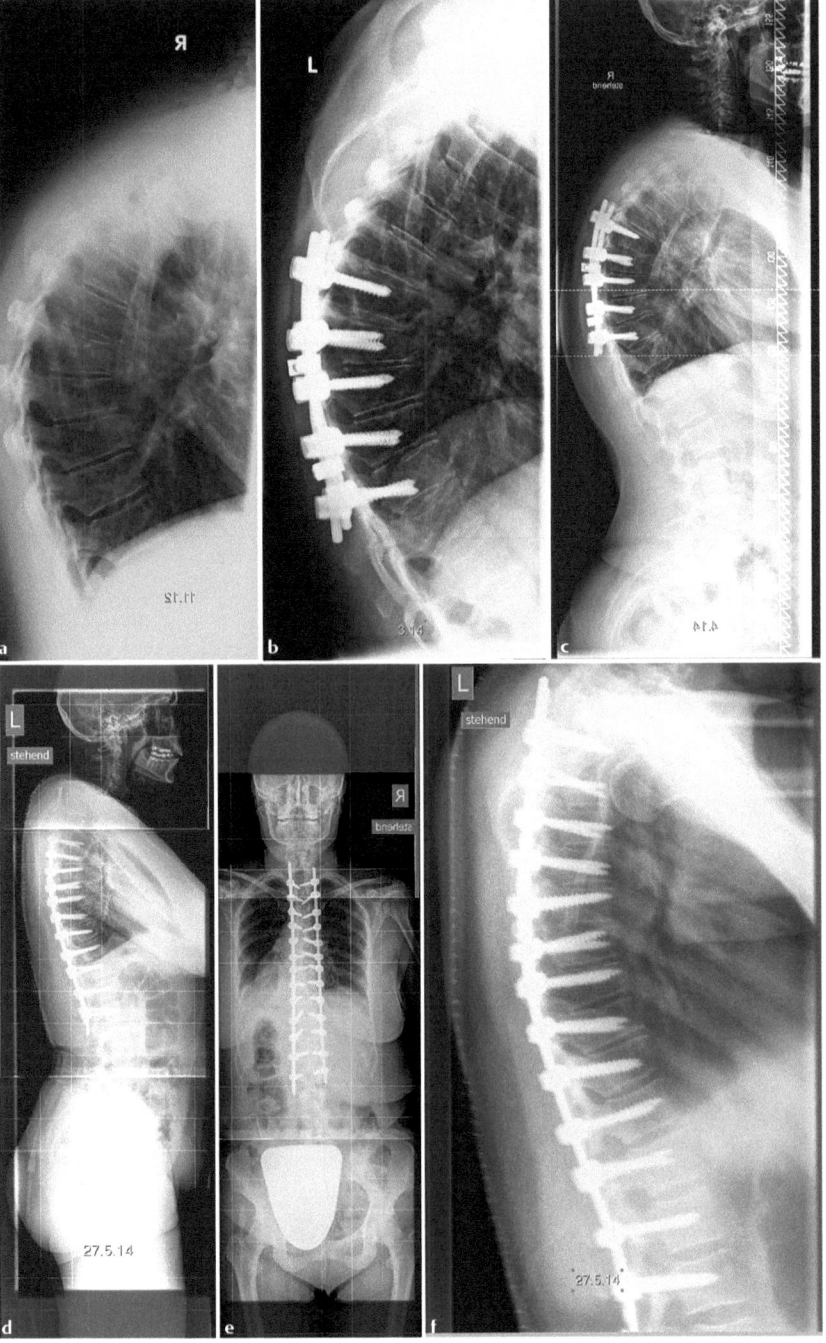

Fig. 5.14 (a) Lateral radiograph of the thoracic spine showing classical type I Scheuermann's hyperkyphosis. (b) Lateral radiograph of the thoracic spine showing a very short fixation over the apex only. This inadequate surgery was performed in another country before being referred. (c) Lateral radiograph of the whole spine showing that there has been no change in the overall thoracic kyphosis which was the reason for surgery in the first place. (d) Lateral radiograph of the whole spine showing a natural sagittal profile after removal of the original metalwork and instrumentation from T1 to L2. (e) PA radiograph post-surgery. (f) Lateral radiograph of the thoracic spine showing fixation in close up.

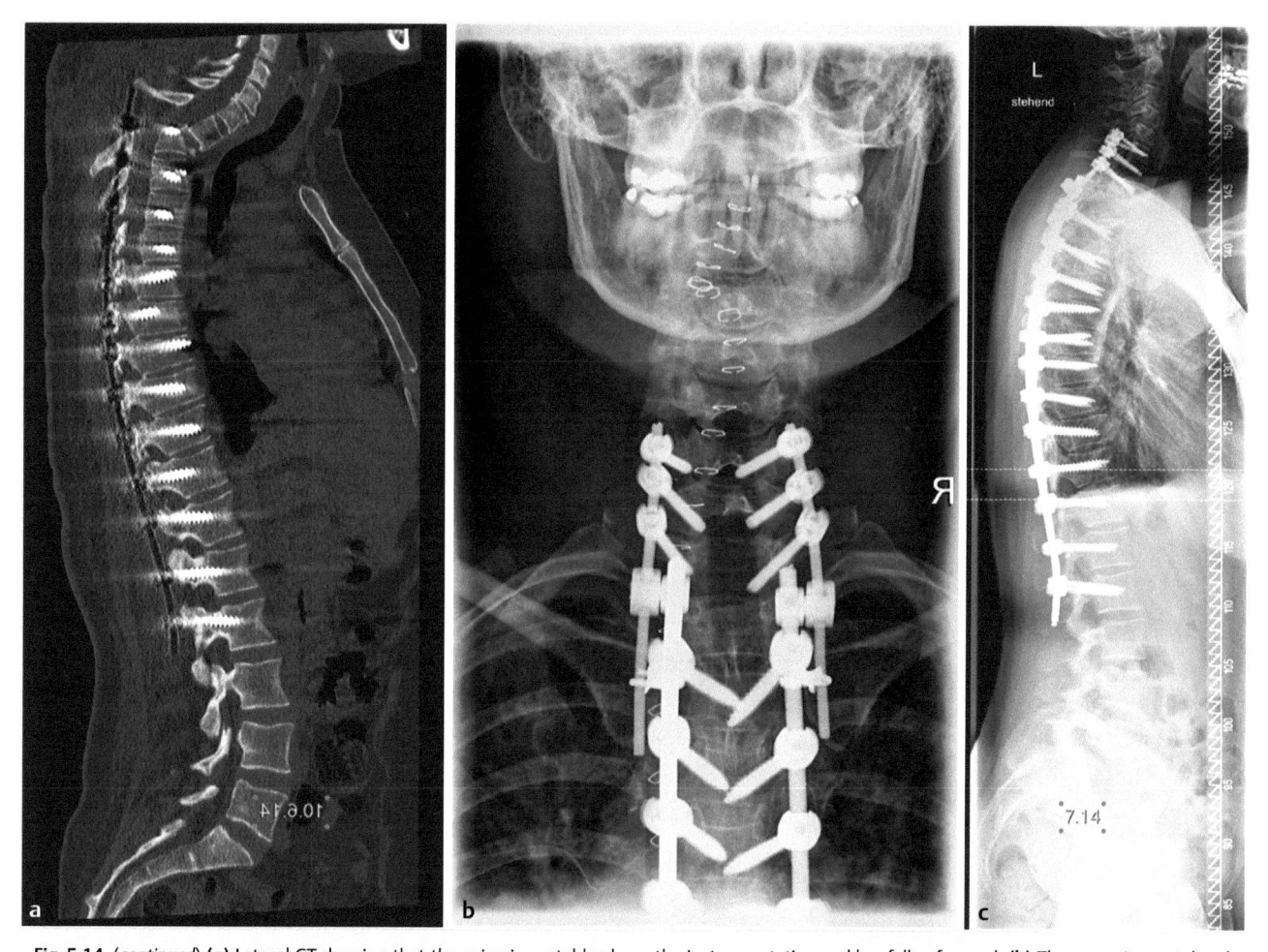

Fig. 5.14 (*continued*) **(g)** Lateral CT showing that the spine is unstable above the instrumentation and has fallen forward. **(h)** The posterior metalwork was extended into the lower cervical spine to maintain a straight cervicothoracic junction. **(i)** Lateral radiograph of the total construct.

compensatory curves to try and restore a natural sagittal profile. An 18-year-old (▶ Fig. 5.15) underwent posterior transpedicular instrumentation 3 years earlier but the instrumentation only extended from T5 to T12 whereas from T3 to L2 would have been minimal preferably one more above and below. The deformity had not only recurred but was even worse than before surgery with a bitterly disappointed young man. The posterior fusion had matured with interbody fusions in some places (▶ Fig. 5.15c). After anterior and posterior osteotomies and reinstrumentation from T2 to L3, an excellent correction was obtained and a natural sagittal profile restored (▶ Fig. 5.15d,e) to a happy lad.

For type II Scheuermann's disease with a more angular and lower kyphosis these often require apical resection of bone as well as multiple disks (▶ Fig. 5.16). A lengthy instrumentation is not necessary for these cases.

The integrity of the spinal cord is only rarely threatened by the kyphosis of Scheuermann's disease and only then when the kyphosis is unusually very severe. In 1980 the Minneapolis group reported their experience of 43 cases of spinal cord compression secondary to kyphotic deformity and only 2 cases were due to Scheuermann's disease, the great majority having congenital kyphoses.[81] Anterior cord compression gave the best results. The American pioneer in this regard was the late Dr. Kenton Leatherman of Louisville, Kentucky, who initially described closing wedge resection for rigid spinal curves and whose report of 67 successful cases is quite unique in the world literature.[61] He always staged his surgery into first stage anterior spinal cord decompression at the apex with the insertion of a strut graft and then posterior instrumentation to stabilize the corrected position (▶ Fig. 5.10).

From the foregoing it can be seen that, although idiopathic scoliosis corrections are excellent, sometimes of the order of 80 or 90%, the general corrections in Scheuermann's kyphosis fall far below that. It would appear that even in very good hands the best corrections that can be achieved are of the order of 50%. Surely it must be the case that the patient deserves the best possible correction and that must be a combination of anterior multiple diskectomy and grafting followed by posterior instrumentation with additional posterior osteotomies as necessary. However, our experience recently of several cases of type I Scheuermann's disease treated by multiple Ponte osteotomies and then transpedicular instrumentation might suggest perhaps that anterior surgery may not be as necessary as originally thought although for kyphosis a sound anterior fusion is a definitive end result. It is however important that sagittal

Scheuermann's Disease

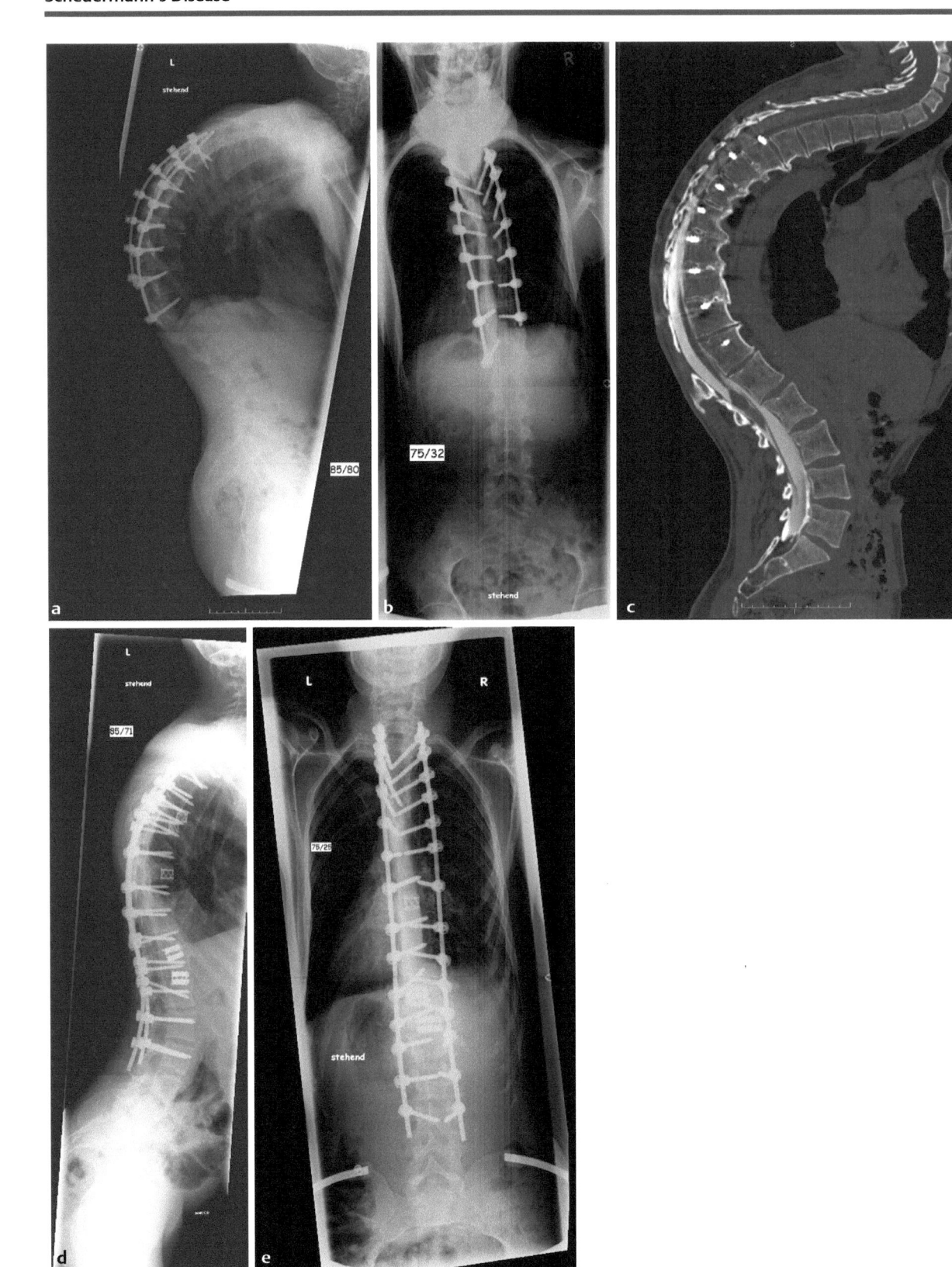

Fig. 5.15 **(a,b)** Revision surgery for type I Scheuermann's disease in an 18-year-old who 3 years previously had undergone posterior fusion with instrumentation that was far too short. **(c)** Lateral CT showing that the kyphosis had worsened to more than 90 degrees with adding on above and below the instrumentation. **(d,e)** Lateral and PA radiographs after osteotomies and reinstrumentation. This lengthy instrumentation should have been done first time round.

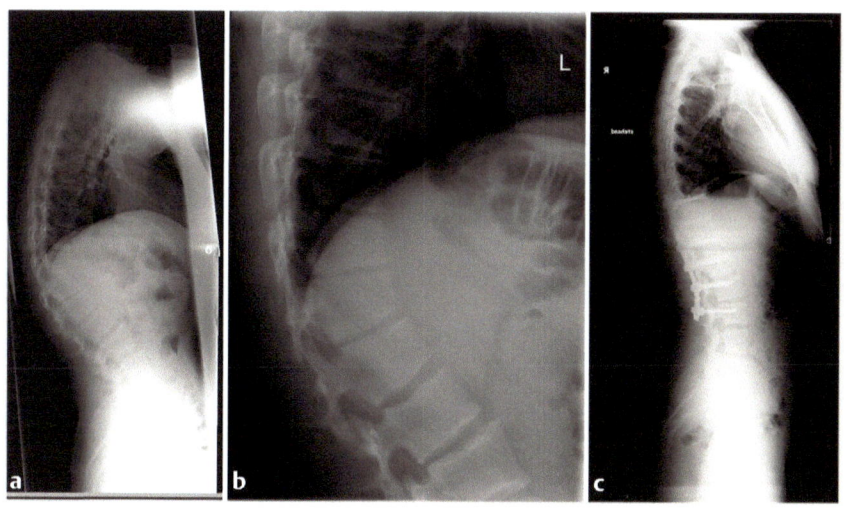

Fig. 5.16 (a) Lateral radiograph of the thoracolumbar spine of a 20-year-old man with type II thoracolumbar Scheuermann's disease. (b) Spot lateral of the thoracolumbar region during the considerable wedging of the apical vertebrae. (c) Lateral radiograph after anterior release and posterior six segment fixation from T9 to L2 showing restoration of a natural sagittal profile.

balance is maintained and that means making sure that the apex of the deformity lies in the center of the instrumentation. It is best to think about this beforehand and look carefully at the standing lateral film against a grid, noting the sagittal stable vertebra.[78]

References

Note: References in **bold** are Key References.

[1] **Sorensen KH. Scheuermann's Kyphosis. Clinical Appearances. Radiography, Aetiology and Prognosis. Copenhagen: Junksgaard; 1964**
[2] **Scheuermann HW. Kyphosis Juvenile (Scheuermanns Krankheit). Fortschr Geb Rontgenstr. 1936; 53:1–16**
[3] **Bradford DS. Juvenile kyphosis. Clin Orthop Relat Res. 1977(128):45–55**
[4] Schanz A. Berlin Klin Wchnschr 1907;44:986. Cited by Sorensen, 1964
[5] Wassmann K. Kyphosis juvenilis Scheuermann—an occupational disorder. Acta Orthop Scand. 1951; 21(1–4):65–74
[6] Micheli LJ. Low back pain in the adolescent: differential diagnosis. Am J Sports Med. 1979; 7(6):362–364
[7] Greene TL, Hensinger RN, Hunter LY. Back pain and vertebral changes simulating Scheuermann's disease. J Pediatr Orthop. 1985; 5(1):1–7
[8] Kehl D, Lovell WW, MacEwen GD. Scheuermann's disease of the lumbar spine. Orthop Trans. 1982; 6:342
[9] Dickson RA, Lawton JO, Archer IA, et al. Bi-planar spinal asymmetry. The pathogenesis of idiopathic scoliosis. J Bone Joint Surg Br. 1984; 66:143–144
[10] Scheuermann HW. . Kyphosis Dorsalis Juvenilis. Ugeskr Laeger. 1920; 82:385–393
[11] Haas SL. Growth in length of the vertebrae. Arch Surg. 1939; 38:245–249
[12] Bick EM, Copel JW. Longitudinal growth of the human vertebra; a contribution to human osteogeny. J Bone Joint Surg Am. 1950; 32 A(4):803–814
[13] Bick EM, Copel JW. The ring apophysis of the human vertebra; contribution to human osteogeny. II. J Bone Joint Surg Am. 1951; 33-A(3):783–787
[14] Larsen EH, Nordentoft EL. Growth of the epiphyses and vertebrae. Acta Orthop Scand. 1962; 32:210–217
[15] Bernick S, Cailliet R. Vertebral end-plate changes with aging of human vertebrae. Spine. 1982; 7(2):97–102
[16] Schmorl G. Die Pathogenese der juvenile Kyphose. Fortschr Geb Rontgenstr. 1930; 41:359–383
[17] Knutsson F. Observations on the growth of the vertebral body in Scheuermann's disease. Acta Radiol. 1948; 30(1–2):97–104
[18] Bradford DS, Moe JH. Scheuermann's juvenile kyphosis. A histologic study. Clin Orthop Relat Res. 1975; 110(110):45–53
[19] Bradford DS, Brown DM, Moe JH, Winter RB, Jowsey J. Scheuermann's kyphosis: a form of osteoporosis? Clin Orthop Relat Res. 1976(118):10–15
[20] Salter RB, Harriw WR. Injuries involving the epiphyseal plate. J Bone Joint Surg Am. 1963; 45:587–622
[21] Aufdermaur M. Juvenile kyphosis (Scheuermann's disease): radiography, histology, and pathogenesis. Clin Orthop Relat Res. 1981(154):166–174
[22] Aufdermar M, Spycher M. Pathogenesis of osteochondrosis juvenile Scheuermann. J Pediatr Orthop. 1986; 4:452
[23] Ippolito E, Ponseti IV. Juvenile kyphosis: histological and histochemical studies. J Bone Joint Surg Am. 1981; 63(2):175–182
[24] Ascani E, Borelli P, Larosa G, et al. Malattia di Scheuermann. I: studio ormonale. In: Gaggia A, ed. Progresi in patologia vertebrale, Vol.5A. Boulogne: Gaggi editore P: 1997
[25] Murray PM, Weinstein SL, Spratt KF. The natural history and long-term follow-up of Scheuermann kyphosis. J Bone Joint Surg Am. 1993; 75(2):236–248
[26] Buckler JMH. A reference manual of growth and development. St Louis: Blackwell, Mosby; 1979:12–16
[27] Gilsanz V, Gibbens DT, Carlson M, King J. Vertebral bone density in Scheuermann disease. J Bone Joint Surg Am. 1989; 71(6):894–897
[28] Willner S. Spinal pantograph - a non-invasive technique for describing kyphosis and lordosis in the thoraco-lumbar spine. Acta Orthop Scand. 1981; 52(5):525–529
[29] Oxborrow NJ, Walder A, Stirling A, Millner PA, Dickson RA. Sagittal spinal profile in normal children: A radiographic study through the growth spurt. J Bone Joint Surg Br. 1998; 80 Supp II:204
[30] Delmas A. Types rachidiens de statique corporelle. Rev Morphophysiol Humaine. 1951; 4(11):26–32
[31] Stagnara P, De Mauroy JC, Dran G, et al. Reciprocal angulation of vertebral bodies in a sagittal plane: approach to references for the evaluation of kyphosis and lordosis. Spine. 1982; 7(4):335–342
[32] Tanner JN. Growth at Adolescence. Oxford: Blackwell; 1962
[33] Roth M. [Idiopathic scoliosis and Scheuermann's disease: essentially identical manifestations of neuro-vertebral growth disproportion]. Radiol Diagn (Berl). 1981; 22(3):380–391
[34] **Deacon P, Berkin CR, Dickson RA. Combined idiopathic kyphosis and scoliosis. An analysis of the lateral spinal curvatures associated with Scheuermann's disease. J Bone Joint Surg Br. 1985; 67(2):189–192**
[35] Dickson RA, Lawton JO, Deacon P, et al. The pathogenesis of idiopathic scoliosis. In: Warner J, Mehta M (eds). Proceedings of the Seventh Phillip Zorab Symposium. 1983: Scoliosis – Prevention. New York: Praeger; 1985:64–79
[36] Lambrinudi C. Adolescent and senile kyphosis. BMJ. 1934; 2(3852):800–804, 2
[37] **Bradford DS, Garica A. Neurological complications in Scheuermann's disease. A case report and review of the literature. J Bone Joint Surg Am. 1969; 51(3):567–572**
[38] Ryan MD, Taylor TKF. Acute spinal cord compression in Scheuermann's disease. J Bone Joint Surg Br. 1982; 64(4):409–412
[39] Yablon JS, Kasdon DL, Levine H. Thoracic cord compression in Scheuermann's disease. Spine. 1988; 13(8):896–898
[40] **Bradford DS, Moe JH, Montalvo FJ, Winter RB. Scheuermann's kyphosis. Results of surgical treatment by posterior spine arthrodesis in twenty-two patients. J Bone Joint Surg Am. 1975; 57(4):439–448**
[41] **Bradford DS, Moe JH, Montalvo FJ, Winter RB. Scheuermann's kyphosis and roundback deformity. Results of Milwaukee brace treatment. J Bone Joint Surg Am. 1974; 56(4):740–758**

[42] Millner PA, Dickson RA. Idiopathic scoliosis: biomechanics and biology. Eur Spine J. 1996; 5(6):362–373
[43] Betz RR. Kyphosis of the thoracic and thoracolumbar spine in the pediatric patient: normal sagittal parameters and scope of the problem. Instr Course Lect. 2004; 53:479–484
[44] Propst-Proctor SL, Bleck EE. Radiographic determination of lordosis and kyphosis in normal and scoliotic children. J Pediatr Orthop. 1983; 3(3):344–346
[45] Boseker EH, Moe JH, Winter RB, Koop SE. Determination of "normal" thoracic kyphosis: a roentgenographic study of 121 "normal" children. J Pediatr Orthop. 2000; 20(6):796–798
[46] Ponte A, Gebbia FE. Non-operative treatment of adolescent hyperkyphosis. Orthop Trans. 1985; 9:108
[47] Ferguson AB, Jr. The etiology of preadolescent kyphosis. J Bone Joint Surg Am. 1956; 38-A(1):149–157
[48] Williams PL, Warwick R, Dyson M, Bannister LH, eds. Grays Anatomy. 39th ed. London: Churchill Livingstone; 1989:467
[49] Winter RB, Hall JE. Kyphosis in childhood and adolescence. Spine. 1978; 3(4):285–308
[50] Dickson RA. Conservative treatment for idiopathic scoliosis. J Bone Joint Surg Br. 1985; 67(2):176–181
[51] Winter RB, Lovell WW, Moe JH. Excessive thoracic lordosis and loss of pulmonary function in patients with idiopathic scoliosis. J Bone Joint Surg Am. 1975; 57(7):972–977
[52] Stagnara P. Cyphoses thorasiques regulieres pathologiques. In: Gaggi I (ed). Modern Trends in Orthopaedics. Boulogne; 1982:268
[53] De Mauroy JC, Stagnara P. Resultats rá long-terme du treitment orthopedic reunion du group d'etude de'las scolios ex enprovance 1978 1: 60
[54] Stagnara P, Perdriolle R. Élongation vertébrale continue par plâtra â tendeurs. Possibilités therapeutiques. Rev Chir Orthop Repar Appar Mot. 1958; 44:57–74
[55] Stagnara PJ, DuPeloux J, Fanchet R. Traitement orthopédique ambulatoir de la maladie de Scheuermann en période d'évolution. Rev Chir Orthop Repar Appar Mot. 1966; 52:585–600
[56] Montgomery SP, Erwin WE. Scheuermann's kyphosis—long-term results of Milwaukee braces treatment. Spine. 1981; 6(1):5–8
[57] Soo CL, Noble PC, Esses SI. Scheuermann kyphosis: long-term follow-up. Spine J. 2002; 2(1):49–56
[58] Riddle EC, Bowen JR, Shah SA, Moran EF, Lawall H, Jr. The duPont kyphosis brace for the treatment of adolescent Scheuermann kyphosis. J South Orthop Assoc. 2003; 12(3):135–140
[59] Axelgaard J, Brown JC, Swank SM. Kyphosis treatment by electrical surface stimulation. Orthop Trans. 1982; 6:1
[60] Taylor TC, Wenger DR, Stephen J, Gillespie R, Bobechko WP.. Surgical management of thoracic kyphosis in adolescents. J Bone Joint Surg Am.. 1979; 61 (4):496–503
[61] Leatherman KD, Dickson RA. Two-stage corrective surgery for congenital deformities of the spine. J Bone Joint Surg Br. 1979; 61-B(3):324–328
[62] Streitz W, Brown JC, Bonnett CA. Anterior fibular strut grafting in the treatment of kyphosis. Clin Orthop Relat Res. 1977(128):140–148
[63] Herndon WA, Emans JB, Micheli LJ, Hall JE. Combined anterior and posterior fusion for Scheuermann's kyphosis. Spine. 1981; 6(2):125–130
[64] Bradford DS. The role of the anterior approach in the management of spinal deformities. In: Dickson RA, Bradford DS (eds). Management of Spinal Deformities. London: Butterworths International Medical Reviews; 1984: 275–302
[65] Gardner AD. 1984. Unpublished data.
[66] Pinto WC, Avanzi O, Winter RB. An anterior distractor for the intraoperative correction of angular kyphosis. Spine. 1978; 3(4):309–312
[67] Rose GK, Owen R, Sanderson JM. Transposition of rib with blood supply for the stabilisation of a spinal kyphos. J Bone Joint Surg Br. 1975; 57:112
[68] Bradford DS. Anterior vascular pedicle bone grafting for the treatment of kyphosis. Spine. 1980; 5(4):318–323
[69] Stagnara P. Traction crânienne par le 'halo' de Rancho Los Amigos. Rev Chir Orthop Repar Appar Mot. 1971; 57:287–300
[70] Leatherman KD, Dickson RA. The Management of Spinal Deformities. London: Wright; 1988:129
[71] Cotrel Y, Dubousset J, Guillaumat M. New universal instrumentation in spinal surgery. Clin Orthop Relat Res. 1988; 227(227):10–23
[72] Griss P, Harms J, Zielke K. Ventral derotation spondylodesis (VDS). In: Dickson RA, Bradford DS (eds). Management of Spinal Deformities. London: Butterworths International Medical Reviews; 1984:193–236
[73] Poolman RW, Been HD, Ubags LH. Clinical outcome and radiographic results after operative treatment of Scheuermann's disease. Eur Spine J. 2002; 11 (6):561–569
[74] Herrera-Soto JA, Parikh SN, Al-Sayyad MJ, Crawford AH. Experience with combined video-assisted thoracoscopic surgery (VATS) anterior spinal release and posterior spinal fusion in Scheuermann's kyphosis. Spine. 2005; 30 (19):2176–2181
[75] Lee SS, Lenke LG, Kuklo TR, et al. Comparison of Scheuermann kyphosis correction by posterior-only thoracic pedicle screw fixation versus combined anterior/posterior fusion. Spine. 2006; 31(20):2316–2321
[76] Arun R, Mehdian SM, Freeman BJ, Sithole J, Divjina SC. Do anterior interbody cages have a potential value in comparison to autogenous rib graft in the surgical management of Scheuermann's kyphosis? Spine J. 2006; 6(4):413–420
[77] Geck MJ, Macagno A, Ponte A, Shufflebarger HL. The Ponte procedure: posterior only treatment of Scheuermann's kyphosis using segmental posterior shortening and pedicle screw instrumentation. J Spinal Disord Tech. 2007; 20 (8):586–593
[78] Cho KJ, Lenke LG, Bridwell KH, Kamiya M, Sides B. Selection of the optimal distal fusion level in posterior instrumentation and fusion for thoracic hyperkyphosis: the sagittal stable vertebra concept. Spine. 2009; 34 (8):765–770
[79] Coe JD, Smith JS, Berven S, et al. Complications of spinal fusion for scheuermann kyphosis: a report of the scoliosis research society morbidity and mortality committee. Spine. 2010; 35(1):99–103
[80] Tsutsui S, Pawelek JB, Bastrom TP, Shah SA, Newton PO. Do discs "open" anteriorly with posterior-only correction of Scheuermann's kyphosis? Spine. 2011; 36(16):E1086–E1092
[81] Lonstein JE, Winter RB, Moe JH, Bradford DS, Chou SN, Pinto WC. Neurologic deficits secondary to spinal deformity. A review of the literature and report of 43 cases. Spine. 1980; 5(4):331–355

Chapter 6

Congenital Deformities

6.1	Etiology of Congenital Spine Anomalies	*154*
6.2	The Clinical Spectrum of Deformity	*159*
6.3	Congenital Bone Anomalies	*159*
6.4	Practice Point	*176*
6.5	Congenital Kyphosis	*182*
6.6	Congenital Lordosis	*191*
6.7	Spinal Dysraphism	*192*
6.8	Congenital Spinal Deformity Syndromes	*197*
Case Gallery		*204*

6 Congenital Deformities

6.1 Etiology of Congenital Spine Anomalies

It is well established that abnormalities of mesodermal development may occur in association with congenital anomalies of the spinal cord and meninges. Various theories have been proposed for the embryological derivation of such deformities of the neurospinal axis. Conditions such as spina bifida and diastematomyelia and anatomical aberrations such as butterfly vertebrae, hemivertebrae, failures of vertebral segmentation, and paravertebral and postvertebral cysts have all been explained in terms of erroneous differentiation of the early embryonic mesodermal and ectodermal cell layers. It is thus not difficult to see how a spinal deformity can arise from such identifiable embryopathic abnormalities.

Associations of deformities of the gut in patients exhibiting congenital defects in either one or both components of the neurospinal axis have alerted investigators to the existence of an intricate relationship between the systems.[1-5] As a result, it is now a commonly held opinion that all types of clinical syndromes with anomalies in both spinal and intestinal structures originate from one basic complex of anomalies and finally become diversified by the modifying effects of growth and repair.

6.1.1 Normal Development of Axial Structures

The early embryo consists of two epithelial cell layers: ectoderm (epiblast) and endoderm (hypoblast). In experiments involving separation, rotation, and recombination of these two layers in duck embryos it has been demonstrated that it is the endoderm that controls the position of the primitive streak in the overlying epiblast and is thus instrumental in establishing the primary (anteroposterior) axis.[6] Mesoderm (primary mesenchyme) cells formed in the primitive streak migrate laterally and anteriorly between the two epithelia, while the notochord extends forward from the anterior end of the streak, at first forming as a flattened structure closely applied to the endoderm, which is the future dorsal wall of the embryonic gut tube. The streak itself remains at the posterior end as the embryo elongates (▶ Fig. 6.1).

The mesoderm cells adjacent to the notochord (paraxial mesoderm) form a series of paired segmental epithelioid blocks, the somites, except in the major part of the cranial region. These cells establish the segmentation of the embryonic body, on which the segmental pattern of the skeletal, muscular, nervous, and vascular systems of the adult trunk is based. The regularity of their pattern and their relationship to the notochord and developing neural tube are therefore of fundamental importance.

The ectoderm overlying the paraxial mesoderm differentiates into the neural plate, which changes shape to form the neural groove then neural tube, coming to lie internally. The whole surface of the embryo is thus formed from ectoderm, which is initially lateral to the neural plate. Following the closure of the neural tube, the epithelial structure of the medial surface of the somites breaks down and the cells are reorganized as mesenchyme. They migrate to surround the notochord, which has by this time separated from the gut wall to form a rod-shaped structure. The segmental pattern of this sclerotomal mesenchyme is retained, but the primordia of the vertebrae thus initiated form in a position that is staggered relative to the part of the somite left behind to form segmental muscle blocks. Thus vertebrae are described as intersegmental in position, whereas the spinal nerves and myotome-derived muscles are segmental.[7,8] The regularity and bilateral symmetry of this arrangement are essential to normal axial development (▶ Fig. 6.2).[9]

According to observations originally based on light microscopy of paraffin sections, the human embryonic notochord differs from its rodent counterpart in being, in its early stages, a hollow structure. The neurenteric canal forms a communication between the amniotic cavity dorsal to the ectoderm and the yolk sac (prior to formation of the gut tube) ventral to the endoderm. This communication from the gut to the dorsal surface of the embryo passing through the midline dorsal structures is a normal but very short-lasting connection and its final location in the fully developed human is at the tip of the coccyx.[2]

6.1.2 Theories of the Developmental Basis of Deformities

Dodds[10] suggests that an abnormally large neurenteric canal, or one that persists too long, would prevent fusion of the converging notochordal and sclerotomal streams. This anomaly could therefore be responsible for the anterior vertebral clefts that most commonly involve the cervicodorsal spine, and for neurenteric connections, cysts, and diverticula, as well as reduplications of the spinal cord. The final location of this neurenteric canal, however, is at the tip of the coccyx, and Bremer[2] suggests that any connection between the intestinal tract and midline dorsal structures above the coccyx is due to the previous existence of an accessory neurenteric canal. He further points out that the former presence of such an accessory canal may be recognized as one of the neurenteric connections mentioned above.

An alternative explanation of this embryonic system interrelationship is presented by Fallon et al,[3] who suggest the notochord, at an early stage of development, becomes intercalated with the endoderm. It is postulated that if the notochord becomes incompletely separated from the endodermal lining then abnormalities of the vertebrae might well occur, since the mesoderm would be unable to surround the notochord completely.

Saunders[11] proposes that a local cleavage of the notochord, for whatever reason, enables endoderm and ectoderm to adhere and form a neurenteric band and/or enteric diverticulum. Such a structure may or may not elongate with growth and so interfere with development of either system by causing traction diverticula, cysts, or strands which may or may not be expressed as vertebral defects. It is an interesting feature of thoracic diverticula and cysts connected with the stomach or intestines that they have a tendency to lie to the right of the vertebral column[3]; this is thought to be caused by a dextrolateral displacement of the embryo's neurenteric connection by the developmental processes of gastric and gut rotation. Bentley and Smith[5] develop this theory further and classify a wide variety of malformations under the general concept of split notochord syndrome. They emphasize that differential growth of gut and vertebral column could lead to wide separation of the areas affected in each.

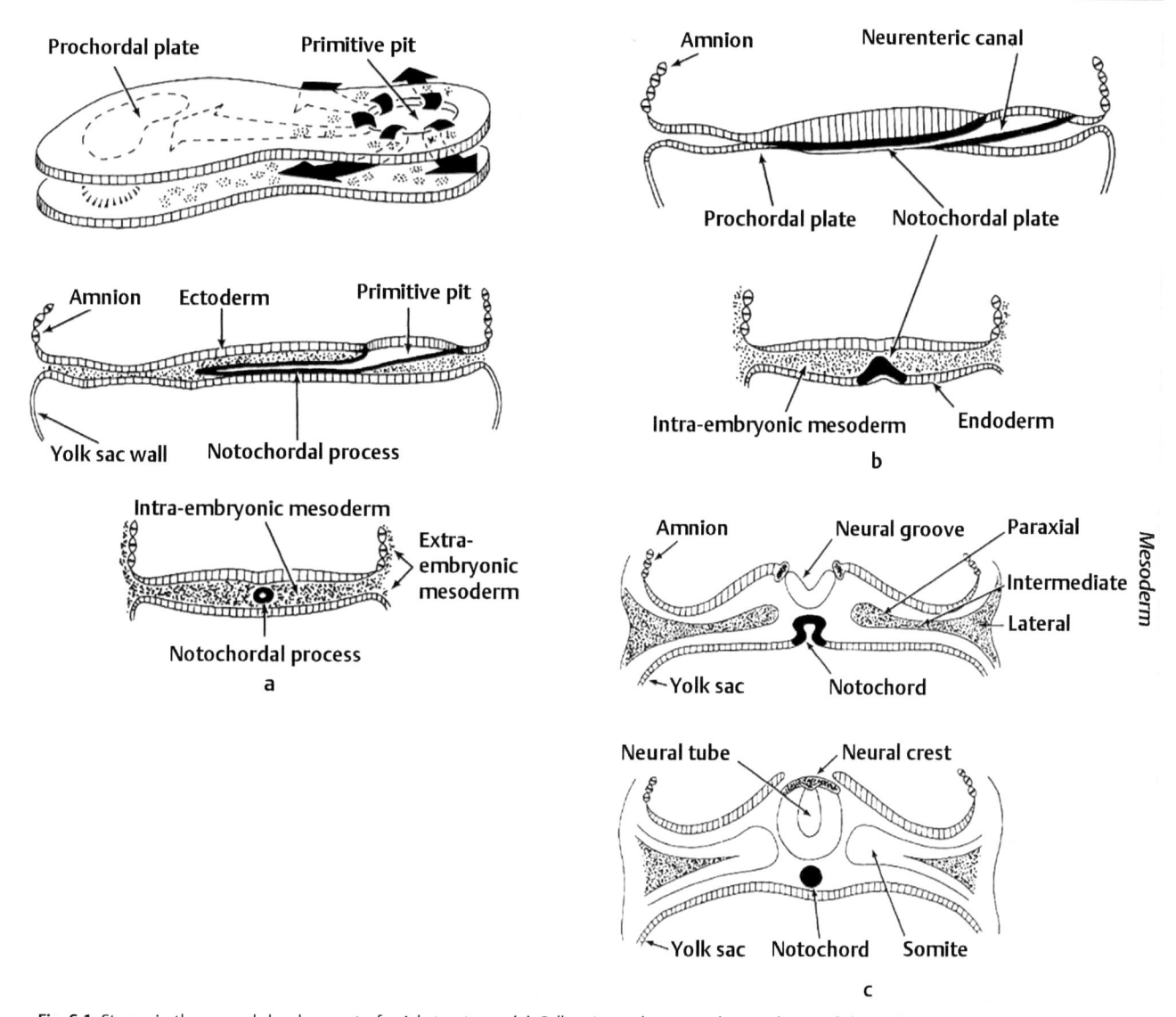

Fig. 6.1 Stages in the normal development of axial structures. (a) Cells migrate between the two layers of the embryonic bilaminar disk to form mesoderm. (b) The notochord flattens forming the notochordal plate which comes to lie in intimate contact with the roof of the endoderm; at this stage a transient connection, the neurenteric canal, exists across the embryonic disk. (c) The notochord reforms and the axial mesenchyme segments to form paired somites.

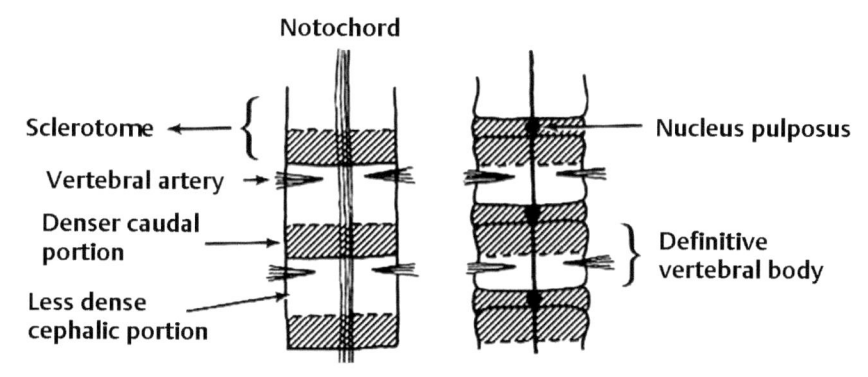

Fig. 6.2 Condensation of the mesodermal somites occurs such that definitive vertebral bodies derive from parts of the adjacent somites.

Beardmore and Wigglesworth[4] propose as a primary event a local endodermal–ectodermal adhesion to occur in the midline of an embryo at a presomite stage between Hensen's node and the prochordal plate. They postulate the adhesion to partially block the cephalad invagination of notochordal material, causing a splitting or diverting to either side of the notochord. In this way various developmental defects of the vertebrae could arise. Prop et al[12] extend this view to the second phase of notochordal growth and suggest that the adhesion might be located in the primitive streak—that is, more caudally.

Although there are some differences in the primary events, the explanations described above have in common the concept of abnormal relationships between notochord and endoderm (including notochordal cleft), and ectodermal–endodermal connections in some stages (▶ Fig. 6.3).

Congenital Deformities

155

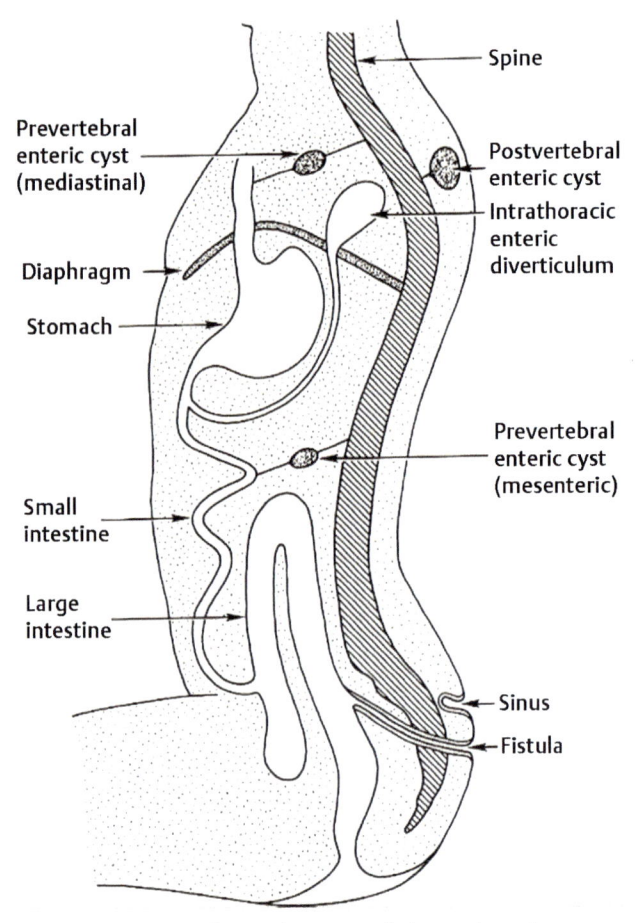

Congenital Deformities

Abnormalities occurring during this crucial, initial period of spinal development can have catastrophic consequences. They are often fatal, although at least they can result in the development of major vertebral deformities with significant neurological impairment. The etiological factors responsible for such abnormalities remain obscure and no single genetic or environmental defect has been identified. Recent work by Smithells et al,[13] however, has highlighted the importance of maternal nutrition with particular regard to vitamin intake in the periconceptual period.

6.1.3 The Pathogenesis of Congenital Vertebral Malformations

Congenital malformations of vertebrae can be divided into failure of formation, failure of segmentation (▶ Fig. 6.4), and the spectrum of abnormalities associated with developmental anomalies of the notochord. Both failure of formation and failure of segmentation can take the form of defects or errors. Failure of formation refers to abnormalities of the vertebral bodies and can be subdivided into (a) a partial or total defect (absence) of the body, and (b) abnormalities in shape. Failure of segmentation refers to abnormalities of the intervertebral disk and can also be subdivided into (a) simple defect (absence) of the disk either totally as in block vertebrae or partially as in a unilateral bar, and (b) errors in disk position or alignment. Many explanations as to how these developmental abnormalities are produced have been proposed, although there is as yet no general agreement as to their origins.

Failure of Formation

Feller and Sternberg[14] postulated that failure of formation (hemivertebra) was due to the lack of a cartilaginous precursor secondary to any underlying problem with the notochord

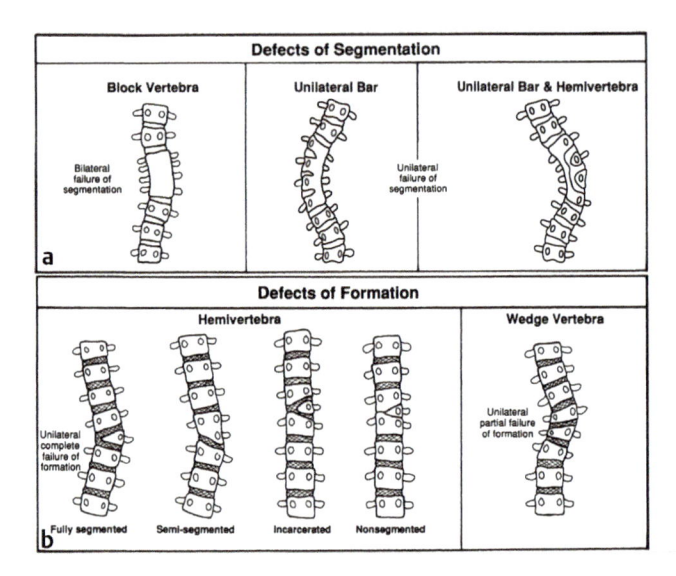

Fig. 6.3 Embryonic adhesions between endoderm and ectoderm at an early stage can give rise to a number of combined anomalies of gut and spine.

Fig. 6.4 Diagram to show the classification of congenital spinal anomalies. (Reproduced with permission from Pediatric Spine, 2nd Edition, Ed S L Weinstein, Lippincott WW, PA 2001; Chapter 7, Table 1, p. 163.)

Congenital Deformities

(▶ Fig. 6.5). Junghanns[15] proposed that a lack of ossification resulting from inadequate vascularization was responsible, although his interpretation was based on the concept that the vertebral body in the early stages of chondrification consisted of two halves separated by a ventrodorsal extension of the perichordal sheath and that ossification centers appeared both dorsally and ventrally. Thus lateral hemivertebrae arose from failure of ossification on one side following failure of fusion of the two chondrification centers. Ventral or dorsal hemivertebrae were thought to arise due to lack of ossification secondary to lack of vascularization.

Although Bardeen[16] described two chondrification centers divided by the perichordal septum, no confirmatory descriptions are given in later papers.[7,17,18] The more recent detailed studies of Tanaka and Uhthoff[9,19] failed to find any evidence to support the mechanism put forward by Junghanns. The vertebral body was found to form as a single cartilaginous structure and defects that were not limited to exactly half or the whole of the body were already present at the stage of chondrification and could not therefore have resulted from failure of ossification. Although failure of formation could arise from abnormal migration of sclerotomic cells, these do not show any morphological differences other than in density. It is now thought that formation defects arise as a result of abnormal differential growth of mesenchymal cells in the stage of resegmentation.

Defects of the vertebral body or anomalies in its shape can result in compensatory growth of adjacent vertebrae. Since ossification centers develop in a normal oval form even in malformed vertebral bodies, the shape cannot be fully determined radiologically until ossification is complete; however, abnormalities in shape can be recognized at much earlier stages.[19]

Failure of Segmentation

The mechanism of failure of segmentation is also controversial. Junghanns did not comment on it; Valentin and Putscher[20] considered that it was due to destruction of the intervertebral disk after it had been formed; Ehrenhaft[21] believed that complete chondrification of the mesenchymal column was responsible; Overgaard[22] thought it arose from regressive changes at the end of the developmental period; and Tsou[23] suggested that it resulted from osseous metaplasia of the annulus fibrosus. Tanaka and Uhthoff[9] describe one 70-mm fetus where failure of segmentation resulted from failure of development of the intervertebral disk before or at the early stages of chondrification. Normally the mesenchymal cells in the dense-celled area start to differentiate into the fibroblastic cells of the annulus shortly after chondrification of the vertebral body has been completed; thus failure of segmentation is due to either complete chondrification of the dense-celled area or its absence altogether (▶ Fig. 6.6).

Junghanns stressed the importance of vascularization in the etiology of developmental abnormalities of vertebrae.[15] Although more recent studies have indicated that defects arise at much earlier stages of development than suggested by him, they have confirmed the crucial role of a normal blood supply. It would appear that abnormalities of formation and segmentation occur during the stage of resegmentation of the mesenchymal vertebral column and are related to abnormalities of the intersegmental arteries. There is no doubt about the relationship between congenital anomalies and a reduction or even absence of local blood supply.

Malformations Associated with Anomalies of the Notochord

The influence of the notochord on vertebral development has been in dispute. Feller and Sternberg[14] described a curvature of the notochord toward hemivertebrae and believed that the notochord was responsible for malformations of the vertebral body.

Schmorl and Junghanns[24] felt that persistent notochordal tissue hinders vertebral development. Tanaka and Uhthoff[19] report one specimen with bifurcation of the notochord in the

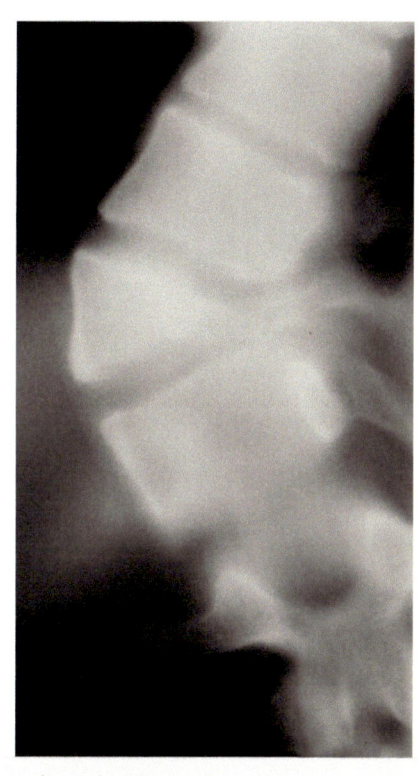

Fig. 6.5 PA radiograph showing a hemivertebra: a unilateral failure of formation.

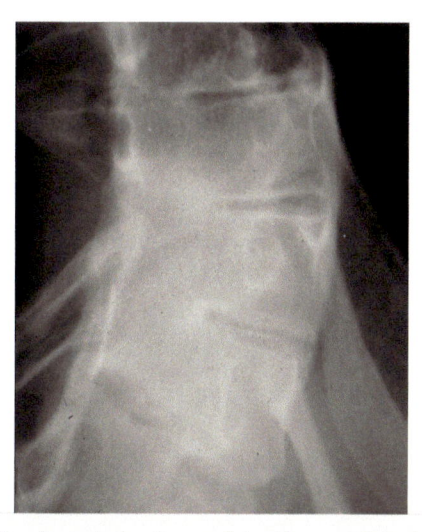

Fig. 6.6 PA radiograph showing a unilateral bar: a unilateral failure of segmentation.

absence of any malformation, although the intersegmental arteries were normally distributed, suggesting that no relationship exists between malformations of the vertebral body and the notochord.

There is, however, an undoubted collection of related developmental abnormalities of the skin of the back, the central nervous system, the spine, and the gut for which there is much evidence, albeit mainly from studies of the embryos of lower vertebrates, that the etiology lies in abnormal development of the notochord. These abnormalities have been collectively referred to by Bentley and Smith[5] as the split notochord syndrome (▶ Fig. 6.7).

Lereboullet[25] described embryos split sagittally with the yolk sac being exposed in the dorsal cleft following artificial insemination of pike ova. Hertwig[26] produced ring embryos with dorsal clefts as a variant of the neurenteric canal by fertilizing postmature frog ova. He appreciated the role of these abnormal communications in the production of combined spina bifida and coined the word diastematomyelia. Clinical cases of combined spina bifida had already been described,[27–29] and Gruber reported cases of spinal defects associated with intestinal fistulae.[29] Johnston[30] and Frazer[31] both reported notochord clefts in human embryos, and Warkanay[5] has experimentally produced changes in mammalian embryos similar to those seen in the frog ring embryos of Hertwig.[26]

According to Bentley and Smith,[5] partial duplication and separation of the notochord leads to herniation of the yolk sac and its adherence to the dorsal ectoderm. The hernia may rupture to produce a fistula that separates the future spine and cord into two halves. Subsequent growth attempts to close and obliterate the fistula meet with a variable degree of success upon which the final deformity depends. Development of the base of skull, vertebral column, and central nervous system as well as the gut may be affected. Sequestration of dorsal ectoderm can produce dorsal dermoid cysts and sinuses, and remnants of the yolk sac may differentiate into tissue characteristic of any part of the gut or its embryological derivatives and persist as posterior enteric remnants in the form of fistulae, sinuses, diverticula, or cysts. Differential growth of the vertebral column and gut leads to wide separation of the affected regions and abnormal fixation of bowel may lead to failure of rotation.

When closure of the defect in the spinal column is incomplete the resultant spinal anomaly can range from a slight widening of the vertebral body to a complete anterior and posterior spina bifida. Minor degrees of anterior spina bifida can produce the radiological appearance of butterfly vertebrae (▶ Fig. 6.8); more severe lesions may incorporate enteric or cutaneous tissues. Hemivertebrae can undergo distorted individual growth, their medial pedicles fusing to form the bony spur characteristic of diastematomyelia. In all these malformations the spinal canal is wider than normal and the meninges may protrude anteriorly or posteriorly where the spine is bifid. When the spinal cord is itself bifid (diplomyelia) then the two halves are separately invested with meninges. The more usual arrangement is for the cord to be divided into right and left halves (diastematomyelia) with no nerve roots arising medially from either half.

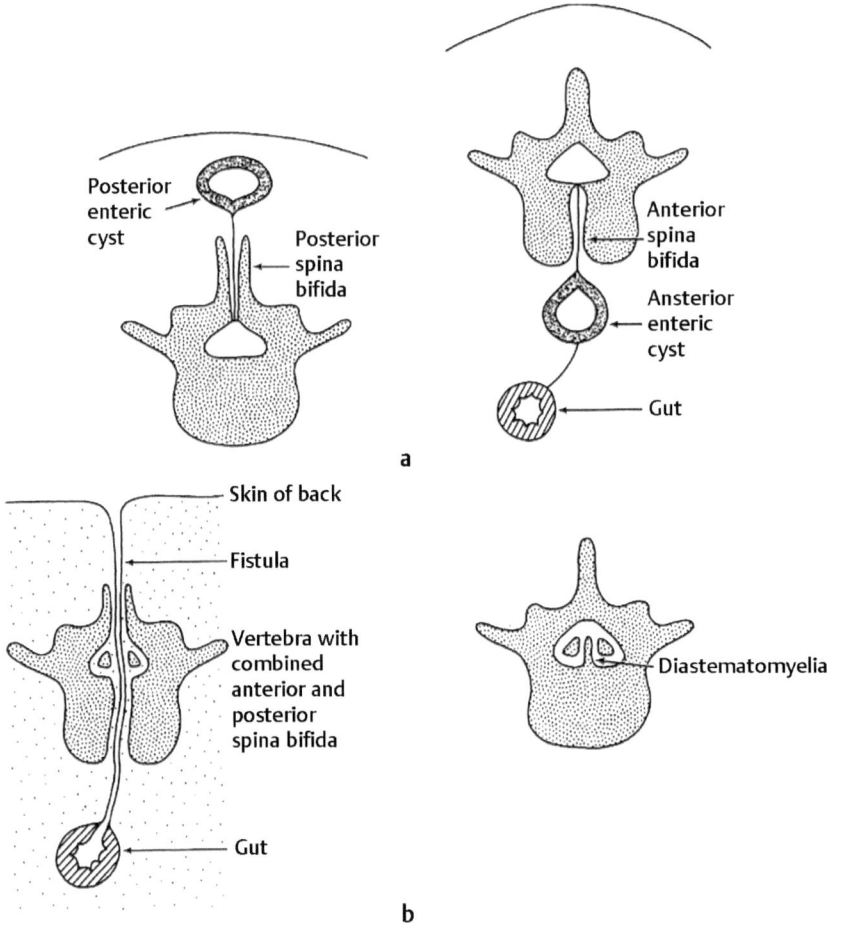

Fig. 6.7 The range of abnormalities attributable to the split notochord syndrome.

Congenital Deformities

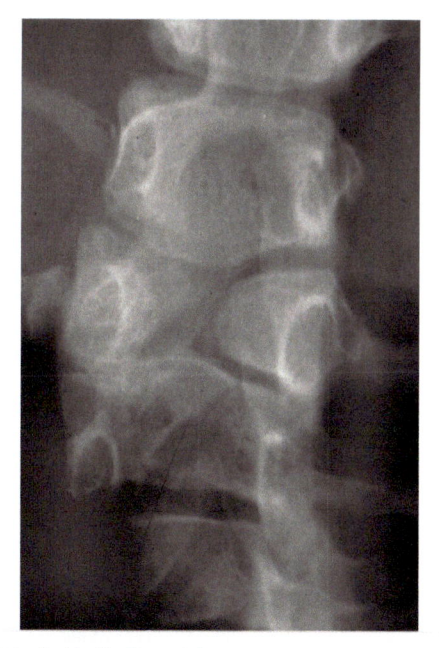

Fig. 6.8 A typical butterfly vertebra.

The more common variety of posterior spina bifida is the result of a separate abnormality occurring much later on in development, although in both types there may be hamartomatous changes in the overlying tissues, usually in the form of a lipoma, an angioma, an area of hypertrichosis or hyperpigmentation, or a dermal pit or sinus (▶ Fig. 6.9). Recently it has been noted that haploinsufficiency of Notch signaling pathway genes in humans can cause these problems and along with short-term gestational hypoxia significantly increases the penetrance and severity of vertebral defects in a mouse model.[32]

6.2 The Clinical Spectrum of Deformity

The term congenital spine deformity implies one that is present at or before birth. This is not strictly true. While the underlying anomaly is most certainly congenital, it does not necessarily produce a spinal deformity at all, and some of those that are produced only manifest themselves years later. The classification of congenital spine deformity is therefore semantically incorrect, as what is being classified is the underlying vertebral anomaly. There are two basic types of congenital spine anomaly capable of producing a spinal deformity: congenital bone anomalies and congenital cord anomalies (myelodysplasia).

6.3 Congenital Bone Anomalies

Two types of congenital bone anomaly commonly produce a deformity: failure of formation and failure of segmentation. The direction of the subsequent deformity is initially entirely dependent on which part of the spine is involved (the side, front, or back). Thus lateral defects produce a scoliosis, anterior defects a kyphosis, and posterior defects a lordosis. Such purely unidirectional deformities are uncommon, as the anomaly and

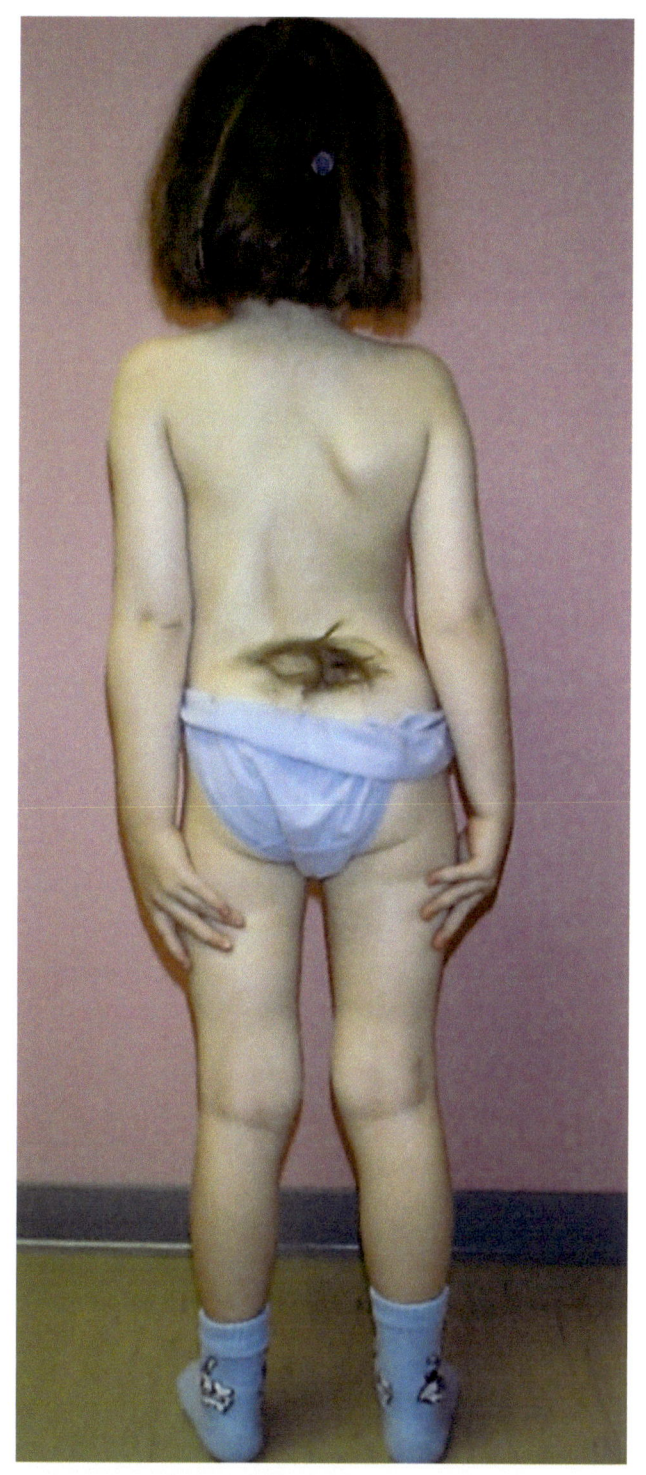

Fig. 6.9 A midline patch of hair is a common accompaniment to an underlying congenital spinal anomaly.

asymmetric growth usually occur in more than one plane. Therefore, a three-dimensional approach to the understanding of the behavior of congenital spine deformities is essential. In addition, thorough knowledge of the pathomechanics of idiopathic scoliosis is necessary so that changes in direction with growth can be understood with congenital and some other etiologies (see Chapter 3).[33–36]

Congenital Deformities

Lordotic deformities are much more common than appreciated, particularly with failures of segmentation and thus with reduction of the growth of the back of the spine; on the concave side they provide the rotational potential in the same mechanical fashion as in idiopathic scoliosis. Rotation with the posterior elements always directed toward the curve concavity testifies to the presence of the lordosis. Moreover, progression from birth creates very serious problems, as chest rotation with diminution of the anteroposterior chest diameter may cause severe cardiopulmonary compromise in exactly the same way as idiopathic scoliosis of early onset. Interestingly, if such areas of congenital lordosis exist in an area that resists the tendency to rotate, such as the cervicothoracic junction or upper thoracic spine, then the rotational effect is translated down into the thoracic spine to produce a secondary deformity. It is therefore not uncommon to encounter an idiopathic-type curve below a seemingly innocuous congenital anomaly higher up. Indeed, this is precisely what has happened, the congenital anomaly producing the necessary essential lesion of biplanar asymmetry[36] (▶ Fig. 6.10).

If the median sagittal plane asymmetry produced is a kyphosis then the spine is protected from rotation. Any associated coronal plane asymmetry can only progress with asymmetric vertebral growth in this plane with very much less of a scoliotic deformity than occurs with idiopathic scoliosis. The spinous processes will, however, be neutral or directed toward the curve convexity, as must occur with an asymmetric kyphosis.

6.3.1 Congenital Scoliosis

Natural History

Just as progression potential is crucial in idiopathic scoliosis so it is in congenital deformities but with the latter there are several different anomaly types to be considered. In general, it can be said that about a quarter of cases are nonprogressive, a quarter are mildly progressive (not more than 30 degrees), and half are significantly progressive (more than 30 degrees). There have been many studies on untreated cases of congenital spinal bony anomalies but, quite naturally, the bigger series have tended to come from the bigger centers, such as, 234 cases from Minneapolis,[37] 315 from Greenville,[38] and 251[39] from Edinburgh. With the two basic types of congenital anomaly—failure of formation or failure of segmentation (▶ Fig. 6.4)—in the former, part or the whole of one side of the vertebra does not develop leaving behind a wedge vertebra or a hemivertebra, respectively.[40] With the latter, a failure of segmentation, whereby the intervertebral disk and of course the growth plates on each side fail to develop either all the way across, or part way giving rise to respectively a bilateral failure of segmentation (block vertebra) or unilateral failure of segmentation (unilateral bar), the latter usually a significantly progressive problem.[37,39] How these are then distributed within the same spine provides detail and prognosis of the problem.

Thus, scoliosis progression potential would appear to depend on the type, site, and extent of the anomaly in the spine and its effect on vertebral growth (worse during the infantile and preadolescent/adolescent growth spurts). If there are multiple congenital anomalies and you are uncertain what the future holds then it is quite reasonable to merely follow the patient up. This 1-year-old had a scoliosis of 33 degrees with a bar on the right at the T4/5 level and a probable bar on the left at the L1–3 level with other obvious anomalies (▶ Fig. 6.11).

Since Kleinberg first described the bad prognosis of the unilateral failure of segmentation,[41] multiple unilateral anomalies have become recognized as the most progressive type.[42] This applies to multiple unilateral failures of either segmentation or formation.[43,44] A particularly sinister combination is the unilateral bar on one side and a hemivertebra on the opposite,[38] the one compounding the other (▶ Fig. 6.4). By contrast balanced anomalies protect against progression,[44] such as, a hemivertebra on one side and a nearby hemivertebra on the other side (hemimetameric shift). Although it is said that solitary hemivertebrae do not tend to produce significant deformities unless they are free (nonincarcerated)[37,39,40] or occur in the lumbar or lumbosacral regions throwing the trunk out of balance this is often not so and they can produce deformities difficult to deal with unless treated early (▶ Fig. 6.10 and ▶ Fig. 6.12).

The most common type of congenital scoliosis encountered is due to a unilateral failure of segmentation followed by a hemivertebra, a bar and contralateral hemivertebra, a block vertebra, and, least common, a wedge vertebra.[39] The anomalies in

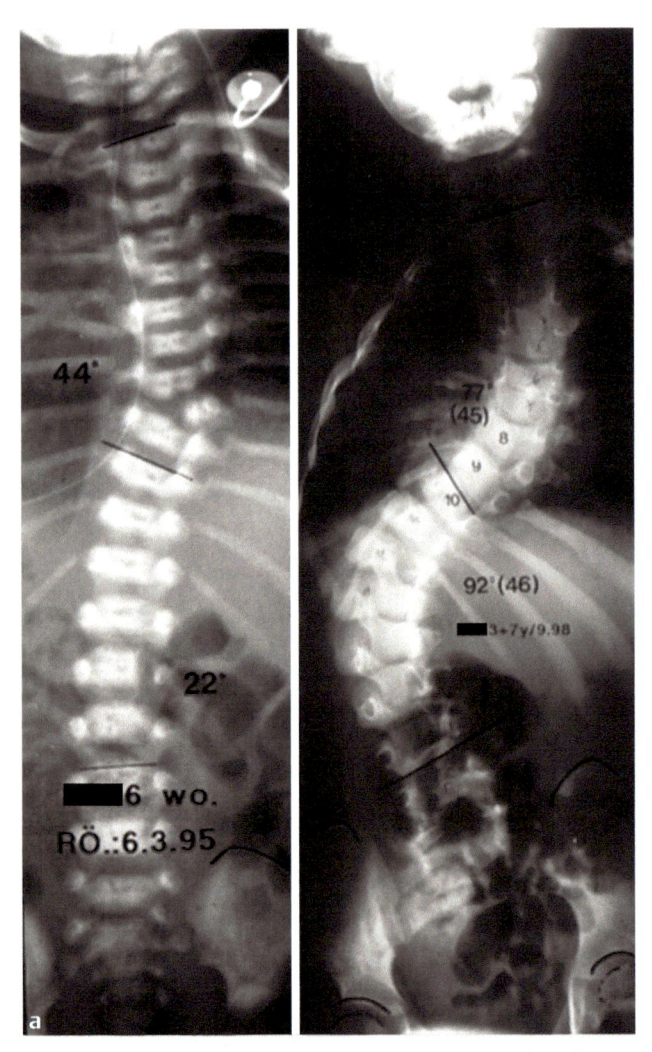

Fig. 6.10 (a) PA radiograph showing a hemivertebra at T8/9 and failures of segmentation above that. (b) Within 3 years these thoracic congenital abnormalities have thrown off a large idiopathic-type curve below.

Congenital Deformities

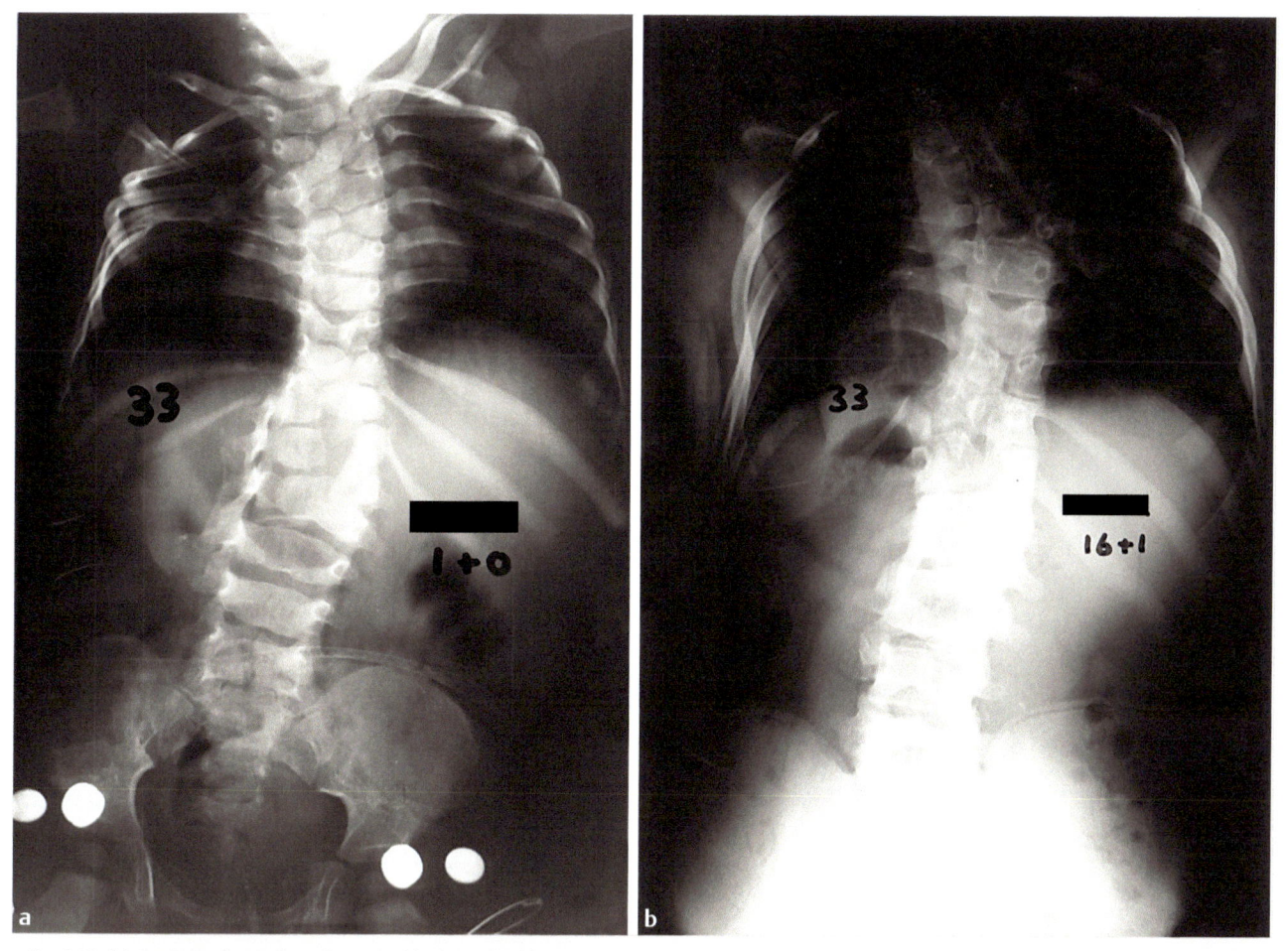

Fig. 6.11 (a) PA X-ray of an infant of 1 year old. The natural history was uncertain and so he was regularly reviewed. (b) At the age of 16 he had the same scoliosis of 33 degrees! Masterly inactivity is amazingly therapeutic.

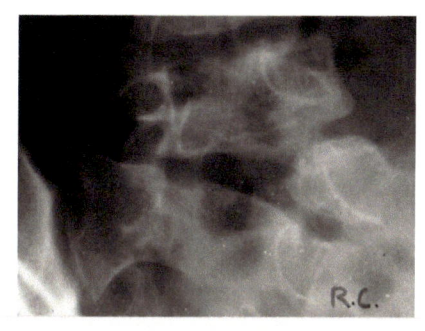

Fig. 6.12 A typical lumbosacral hemivertebra which immediately throws off a left-sided curve above.

descending order of progression potential are, however, bar and contralateral hemivertebra, bar only, hemivertebra, wedge vertebra, and block vertebra.[39] Girls are more often affected than boys and appear to have a worse progression potential. Progression is more obvious if the anomaly exists low in the thoracic region or in the thoracolumbar region, and least obvious high in the thoracic region.[37,39,40] Once a deformity starts progressing it never stops during growth. Deformities presenting shortly after birth have a worse prognosis and progressive deformities of all types tend to deteriorate more during the preadolescent/adolescent growth spurt. However, about a third of cases have multiple anomalies and are difficult to classify[37,39,40] (▶ Fig. 6.13).

Asymmetric growth in the coronal plane has been regarded as the most important factor governing progression potential.[37,39,40] Indeed it would appear obvious that no growth is possible on the side of the bar while some growth is still available on the concave side of a hemivertebra, but is that the sole reason why the former has the worse prognosis? Moreover, it is well known that not all radiographically similar deformities behave in the same way.[44] In order to fully understand progression potential it is necessary, as it was with idiopathic scoliosis, to encompass the median sagittal plane and consider the spine in all three dimensions. While the anomalies producing congenital scoliosis have been exhaustively classified and monitored in the coronal plane, it is the biomechanical effect of the sagittal plane which holds the key.

The Importance of the Sagittal Plane

A clue to the importance of this plane is derived from the observation that deformities associated with failures of segmentation have a severe progression potential. When an area of the spine

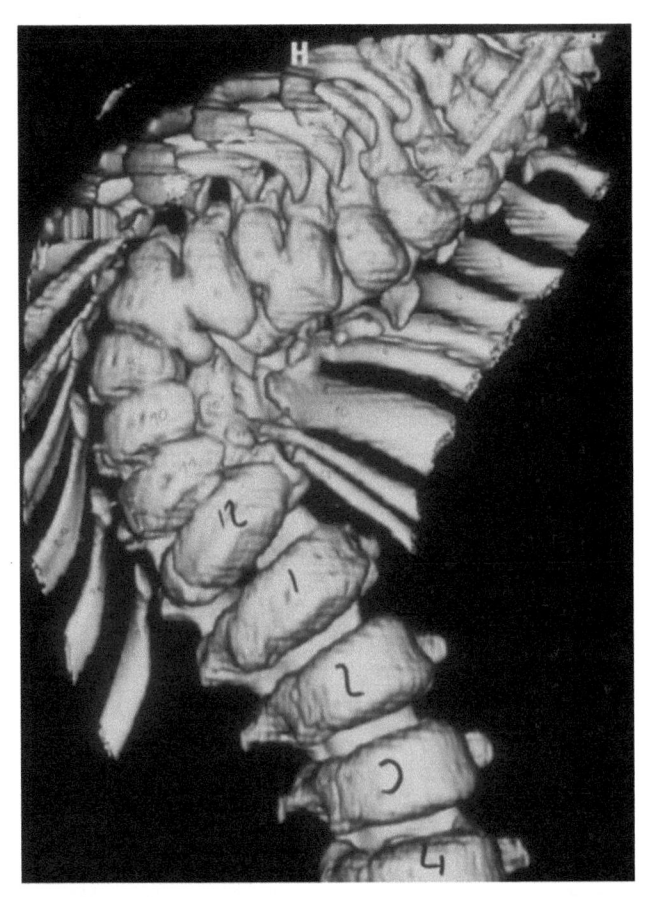

Fig. 6.13 Multiple congenital anomalies nicely demonstrated by 3D CT scanning. It looks as though there is a hemivertebra at T9 and above that two block vertebrae. Meanwhile the apex on the concave side shows clearly a rib fusion which means there is a failure of segmentation opposite the hemivertebrae.

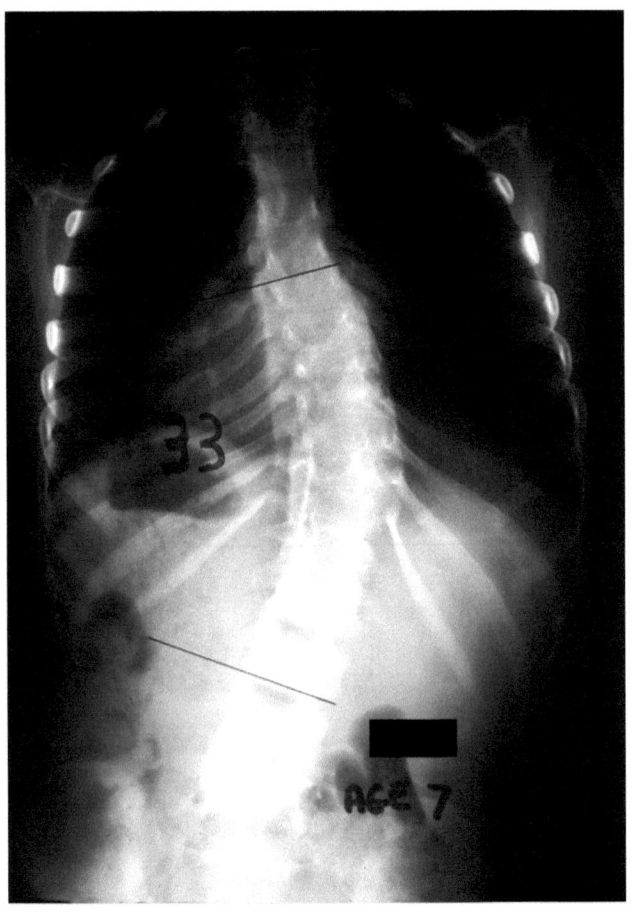

Fig. 6.14 PA radiograph showing that, from T11 to L1 on the left side, a posterior plaque is seen. Note there is no rib fusion that would occur with a vertebral body failure of segmentation, because ribs are derived from the costal processes of the vertebrae.

fails to segment it can do so both at the front and at the back and, indeed, evidence of a posterior plaque is commonly seen radiographically (▶ Fig. 6.14), particularly in the older child when ossification is more advanced. If this segmentation failure is unilateral then the more obvious coronal plane anomaly is compounded by a posterior tether, thus the same biplanar mechanism exists as in idiopathic scoliosis.[36] This is verified by the fact that the spine rotates in a constant direction with the posterior elements directed toward the curve concavity (concordant rotation), which can only occur with a rotated lordosis. The more levels that are affected then the more both components of the deformity are augmented and the more serious is the rotational progression. The reason why not all patients with seemingly the same radiographic anomaly have the same rate of progression is not because of differential growth in the frontal plane[44] but because the more important posterior tether is clearly variable with the degree of rotational instability more or less pronounced.

Conversely, failures of formation tend not to have the same "tethering" effect posteriorly and, thus, while the deformity may progress in the coronal plane, it is less often associated with rotation and so progression potential tends to be less marked. However, when a failure of segmentation is sited opposite to a failure of formation (▶ Fig. 6.13)—a notoriously progressive situation[37,39,41]—then the biplanar asymmetry so produced facilitates a marked degree of rotational progression.

It has also been stated that a bilateral failure of segmentation should theoretically not produce a scoliosis[37] and yet sometimes, apparently surprisingly, a curvature is seen. This is due entirely to the sagittal plane. Two, or more, vertebrae that are fused together before birth do not develop a normal sagittal shape and this area also represents a region of stiffness. In the thoracic region a normal kyphotic shape is essential so that the axis of spinal rotation is anterior to the vertebral bodies in order to protect them from rotation.[36] With block vertebrae the axis is now sited more posteriorly and, as the block is not always symmetrical in the coronal plane, this latter provides directional instability to the block and thus a rotational lordoscoliosis is produced in exactly the same fashion as with idiopathic scoliosis. It is therefore not uncommon to encounter an apparently idiopathic deformity with a disk space that is absent or difficult to visualize to which the semantically incorrect term congenital idiopathic scoliosis would appear very appropriate (▶ Fig. 6.15). As we have seen, if the area of congenital fusion is cervicothoracic and resists rotation locally, then rotation can be translated lower down the spine, as not uncommonly occurs with the Klippel Feil syndrome.

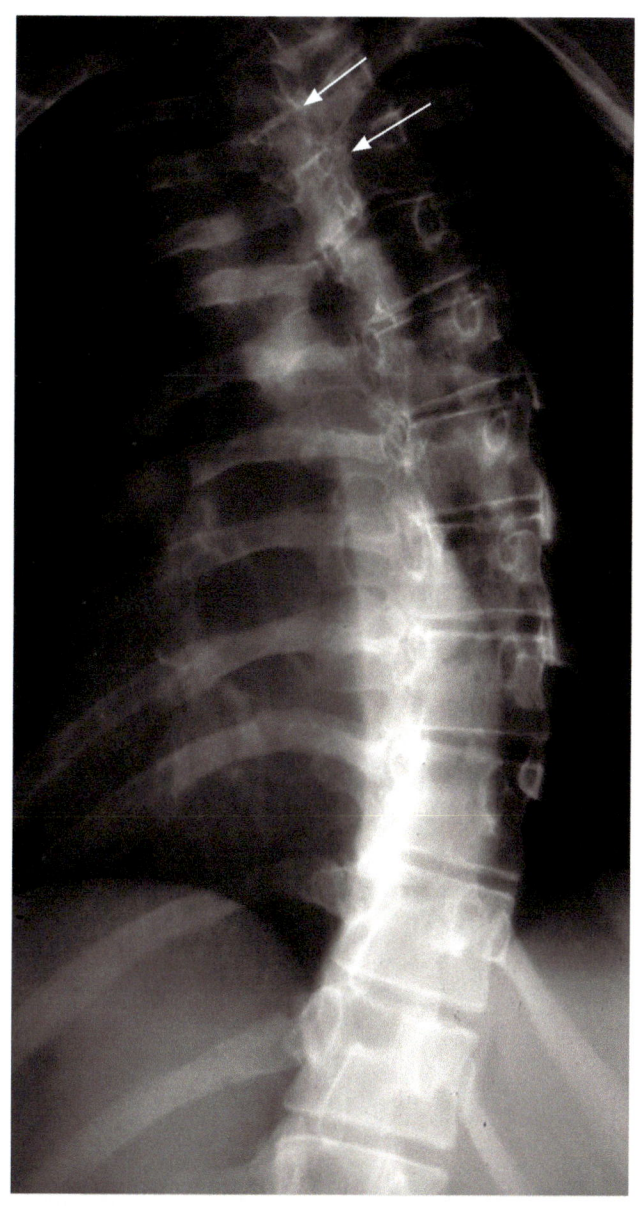

Fig. 6.15 Congenital idiopathic scoliosis. At T3//4 there is a failure of segmentation bilaterally (arrows) and this generates an idiopathic-type curve below.

lordotic sagittal plane problem by tethering posterior spinal growth in bone.

In 1986 McMaster published 104 patients with 154 hemivertebrae that had produced scoliotic curves; 65% were fully segmented, 22% semi-segmented, and 12% were incarcerated.[40] Again there were almost twice as many females as males. The hundred diagnosed before skeletal maturity were then followed for a mean of 5 years. The 65% fully segmented hemivertebrae were evenly distributed throughout the spine with equal numbers on each side and were usually triangular in shape with normal disk spaces above and below. These were two relatively normal vertebrae above and below which became slightly wedge-shaped during growth.

The 34 semi-segmented hemivertebrae were most common in the lumbar region and tended to be single. In some cases it wasn't until after the first year or two of life that ossification showed these hemivertebrae to be semi-segmented.

McMaster concluded that incarcerated and semi-segmented hemivertebrae do not need treatment and fully segmented hemivertebrae may require treatment according to site and number and the stopping of growth on the overgrowing side should be the aim of treatment, but, of course, fusion was the only surgical technique used in those days.[40]

Minor degrees of anterior spina bifida can produce the appearance of butterfly vertebra (▶ Fig. 6.8).

Finally, it is becoming more common for patients to be referred prenatally with a hemivertebra visualized on ultrasonography (▶ Fig. 6.16). Wax et al described 19 fetuses with a hemivertebra diagnosis at a mean gestational age of 20 weeks and those fetuses had additional anomalies, often syndromic, that affected prognosis.[45] They were often delivered before term and had either growth restriction or higher mortality rates.

Treatment

Back in the Dark Ages* the Milwaukee brace was prescribed, unsuccessfully of course, in the nonoperative treatment of congenital scoliosis.[46] Not long after came the results of spinal arthrodesis for congenital spinal deformity in patients younger than 5 years of age.[47] At this time in the late 1970s and even early 1980s the only surgical treatment prescribed by these centers was a big posterior fusion mass to try and stop these deformities from progressing. Of course what a posterior fusion in situ was doing was to try and solidify in bone the preexisting deformity with no correction at all and indeed a distinct possibility of worsening the deformity by posterior bony tether.[48,49] This was rather like carrying out a posterior fusion for clubfoot. The proponents concluded that early spine fusion for selected difficult deformities appeared to be a highly satisfactory procedure[47] and refuted the experience of Leatherman and Roaf that such fusions would become a posterior tether facilitating further deformation[48,49] (▶ Fig. 3.16). Thus it was that early posterior fusion in situ with as big a fusion mass as possible became the Holy Grail to be sought by all treating such deformities at that time and still perceived in some quarters as the gold standard.

It is quite clear that not only is the thoracic spine the most common location for progressive anomalies it is also the most common site for progression, in the Minneapolis series 17 of the 28 thoracic curves progressing to a maximum of 93 degrees.[37] In the Edinburgh series hemivertebrae and bars were again particularly prevalent in the thoracic spine: 18 in the thoracic spine and 10 in the thoracolumbar spine. Meanwhile hemivertebrae were common in the lumbar and lumbosacral areas: 19 lumbar and 12 lumbosacral. Of course the reason why there were so many untreated congenital anomalies to study was that nonoperative treatment in the form of casts, casts and braces, or braces alone were, like with idiopathic scoliosis where at best vertebral growth is normal, quite ineffective and the alternative of posterior fusion in situ was at least uncertain and often damaging by adding to the

___

*Dark Ages, 500–1000 AD.

Congenital Deformities

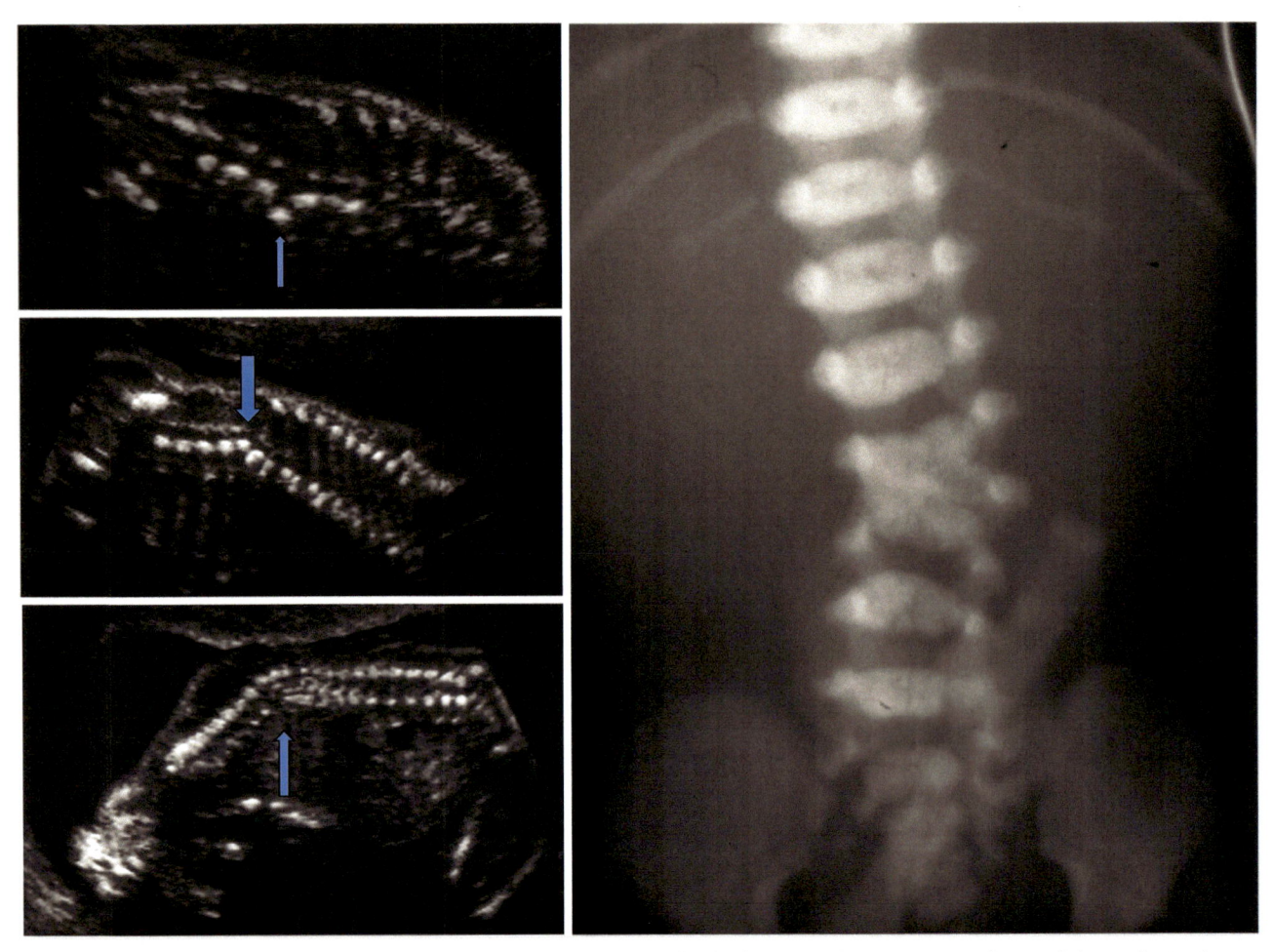

Fig. 6.16 A hemivertebra visualized on a prenatal ultrasound scan. (With grateful thanks to Dr. Mike Weston, Consultant Radiologist, the Leeds Hospitals.)

Meanwhile back in the 1950s, Robert Roaf from Oswestry, England, an orthopaedic intellectual giant of his time, conceived the concept of the treatment of progressive scoliosis by unilateral growth arrest. Most of the 180 patients he reported in 1960 were idiopathic although there were several congenital cases.[49] His main object of treatment was to "correct the disfigurement and hopefully restore a normal appearance." "Hence over a number of years I have tried to control progressive deformity by inhibiting growth on the convex side." He added, "for many years I tried posterior spinal fusion but did not succeed in controlling the deformity."[49] "There are two reasons for this," he said: "the usual area of posterior fusion for lordoscoliosis with rotation lies in the concavity of the curve and by acting as a tether it accentuates the inhibition of growth and even increases the deformity" and (2) "the new bone of the fusion is no less plastic than the rest of the child's skeleton so that if the deforming forces are strong it tends to bend with growth." If learning, and indeed established, spinal deformity surgeons want to understand the importance of the sagittal plane, then Roaf's papers are a must-read starting point. It is disappointing/somewhat annoying that his hugely important work is not more internationally known.

This led him to the more logical step of combining anterior and posterior convex growth arrest but this of course depended upon there still being growth potential on the concave side, not necessarily the case with congenital scoliosis. Improvement wasn't great but the majority of his patients improved by up to 20 degrees,[49] a whole lot better than posterior fusion in situ which of course could never lead to curve improvement.

This concept of trying to stop growth on the anteroconvex side of the spine soon caught on and in 1981 Winter reported on 10 children with anterior and posterior hemiarthrodesis with two improvements and the rest nonprogressive.[50] Winter and colleagues went on to report on 13 patients with progressive congenital scoliosis treated by anterior and posterior hemiarthrodesis and hemiepiphysiodesis.[51] They admitted after all that the Holy Grail of early bilateral posterior fusion was not the universal panacea and had mixed results, sometimes arresting progression and at other times, despite a solid fusion the curve progressed, the solid fusion mass bending under the forces of growth just as Roaf had predicted.[49] Curve progression was altered in all cases and two patients showed evidence of improvement but longer follow-up was necessary.

Just as Roaf had found out that the ideal patient had a pure scoliosis, that is, with no significant lordosis,[36] and so with these simple deformities lying only in the coronal plane then clearly stopping growth on the convex side might allow the concave side to catch up. The results were however not reliable and only a few other centers followed suit.[52]

Meanwhile Andrew and Piggott reviewed Roaf's long-term results[53] and found them to be unsatisfactory but this really was because the majority of Roaf's cases were infantile progressive idiopathic lordoscolioses and not simple hemivertebrae. By the time the logic of the growth arrest procedure could catch up, the biomechanics of the rotational lordosis had overwhelmed the deformity.[36]

The fundamental difference between deformities of congenital origin and those that are idiopathic is that the former are rigid from an early stage and this is because there is asymmetric deformation of vertebral shape at the keystone curve apex. Unlike its idiopathic counterpart, there is no inherent slack to be taken up by instrumentation and so the objective of surgery is to address the curve apex. If the problem is of a hemivertebra then excision of this misshapen vertebra suffices but if the anomaly also incorporates failure of segmentation then the whole anomaly can be excised in toto at the apex in wedge shape fashion. If this is not done until the secondary deformity of a long scoliosis is established then the entire structural curve needs to be corrected and fused as Leatherman clearly pointed out[54] (▶ Fig. 6.10). Hence the attraction of dealing with the problem before secondary deformation develops above and below a curve. In this regard hemivertebrectomy at a very young age has become the optimal option.

Although we recognize the pioneering contributions of Royle,[55] Compere,[56] Von Lackum and Smith,[57] and Wiles,[58] the really important advances were made by Roaf in Liverpool[59] and Leatherman in Kentucky.[48] Roaf and Leatherman understood better than anyone else at the time about the three-dimensional nature of structural scoliosis and as regards rigid curves Roaf stated "obviously the rational approach to the problem is to excise a wedge of bone from the apex of the curve" (▶ Fig. 4.10, ▶ Fig. 6.17, and ▶ Fig. 6.18). He likened this to the correction of a pes cavus. It differed from previous descriptions, such as the relatively minor procedure of Royle in excising an accessory hemivertebra, and encompassed apical wedge resection for a rigid deformity of any etiology. However, just like the previous paper it was largely ignored by the major scoliologists at the time who did not seem to read all that widely, at least internationally. It certainly is another must-read paper, that any scoliosis surgeon should study particularly if proposing to carry out an osteotomy.

The *American Journal of Bone and Joint Surgery* turned down Leatherman's life's work (editorial boards have a lot to answer for) and so it was sent to the *British Journal of Bone and Joint Surgery* who were delighted to accept this distinguished man's pioneering work and moreover was selected by Professor James (President of the British Orthopaedic Association [B.O.A.] at that time) to be the opening paper of the annual meeting of the B.O.A. in Liverpool in 1977.

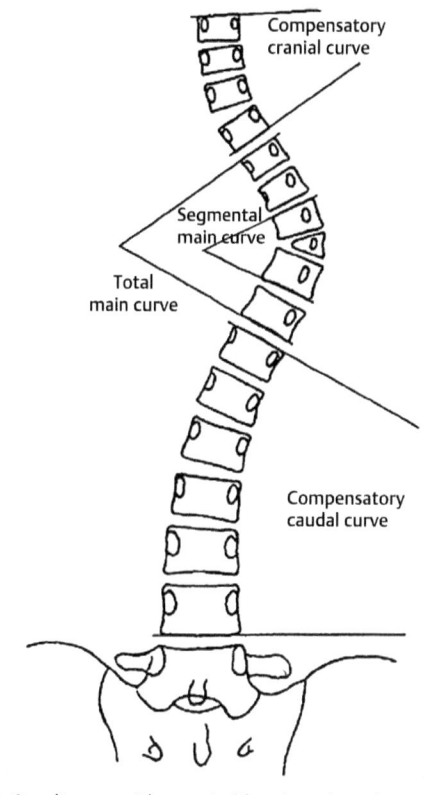

Fig. 6.17 Our diagram with an apical hemivertebra; the segmental curve is the important one.

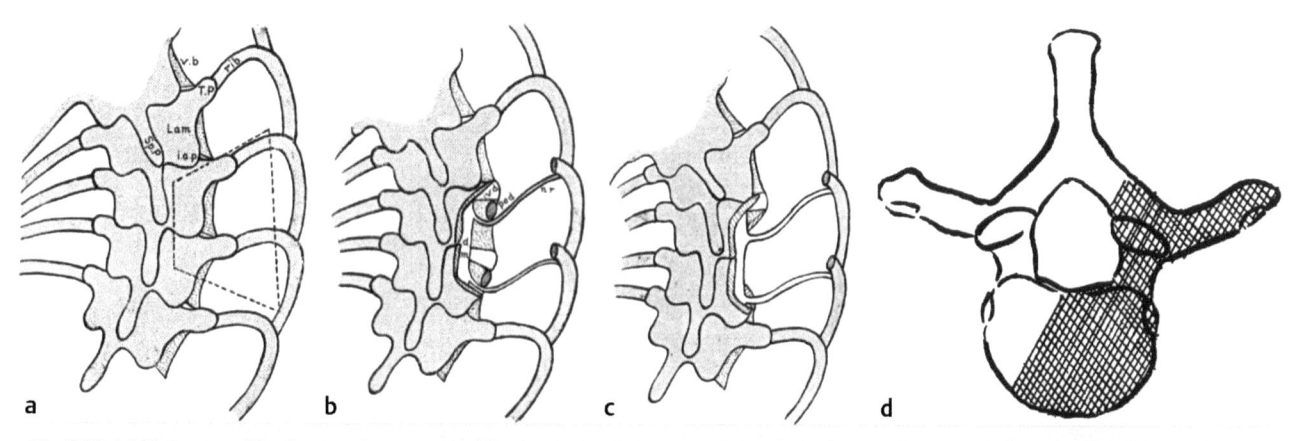

Fig. 6.18 (a) First stage of Roaf's operation: removal of laminae, transverse processes, and vertebral end of two ribs. (b) Exposure of cord, nerve roots, and vertebral bodies and discs. (c) Removal of most of the vertebral bodies and disks and pedicle. (d) Cross section showing the amount of vertebra removed. (Reproduced with permission and copyright © of the British Editorial Society of Bone and Joint Surgery, Roaf R. Wedge Resection for Scoliosis. J Bone Joint Surg (Br) 1955;1:97–101.)

Congenital Deformities

Unfortunately for Roaf the only way he could close his wedge was by the use of a corrective plaster jacket as no instrumentation was available at that time. Notwithstanding, excellent corrections were obtained and in one illustrated case in his classic paper a curve was corrected from 70 degrees to 10 degrees! Look at the pictures. In all, 16 cases were described with no complications. Roaf's vertebral excision was however incomplete in that he left behind the concave third of the vertebra. This of course acted as a hinge so that there wasn't complete instability at the osteotomy site prior to reduction and plaster jacket application. Being a wedge resection this technique could be applied to deformities other than a single hemivertebra. Moreover, being a closing wedge osteotomy the spinal cord was not unnecessarily stretched.

Then in Hong Kong Hodgson, following his great experience of anterior spinal fusion for tuberculosis,[60] turned his attention to the correction of fixed spinal curves. He favored an opening wedge osteotomy but this stretched the spinal cord at the apex of the deformity and resulted in an unacceptable level of paralysis.[61] In South Africa George Dommisse carried out 68 of Hodgson's circumferential osteotomies but there were four paraplegias.[62] Meanwhile in Louisville, Kentucky, Leatherman had successfully carried out resection of vertebral bodies anteriorly for years[48] and, unlike Roaf's this was a complete wedge. But at that stage he had no reliable metalwork, other than staples, to secure his wedge resection after closure. Then with the introduction of Harrington instrumentation, and in particular the Harrington compression system, he now had a method of closing his wedge and securing it rigidly (▶ Fig. 6.19). He then reported all of 67 cases of anterior and posterior wedge resection for rigid spinal curves in 1979 with excellent results.[54] ▶ Fig. 6.20 and ▶ Fig. 6.21 demonstrate Leatherman's brilliance.

This was revolutionary stuff (unnecessarily radical and potentially dangerous) as the critics were quick to inappropriately point out, at a time when the perceived wisdom was a simple posterior fusion in situ. Leatherman staged his procedure with 1 or 2 weeks between the anterior first and posterior second stages simply because he felt that to do it all at once might be too much for the patient (and the surgeon) but soon one-stage resections were reported.[63] These Leatherman procedures tended to be carried out on established congenital deformities of some magnitude simply because early referral was not common plus the fact that many had had a tethering posterior fusion in situ beforehand. Leatherman already knew that the natural history of a solitary hemivertebra was unpredictable and could cause severe and relentless progression long before others appreciated that[64] (▶ Fig. 6.10). That was why the lower age limit in his series of 60 cases was 2 years and 3 months thus showing Leatherman's understanding of trying to remove hemivertebrae and so "altering the deforming forces in the growing spine" which indeed was his life's mission statement.

Of course with the use of anterior and posterior techniques in wedge resection, this mandated an approach through the chest, abdomen, or both and it was not long before there were reports of hemivertebra resection through a single posterior approach.[65-67] Nakamura started posterior wedge resections in 1984, but he used Harrington instrumentation and in particular the compression system like Leatherman had done to close his wedge.[66] Furthermore these tended to be older children and in Karlsbad our goal was to perform the posterior hemivertebra resection in the first 2 years of life before the deforming effect of the hemivertebra had exerted its secondary damage with growth. In 1991 in Karlsbad we began to put into practice this exciting concept[68] and in 2002 J.H. reported upon his 21 consecutive hemivertebra cases dealt with by posterior resection, transpedicular instrumentation, and short segment fusion but with a mean age of almost 6 years and the youngest being 1 year and 2 months. All these 21 patients achieved excellent corrections of more than 60%, down to a Cobb angle of 15 degrees or so (▶ Fig. 6.22).

It was clear, in parallel with this clinical experience, that first of all the feasibility of pedicular screw instrumentation in the very young had to be validated. Inherent with this approach

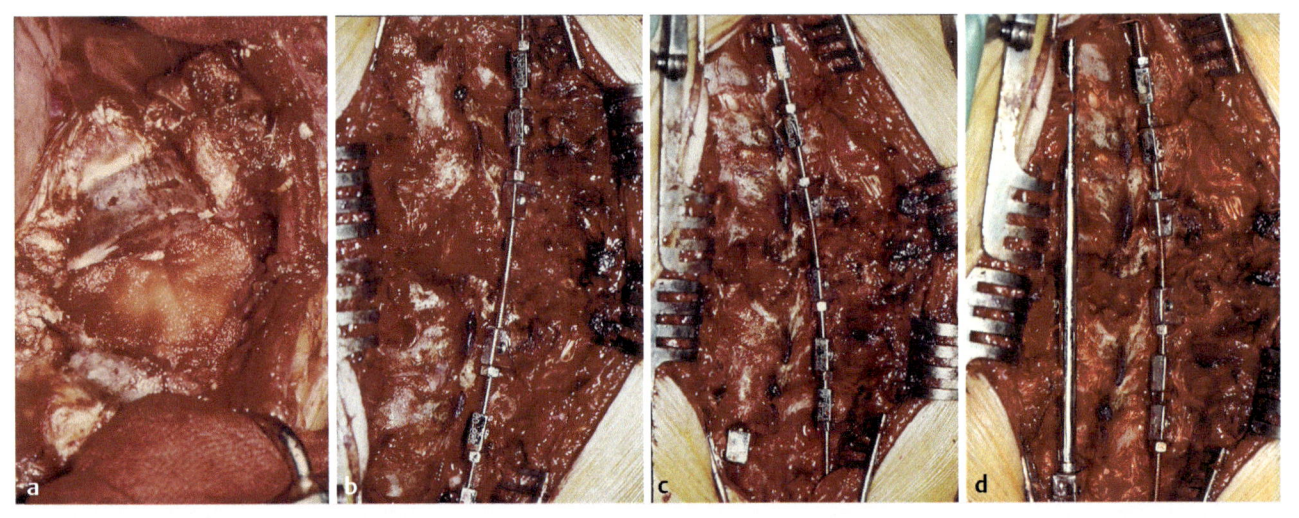

Fig. 6.19 Leatherman's wedge resection. (a) A wedge has been removed anteriorly leaving behind only the concave pedicle and facet joint; a hemostatic agent fills the gap. (b) The posterior part of the wedge has been removed including the concave facet joint and pedicle and a compression system has been inserted on the convex side. (c) The compression system has been tightened to close the wedge. (d) A distraction rod has been inserted on the concave side to aid correction and stability. A posterolateral spinal fusion with abundant iliac crest bone graft completes the procedure.

Congenital Deformities

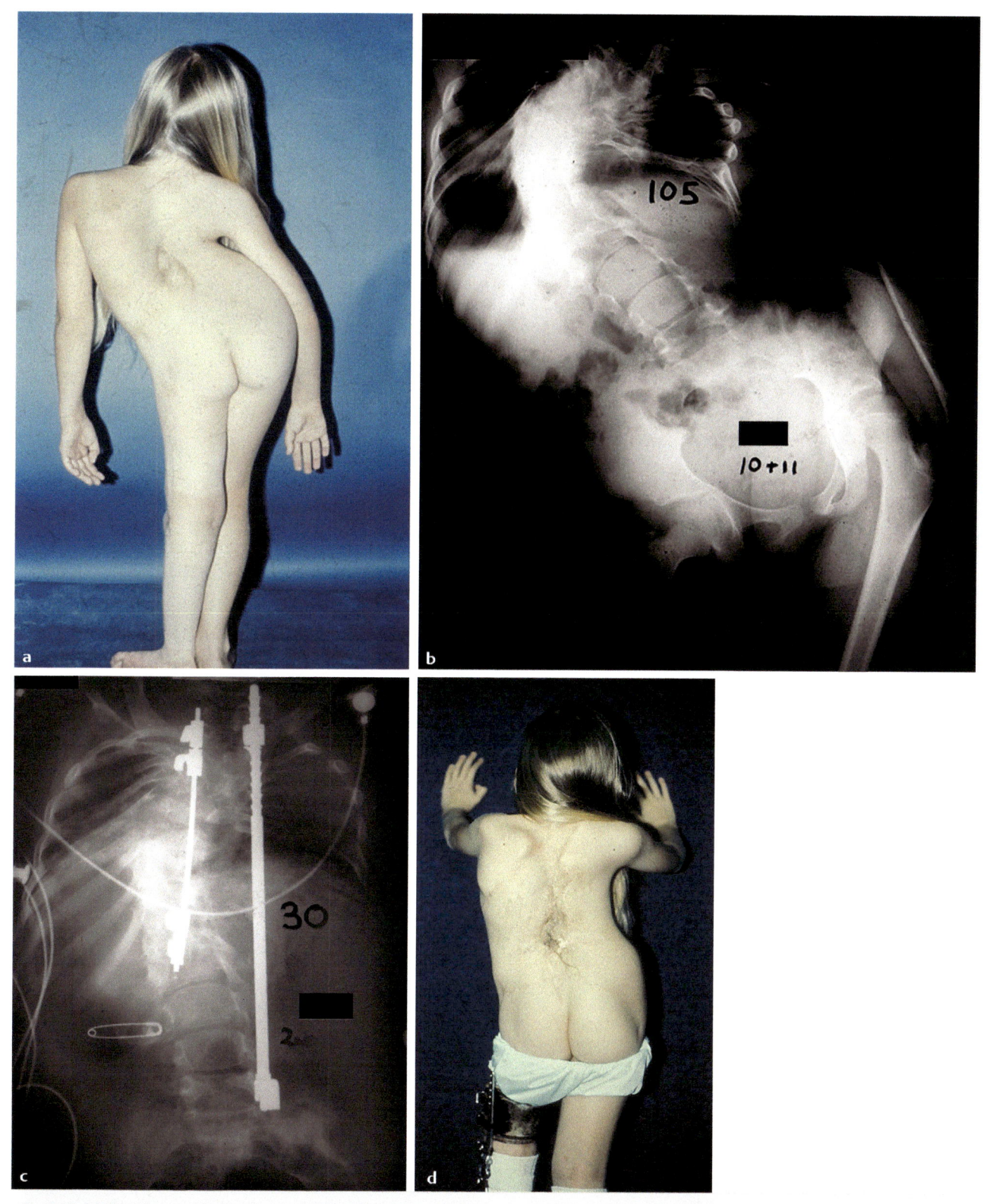

Fig. 6.20 (a) This 10-year-old girl with spina bifida with ambulatory ability has a severe congenital bony scoliosis above her spina bifida area and needs a stick to prevent her falling over. **(b)** PA radiograph demonstrating the severe congenital scoliosis due to mixed anomalies and a marked pelvic tilt. **(c)** PA radiograph showing a superb correction having taken as much of a wedge as we felt safe. **(d)** A well balanced spine without pelvic obliquity.

would be that surgery would only have to be localized to the primary area of deformation with short segment fixation and fusion. Two particularly important questions arose when considering pedicular screw fixation in 1- or 2-year olds: the first being the size of the pedicles at this age and would they be big enough in the thoracic and lumbar spine to accept a

Congenital Deformities

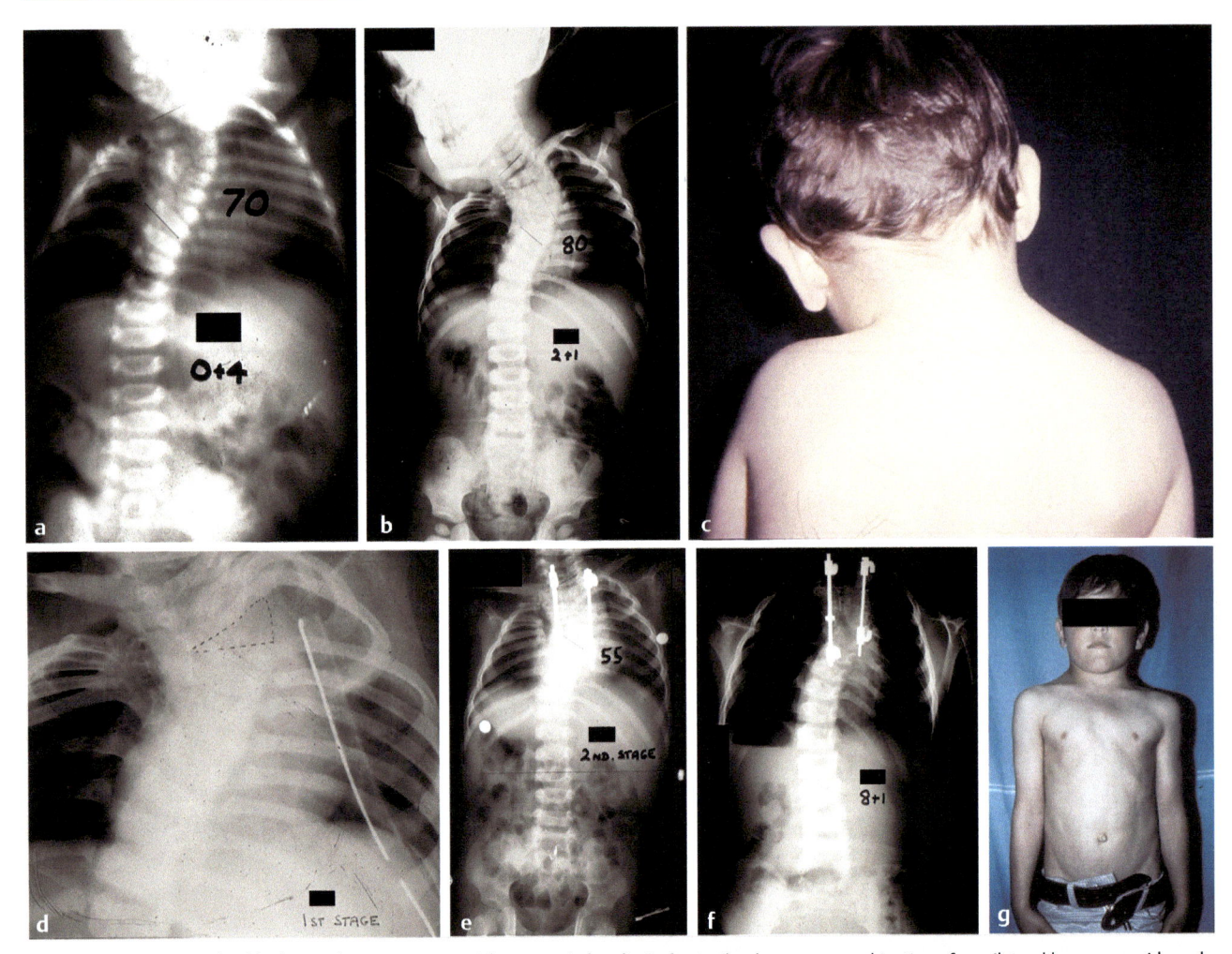

Fig. 6.21 (a) A 4-month-old infant with a severe upper right congenital scoliosis due to the dangerous combination of a unilateral bar on one side and a hemivertebra on the other. (b) No treatment was sought and by the age of 2 the deformity had worsened considerably. (c) Back view of the little boy confirms the severe deformity. (d) After the first stage high thoracotomy and anterior wedge removal. (e) After the second stage there has been a good correction of the deformity and excellent spinal alignment. The compression system on the left has been inserted in distraction mode, a useful modification when you want a small implant. (f) PA radiograph at the age of 8 showing a solid fusion and maintenance of the corrected position. (g) At age 8 the head, neck, and torso are perfectly aligned. No one else was doing this in the late 1960s.

pedicular screw and if so what would be the best screw diameter.[69] Second there might be concerns about vertebral growth after screw insertion and we did not want any vertebral body growth retardation or any spinal canal narrowing. We knew something about the morphometric characteristics of pedicles in young children from the work of Ferree[70] but their youngest child was 3 years of age and only lumbar pedicles were looked at. However, Zindrick had looked at anatomical specimens of immature spines and looked at pedicle morphology from T1 to L5 but again his youngest specimen was already 3 years of age.[71] Ferree's pedicular diameters ranged from 6 to 12 mm and Zindrick's from 3 to 8 mm. Of the first 19 consecutive patients whom we reported using pedicle screws in 1- and 2-year-old children, the first 11 were in conjunction with a small plate and rod system (from use in the cervical spine) (▶ Fig. 6.22) but we then developed a new screw/rod system in 1998 and applied it to a further eight children. These were polyaxial titanium screws of diameter 3.5- and 3-mm rods (baby-Moss-Miami) which ideally fitted the dimensions of small children in the thoracic and lumbar spines (▶ Fig. 6.23).

We found no neurological complications with their use. A monosegmental fusion was performed in all cases. Long-term follow-up of instrumented cases showed no significant retardation of growth in the instrumented vertebrae compared to the adjacent ones and CT showed no major spinal canal stenosis[69] (▶ Fig. 6.24 and ▶ Fig. 6.25).

We then reported posterior hemivertebra resection with transpedicular instrumentation in 28 children aged 1 to 6 years with 12 thoracic cases, 12 thoracolumbar, and 4 lumbar.[72] In eight cases there was an associated unilateral bar that was divided after hemivertebra resection (▶ Fig. 6.26). There were no neurological complications and no significant growth retardation of the pedicles on scanning and nor was there any evidence of spinal canal stenosis. In two patients with severe pseudokyphosis a convex pedicle was overloaded and broke requiring temporary one level additional segment instrumentation and two patients required further surgery—one because of bar formation at the operative site and one because of a new bone mass at the site of the resected hemivertebra. All patients had an excellent final clinical result with a Cobb angle of 45 degrees

Congenital Deformities

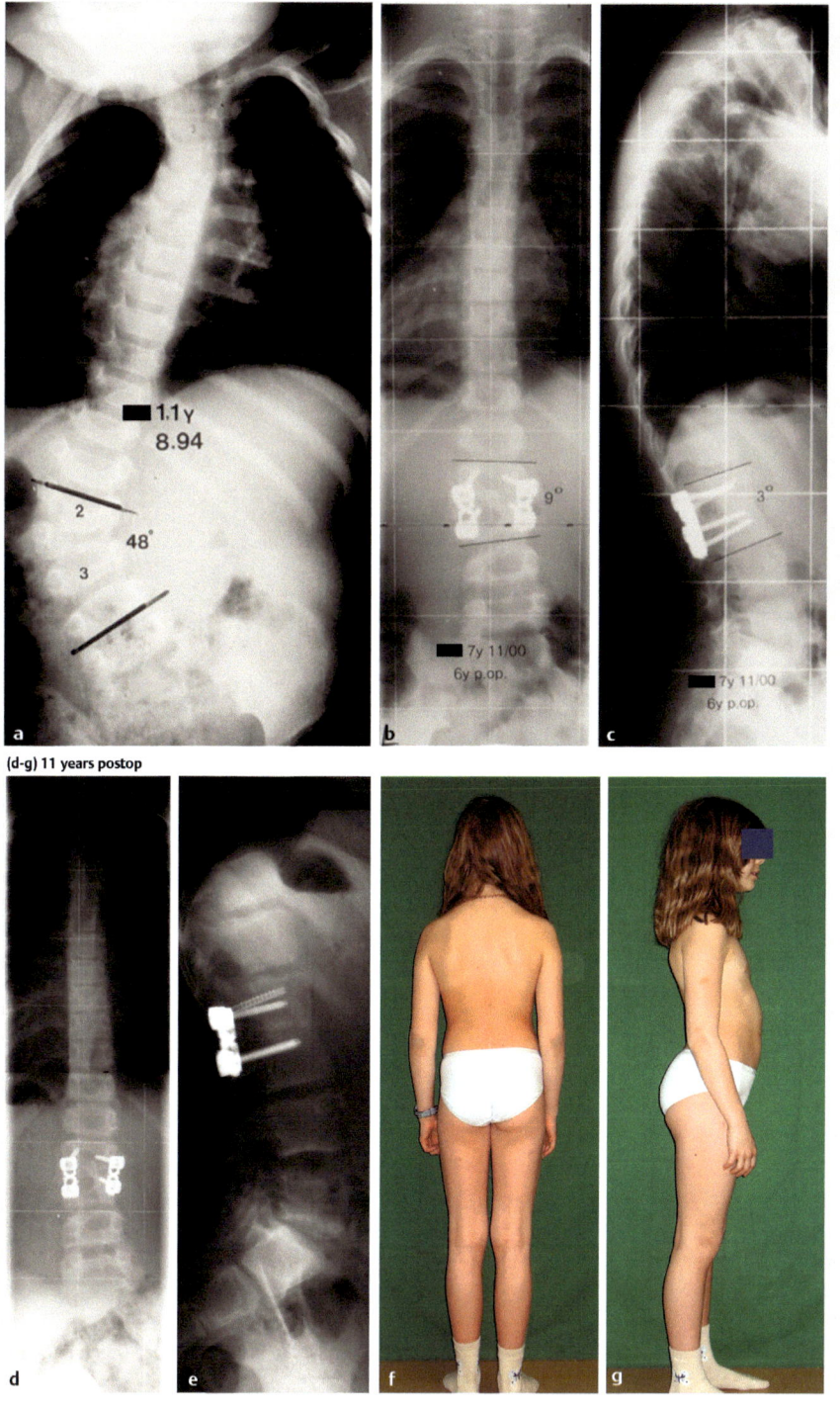

Fig. 6.22 (a) Preoperative radiograph of a 14-month-old girl with a fully segmented hemivertebra, causing a scoliosis of 48 degrees. (b) After resection of the hemivertebra and transpedicular instrumentation with a cervical plate system there is nearly complete correction in the frontal plane. (c) And in the sagittal plane. (d–g) Age 11 years there is maintenance of the corrected position and no visible clinical deformity.

(d-g) 11 years postop

reduced to 13 degrees after 3.5 years of follow-up. Complete correction of the local deformity with a short segment fusion allows for normal growth of the unaffected parts of the spine.[72]

Others were tackling the problem of hemivertebrae at an early age somewhat differently. In 2005 the Boston group reported on 18 children under the age of 8 with a congenital spine deformity who had been treated with reduced size instrumentation and short segment fusion with excellent and safe curve correction with a minimum of 3 years of follow-up.[73] This was however done through both an anterior and posterior combined approach as did Xu in China.[74]

Garrido et al performed a short anterior instrumented fusion along with a posteroconvex noninstrumented fusion[75] while Elsabaie et al carried out an anterior single stage partial vertebrectomy with instrumentation reporting good results in 12 children with a mean age of just less than 3 years with corrections from 48 degrees down to 17 degrees.[76] The advantages of a one-stage posterior hemivertebra resection with transpedicular instrumentation were also noted in China with Yu from Nanjing reporting on 27 consecutive cases with a mean age of 5.5 years but with an average of more than four segments.[77] Then Peng from Guangzhu reported on 10 patients under the

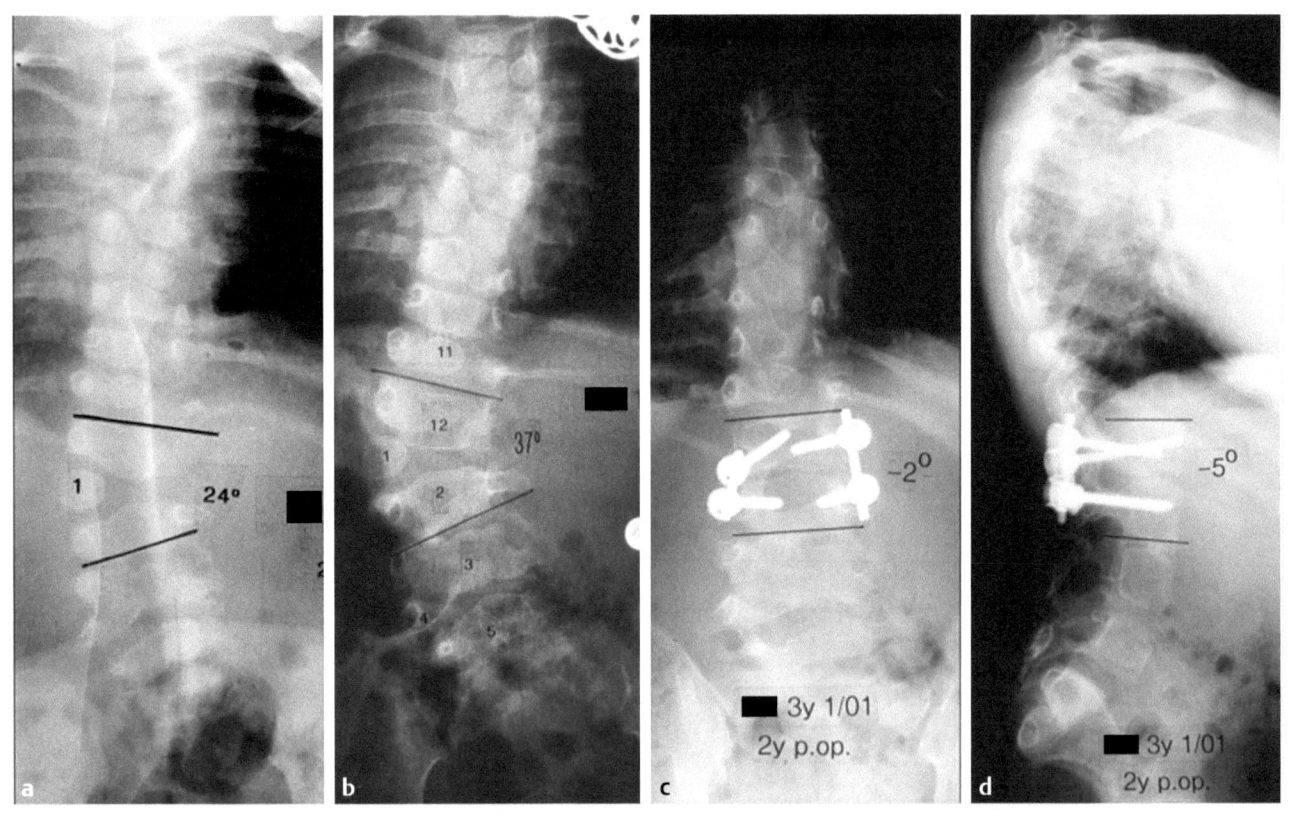

Fig. 6.23 Baby Moss-Miami. **(a,b)** A 3-month-old child with multiple congenital anomalies of the spine but balanced in the thoracic spine with a midlumbar fully segmented hemivertebra showing rapid progression within the first year. **(c,d)** Two years after resection of the hemivertebra and instrumentation with a transpedicular screw rod system. (Reproduced with permission from Lippincott WW. Spine 2002;Vol 27(10):116–1123, Figure 4, p. 1121.)

age of 5 with a unilateral posterior approach with a single rod and pedicle screws. At follow-up averaging 3.5 years there was a 63% segmental curve angle correction (▶ Fig. 4.10 and ▶ Fig. 6.17). It was recommended as less traumatic, simple, and safe.[78]

In 2009 Lenke et al reported on 35 patients treated by posterior only vertebral column resection (VCR) carried out between 2000 and 2005 for both congenital scoliosis and kyphosis producing what they described as "dramatic radiographic and clinical corrections."[79] Perioperative spinal cord monitoring was regarded as being mandatory as there were two temporary monitoring problems that reverted to normal after "prompt surgical intervention." There were several different patient categories including both severe scoliosis and kyphosis but the average patient age was beyond 10 years therefore not focusing on the very young.

Then in 2011 a multicenter comparison of three surgical techniques was reported by Yasnay et al.[80] Hemivertebra resection with instrumented fusion was compared with instrumented fusion without hemivertebra resection or hemiepiphysiodesis or in situ fusion. Seventy-six patients were studied in all with a mean age of 8 years. The instrumented fusion with hemivertebra excision group were youngest (mean age 5 years) but with a much better correction at 73%. However, there was a higher neurological complication rate although all such patients made a complete neurological recovery. There was also a higher instrumentation problem rate requiring revision surgery.

Then in 2009 we published our experience of 41 very young children (mean age 3.5 years) followed up for more than 6 years. Group 1 comprised 28 children with hemivertebrae only who underwent posterior hemivertebra resection and pedicular instrumentation while group 2 comprised 13 children with a contralateral bar who required hemivertebra resection plus additional osteotomy of the bar and/or rib fusions. In group 1 the main (segmental) curve was reduced from 36 to 7 degrees while in group 2, with bigger initial curves, the main curve reduced from 70 degrees to 23 degrees.[81]

Thus it can be seen that apical wedge resection carried out from a purely posterior approach with the use of pedicular instrumentation can be utilized to deal with not only simple solitary hemivertebrae but also more complex deformities including those with concave bar formation (▶ Fig. 6.26) or multiple hemivertebrae (▶ Fig. 6.27). This case shows the importance of checking on the sagittal plane after posterior instrumentation. We only fuse the area of the congenital deformity and so the posterior instrumentation covers several segments above and below so as to control the deformity in the frontal plane. The posterior instrumentation does however stop spinal growth at the back of the spine and so continuing anterior growth can cause an increasing thoracic lordosis that will hinder correction in the frontal plane. Moreover, if the lordosis is unchecked, patients find the displeasing cosmetic effect just as bad as a rib hump. Controlling growth of the structural curve above and below the area of the congenital anomaly which we have fused is extremely important, particularly during the

Congenital Deformities

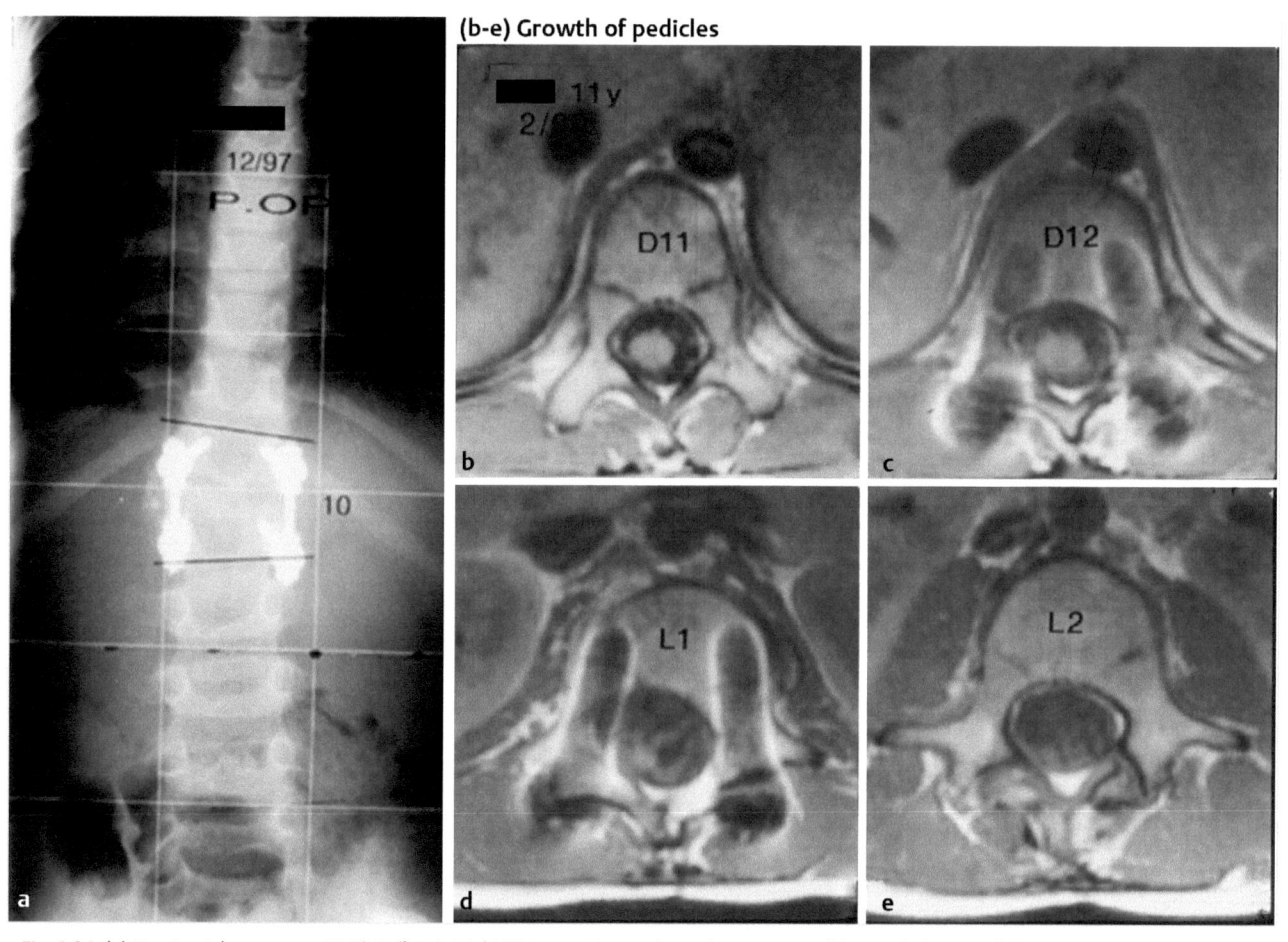

Fig. 6.24 (a) Hemivertebrectomy at T12/L1. (b–e) Axial MRI scans 11 years later showing no problem with the size of the central canal and therefore no spinal cord problems. (Reproduced with permission from Lippincott WW. Spine 2002;Vol 17:1791–1799, Figures 5 and 7.)

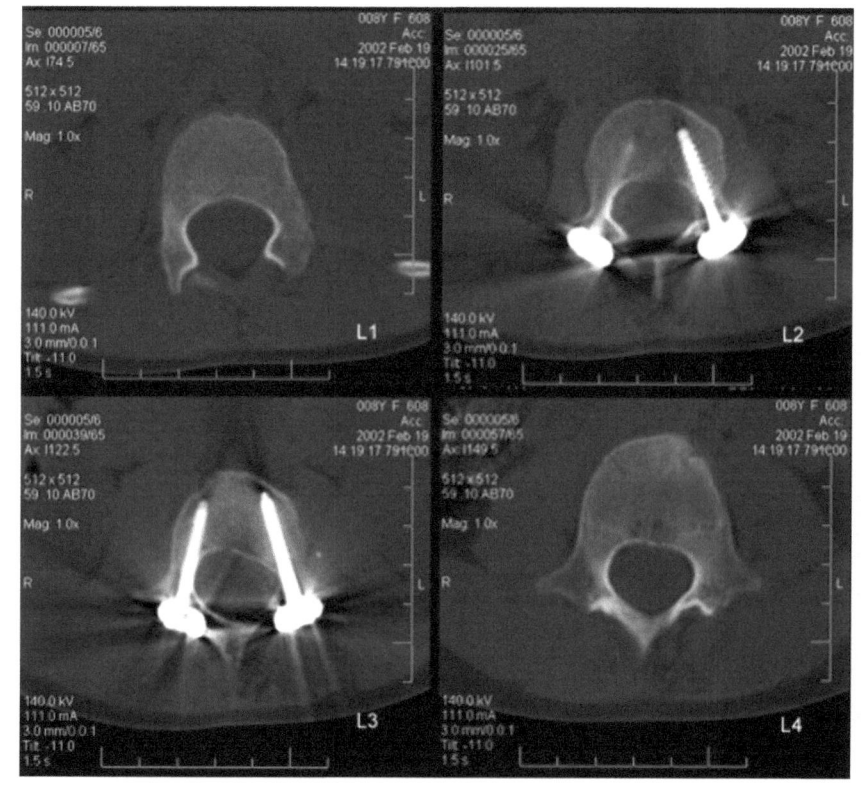

Fig. 6.25 Axial CT scan 8 years after hemivertebrectomy at L2/3 showing normal pedicular and vertebral growth 8 years postoperatively.

Congenital Deformities

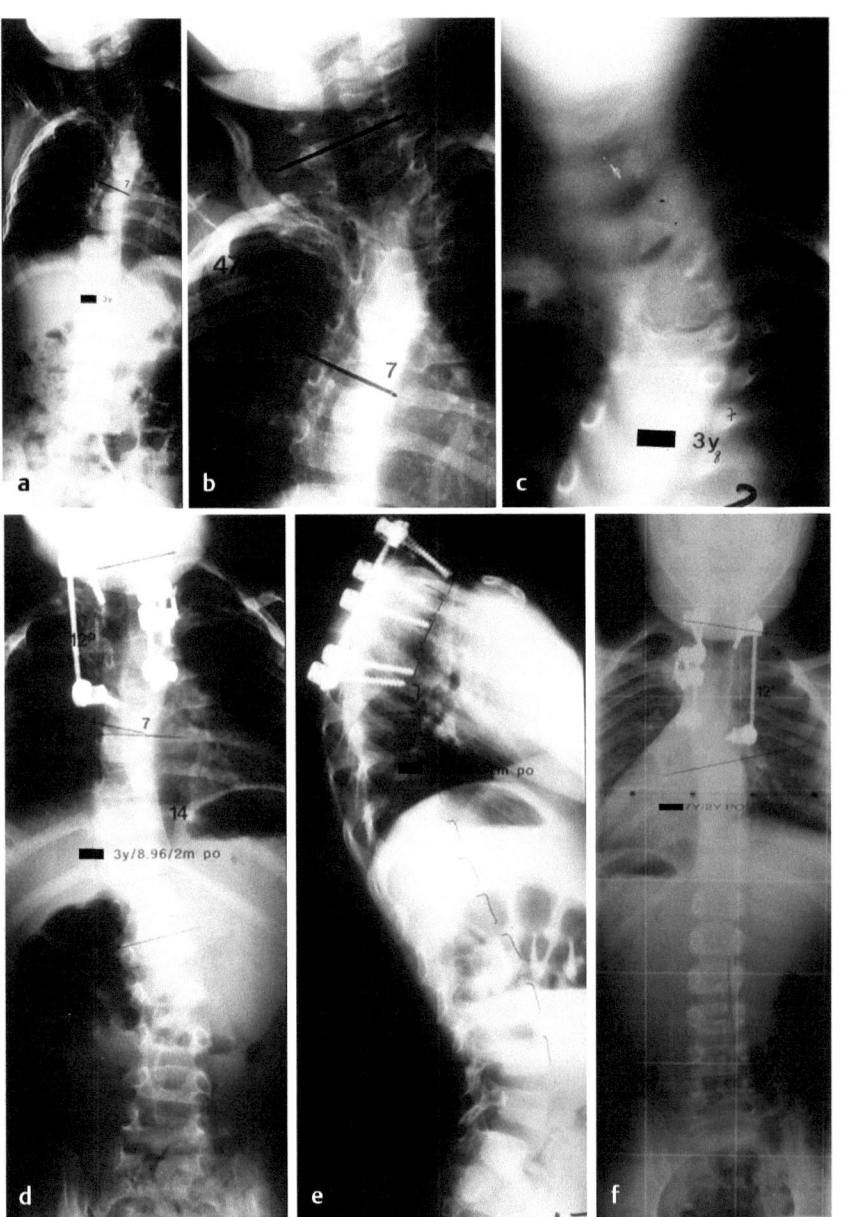

Fig. 6.26 (a–c) Double hemivertebrae with a contralateral bar in a 3-year-old girl; worst case scenario regarding prognosis. (d,e) After hemivertebra resection and division of the bar a good correction was obtained. (f) Four years later the correction is maintained and there is a solid fusion.

preadolescent/adolescent phase of increased growth acceleration. When this period has been safely negotiated then the whole structural curve must be fused, otherwise there will be a situation of a mobile deformity versus rigid metalwork that is bound to lead to ultimate metalwork breakage or loosening. Therefore, it is important that these patients are followed up until spinal maturity.

To reiterate, the important concept of early apical resection is to remove the deforming force before it creates either a primary local scoliosis or any secondary scoliogenic effect elsewhere in the spine (▶ Fig. 6.10 and ▶ Fig. 6.14). Thus many of these potentially difficult deformities can be dealt with by a one-level localized short segment spinal fusion in the very young. Don't wait and see what happens.

Congenital anomalies in the neck and cervicothoracic junction require special attention if they are to be dealt with surgically. Obviously the pathological bony deformity should be clearly established by whatever imaging techniques. Then, when there are congenital bony anomalies there is an increased incidence of associated vascular anomalies with particular reference to the vertebral arteries. ▶ Fig. 6.28 shows the normal arterial anatomy from the root of the neck upward. The vertebral artery normally arises from the first part of the subclavian artery and then passes upward through the transverse process foramina from the sixth cervical vertebra upward. The vertebral artery may however enter the transverse foramina at the fourth, fifth, or seventh cervical vertebrae and may itself arise from the common carotid artery rather than the subclavian. It is mandatory therefore to perform angiography/arteriography to determine the arterial situation prior to surgery (▶ Fig. 6.29). Furthermore, you have to anticipate that there is a risk of damage to the vertebral artery and so you have to know whether the contralateral vertebral artery can take over the blood supply to the brain. For this purpose, an occlusion test is performed bilaterally. A vascular catheter has to be inserted into the vertebral artery on one side and by opening a balloon at the tip of

Congenital Deformities

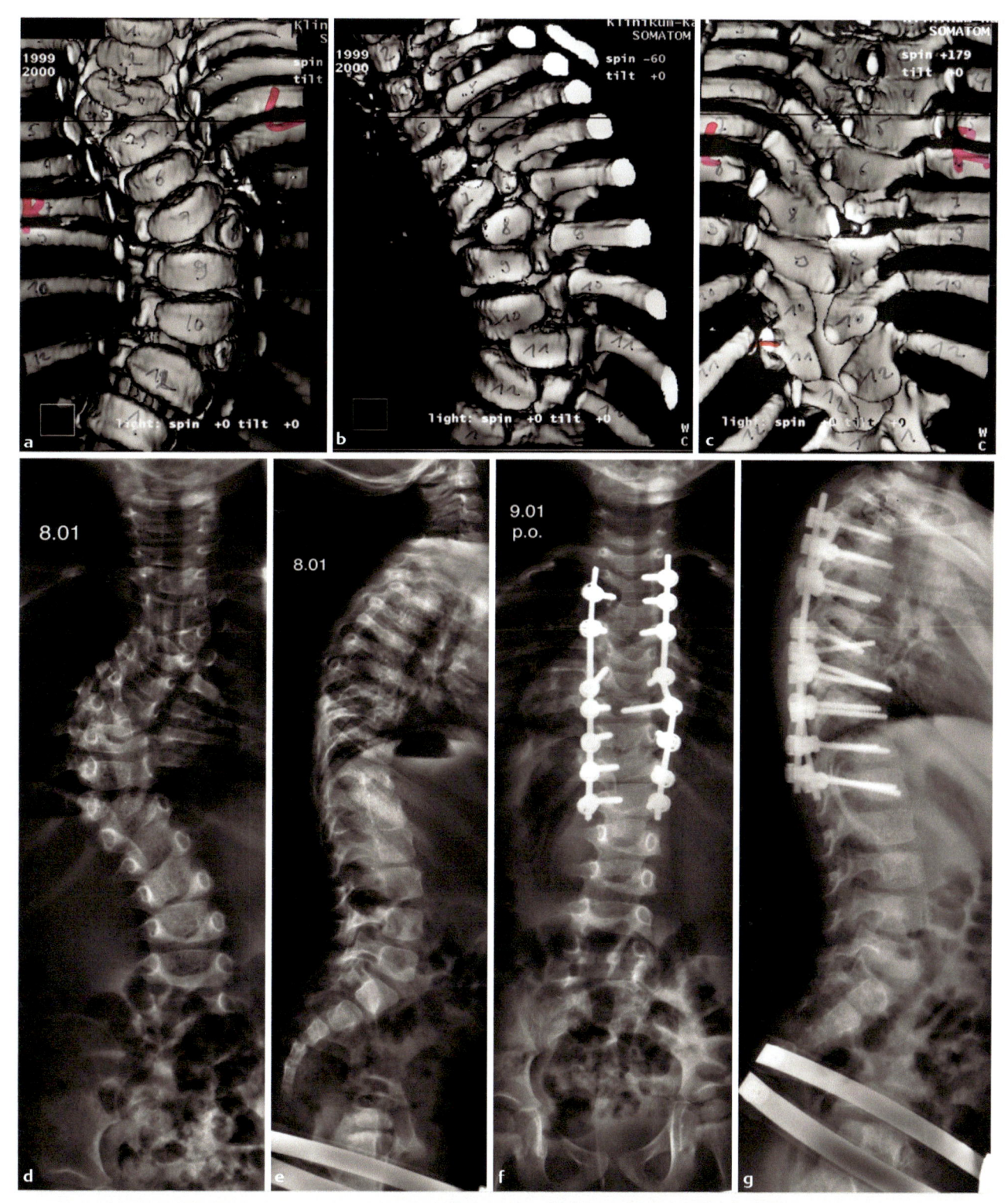

Fig. 6.27 (a–c) Reformatted 3D CT scans showing multiple thoracic hemivertebrae: one on the right at T4, one on the left at T8, and again on the left at T11. (d,e) PA and lateral radiographs showing 80 degree left thoracic curve with significant rotation (note the rib asymmetry). Also note the apical lordosis on the lateral view. (f,g) PA and lateral radiographs after resection of the hemivertebrae and instrumentation, the spine is straight in the frontal plane and a natural kyphosis in the lateral plane.

▶

Congenital Deformities

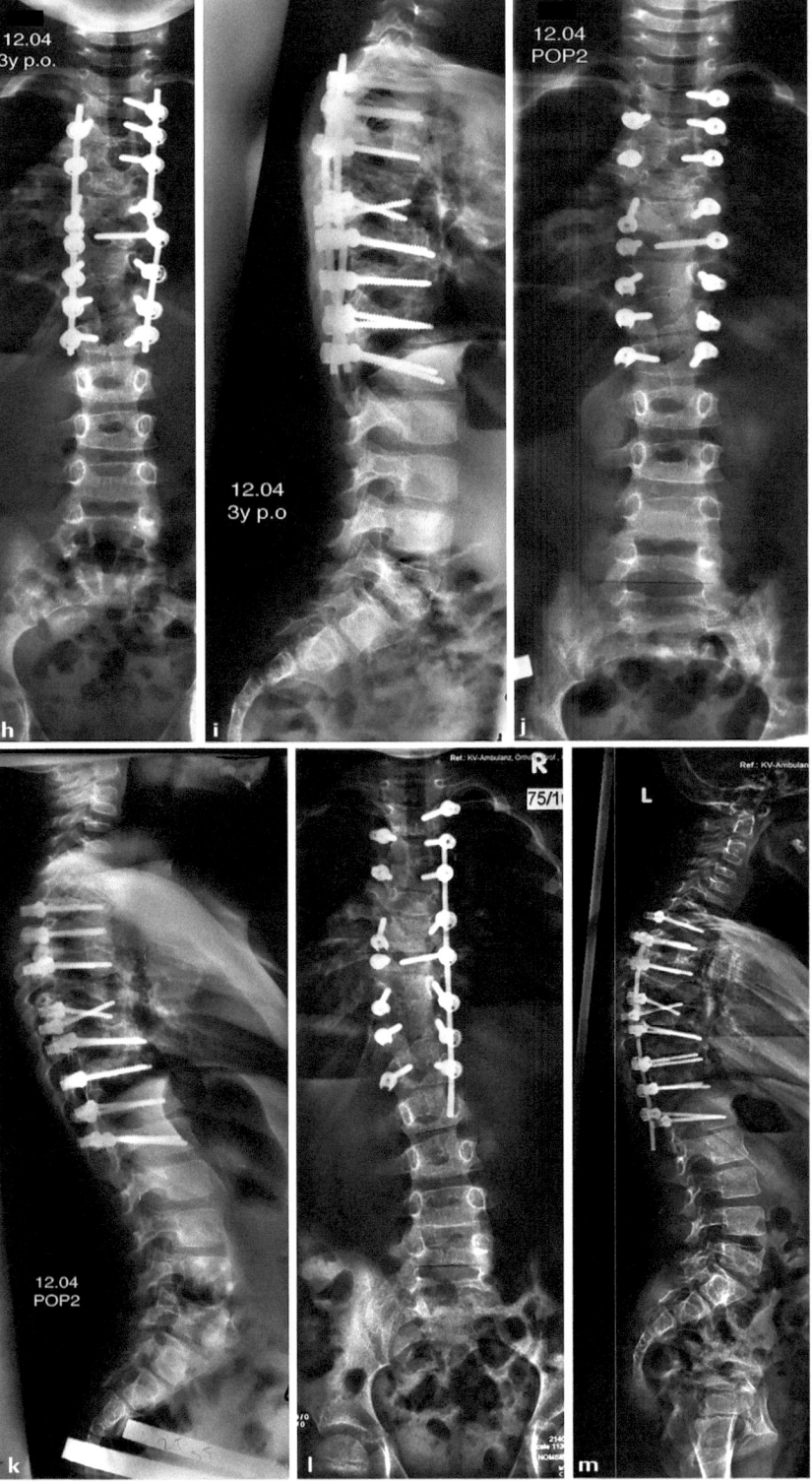

Fig. 6.27 (*continued*) **(h,i)** PA and lateral radiographs three years after surgery showing that a natural kyphosis that was present immediately after surgery has developed into a thoracic lordosis. The posterior metalwork has restricted posterior growth and allowed the front of the spine to continue. **(j,k)** PA and lateral radiographs after removal of the rods but we left the screws. **(l,m)** PA and lateral radiographs after insertion of the right rod just to control the frontal plane while the lateral radiograph shows restoration of a normal kyphosis.

the catheter you perform a temporary occlusion of the artery. Then you have to observe the patient for 5 to 10 minutes to determine whether a neurological deficit occurs. Then you know perfectly whether the contralateral artery is sufficient enough to provide the blood supply of the brain (▶ Fig. 6.30). Without performing this occlusion test you should never resect a hemivertebra in the cervical spine or the cervicothoracic junction. Once this has been done then the vertebral resection can be confidently carried out.

Later in this chapter we consider conditions/syndromes in which congenital spinal anomalies are not uncommon. Marshall-Smith syndrome is, however, a condition of overgrowth, accelerated skeletal maturation, dysmorphic facial features, respiratory difficulties, and some degree of psychomotor

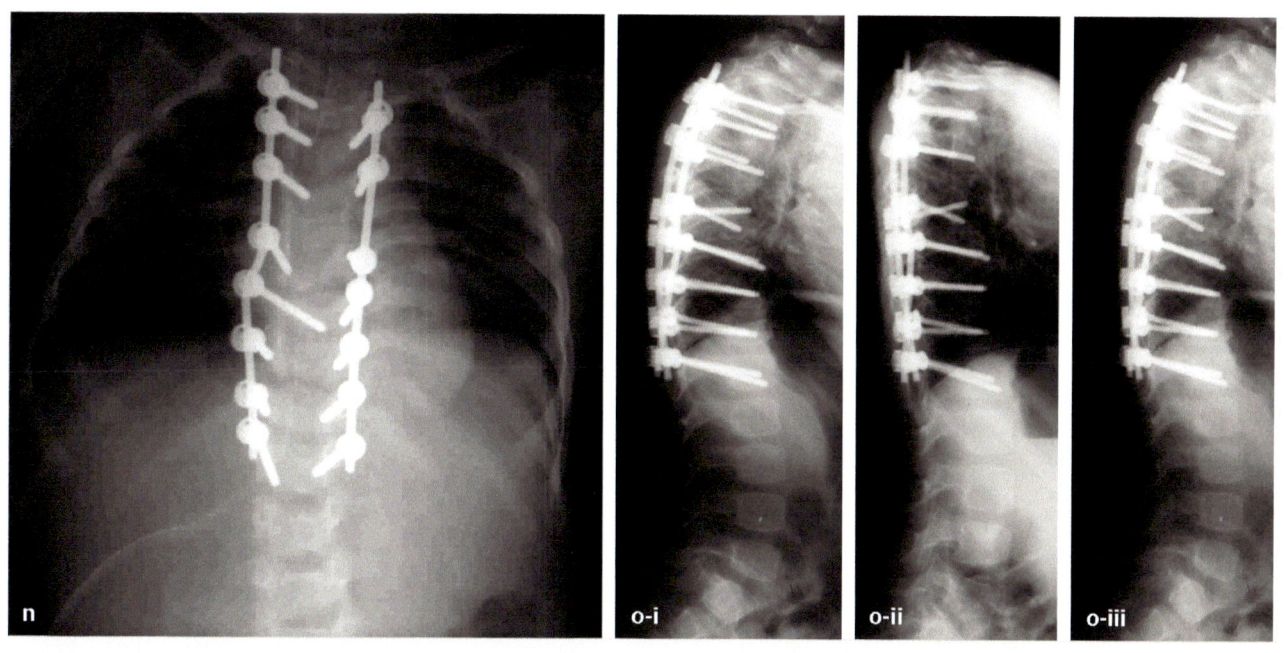

Fig. 6.27 (*continued*) **(n)** PA radiograph after insertion of the second rod. **(o)** Composite lateral radiographs showing initial kyphosis followed by the development of a significant lordosis and then restoration of a normal thoracic kyphosis.

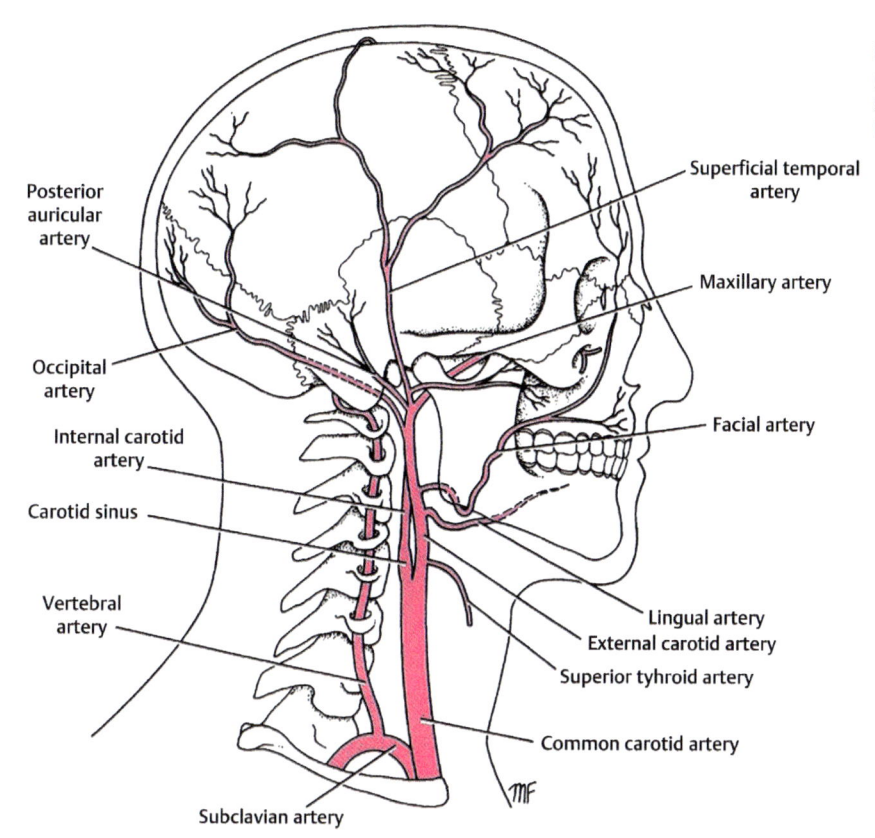

Fig. 6.28 Vascular anatomy. (Reproduced with permission from Clinical Anatomy, 7th edition, Ed Snell RS, Lippincott, Williams and Wilkins, 2004, Figure 11.12, p. 737.)

retardation collectively described as an osteochondrodysplasia with connective tissue abnormalities. The syndrome was first described in 1971[82] and since then about 50 children and adults have been diagnosed. The problem gene is *NF1X*. This young girl happened to have a congenital spine anomaly in association with the Marshall–Smith syndrome (▶ Fig. 6.31). The radiographs show a severe congenital scoliosis in the upper mid-thoracic spine. There is so much rotation that the AP and lateral Cobb angles are very similar (see Chapter 3) and the clinical appearance shows a severe deformity. After posterior pedicle subtraction osteotomies and pedicular instrumentation the deformity was nicely corrected. Unfortunately, because of

Congenital Deformities

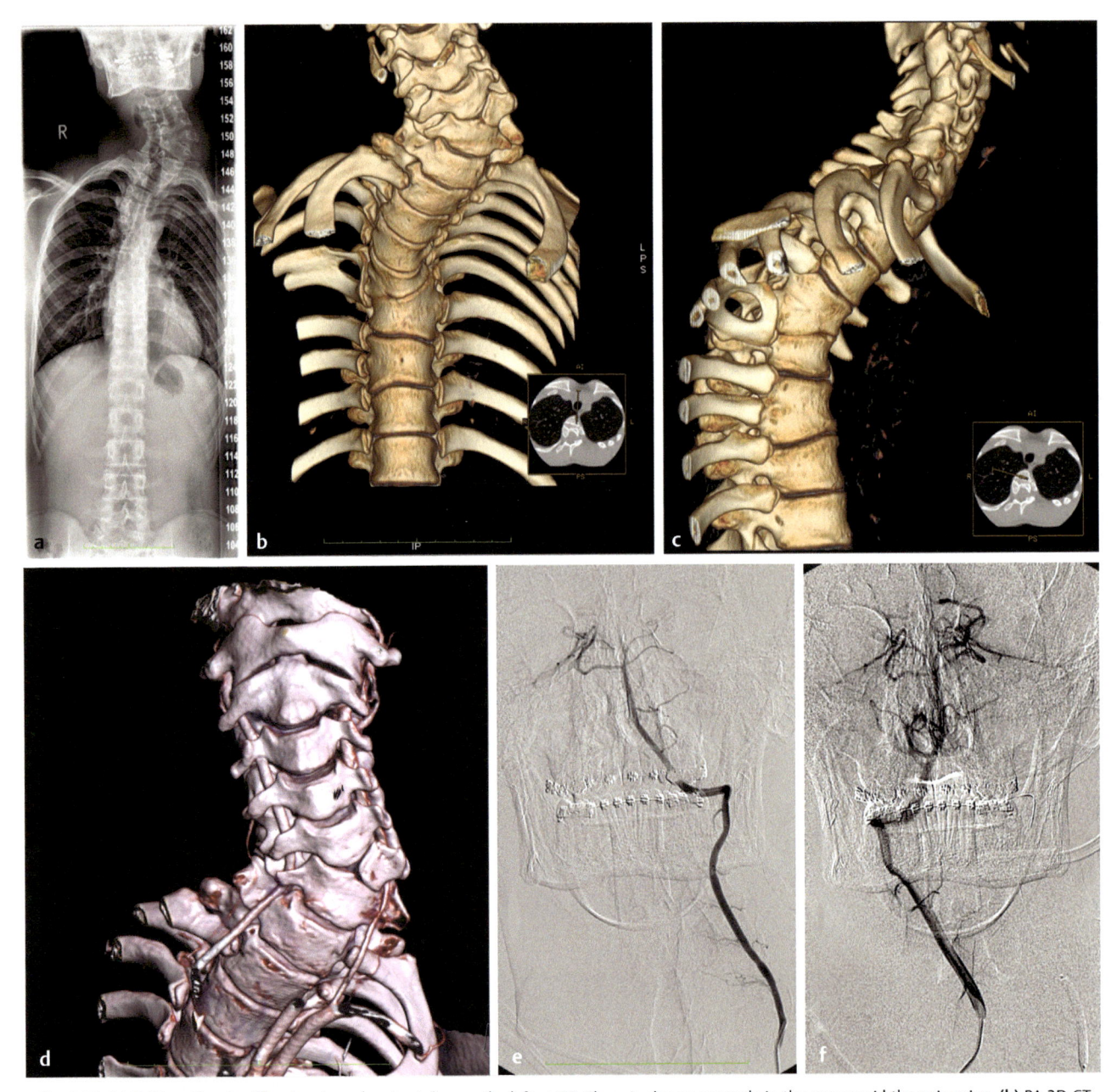

Fig. 6.29 (a) Full length spine film showing a hemivertebra on the left at C6. There is also an anomaly in the upper-mid thoracic spine. (b) PA 3D CT scan of the upper spine very nicely showing the hemivertebra at C6 on the left. (c) Lateral 3D CT view showing that two of the upper thoracic vertebrae are fused together with resultant kyphosis. (d) AP frontal angiography CT showing the vertebral arteries entering the transverse process foramen through C6 but being a little compromised at C7 particularly on the left. (e) A balloon-catheter has been inserted into the left vertebral artery and an occlusion has been performed before it forms the basilar artery with its namesake on the right side. (f) At the same time there is also a catheter in the right vertebral artery and during the occlusion of the left vertebral artery contrast medium is injected into the right vertebral artery; the blood flow demonstrates that there is a perfect blood supply of the brain. Meanwhile the patient is checked clinically and by spinal cord monitoring (SCPs and MEPs). Therefore, we know very precisely if the potential damage to the left vertebral artery will be a problem for the patient.

the straightening effect of the posterior instrumentation in the sagittal plane the spine above kyphosed and so the instrumentation had to be extended upward.

6.4 Practice Point

Surgical technique for hemivertebra resection and pedicular instrumentation by a posterior approach is described here.[81]

6.4.1 Preoperative

Precise imaging is necessary. Focus views, CT, and three-dimensional CT reconstruction and tomography may all be required to identify the shape and position of the hemivertebrae and the adjacent vertebrae, the anatomy around the pedicles, and the posterior parts of the vertebrae. These also provide information on any synostosis of the vertebrae or the ribs. MRI is essential to ensure normality of the spinal cord.

Congenital Deformities

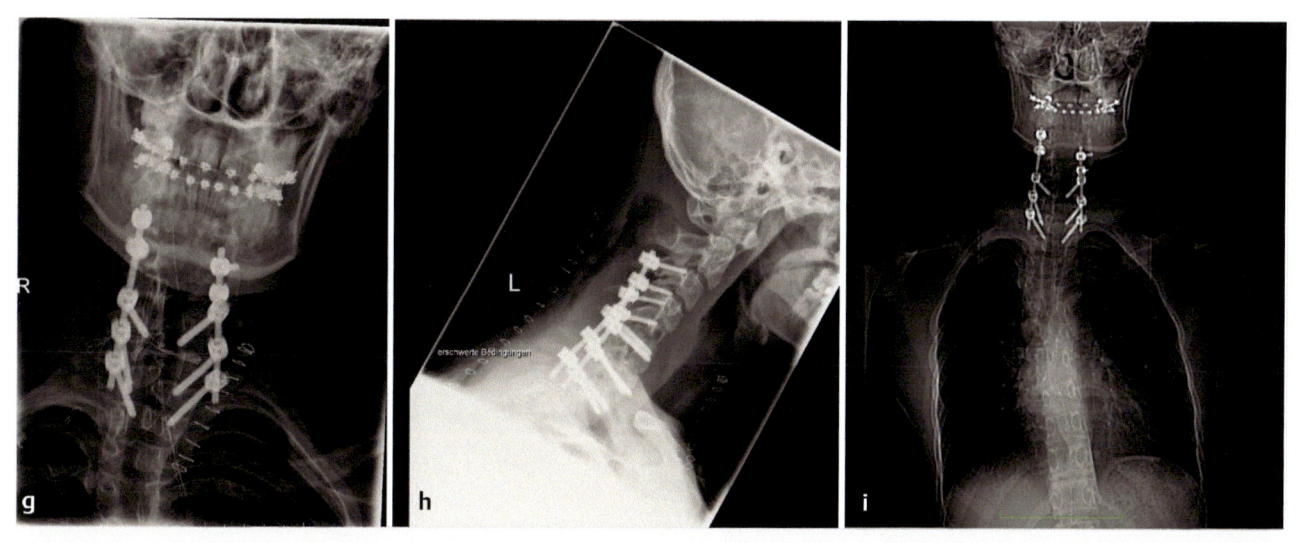

Fig. 6.29 (*continued*) **(g,h)** AP and lateral radiographs after hemivertebra resection and fusion. **(i)** Longer length postoperative spinal X-ray showing a well corrected and balanced spine in the frontal plane. The upper-mid thoracic kyphosis was not deemed significant enough to warrant correction.

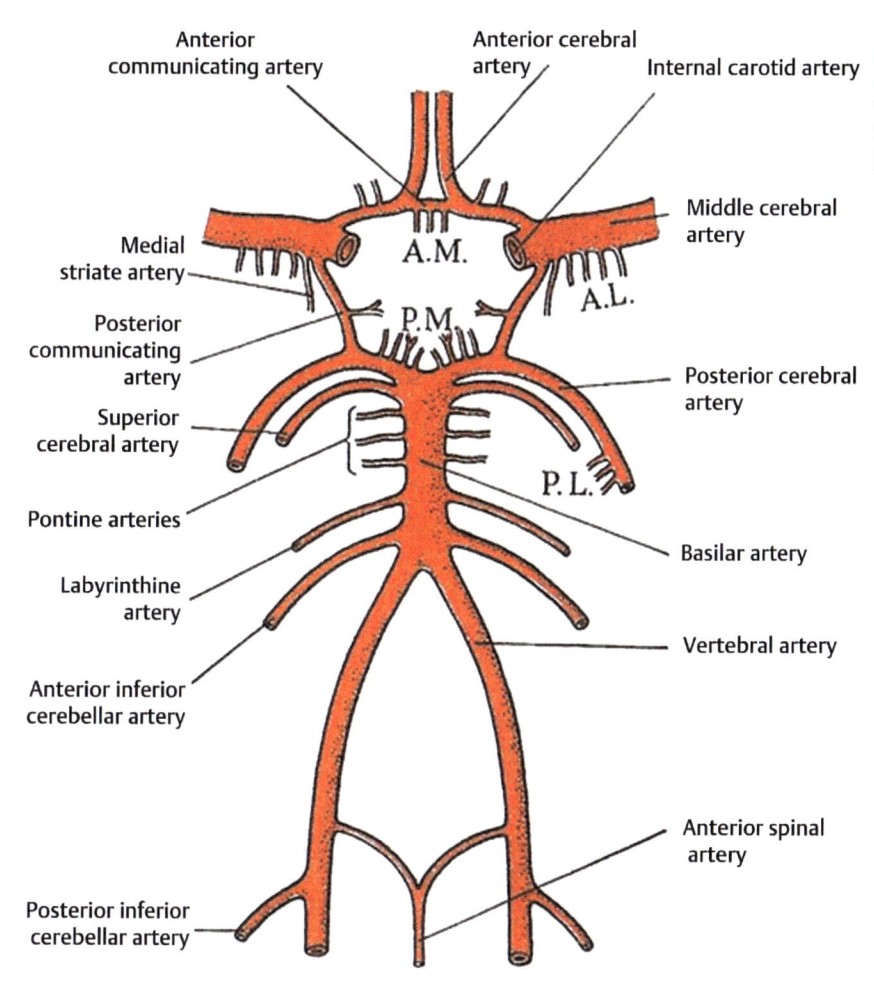

Fig. 6.30 The circle of Willis. (Reproduced with permission from Gray's anatomy. Williams PL, Warwick R, Dyson M, Bannister LH (eds). Churchill Livingstone, Edinburgh 1989: Fig 6.84a p748.)

Congenital Deformities

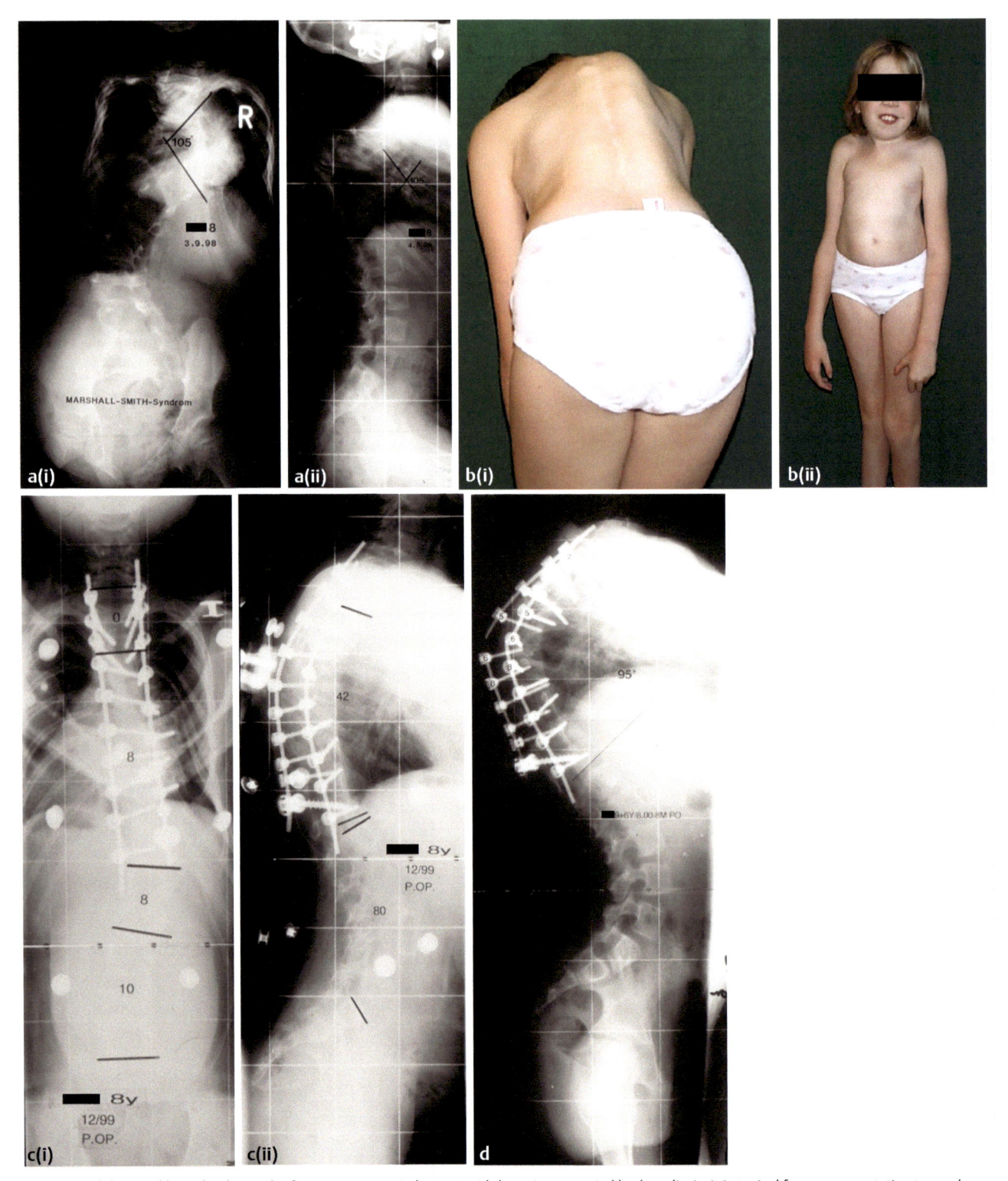

Fig. 6.31 (a) PA and lateral radiograph of a severe congenital upper-mid thoracic congenital lordoscoliosis. It is typical for a severe rotation to produce a big pseudokyphosis. (b) Clinical appearance of this deformity which has significantly shortened the trunk. (c) After pedicle subtraction osteotomies there has been a nice correction. (d) X-ray 8 months after surgery show that the rather slender metalwork has failed under tension.

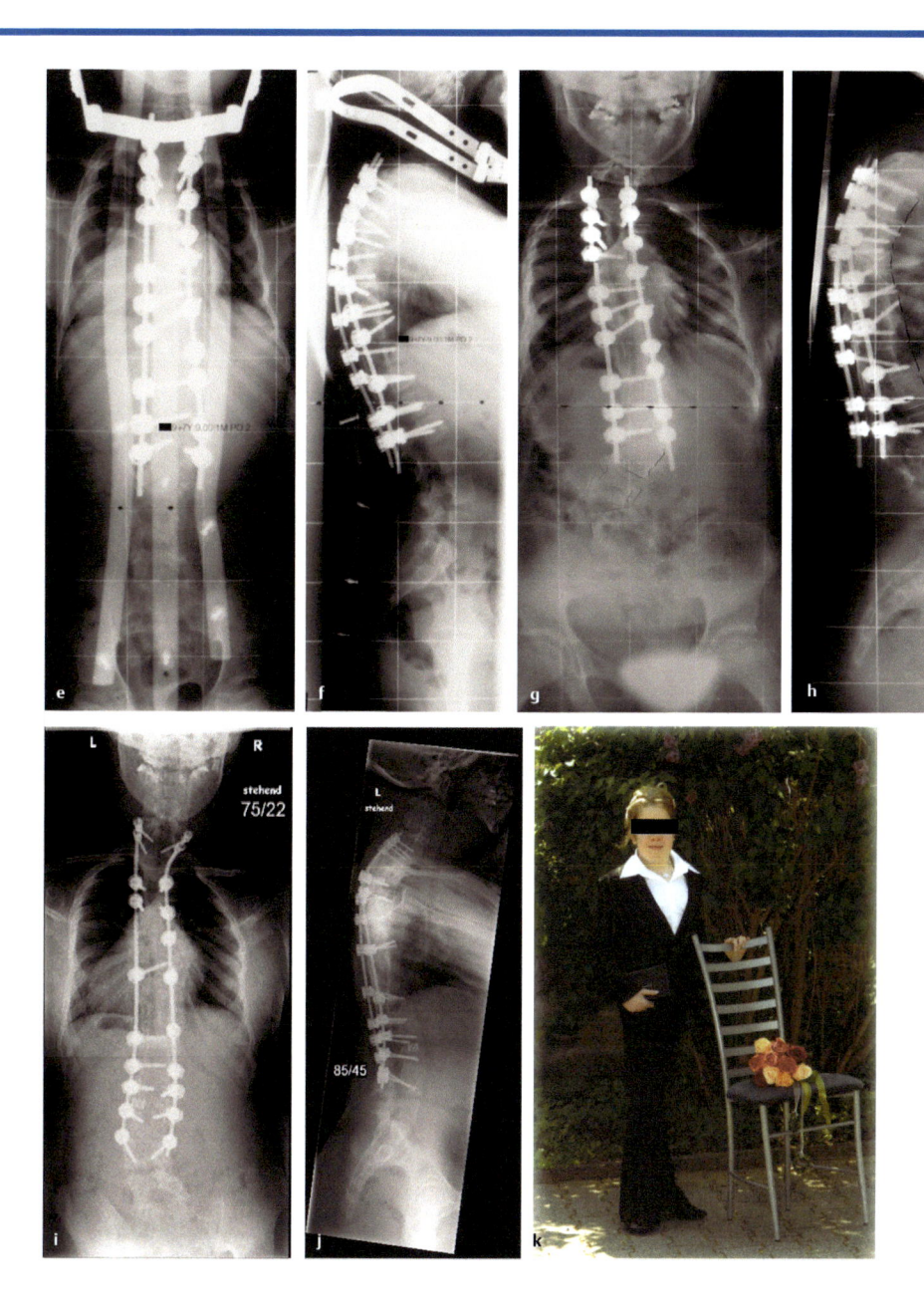

Fig. 6.31 (continued) **(e,f)** PA and lateral radiographs after re-instrumentation with wider bore metalwork supported in the postoperative phase with a CTLSO. **(g,h)** PA and lateral radiographs 5 years later showing a sustained correction of the deformity but the lateral view shows that the spine above the instrumentation has drifted forward into kyphosis. **(i,j)** PA and lateral radiographs showing extension of the metalwork to correct progressive kyphosis. **(k)** An extremely contented young lady.

6.4.2 Surgical Technique

Hemivertebra Removal

The spine is exposed at the level of the hemivertebra and the adjacent vertebrae (▶ Fig. 6.32). The posterior elements are carefully exposed at the affected levels including the laminae, transverse processes, facet joints, and, in the thoracic spine, the rib head on the convex side (▶ Fig. 6.32a). The entry point for the pedicle screws in the lumbar region is the base of the transverse process at the lateral border of the superior articular facet. In the thoracic region the entry point is at the superior margin of the transverse process, slightly lateral to the lower lateral edge of the articular facet. These entry points in the vertebrae adjacent to the hemivertebra are marked by fine needles (▶ Fig. 6.32b) and their positions checked by an image intensifier in the AP view (▶ Fig. 6.32c). The tips of the cannulae should project on to the oval of the pedicles ideally slightly lateral to the center. The bone at the entry point is then opened with a sharp awl or a small bur and a 2-mm drill is used to advance through the pedicle into the vertebral body. The direction of the drill hole is in the sagittal plane perpendicular in the lumbar spine and about 10 degrees caudally in the thoracic region, converging 10 to 15 degrees in the transverse plane. These drill holes are marked with K-wires and their correct position checked with image intensification. These holes are then tapped and 3.5-mm screws inserted (▶ Fig. 6.33).

The posterior elements of the hemivertebra (the laminae, transverse processes, the facet joints, and the posterior parts of the pedicle) are removed. The spinal cord and the nerve roots around the hemivertebra are identified. In the thoracic spine after rib head and transverse process resection in the convexity, the lateral and anterior part of the hemivertebra is exposed (▶ Fig. 6.34), intrathoracically and extrapleurally in the thoracic spine and retroperitoneally in the lumbar spine. The remnants

Congenital Deformities

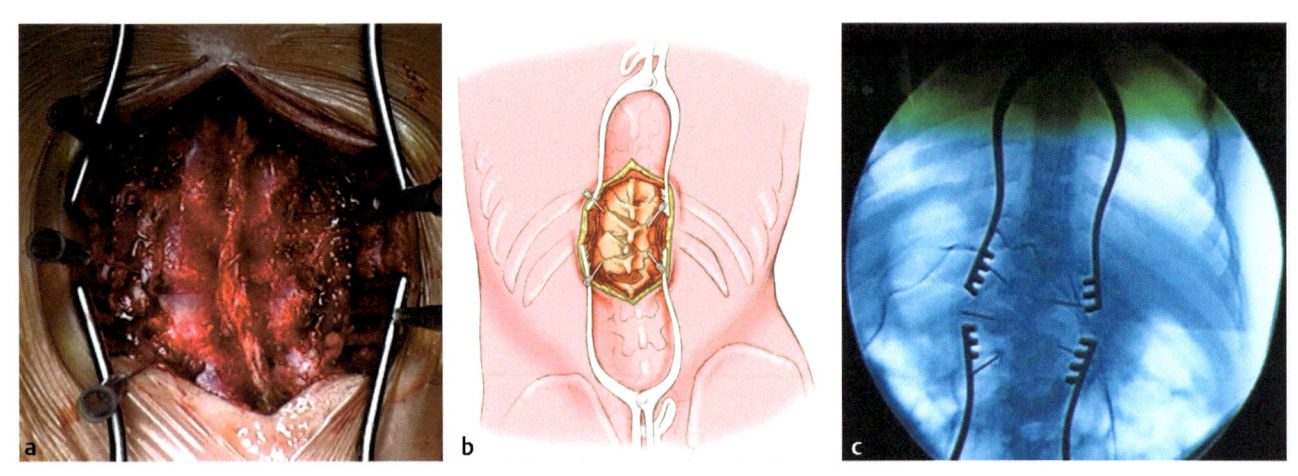

Fig. 6.32 Exposing the hemivertebra and adjacent vertebrae (a) and identifying the pedicles (b,c).

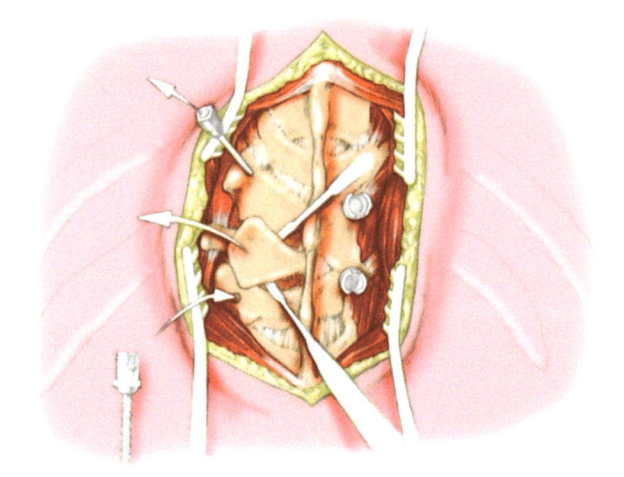

Fig. 6.33 Insertion of screws and removal of posterior elements.

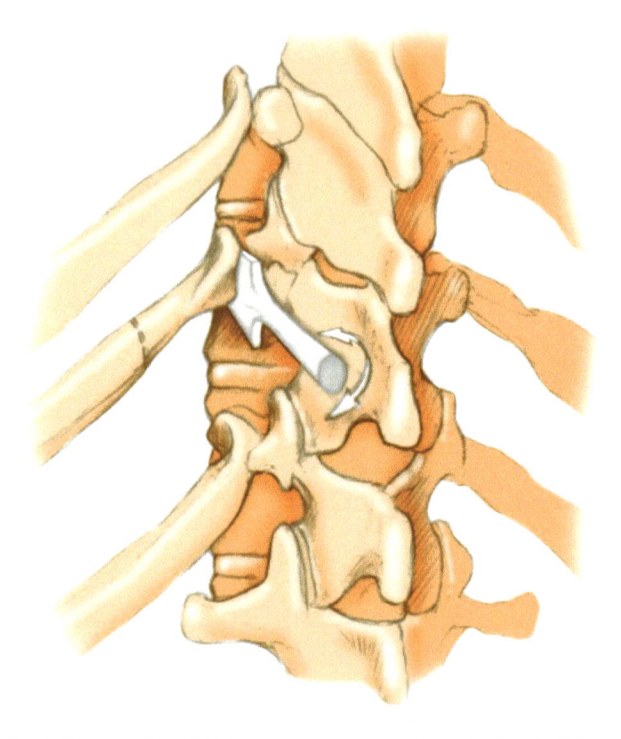

Fig. 6.34 Resection of rib heads gives access to the lateral wall of the hemivertebra.

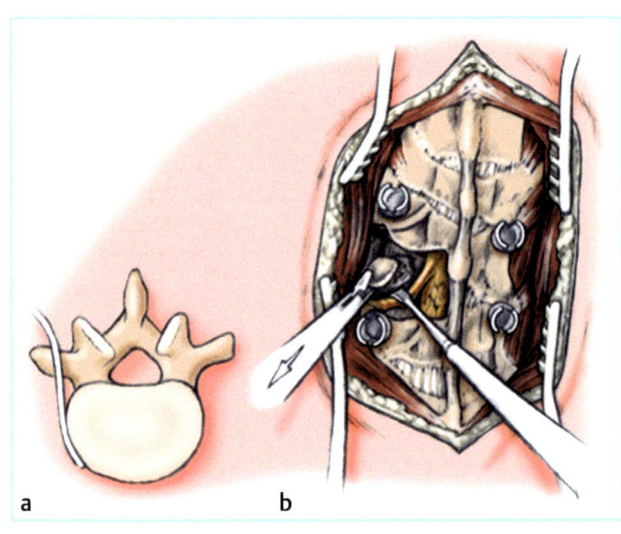

Fig. 6.35 Resection of pedicles (a) and placement of spatula (b).

of the pedicle and vertebral body of the hemivertebra are removed using the microscope (▶ Fig. 6.35, ▶ Fig. 6.36, and ▶ Fig. 6.37). The disks adjacent to the hemivertebra are removed and the end plates are cleared of any soft or cartilaginous tissue down to bleeding bone (▶ Fig. 6.38). It is important that disk removal goes right across to the contralateral side. If there is a concave bar it should now be divided (▶ Fig. 6.39).

The instrumentation is then completed and compression is applied on the convex side until the gap left after the resection closes completely under direct vision (▶ Fig. 6.40 and ▶ Fig. 6.41). If there is a small gap remaining, then cancellous bone is used to fill this. If there is real kyphosis present, that is, more of a dorsal hemivertebra than a lateral one, it may be necessary to add a titanium mesh cage anteriorly as a fulcrum to

Congenital Deformities

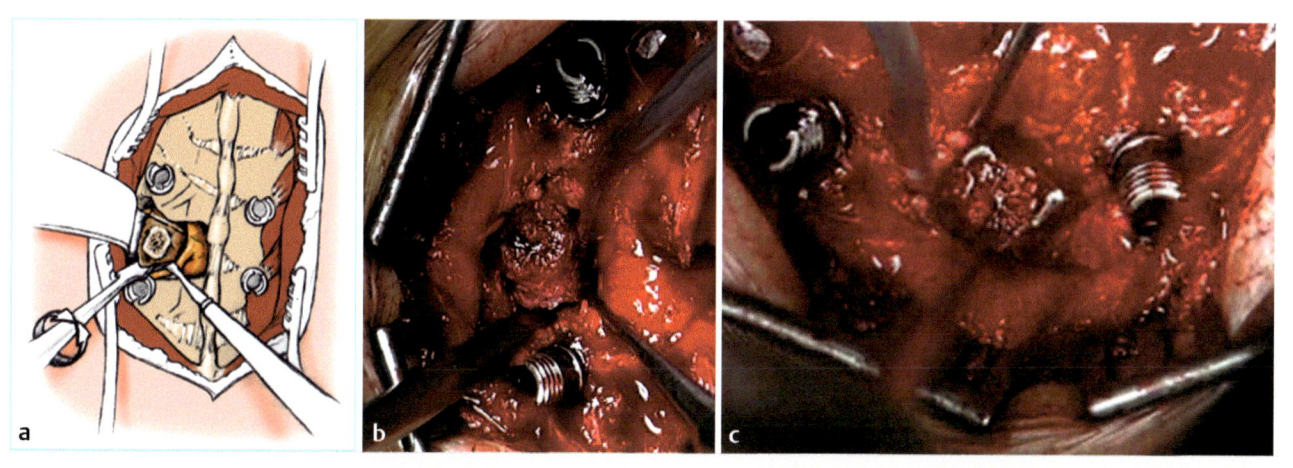

Fig. 6.36 Resection of body of hemivertebra.

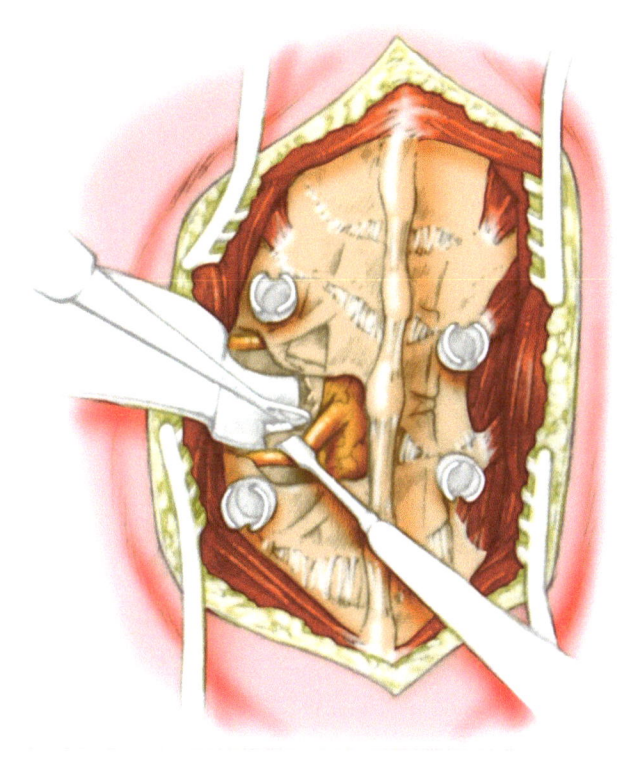

Fig. 6.37 Removal of the anterior part of the hemivertebra.

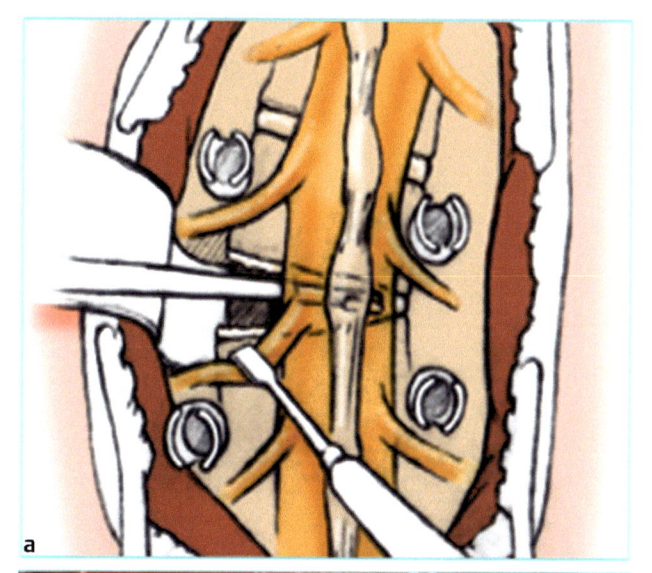

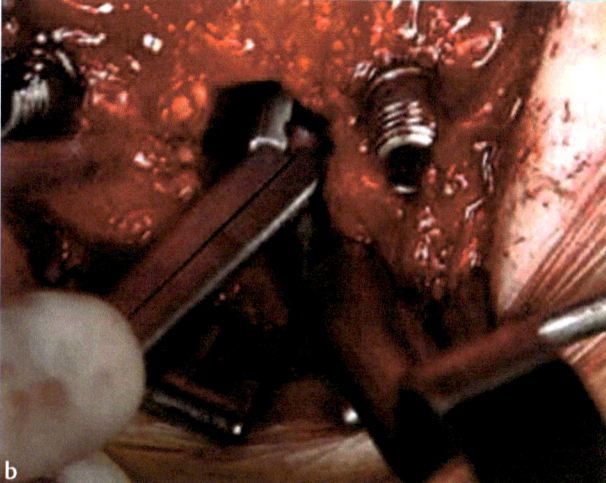

Fig. 6.38 Removal of the adjacent disks.

achieve lordosis (▶ Fig. 6.42). In cases of single hemivertebrae nothing further is required.

High compressive forces should not really be necessary but if so, especially in cases with pronounced kyphosis, then one or two additional segments can be temporarily included into the instrumentation to avoid pedicular overload and subsequent fracture. If absolutely necessary, the additional metalwork can be left in permanently. However, 3 months after the primary surgery, the instrumentation can be shortened down to the single level so as to release joints to regain movement.

All this is performed under careful electrophysiological spinal cord monitoring.

Congenital Deformities

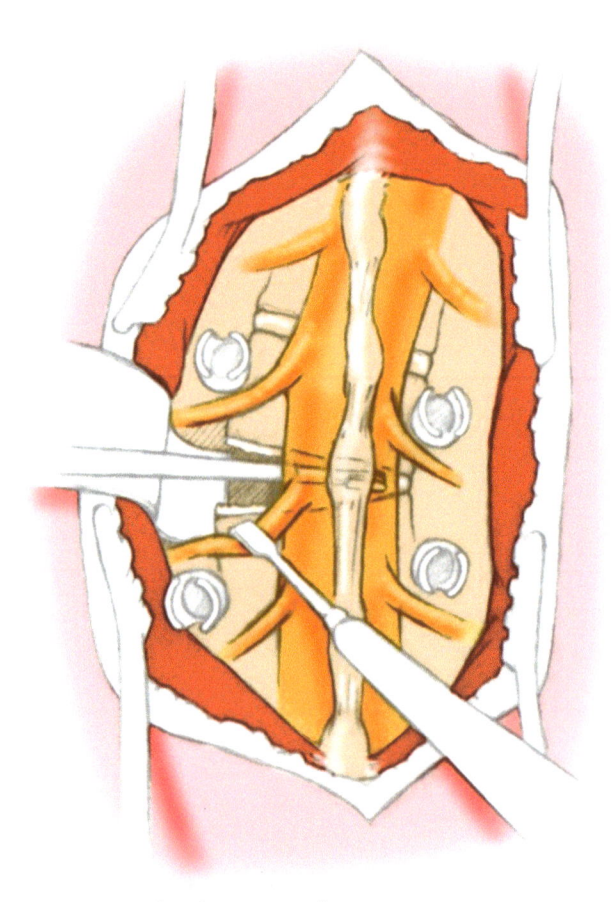

Fig. 6.39 Dividing the concave side.

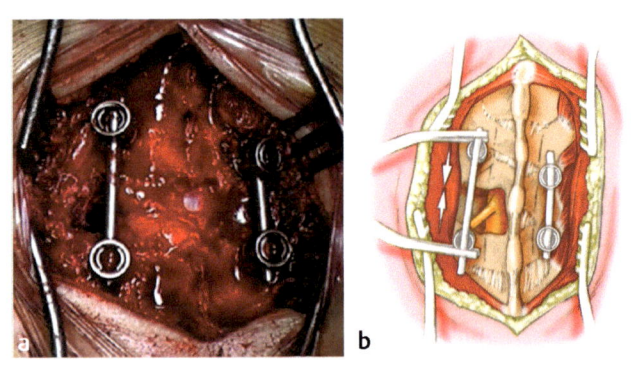

Fig. 6.40 Application of the rods into the screw heads.

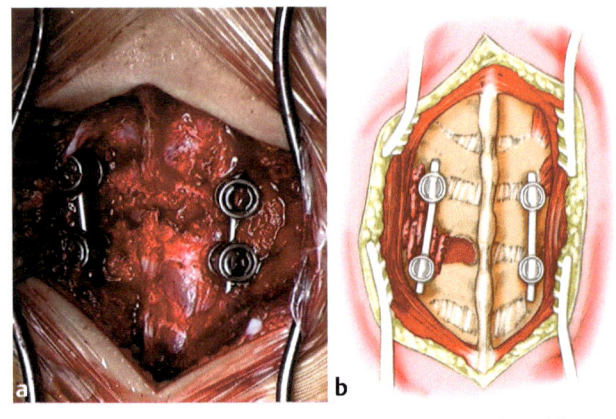

Fig. 6.41 Application of compression forces plus posterolateral fusion.

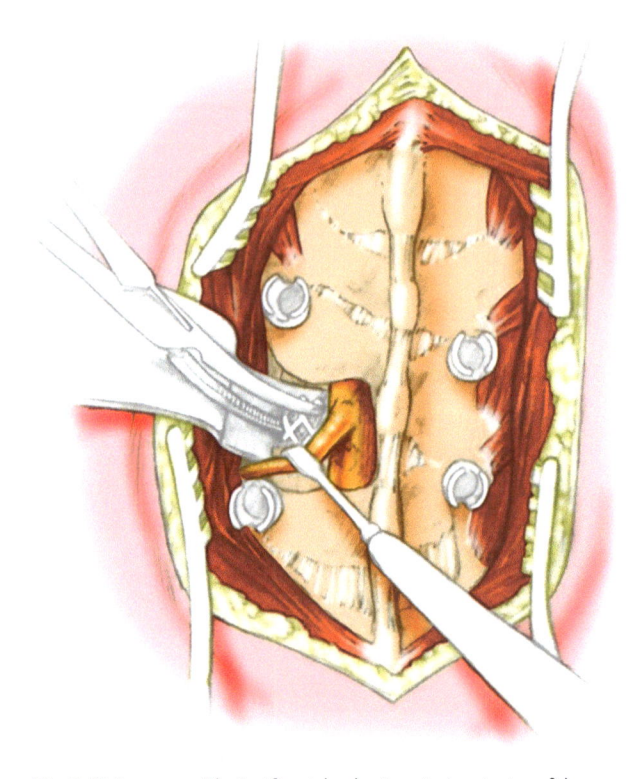

Fig. 6.42 In cases with significant kyphosis anterior strut graft/cage may be necessary.

6.5 Congenital Kyphosis

Congenital kyphoses, and of course any other kyphoses, are rotationally stable because of the anteriorly situated axis of spinal rotation (▶ Fig. 3.4); therefore, progressive rotational scoliosis does not occur in association with these kyphoses. If the kyphotic process is asymmetric, affecting more the right or left of the involved vertebra or vertebrae, then a minor scoliosis may be seen on the PA radiograph but with the spinous processes either central (not rotated) or directed to the curve convexity, as occurs in Scheuermann's disease (see Chapter 5). The problem of congenital kyphoses is therefore not so much one of deformity, although kyphoses of any origin can be ugly if severe enough, but of the danger of paralysis.[83-91] This pertains to kyphoses due to failures of formation (▶ Fig. 6.43) and does not occur if the deformity is due solely to a failure of segmentation (▶ Fig. 6.44); the latter is often associated with lumbar pain, possibly due to the compensatory lumbar hyperlordosis. This is because the deformity due to a segmentation failure is less angular but the most important factor with dorsal hemivertebrae appears to be the potential for local spinal instability. Because kyphoses due to dorsal hemivertebrae only progress at a rate of about 7 degrees per year,[87] the pressure backward onto the front of the spinal cord is relatively gradual and the cord is able to adapt and maintain normal function for a surprisingly

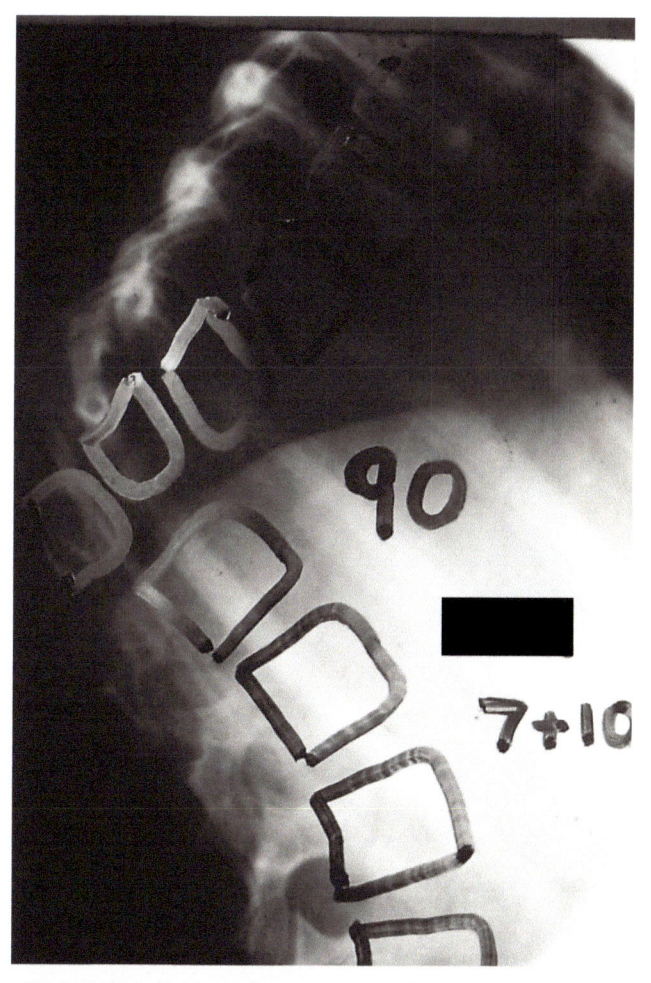

Fig. 6.43 Dorsal hemivertebra.

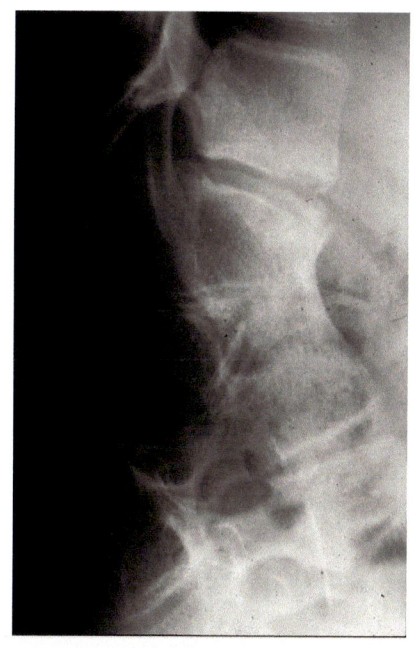

Fig. 6.44 Anterior bar with hemivertebra behind.

long time. Therefore, temporal considerations are of the utmost importance. Indeed, when anterior decompression is required for significant kyphosis it is always quite remarkable how the cord can still be functioning in an area of the spine with so little space available—when it can resemble a very thin ribbon of tissue or cannot in fact be clearly visualized at all until during/after decompression. Therefore, repeated neurological observations are crucial in such patients and even subtle changes take on great import.

Twenty percent of patients seen with dorsal hemivertebrae develop signs of impending paraplegia,[87,88] usually during the adolescent growth spurt. Those with dorsal hemivertebrae in the upper thoracic or thoracolumbar regions are most liable. Particular attention should be paid to local spinal stability and while the anterior failure of segmentation (▶ Fig. 6.44) can produce a progressive kyphosis the front of the spine is effectively strutted, and this may be why paralysis does not occur in such cases.[90] In contradistinction, failures of formation do not have such a mechanical benefit and often display subluxation (▶ Fig. 6.43) or even spondylolisthesis locally.[90–92] Although the most severe examples are uncommon and are so significant in their neurological effect as to present at birth,[92–94] the importance of spinal stability should not be underestimated and must be an important factor in tilting the dorsal hemivertebra patient over the neurological brink.

6.5.1 Natural History

Although von Rokitansky was thought to have first described congenital kyphosis back in the middle of the 19th century,[95] and although there were others in various European languages describing case reports, the main issue at that time was whether these kyphoses were tuberculous rather than congenital. However, in the Edinburgh medical journal almost 100 years ago, Grieg described a congenital failure of formation of the first thoracic vertebra.[84] The importance of the difference between those due to failure of formation and those due to failure of segmentation was described by Von Schrick.[96] Then James in Edinburgh in 1955 described 21 patients with congenital kyphoses most of which were at the thoracolumbar junction, the rest being in the upper thoracic spine.[85] There were five paraplegics and early posterior fusion was recommended.

However, once again, it was the major scoliosis centers in Minneapolis[87] and in Edinburgh[97] that described congenital kyphoses in sufficient numbers to be of meaningful value. In 1973[87] Winter described 130 patients with congenital bony kyphoses, making a point of excluding those with rib hump deformities and those with more scoliosis than kyphosis, leaving him with 68 pure kyphoses and 62 kyphoscolioses. As with other congenital spinal anomalies there were almost twice as many females as males and other important congenital anomalies were also present (see later). It was pointed out embryopathologically that it was failure of the cartilage model to form, rather than ossification thereof, and the more body or bodies to form dysplastically the more severe the kyphosis. Failure of formation was the most common cause and occurred in 86 patients. Those that had an associated scoliosis tended to be due to failure of vertebral body formation whereas failures of segmentation were more symmetric. As with congenital scolioses some cases could not be precisely categorized. Winter recommended that congenital kyphoses should be classified

Congenital Deformities

according to Von Schrick[96] into three types: type I, congenital failure of vertebral body formation; type II, congenital failure of vertebral body segmentation; and type III, mixed. There were 86 type 1 deformities, more than half of which occurred at the thoracolumbar level and most of the rest above. There were 19 type II kyphoses with again the majority at the thoracolumbar level. Winter made three generalizations: significant progression was usual, severe deformity was frequent, and even qualified orthopaedic surgeons were unaware of the importance of the condition. Type I lesions were angular, more severe, and progressed most rapidly and, not surprisingly, paraplegia only occurred in type I lesions. Paraplegia, if it did occur, tended to do so in the pre-adolescent growth period. In 1999 McMaster reported on 112 patients attending Edinburgh with congenital kyphosis or kypho-scoliosis.[97] They used the same Von Schrick classification. In two-thirds of their cases the kyphosis was thoracolumbar while maximum progression again occurred during the preadolescent growth spurt.

McMaster's classification and accompanying diagrams are extremely helpful in appreciating the geometry of the different basic anomalies (▶ Fig. 6.45). Of the 68 anterior failures of vertebral body formation half were posterolateral quadrant single hemivertebrae, four were single posterior hemivertebrae, and 15 were butterfly or sagittal cleft vertebrae. Of the 24 failures of segmentation, 15 were anterior unsegmented bars and 9 anterolateral unsegmented bars.

The posterolateral quadrant hemivertebrae were due to a failure of formation of the anterior and unilateral portion of the vertebral body leaving the posterolateral fragment of bone attached to the pedicle and neural arch behind and this posterolateral fragment of bone could range in size from complete absence of the body to a tapering of the vertebral body toward the anterior longitudinal ligament. Progression before the age of 10 was 2.5 degrees a year and twice that after the age of 10. It would appear that one patient developed paraparesis and five paraplegia, with only one not responding to surgical treatment. Clearly the spinal cord must be decompressed at the earliest opportunity.

Of the eight patients with a posterior hemivertebra, one had a 40-degree kyphosis with forward subluxation of the eleventh thoracic vertebra on the twelfth producing a bayonet type of deformity. This was described as congenital vertebral displacement. One of the four patients with two adjacent hemivertebrae became paraplegic but again responded to treatment.

There were 15 patients with single butterfly vertebrae (▶ Fig. 6.8)—that is, partial or complete failure of formation of the anterior and central portions of the vertebral body leaving two posterolateral fragments of bone attached to the neural arch, wedged anteriorly and medially, and separated by a sagittal cleft. All these anomalies occurred at the thoracolumbar junction. In 10 patients a pure kyphosis was produced progressing before the age of 10 years at 1.5 degrees per year.

The 24 patients with type II segmentation anomalies produced a kyphosis or kyphoscoliosis according to the degree of asymmetry. The extent of the bar was 3.5 vertebrae on average.

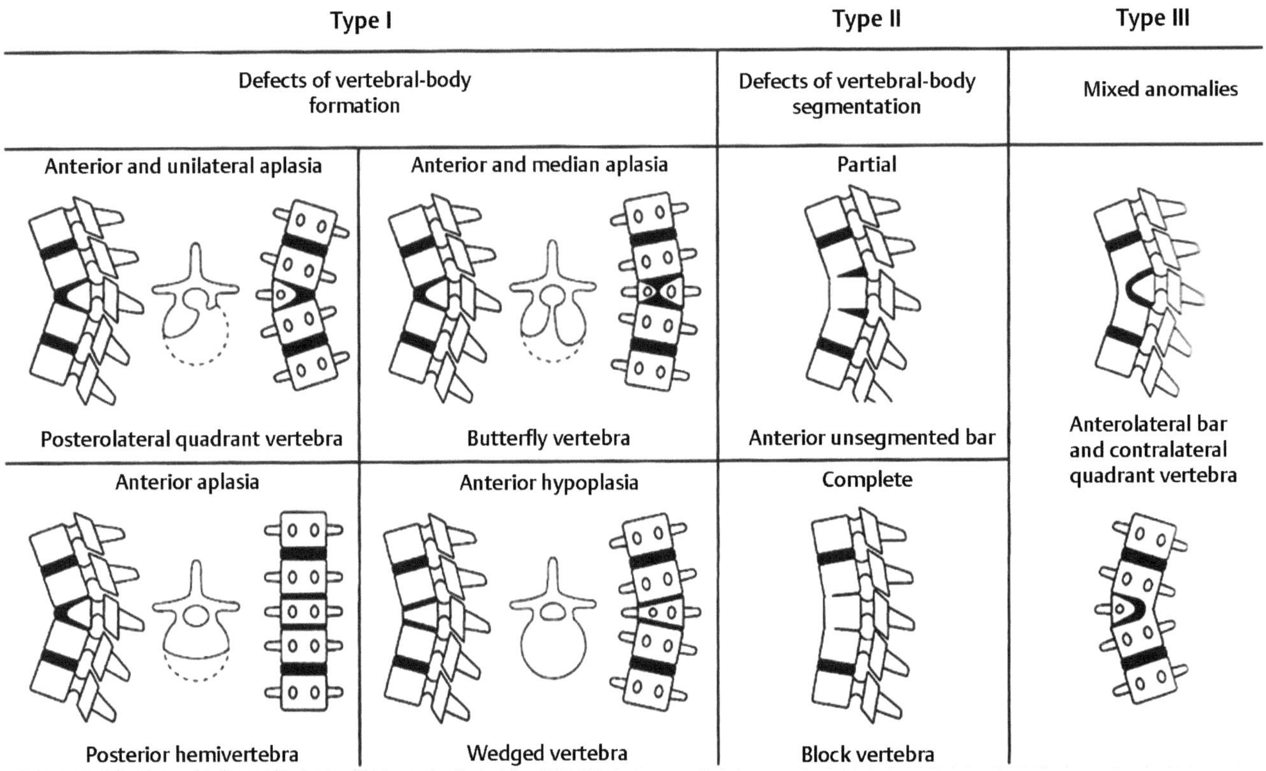

Type I		Type II	Type III
Defects of vertebral-body formation		Defects of vertebral-body segmentation	Mixed anomalies
Anterior and unilateral aplasia	Anterior and median aplasia	Partial	
Posterolateral quadrant vertebra	Butterfly vertebra	Anterior unsegmented bar	Anterolateral bar and contralateral quadrant vertebra
Anterior aplasia	Anterior hypoplasia	Complete	
Posterior hemivertebra	Wedged vertebra	Block vertebra	

Fig. 6.45 Congenital kyphosis type 1 results from defects in vertebral body formation, Type II from defects in segmentation and congenital kyphosis type III results from mixed anomalies. (Reproduced with permission from The Spine, Eds Herkowitz HN, Garfin SR, Baldeston RA, Elsmont FJ, Bell GR, Rothman Simeone, 6th edition, Elsevier 2011, Chapter: The Child's Spine, p. 460.)

Congenital Deformities

Progressive paraparesis of the lower limbs occurred in 11 of the 112 patients, seven with a posterolateral hemivertebra, two adjacent posterolateral quadrant hemivertebrae, one with two adjacent posterior hemivertebrae, and four that were unclassifiable.[97] Neurological deterioration occurred between the ages of 8 and 11 years. Removal of these dangerous hemivertebrae should be carried out as soon as diagnosed (▶ Fig. 6.46).

The importance of instability in association with a posterior hemivertebra, which had been raised by Winter,[87] was then shown by Weinstein in 1998[98] when he described two cases of an atypical congenital kyphosis in which a hypoplastic lumbar vertebral body lay in the spinal canal because of short pedicles with no posterior element defects. The first was an 18-day-old boy with a congenital cardiac anomaly at birth and a palpable bony prominence in the thoracolumbar region. At 15 months of age the spinal canal was shown to be narrow due to short L2 pedicles and an operation was advised. Combined differential anterior and posterior fusion (short anterior and longer posterior) was shortly thereafter carried out. At the age of 5.5 years, the kyphotic deformity had reduced from 25 to 15 degrees and the spine was solid with an excellent cosmetic result and no neurological deficit. The second case was much the same except it involved the first lumbar vertebra and again did very well following similar anterior and posterior differential surgery.

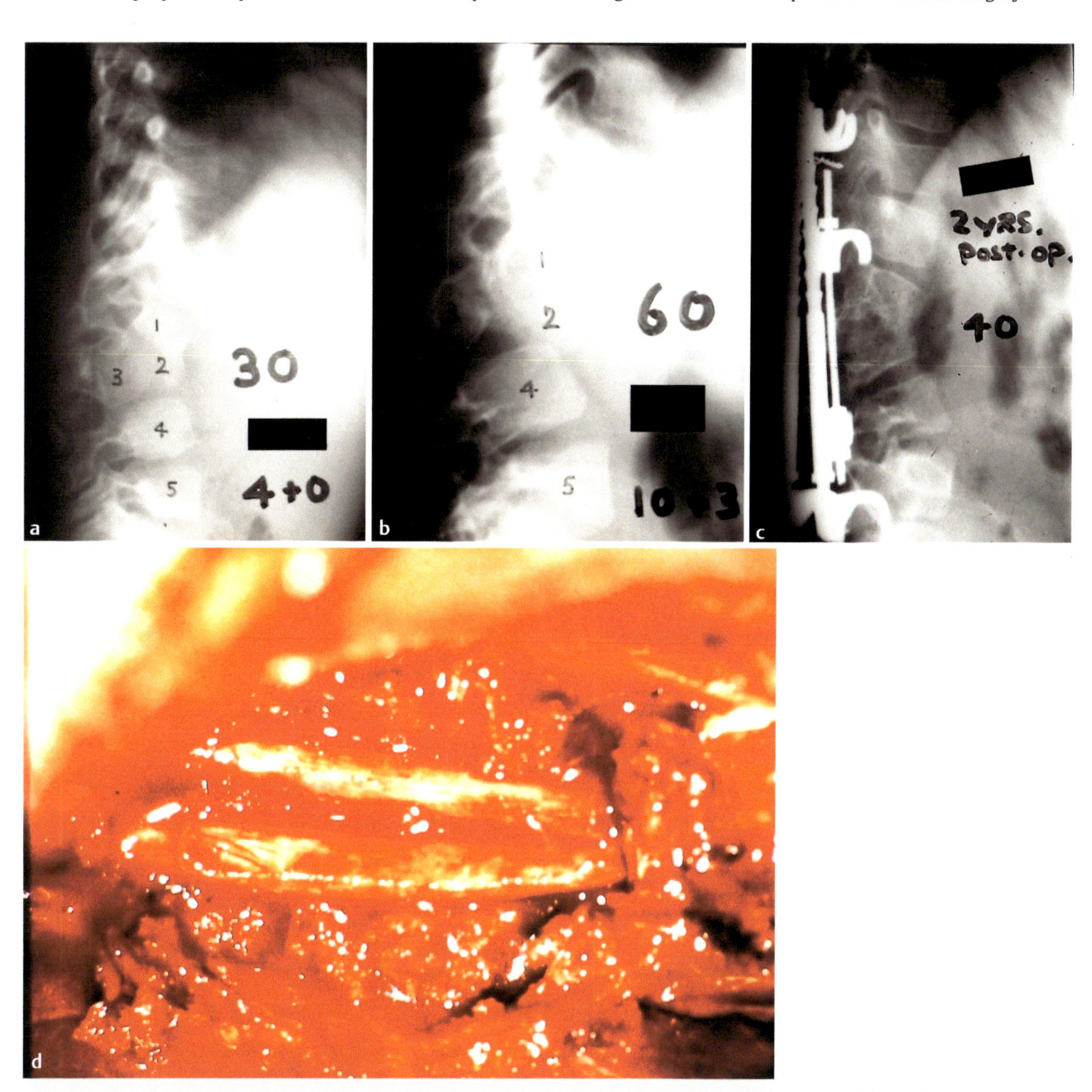

Fig. 6.46 (a) Lateral radiograph of the lumbar spine showing a dorsal hemivertebra at L3 with 30 degrees of kyphosis at the age of 4. (b) By the age of 10 kyphosis measured 60 degrees and there were upper motor neurone symptoms developing. (c) lateral radiograph after removal of the hemivertebra with anterior strut grafting and posterior metalwork. (d) Shows what a strut graft should look like. Of course only one strut is load-bearing but the other incorporates with the help of surrounding iliac bone.

Congenital Deformities

Then McMaster from Edinburgh reported five children with segmental subluxation of the spine in association with a developmental thoracolumbar kyphosis presenting at a mean age of 1.5 years.[99] He thought the spinal deformity seemed to be more developmental than congenital with the anterior vertebral wedging secondary to localized instability. He suggested the term "infantile developmental thoracolumbar kyphosis with segmental subluxation of the spine" to differentiate this type of deformity from congenital displacement of the spine in which the congenital vertebral anomaly does not resolve. This type of developmental kyphosis may carry the risk of neurological compromise. Dubousset[100] divided anterior vertebral body formation defects into types I or II, the latter being where there was a dislocated canal and a step off deformity giving rise to a bayonet type appearance in the frontal plane, rather like Weinstein's. However, with McMaster's cases unlike Weinstein's, there was no segmental narrowing due to short pedicles. Only posterior arthrodesis was required to correct the deformity. Then Weinstein reported seven cases of thoracolumbar kyphosis due to lumbar hypoplasia that spontaneously resolved.[101]

Although we have successfully treated such a case by differential growth arrest we would prefer to be more certain about the outcome by removing the offending hemivertebra and thus thoroughly decompressing the spinal cord followed by short segment fusion to deal with the instability.

Unfortunately, patients sometimes do not present with simple single dorsal hemivertebrae early in their natural history and can present much later with more complex congenital kyphoses involving more than one hemivertebra, particularly in awkward situations like the cervicothoracic junction or upper thoracic spine. They still require anterior cord decompression by removal of the hemivertebra and insertion of an anterior strut (cage or bone) synchronous combined with posterior instrumentation (▶ Fig. 6.47). For solitary hemivertebrae without too much kyphosis then, like anywhere else in the spine, a straightforward anterior approach is appropriate. However, when there is more than one hemivertebra the degree of

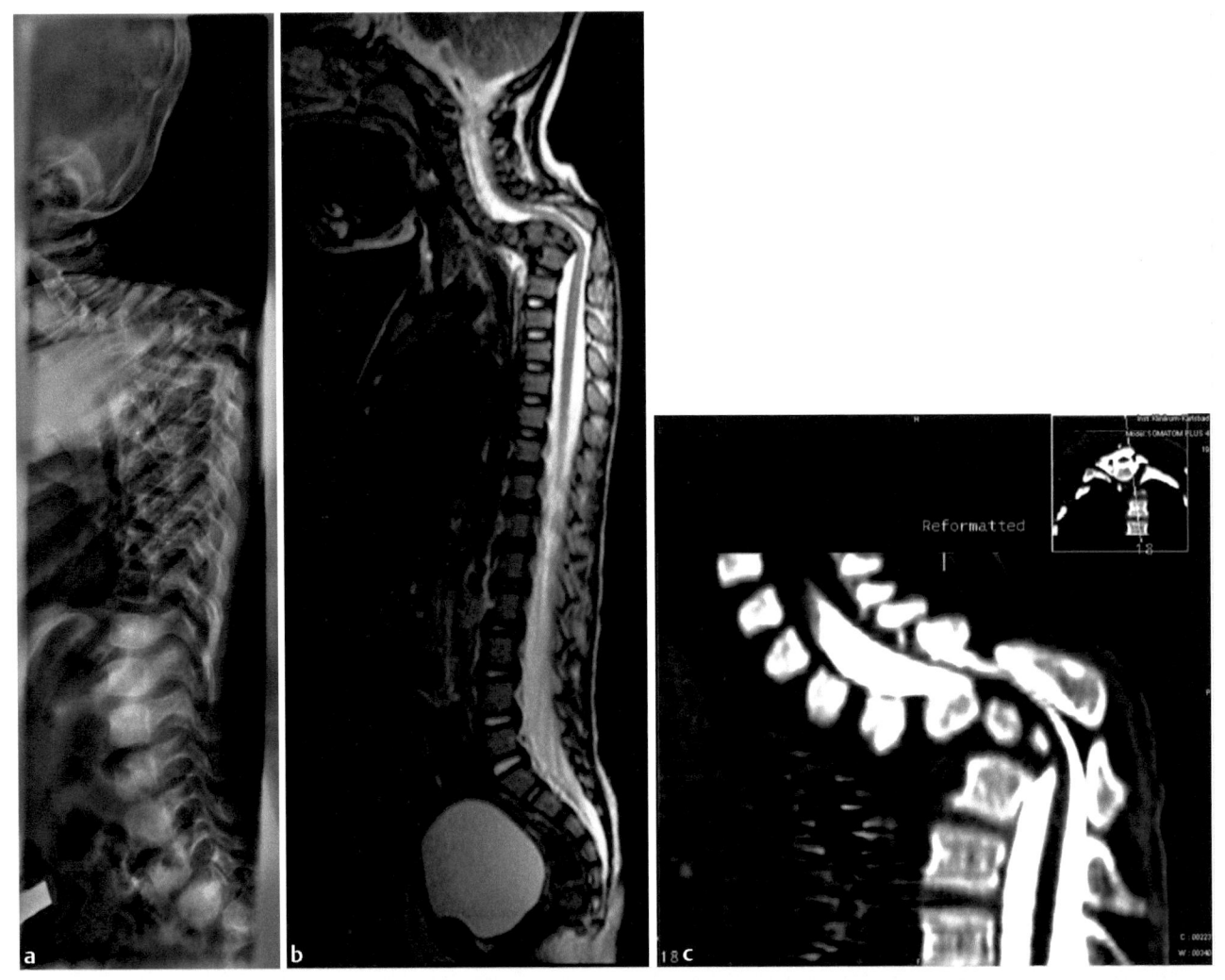

Fig. 6.47 (a) Lateral radiograph showing a severe upper thoracic kyphosis, the nature of which is not accurately delineated on plain films. (b) A sagittal T2 MRI beginning to show the nature of the bony deformity with more than one hemivertebra effacing the spinal cord. (c) Reformatted scan showing that there are two hemivertebrae at the apex of the kyphosis.

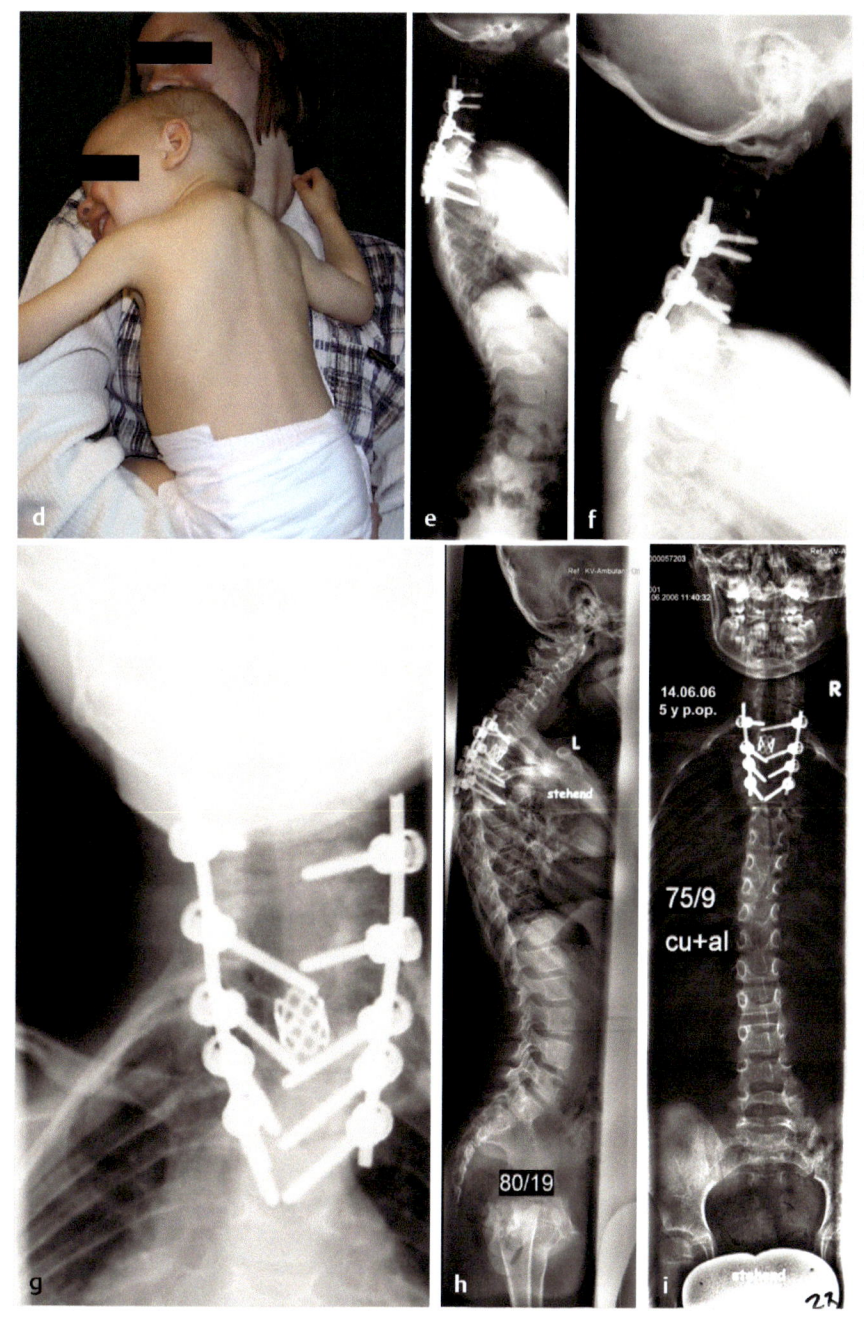

Fig. 6.47 (continued) **(d)** Clinical photograph of this infant; the severe kyphosis is clearly visible. **(e)** A full length lateral radiograph showing the length of the construct and the anterior cage replacing the hemi-vertebrae at the apex which had been resected. **(f)** Lateral and **(g)** AP close up views. **(h,i)** Lateral and PA views 5 years postoperatively with maintenance of an excellent correction. Now after fusion the prominent upper two screws have been removed.

kyphosis is so severe that there is no obvious direct anterior approach but the cord can still be decompressed by doing a high thoracic costotransversectomy, removing first, second, and third ribs. This gets you first to the side of the spine and then you can go round the front to make sure important vessels are clear of bone excision. The fact they usually fall away into the concavity helps. ▶ Fig. 6.47 is a good example of such a case with the cord being significantly compressed behind the hemivertebrae. It is important first of all to get good pedicular screws into the back. Then the costotransversectomy carried out over how many ribs that are required to be removed is followed by removal of the hemivertebrae and therefore direct anterior decompression of the spinal cord. Then in a simultaneous anterior and posterior maneuver the kyphosis is corrected and the anterior deficit replaced by a cage of appropriate length.

6.5.2 Congenital Cord Deformities

This refers to spina bifida and there are four basic embryopathological types: (1) spina bifida occulta, (2) meningocele, (3) myelomeningocele, and (4) myelocele (▶ Fig. 6.48).

Treatment of the myelodysplastic spine presents one of the greatest therapeutic challenges in the entire field of spinal surgery. However, this does not imply that the challenge should necessarily be accepted. The results are all too frequently disappointing and the rate of significant complications is higher than with any other type of spinal deformity except possibly cerebral

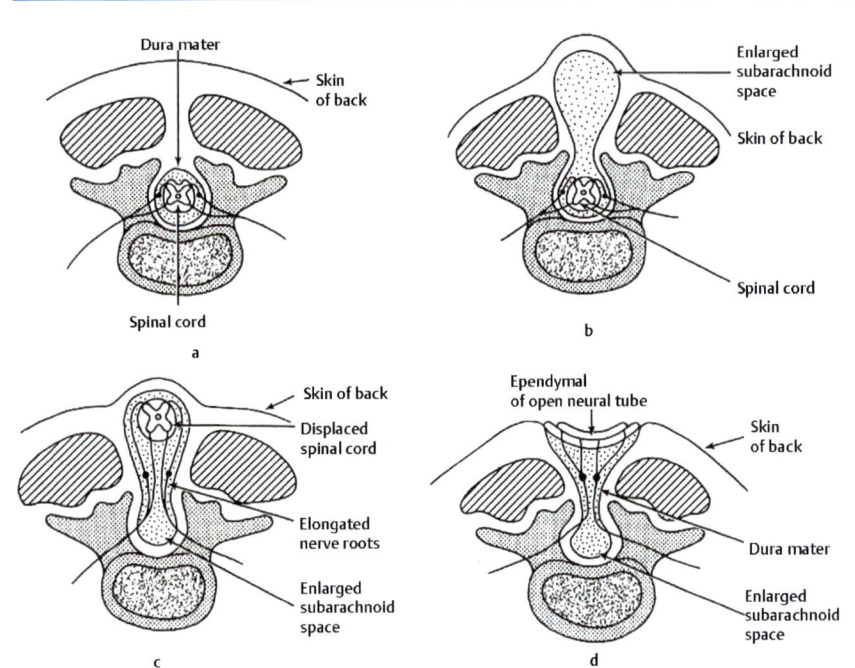

Fig. 6.48 The four categories of severity of spina bifida: **(a)** spina bifida occulta, **(b)** meningocele, **(c)** myelomeningocele, and **(d)** myelocele.

palsy. Nonetheless, a philosophy of management has developed over recent years with the appropriate indications becoming clearer. With so many life-threatening issues at stake in areas outside the musculoskeletal system, treatment of the deformed spine must be placed in its proper setting so that the very concerned parents will not be under the misapprehension that a straighter spine will be a universal panacea for the other problems. Therefore, only with great responsibility, understanding, and experience can the deformity of the spine within the context of the entire spina bifida patient be tackled effectively (much like the cerebral palsy child).

Scoliosis

It is important to appreciate that the spina bifida syndrome represents a spectrum of handicap extending from the virtually normal individual, with perhaps minor weakness of a muscle group in one lower extremity, to the most severely disabled who are incontinent nonwalkers with a high neurological lesion, often accompanied by significant cerebral impairment because of the associated hydrocephalus. The therapeutic approach must therefore be very flexible, and at the mild end of the spectrum would be the lower level spinal lesion with preservation of walking ability and that can be threatened by a severe scoliosis. It is important to recognize those whose scoliosis is attributable to a severe congenital bony anomaly[102–105] (▶ Fig. 6.20) and then to differentiate those whose deformity comes down to a level square pelvis but is threatening walking potential (▶ Fig. 6.49) from those more severely paralytic with the more typical C-shaped lordoscoliosis with pelvic obliquity (▶ Fig. 6.50 and ▶ Fig. 6.51).

It is important to appreciate the crucial role that pelvic obliquity plays in all this. In an effort to rationalize the deforming forces responsible for the production of a scoliosis, Raycroft and Curtis considered suprapelvic, transpelvic, and infrapelvic factors[102] (▶ Table 6.1). This needs to be appreciated by both scoliosis surgeons and pediatric orthopaedic surgeons.[104] They noted that the neurological deficit was seldom symmetrical as far as the spinal muscles were concerned and, together with frequent episodes of meningitis and soft tissue contractures, referred to these as *suprapelvic* factors. There is only one possible cause of *transpelvic* pelvic obliquity and that is the asymmetric action of the iliopsoas, the only muscle to cross the pelvis from spine to lower extremity. Asymmetric muscle action around the hip joint, typified by the wind-blown appearance of the lower extremities with one abducted and one adducted, is the *infrapelvic* mechanism (▶ Fig. 7.1).

Far too much therapeutic attention has been directed toward transpelvic and infrapelvic factors, when the chief factor responsible for the pelvic obliquity lies above the pelvis in the form of the scoliosis itself: suprapelvic pelvic obliquity. Therefore, operations designed to correct suprapelvic pelvic obliquity by rerouting musculature about the hip are destined to failure. Only by attention to the scoliosis itself is the pelvic obliquity properly corrected and stabilized.

Functional considerations are the only relevant matters in these children and for those with walking ability their gait pattern should be analyzed carefully as some children require very considerable lumbopelvic movement to preserve their ambulatory ability. Therefore, a fused spine, even though it is straight or straighter, can do them a disservice. This can be quite a difficult decision but more often than not it is the spinal deformity that is causing the walking difficulties and therefore such patients do merit surgical consideration. For the child who only has sitting function then maintenance of sitting stability is crucial. As suprapelvic pelvic obliquity due a long C-shaped thoracolumbar paralytic curve increases so the child has to use their upper extremities to maintain their sitting position which in turn denies them the upper extremities' prehensile function. Therefore, correcting pelvic obliquity and allowing them to continue using their arms and hands is the prime indication for

Congenital Deformities

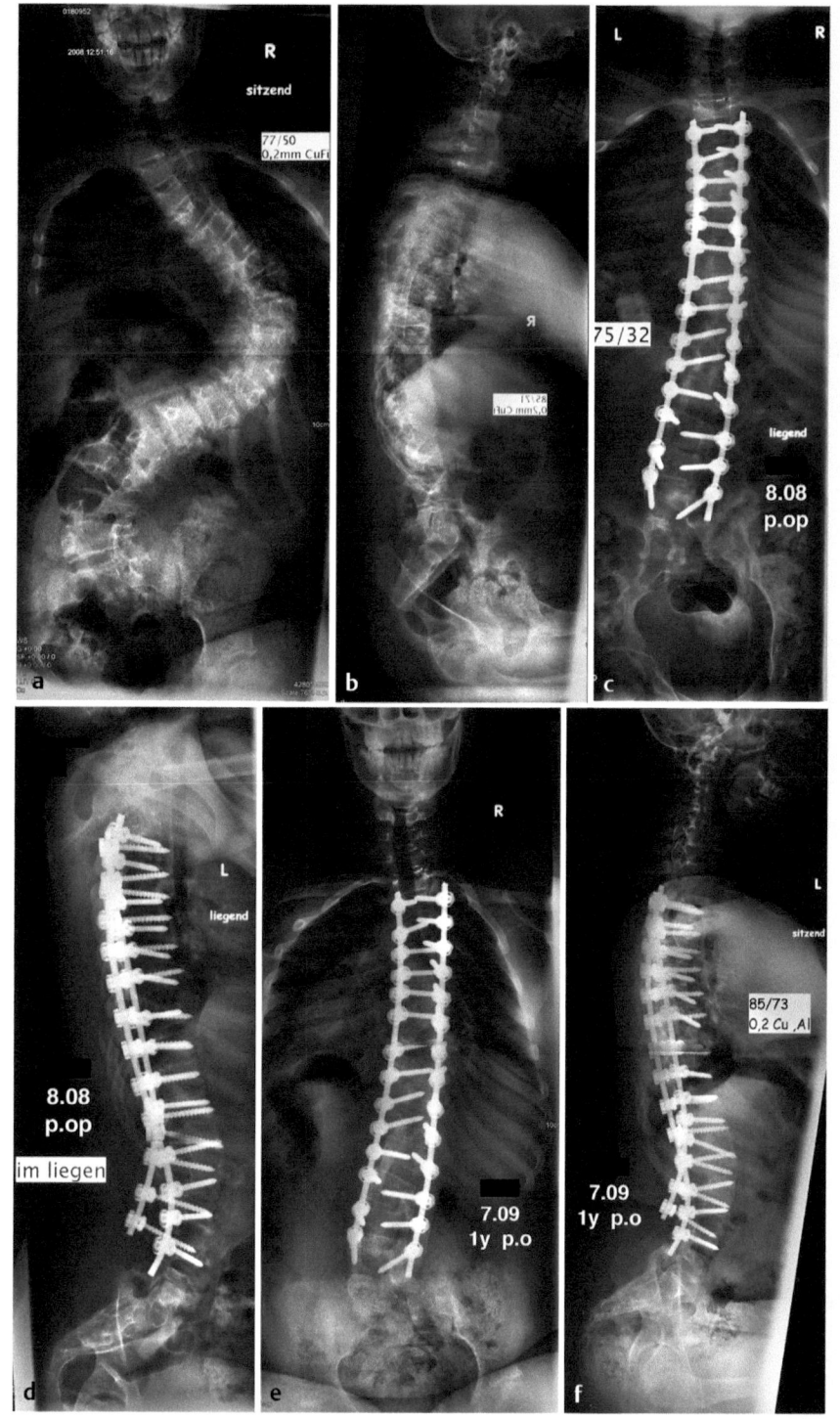

Fig. 6.49 (a) PA radiograph of this 12-year-old ambulatory spina bifida patient with principally a severe right lower thoracic lordoscoliosis above a fixed compensatory curve down to the sacrum with the absence of posterior elements. (b) Lateral radiograph showing the flat spinal appearance of a lordoscoliosis. (c) The curve was not thought flexible enough to respond to instrumentation alone and so the apical vertebral bodies (T7 and T8) were resected and the deformity corrected with transpedicular metalwork. (d) Lateral radiograph showing maintenance of a good lateral profile. (e,f) AP and lateral views a year after surgery. There was well preserved walking ability and excellent correction and fusion down to a solid L5 base without instrumentation into the pelvis.

surgical stabilization in these severely affected individuals (▶ Fig. 6.50g). It is important to treat the scoliosis early because it would appear that the scoliosis can threaten walking or sitting if the curve reaches only 40 degrees and the pelvic obliquity 25 degrees.[105] If this is associated with a high level of neurological loss then functional deterioration is certain along with a reduction in quality of life and so treatment should most definitely be prescribed. For the walking patient their main curvature does not go down to the pelvis and so these spines can be dealt with by posterior transpedicular instrumentation down to the lowest end vertebra leaving the lower part of the lumbar spine (▶ Fig. 6.49) and the sacrum mobile so as not to impede walking potential. Don't go down to the pelvis if you don't need to. However, with the sitter significant weight gain with increasing age is the norm and the spine readily collapses into a significant deformity with associated pelvic obliquity. In the evolution of surgical treatment for such patients we learned that either posterior instrumentation or anterior instrumentation alone was insufficient and could not deal with the

Congenital Deformities

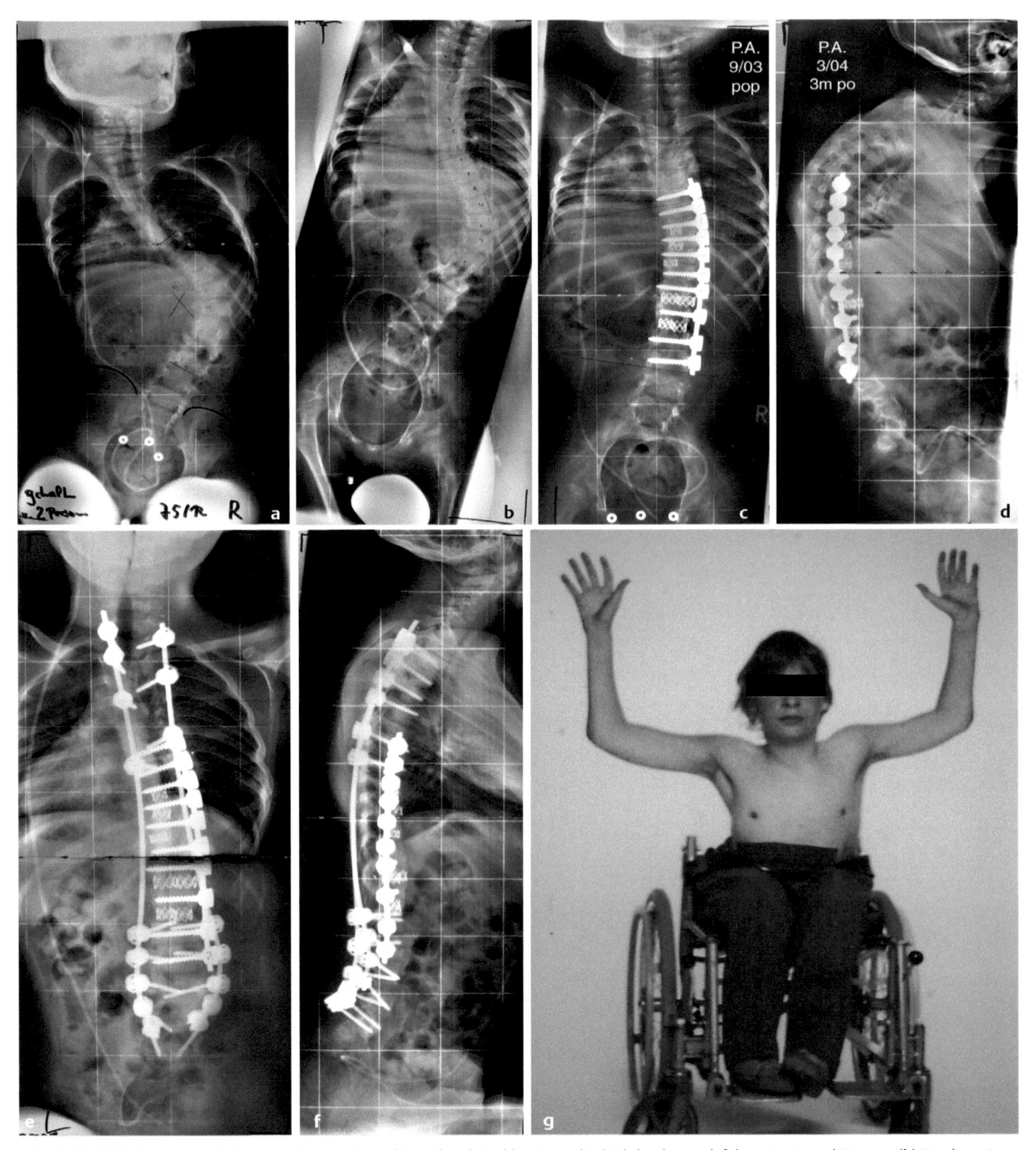

Fig. 6.50 (a) Collapsing paralytic curve down to the pelvis with pelvic obliquity in this high level spina bifida patient aged 9 years. (b) Bending view showed distinct curve rigidity and so an anterior approach was performed. (c) PA view after multiple discectomy and cage replacement with anterior instrumentation showing a good correction in the frontal plane. (d) Lateral view showing correction of the curve with maintenance of a good lateral profile but with a few segments of real kyphosis above. (e) After second stage posterior instrumentation up to T1 to maintain good frontal and (f) lateral profiles. (g) Hands up: this is the primary objective for scoliosis in sitting patients who have lost their sitting stability and require their arms to hold themselves up. After successful surgery the hands are liberated to carry out their intended prehensile function.

unfavorable biomechanical challenge and so it became established, rather like the severe cerebral palsy case, that such spines needed both anterior and posterior instrumentation for reliable results. As the sacrum is the lowest end vertebra in these long C-shaped collapsing curves, then fusion down to the pelvis is mandatory (▶ Fig. 6.50). Both fixation and fusion to the pelvis is not easy. The Galveston fixation technique is the best construct for this purpose. It was first introduced as an adjunct to Luque L rod instrumentation whereby fixation of the shorter limb of the L was

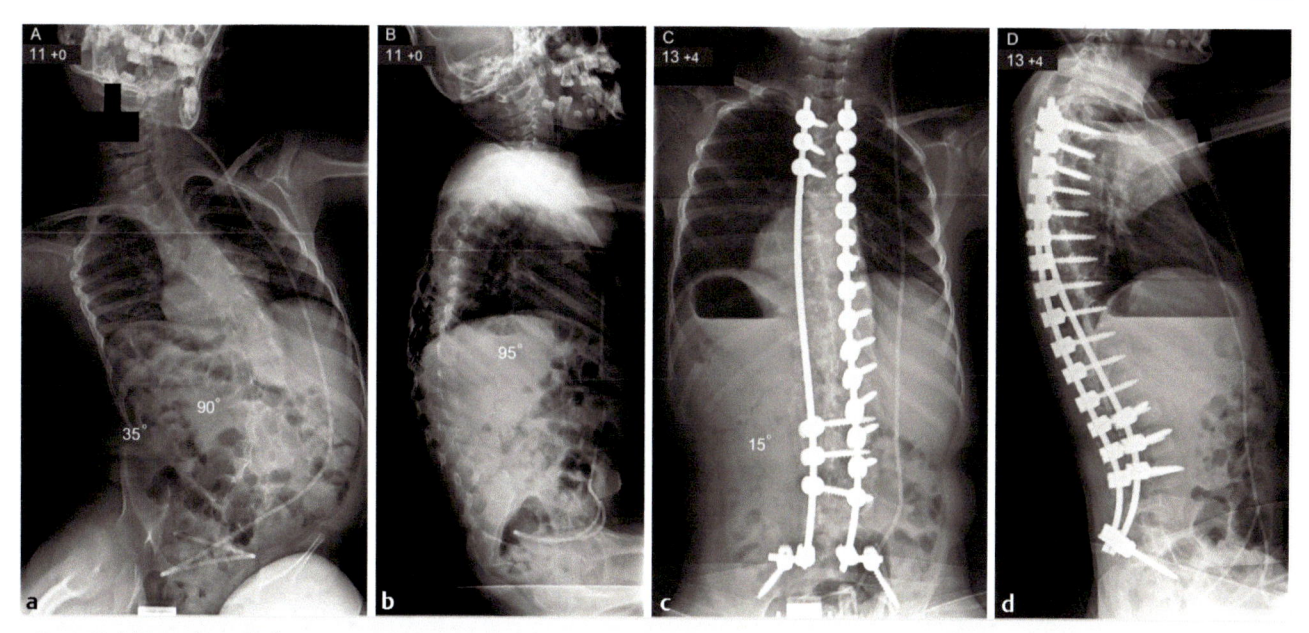

Fig. 6.51 (a) PA radiograph showing typical long C-shaped paralytic lordoscoliosis with pelvic obliquity in a high grade spina bifida patient. (b) A lateral radiograph showing the pseudokyphosis of a significantly rotated lordoscoliosis. (c) PA radiograph showing an excellent correction of both the scoliosis and pelvic obliquity. Note the Galveston pelvic construct. (d) Lateral radiograph postoperatively showing restoration of a natural sagittal profile. (Courtesy of and thanks to Professor Thanos Tsirikos, our colleague and friend who now runs the Edinburgh Scoliosis Clinic.)

Table 6.1 Causes of pelvic obliquity

Suprapelvic factors
Muscle imbalance—paralytic scoliosis
Asymmetrical involvement
Soft tissue contracture
Transpelvic factors
Psoas muscle—hip flexion contracture
Lordosis
Infrapelvic factors
Hip abduction/adduction
Wind blown
Dislocated hip—high side
Exaggerated spine deformity

made much stronger when passed intraosseously across the iliac wing.[106] Nowadays with modern pedicular instrumentation there are screw accessories for this purpose (▶ Fig. 6.51). It is important to realize that only 60% of spina bifida deformities are paralytic in nature while all of 40% are due to congenital bony deformities and require a quite different treatment strategy (▶ Fig. 6.20).

The Congenital Kyphosis of Myelomeningocele

All too frequently the mode of presentation to the scoliosis surgeon is such a severe deformity that the anterior thighs and anterior abdominal wall are closely approximated and so that for the head to be upright there has to be compensatory hyperextension in the thoracic and cervical spine often achieved by the patient leaning both upper extremities on the knees which of course denies the hands their important prehensile function (▶ Fig. 6.52). Of course getting the patient comfortable in a wheelchair is very difficult with the prominent kyphotic bend in the back but because the spinal cord is redundant from at least the waist down then the kyphosis can be resected (kyphectomy). All the structures in front of the vertebral bodies are contracted which includes anterior wedging of the apical vertebra/e, the annulus fibrosus of the disks, the anterior longitudinal ligament, the iliopsoas muscle, and sometimes even the anterior abdominal wall as Hoppenfield so beautifully demonstrated (▶ Fig. 6.53).[107] Once the gibbus has been excised then a lengthy posterior transpedicular construct down to the sacrum is necessary for a sustained correction (▶ Fig. 6.54). It is extraordinary how grateful patients are to be able to sit comfortably in their wheelchair. The bony kyphosis is also compounded by gravity. Posterior instrumentation initially was the Dwyer apparatus applied to the back of the spine[108] but nowadays it is possible to obtain an extremely good correction following kyphectomy using posterior pedicular instrumentation (▶ Fig. 6.54).

6.6 Congenital Lordosis

Congenital lordosis is rare because only if the lordosis is perfectly symmetrical can progressive rotation be avoided. These cases represent the end of a 90-degree spectrum. At one end is the coronal or transverse plane deformity which does not rotate because there is no median plane asymmetry, while at the other is the pure lordosis or pure median plane asymmetry which does not rotate because there is no coronal plane or transverse plane component to provide directional instability.

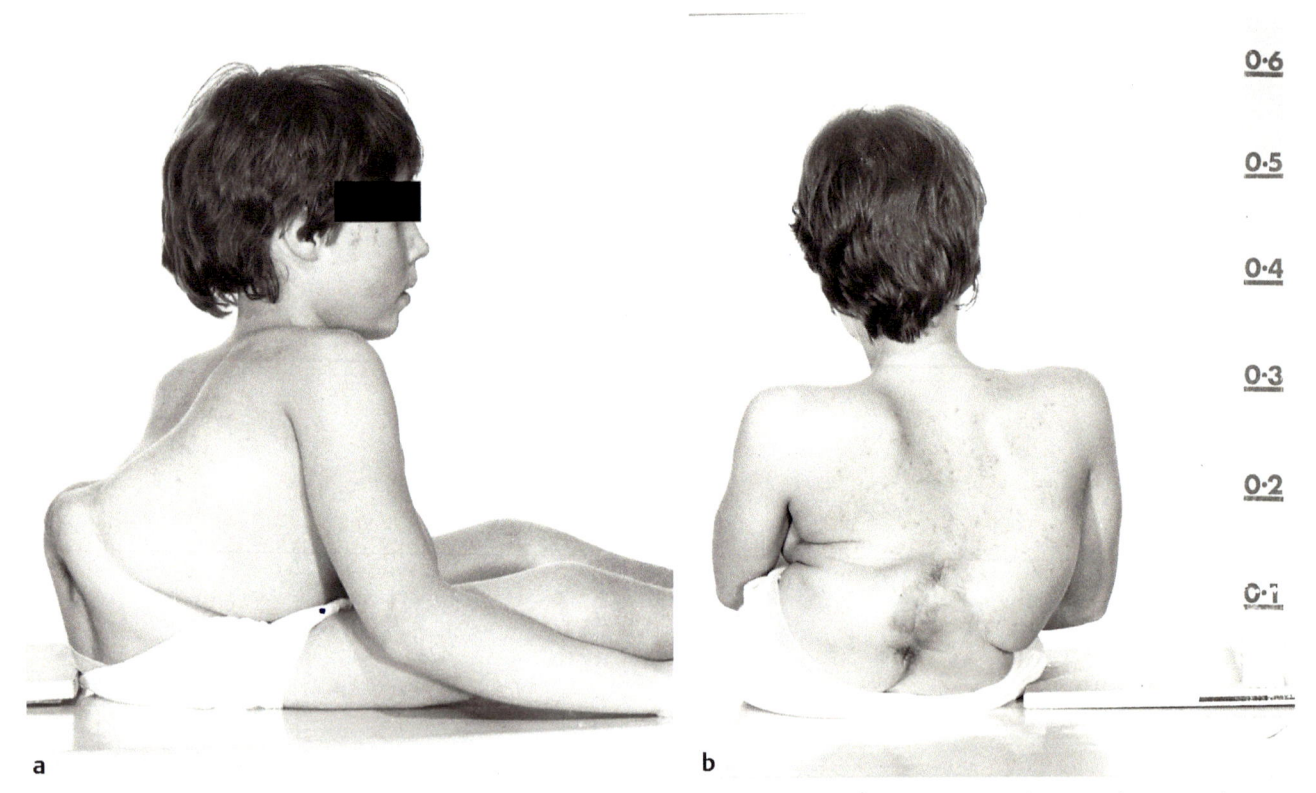

Fig. 6.52 (a) Sideways view showing the fully developed congenital kyphosis of myelomeningocele. (b) Above the kyphotic area there is a scoliosis in association with a compensatory lordosis above.

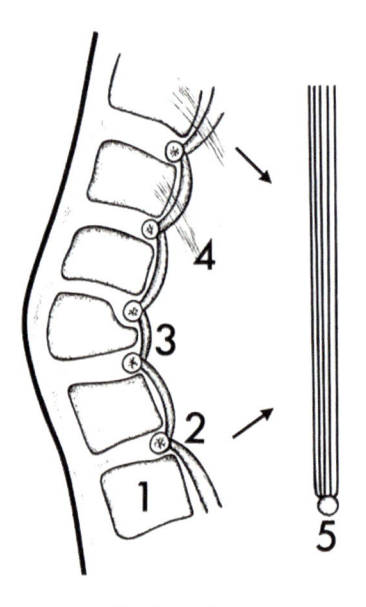

1. Vertebral Body
2. Annulus Fibrosus
3. Anterior Longitudinal Ligament
4. Ilio-Psoas
5. Rectus Abdominis

Fig. 6.53 A diagram showing all the tight structures with the congenital kyphosis of MM.

6.7 Spinal Dysraphism

The term spinal dysraphism, coined by Lichtenstein,[109] was originally used to describe all varieties of spina bifida together with other sources of cord tethering. We now consider spina bifida separately and use the word dysraphism for cord tethering, although coexistence is not uncommon.

The word diastematomyelia was coined by Hertwig in 1892[26] and first used in a clinical context by Ollivier in 1827.[110] This refers to a midline spike of bone or fibrous tissue or both that divides the cord into two (▶ Fig. 6.55). There is however only one dural sac[111] in contrast to the two sacs seen in the rare true cord reduplication (diplomyelia).

The term dysraphism refers to a number of embryopathological conditions that have the common denominator of being a possible source of spinal cord tethering.[112–119] The conditions are multivarious but the more common ones are diastematomyelia, tethered conus (conus extending abnormally low) (▶ Fig. 6.56 and ▶ Fig. 6.57), intraspinal lipoma (▶ Fig. 6.58), teratoma, dermoid and neurenteric cyst, and spinocutaneous fistula.[120–122] While spina bifida is equally common in females and males, spinal dysraphism is more than twice as prevalent in females.

In 1973 Gillespie reported the Boston experience of intraspinal anomalies in association with congenital scoliosis.[120] They reported on 31 cases, 17 of whom had a diastematomyelia and 14 a miscellaneous group of developmental tumors. They recommended preoperative spinal cord imaging (myelography in those days) in association with congenital scoliosis and that neurosurgical management of the intraspinal lesion should precede spinal fusion for the scoliosis.

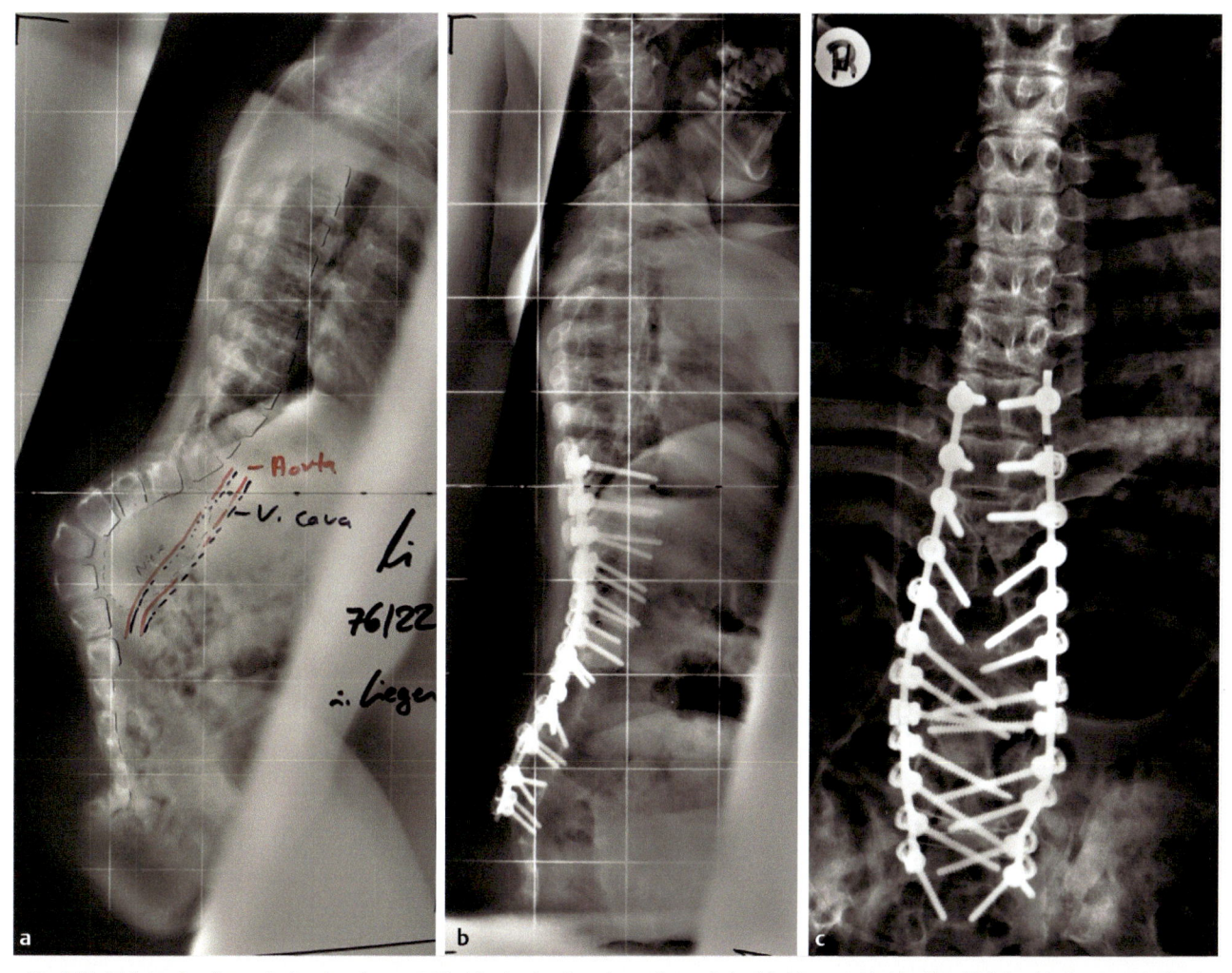

Fig. 6.54 (a) Lateral radiograph showing the congenital kyphosis of myelomeningocele in this 11-year-old girl with a high level lesion at waist level. The position of the great vessels is marked out. (b) Lateral view showing that the gibbus has been resected, the spine fixed down to the pelvis with transpedicular instrumentation, and a good correction obtained. (c) PA view of the construct. Note the pedicular widening in the lower lumbar spine typical of spina bifida. Sitting stability and hand function were restored.

Then in 1974 Winter described the Minneapolis experience of diastematomyelia and reported on 27 cases.[121] There was a 5% prevalence rate of diastematomyelia in association with congenital scoliosis. The other lesions were dermal sinus, dermoid cyst, neurenteric cyst, fibrous band, lipoma, and intradural angioma. While 11 patients had a hairy patch (▶ Fig. 6.9), 7 patients had no cutaneous lesion; 12 patients had a significant foot deformity, mostly club foot (▶ Fig. 6.59). Winter reminded us that the interposed midline septum could be bone, cartilage, fibrous tissue, or a combination thereof. Nearly all patients had associated widening of the interpedicular distance at the site of the septum and 25 had spina bifida; 19 of the lesions were located in the lumbar spine and only 8 in the thoracic spine.

Then in 1984 McMaster reported the Edinburgh scoliosis clinic experience of occult intraspinal anomalies in association with congenital scoliosis.[122] Of 251 patients with congenital scoliosis, occult congenital intraspinal anomalies were diagnosed in 46 (18%) and diastematomyelia was the most common anomaly, in 41 patients (16%). By far the highest prevalence (just more than half) occurred in association with a unilateral unsegmented bar with a contralateral hemivertebra. A total of 30 patients had neurological abnormalities, usually affecting one lower extremity (▶ Fig. 6.60). Neurological deterioration occurred in nine of these patients before the age of 5 years and excision of the anomalies stopped neurological progression.

In those that present with neurological involvement, lower extremity abnormalities and micturition disturbances are the most obvious, the former presenting to orthopaedic surgeons and the latter to neurosurgeons.[122]

There are four usual modes of presentation: visible cutaneous abnormalities over the back, abnormalities of the lower extremity, disturbances of micturition, and the patient with a scoliosis in whom investigations preparatory to spinal surgery indicate the presence of spinal cord tethering. The cutaneous abnormalities are always in the midline, are usually in the nature of abnormal hair-bearing skin, a skin dimple, sinus or fistula, a congenital scar, or a flat capillary nevus. There may only be a limp due to unequal size of the legs in all dimensions. The clinical differential diagnosis of the foot deformity is important and may mimic to the uninitiated the appearances of old

Congenital Deformities

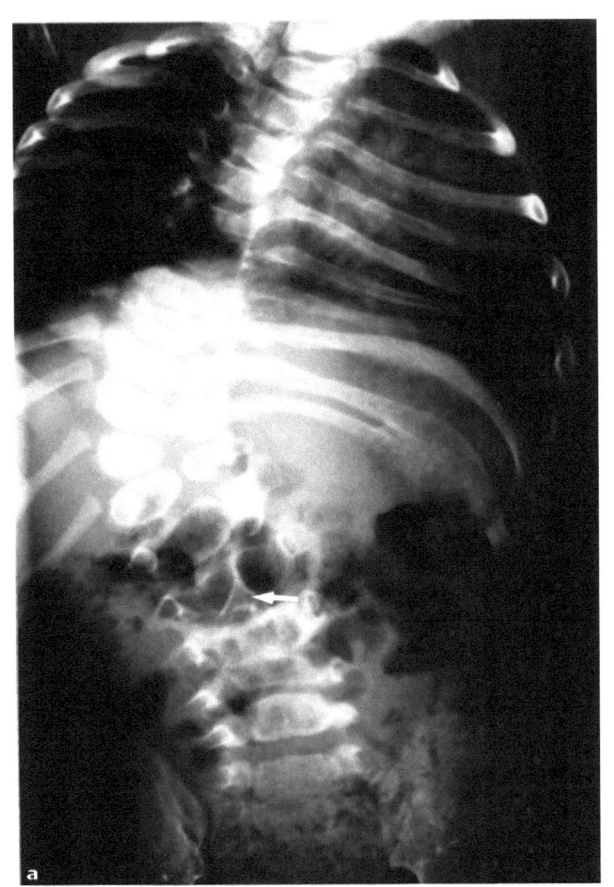

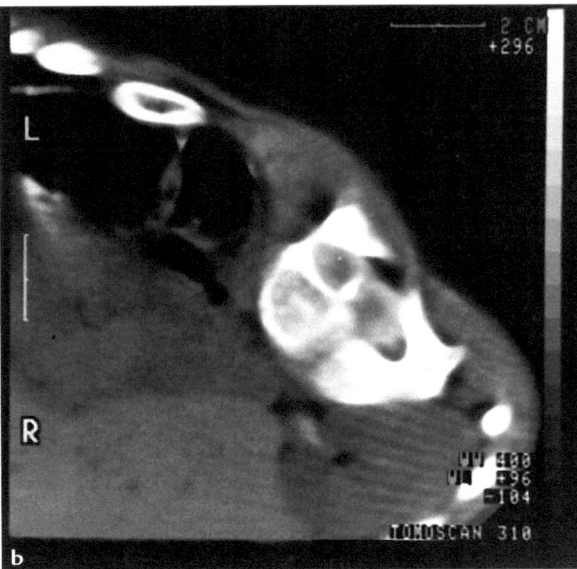

Fig. 6.55 (a) PA view of a thoracolumbar curve with several congenital anomalies from the lower thoracic spine downward. Note the marked interpedicular widening at the L1/2 level and the central spike of bone (*arrow*) being the diastematomyelia. (b) CT myelogram/tomogram showing the two halves of the cord and the bony spike in between.

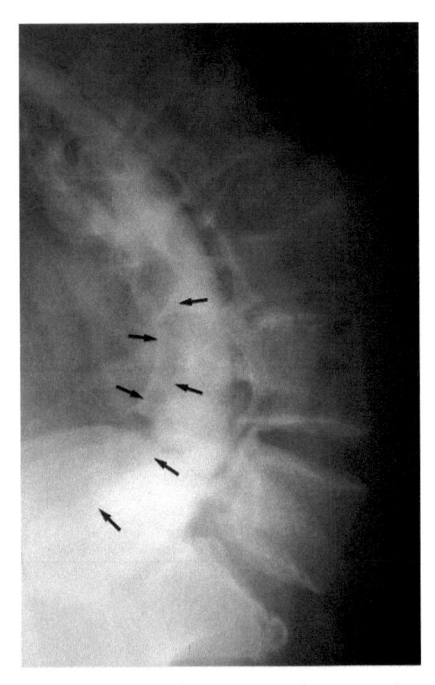

Fig. 6.56 Lateral myelogram showing a very low conus (*arrows*) in this young adult with a cord extending down to S1.

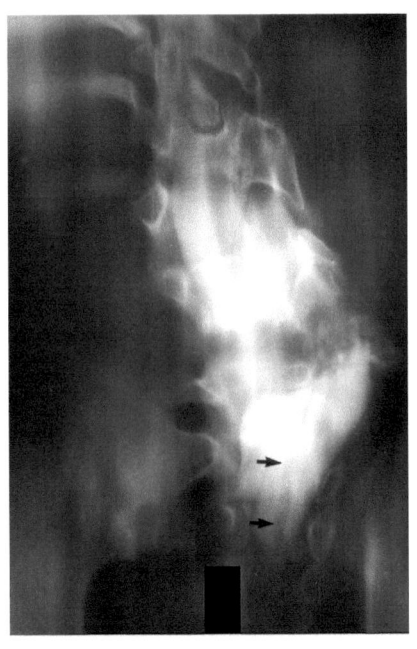

Fig. 6.57 Posteroanterior myelogram/tomogram of a complex congenital lumbar anomaly. The filum terminale (*arrows*) is visible and thus thickened and shortened.

poliomyelitis, cerebral palsy, or Friedreich's ataxia. Interestingly, the lower limb abnormalities and micturition disturbances seldom occur together.[114] Neither situation usually presents until the second or third year of life, when continence and normal ambulation should both have been achieved. The uncommon spinocutaneous fistula is a very serious condition presenting with meningitis of which there may be recurrent attacks. Even if the fistula is closed, meningeal fibrosis and tethering from the inflammatory episodes provide a secondary source of cord tethering. Early reports about spinal dysraphism tended to come from a neurosurgical background with discussion as to the merits or otherwise of surgical release.[113-116] Then reports

Congenital Deformities

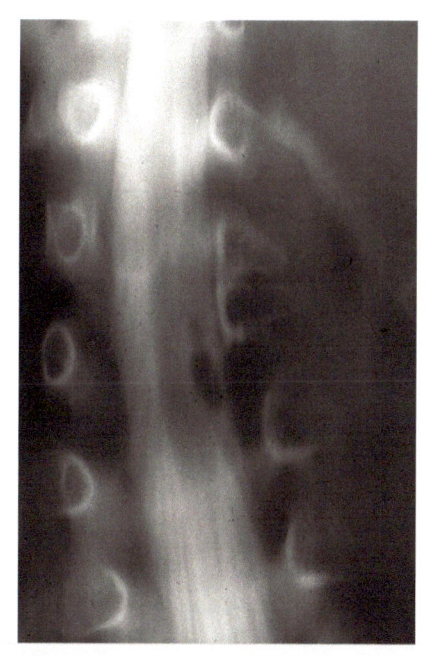

Fig. 6.58 PA myelogram showing an intradural lipoma.

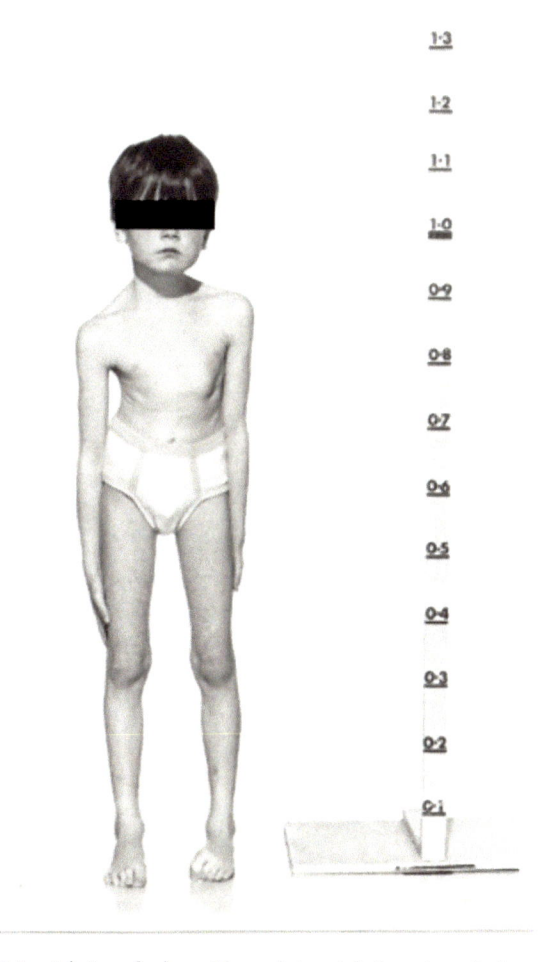

Fig. 6.59 Frontal view of a boy with an obvious left thoracic scoliosis with a high left shoulder and lower thoracic recession on the concave side. On the left side there is a talipes equinovarus that persisted despite standard club foot treatment, typical for a neuropathic clubfoot.

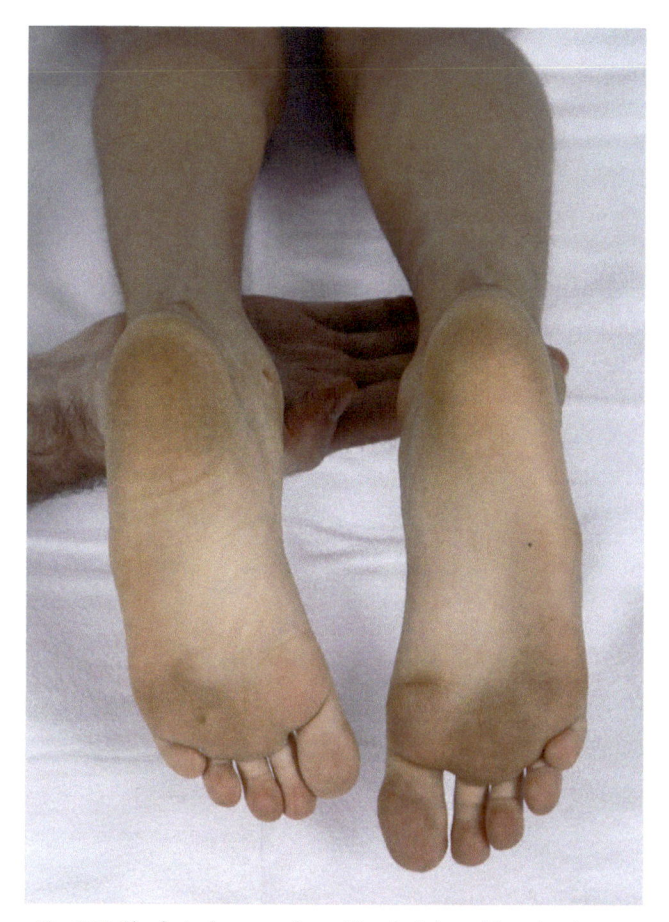

Fig. 6.60 The feet of a young boy with spinal dysraphism showing a wasted left calf and a smaller left foot.

from the big centers tended to focus on whether or not surgical release was necessary before surgical correction of a spinal deformity.[121,122] Interestingly there is still a debate about whether the isolated tether should be routinely released neurosurgically, but scoliosis surgeons certainly favor having the cord tether dealt with before corrective surgery.

Minimally invasive techniques for spinal cord untethering have been described more recently[123] and have been shown to be just as safe and effective as through a mini-open approach.[124] There is of course nothing new in spinal surgery and in the previous textbook there is a description of the use of a mini arthroscope to look down the dura to inspect the filum[125] (▶ Fig. 6.61). Concurrent tethered cord release and spinal fusion for correction of scoliosis has also been shown to be just as safe and effective as a staged procedure.[126] Whether tether release does have an effect on halting the progression of scoliosis is more uncertain. Improvement in size of curvatures or at least a diminution in rate of progression has been noted following release of a tethered spinal cord.[127]

195

Congenital Deformities

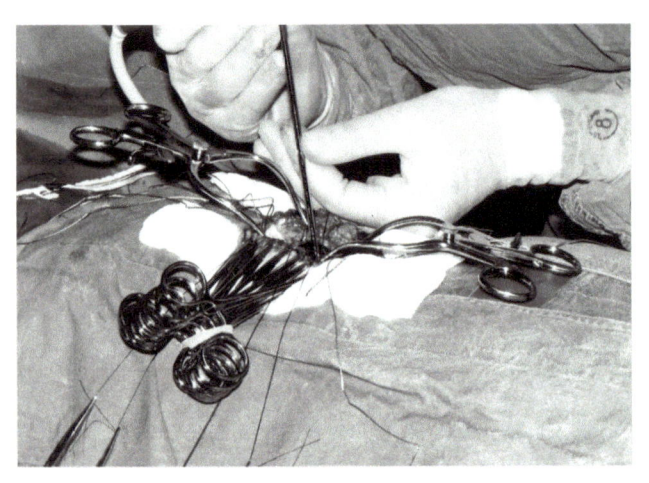

Fig. 6.61 Using a mini-arthroscope to look down the spinal canal to see if the filum is thickened.

In patients with spinal dysraphism the spinal column is never radiographically normal. The most important feature is local widening of the spinal canal as evidenced by an increased interpedicular distance (▶ Fig. 6.55a) but no pedicular thinning unless an expanding intradural lesion such as a dermoid cyst is present. The local neural arches are either cleft or fused and the adjacent bodies have failed to segment to a variable degree. In less than a third of cases is a bony spur visible, indicative of a bony diastematomyelia. MRI/myelography shows the anomaly excellently (▶ Fig. 6.55b) but a complete diagnosis is never possible until surgical exploration has been undertaken.[113] Nevertheless, the location of a diastematomyelia or lipoma is revealed, although not always to its full extent. Importantly, the position of the conus can be identified so that additional tethering can be diagnosed and if the filum terminale is visible then it is always abnormally thick (▶ Fig. 6.57). Because a diastematomyelia is present in so many patients with congenital spinal deformities, a careful neurological examination of the lower extremities is essential in all cases, followed by MRI to exclude a source of spinal cord tethering. This is particularly important if the patient is to undergo surgical instrumentation. However, for any congenital spinal anomaly, from an isolated hemivertebra right through to complex hemivertebral patterns, there is a similar rate of intraspinal anomalies detected by MRI and similar rates therefore of required neurosurgical intervention. The history and physical examination are not a predictor of spinal anomalies and so all patients with a congenital scoliosis must have MRI evaluation.[119]

6.7.1 Tethered Conus

The tethered conus as a source of neurological problems in patients with spinal dysraphism is much more important than generally appreciated. Approximately half the patients operated on for spinal dysraphism have a tethered conus as the most important abnormality.[114] While the conus medullaris is normally sited behind the first lumbar vertebra, the filum terminale extends downward through the cauda equina to the termination of the dural tube and then onward to the periosteum on the back of the coccyx. It is continuous with the pia mater at the end of the conus and is about 18 cm in length. Shortening of the filum in association with a low conus is important both historically and practically (▶ Fig. 6.55 and ▶ Fig. 6.56). In 1894 Arnold described cord tethering,[128] and a year later Chiari demonstrated that cord tethering and differential growth could pull the brain down into the upper spine with blockage of the aqueduct of Sylvius and subsequent hydrocephalus.[129] Thus the Arnold-Chiari syndrome was established and this was further described by Lichtenstein[130] and Steele.[131] Garceau demonstrated that the Arnold-Chiari syndrome of cord traction could be relieved by section of a tight filum terminale. He successfully treated a case of paraplegia due to congenital kyphosis by this means.[132] As the simplest of all operations for spinal dysraphism is section of the filum terminale, then the filum and the position of the conus should be scrutinized on the MRI.[125]

The results of dividing a tight filum are generally good and Cornips et al in 2012 published the surgical status in 25 cases.[133] Neurological status improved in 20 cases and stabilized in 5. A total of eight children presented with a scoliosis of which three improved, four stabilized, and one worsened. The patients' ages were between 2 and 18 years and there was a 2:1 female to male gender ratio.

Hajnovic and Trnka reported their series of 22 patients treated surgically for a tight filum and focused on the time period between onset of symptoms and treatment. Interestingly the results were not quite as good as one might expect.[134] A total of 9 of the 22 patients showed improvement of symptoms, 2 of them to normal; 11 remained unchanged without further progression and 2 patients worsened. There was a direct correlation between the time lag from onset to treatment and outcome. They concluded that virtually all patients operated within the first year will show a subsequent improvement of symptoms.

Colombo and Motta then reported on the orthopaedic problems in patients with Chiari 1 malformations as well as treatment.[135] Scoliosis was the most common deformity and interestingly asymptomatic scoliosis tended to be single curves convex to the left while symptomatic scoliosis (pain, stiffness) tended to be double curves. Suboccipital craniectomy gave the best chance for syrinx reduction and scoliosis improvement particularly in children under 10 with a Cobb angle of less than 30 degrees.

Increasing neurological loss in the spina bifida patient also appears to be much more important than traditionally thought, and while spina bifida patients with inadequate quadriceps musculature inevitably become wheelchair-bound, this natural passage from splints and callipers to wheelchair may disguise true evidence of neurological deterioration. This occurs in patients with the Arnold-Chiari malformation producing hydrocephalus which has spontaneously arrested and the problem has been defined as a communicating hydrosyringomyelia.[136] This was noted in 14 out of 15 such patients in whom ventricular decompression and shunting improved function. Therefore, it is particularly important to evaluate carefully these difficult spina bifida patients to ensure that it truly is the spinal deformity and not a more subtle reason for functional deterioration. It is perhaps surprising that differential growth of bone and neural tissue in patients with spina bifida does not produce more evidence of progressive neurological deterioration with time. Presumably, temporal factors are again important in that very gradual changes in cord tension can be tolerated with no significant change in neurological function whereas the more rapid tension of a distraction operation can have catastrophic consequences. Interestingly, some patients would appear to have been inadvertently saved from the consequences of neurological tension by spontaneous transposition of the spinal cord herniating through the posterior element deficiencies.[137,138]

6.8 Congenital Spinal Deformity Syndromes

A congenital spine deformity may occur as part of a syndrome affecting many other sites and systems and perhaps the most important thing that can be done for a child with a congenital spine deformity is a thorough evaluation of the other areas where problems may occur. This is particularly relevant when the congenital vertebral anomaly involves the cervical spine.

6.8.1 Klippel-Feil Syndrome

Any congenital failure of segmentation affecting the cervical spine, or cervicothoracic junction, is now referred to as the Klippel-Feil syndrome, and indeed that is what was described by Klippel and Feil in 1912.[139] The triad of a short neck, low hairline, and restricted range of cervical spine motion was not described until 8 years later[140] (▶ Fig. 6.62). Winter with his great interest in the subject of congenital spine deformities has found descriptions of this condition dating back to the early part of the 18th century.[141] The presence of a scoliosis and Sprengel's deformity of the shoulder are the most common musculoskeletal consequences.[142-144]

There are two types of scoliosis occurring in the Klippel-Feil syndrome, a local deformity occurring in the cervical or cervicothoracic region and an idiopathic type of curve occurring secondarily in the thoracic spine below (▶ Fig. 6.15).

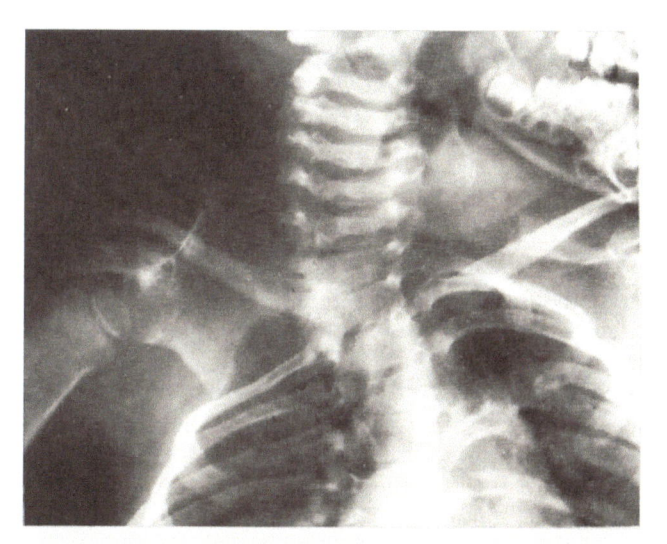

Fig. 6.62 Congenital cervicothoracic bony anomalies characterizing the Klippel Feil syndrome.

The local scoliosis is usually cervicothoracic or upper thoracic but it can be midcervical or even upper cervical, the latter being usually caused by failures of formation rather than failures of segmentation. The scoliosis occurring secondarily in the thoracic region is a rotated lordoscoliosis typical of the idiopathic deformity. This is caused by a failure of segmentation affecting both the coronal and sagittal planes, such that the resulting lordosis is the most important factor precipitating rotation which occurs in the same direction as an idiopathic scoliosis with the posterior elements directed toward the curve concavity. Often by the time the patient seeks clinical help it is the thoracic lordoscoliosis which is the cause of the deformity, but careful radiographic scrutiny of the cervical and upper thoracic spine reveals the primary abnormality.

The cosmetic problem of the scoliosis is compounded by the presence of Sprengel's elevated scapula deformity (▶ Fig. 6.63) and, combined with the rigid short neck and low hairline, often gives rise to a very unfavorable appearance. Fortunately, the local cervical scoliosis seldom requires treatment in its own right but the thoracic lordoscoliosis below frequently does. In the assessment of these patients it is therefore important to differentiate the presence of a deformity from any functional impairment from it and then to establish of which of the problems the patient is complaining. Moreover, treatment for the Sprengel's deformity is difficult and not without risk, particularly to the brachial plexus, such that the patient, the deformity, and treatment all have to be carefully titrated one against the other before a decision in favor of treatment is made.

Early procedures to bring down the Sprengel's shoulder involved scapular osteotomy or subperiosteal freeing of the entire scapula with the excision of any omovertebral bone present.[145,146] In order to avoid plexus damage, a two-stage procedure with interval skeletal traction was devised.[147] This was followed by the concept of extraperiosteal release with resection of the supraspinous portion of the scapula along with the omovertebral bone.[148] Jeannopoulos found that satisfactory results could only be obtained in 50% of patients and that bad results followed subperiosteal resection with scapular winging and sternoclavicular joint instability.[149] He recommended operating on children between the ages of 2 and 5 years and keeping the surgical attack outside the periosteum. To this has been added release of the origins of the trapezius and medial scapular muscles from the spine,[150] along with tenderization of the clavicle in order to reduce the problems of plexus palsy.[151] Digennaro recently reported the 25-year experience of the surgical treatment of Sprengel's shoulder from the Rizzoli Institute.[152] There were 56 children and they concluded that a modified Green procedure combined with resection of the superomedial portion of the scapula provided the best cosmetic and functional results. It would appear that the disadvantage of postoperative scarring outweighs the relatively modest gain in cosmesis. We have found, however, that in patients with the classic triad, where the Sprengel's deformity is bilateral and the shoulder girdles are protracted, that simple excision of the middle third of the clavicle can provide some shoulder retraction with an improvement in appearance as the result of a relatively minor surgical intervention with minimal scarring.

The other musculoskeletal problem of significance in these patients is cervical spine instability occurring in the hypermobile areas above the fused segments; this occurs in about 5% of

Congenital Deformities

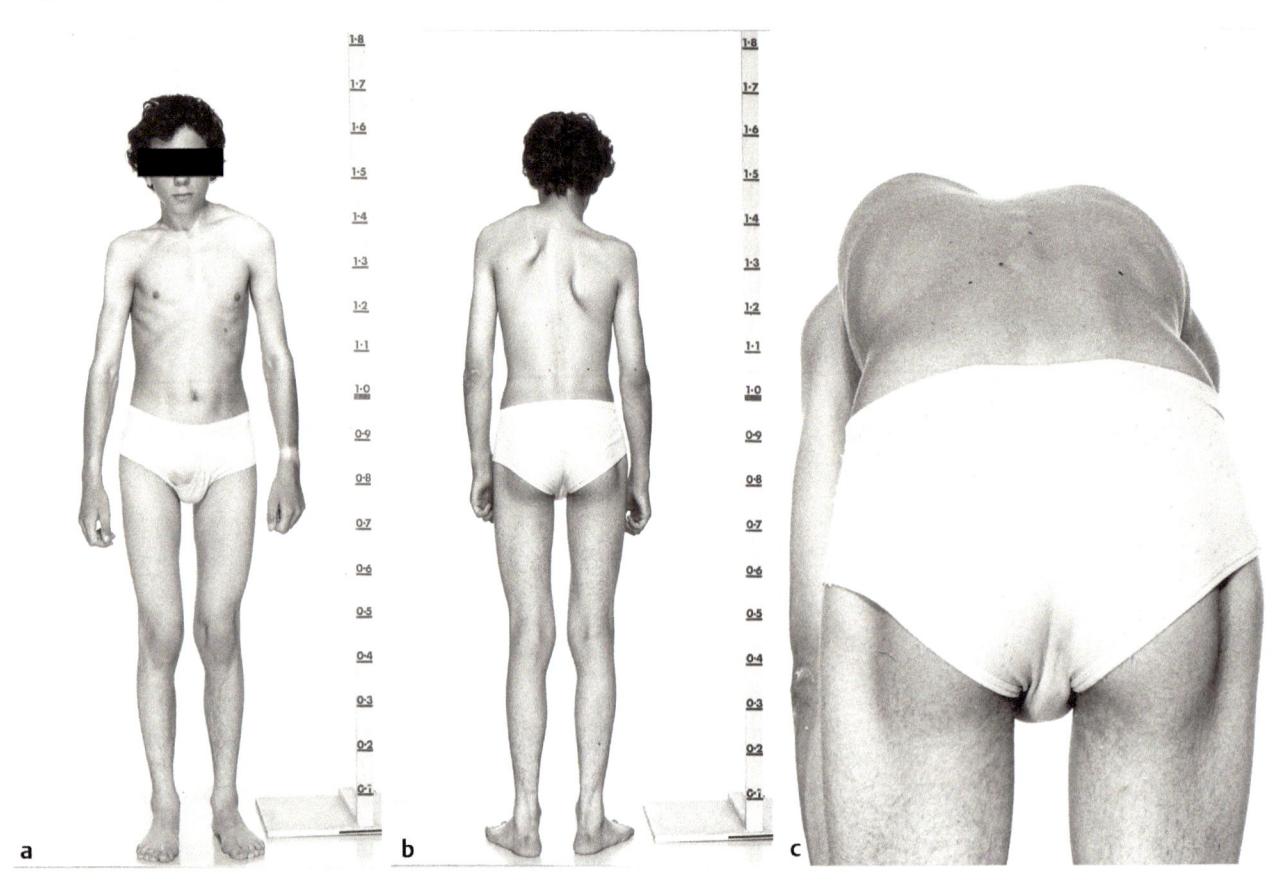

Fig. 6.63 Sprengel's elevated left shoulder. (a) Front view. (b) Back view showing how high the left scapula is. (The scapulae develop from mesenchyme in the neck and then migrate down to their final position.) The congenital insult halts the normal descent and so there is a high shoulder on the affected side. (c) Forward bending view showing the associated upper thoracic scoliosis.

such patients.[143,153–156] A careful neurological examination is therefore a very important part of the evaluation of these patients. Perhaps the most important nonmusculoskeletal problem with the Klippel-Feil syndrome is the high prevalence rate of genitourinary anomalies.[43,148,157–160] In one study the majority of intravenous pyelograms were abnormal.[157] Indeed, there is a surprisingly high prevalence rate of genitourinary anomalies in congenital scoliosis not associated with the Klippel-Feil syndrome.[160] The alimentary tract should also be carefully evaluated as the commonest gastrointestinal problem in congenital deformities is tracheoesophageal fistula. Other less common problems in the Klippel-Feil syndrome include hearing defects, cardiac problems, and synkinesia.[143]

6.8.2 VACTERL Association

This acronym refers to an aggregation of congenital anomalies in different body systems that occur more frequently than expected by chance although not pathogenetically related. It starts with V for vertebral anomalies, then anal atresia, cardiac defects, tracheoesophageal fistula, renal anomalies, and limb defects. It used to be referred to as the VATER association but became VACTERL with the addition of cardiac and limb anomalies. The R in VATER association originally referred to radial dysplasia and so the capital R referred to both renal and radial congenital problems whereas the acronym VACTERL clearly differentiates the two.[161]

6.8.3 Thoracic Insufficiency Syndrome

Although there are a number of syndromes that can be associated with thoracic insufficiency particularly in the infantile and juvenile years, such as severe early-onset idiopathic or neuromuscular disease, the term thoracic insufficiency syndrome is most commonly associated with multiple congenital spinal and rib anomalies usually described as spondylocostal dysplasia. Von Rokitansky is generally regarded as providing the first description of this syndrome which has a high mortality due to associated lung dysfunction.[162] In 1938 Saul Jarcho and Paul Levin reported thoracic insufficiency cases due to vertebral and rib anomalies and the condition of spondylocostal dysostosis or dysplasia (SCD) is referred eponymously as the Jarcho-Levin syndrome.[163] However, 30 years later, in 1966, Norman Lavy reported from Indiana University a similar syndrome in a family from Puerto Rico.[164] Soon after Moseley from New York reported a similar case and this was when the term spondylothoracic dysplasia (STD) was first used.[165] This gave rise to confusion between the two similar clinical syndromes that caused thoracic insufficiency but SCD and STD are different genetically —the former linked to genes such as *DLL3* and the latter to the *MESP2* gene, both associated with the Notch pathway. STD has become known eponymously as the Lavy-Moseley syndrome and while SCD causes mild to moderate respiratory insufficiency, STD is associated with more severe respiratory compromise although a quarter may survive into adult life.

Ramirez looked at the natural history of thoracic insufficiency in association with STD in 28 patients.[166] Eight died in the neonatal period and the survivors had less than 30% of predicted forced vital capacity and forced expiratory volume with CT lung volume 28% of the predicted. The thorax was severely shortened posteriorly, averaging less than a quarter of the predicted normal length. The thoracic spine was composed predominantly of block vertebrae. The survivors showed an impressive clinical tolerance of restrictive lung disease and could have a good quality of life.

Clinically we all observe that respiratory function is markedly worsened in these children by the unsupported sitting position but with the child lifted to open up the chest cavity function can be seen to improve straightaway. Concerns about interfering with the spine instrumentally at a very young age in terms of inducing premature fusion to mention but one led to the development of instrumenting the chest wall itself on the concave side of the scoliosis so as to prop up the compressed hemithorax. The notion was that if the instrumentation was to be applied to the rib cage then the spine would be protected from insult. Campbell from San Antonio obliged by developing a chest wall distractor so that there could be lengthening of the concave hemithorax by way of an opening wedge thoracostomy.[167] This chest wall distractor was unnecessarily lengthened in name to a vertical expandable prosthetic titanium rib—thankfully shortened to the acronym VEPTR (▶ Fig. 6.64). Then at 4- to 6-month intervals or so the device could be lengthened to maintain Cobb angle correction, improve lateral deviation of the spine and thoracic spinal height, as well as physiological measures of pulmonary status. This was used first in San Antonio in 1989 and was not introduced into Europe until 2002.[168] In 2004 Campbell reported his first 27 patients with a 6-year follow-up.[167] Although the mean age was 3.2 years the range was down to 7 months and the oldest was 7.5 years. They managed to reduce the mean Cobb angle from 74 degrees down to 49 degrees at follow-up and increase the thoracic spine height at 0.7 cm per year. The vital capacity at follow-up was 58% for patients under the age of 2 and 36% for older patients.

Hell described the European experience in Germany of 15 children with similar results[168] and felt that the VEPTR instrumentation was a safe and efficient method for treating thoracic insufficiency syndrome in young children with severe scoliosis. In Great Ormond Street, London, 13 cases of SCD were described along with their management,[169] stressing the importance of repeated postnatal chest physiotherapy but also pointing out that the diagnosis can be made prenatally by ultrasound allowing genetic counseling and quantifying risks to siblings. Others followed the VEPTR trail and the Boston group reported their results of 31 patients.[170] Thirty had their spinal deformity controlled and allowed growth to continue at rates similar to normal. They felt that VEPTR should be considered early in growth before the deformity becomes severe but noted the complications of metalwork migration, infection, and brachial plexus palsy.

There are some dreadful cases when the thoracic dysplasia is so bad that the child can asphyxiate and Fette reported a case of a newborn female with such severe asphyxiation that VEPTR was warranted promptly.[171] The infant survived to be discharged home.

Groenefeld reported the problem of ossification in almost 50% of children treated with VEPTR instrumentation at a follow-up of 4.5 years.[172]

Then Campbell published in 2013 his thoughts about his past experience and the future of VEPTR principles.[173] VEPTR was thought to be an important first step toward improving the quality of life and longevity in children with thoracic insufficiency syndrome but much work remained to advance the instrumentation design and its usage.

Perhaps the most important decision or consideration is when, having achieved what VEPTR instrumentation was supposed to do, spinal instrumentation should take over and be the definitive treatment for the scoliosis in association with these complex dysostoses/dysplasias (▶ Fig. 6.65).

6.8.4 Conditions Associated with Congenital Spine Deformities

Limb and facial malformations also occur in association with congenital spinal deformities and some are recognized eponymously as syndromes. The pterygium syndrome involves odontoid hypoplasia, limb pterygium (web formation), and a congenital spinal deformity,[174] while the Holt-Oram syndrome

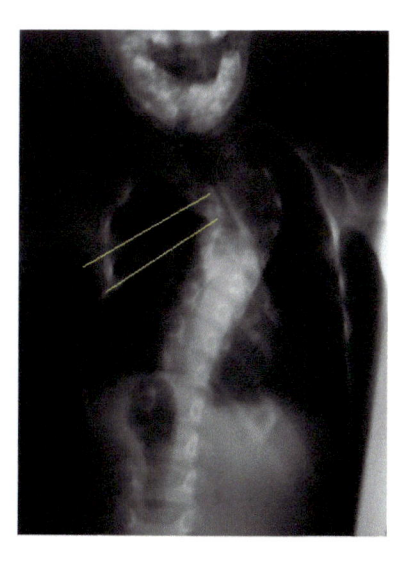

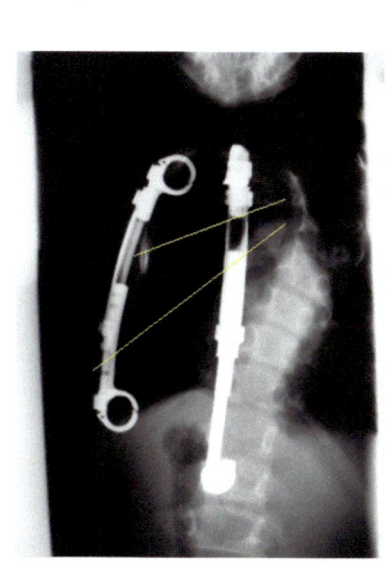

Fig. 6.64 The use of the VEPTR instrumentation for a severe upper thoracic congenital scoliosis, one distracting the ribs and the other distracting the spine.

Congenital Deformities

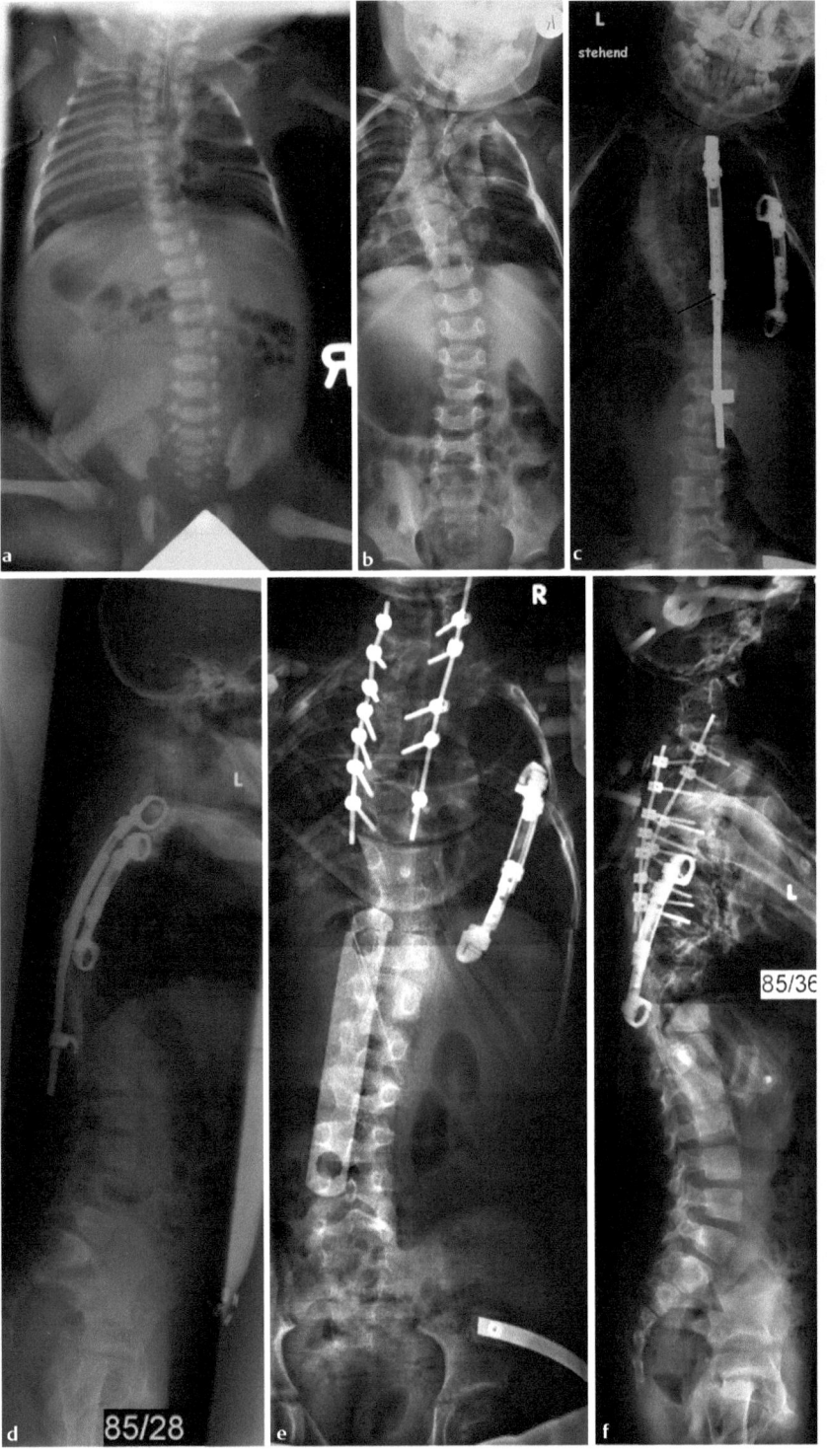

Fig. 6.65 Multiple upper thoracic congenital spine deformities with rib fusions restricting right sided lung function **(a)** at 3 months, **(b)** at 3 years. **(c,d)** PA and lateral radiographs after insertion of the VEPTR instrumentation. **(e,f)** PA and lateral radiographs after AVR and posterior instrumentation. The remaining VEPTR was subsequently removed.

includes upper limb defects and cardiac-septal defects, sometimes in association with a spinal deformity.[175] Goldenhar considered that a malformation of the ear was probably the commonest associated anomaly with a congenital spine deformity and dysplasia of ear, eye, face, and spine describes this syndrome.[176] More recently, three types of facial malformations have been shown to have a relationship to congenital spine deformity, usually mild, hemifacial dysplasia (Goldenhar's syndrome)[177] (▶ Fig. 6.66), mandibulofacial dysostosis (Treacher Collins syndrome),[178] and craniofacial dysostosis with or without syndactyly (Apert's or Crouzon's syndromes, respectively)[177–179] (▶ Fig. 6.67 and ▶ Fig. 6.68). In Larsen's syndrome[180] there are multiple congenital dislocations associated with the characteristic facial abnormality (▶ Fig. 6.69). The eyes are widely spaced and there is a prominent forehead with a depressed nasal bridge. Congenital cervicothoracic vertebral anomalies are common in this syndrome,[180] and severe spinal deformities, either in the form of a rotated lordosis or severe kyphosis, can be

Congenital Deformities

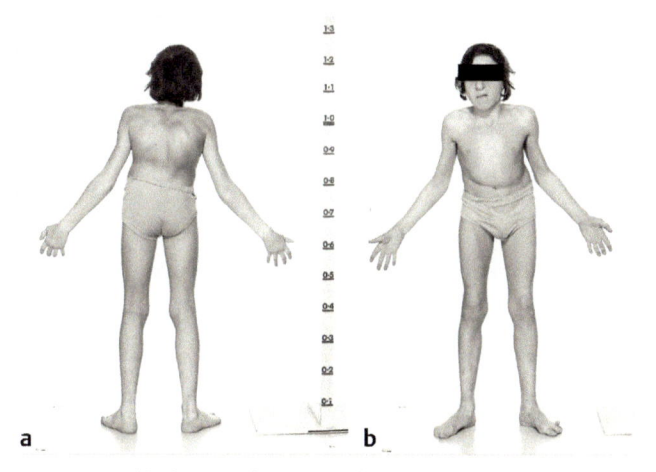

Fig. 6.66 Goldenhar's syndrome (hemifacial dysplasia).

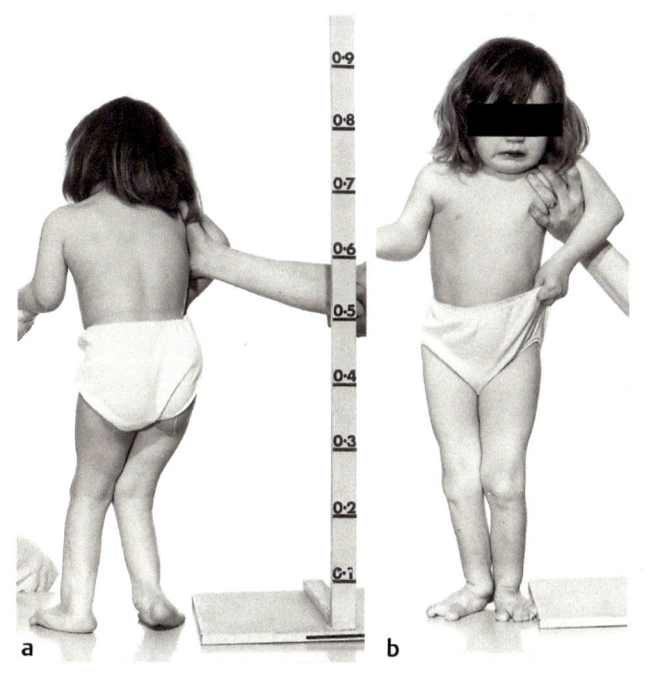

Fig. 6.67 Apert's syndrome (craniofacial dysostosis with syndactyly).

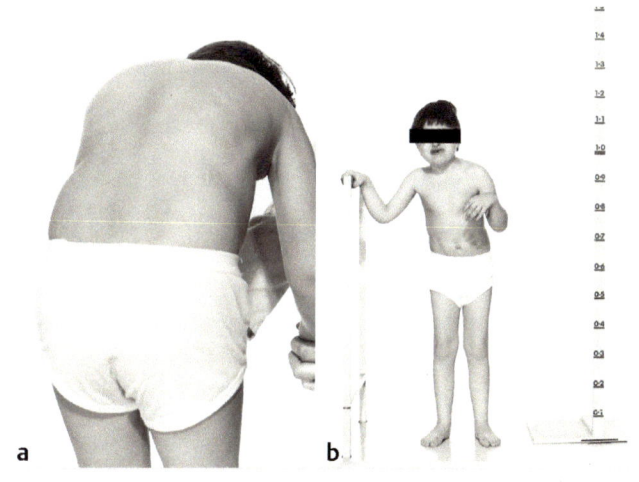

Fig. 6.68 Crouzon's syndrome (craniofacial dysostosis without syndactyly).

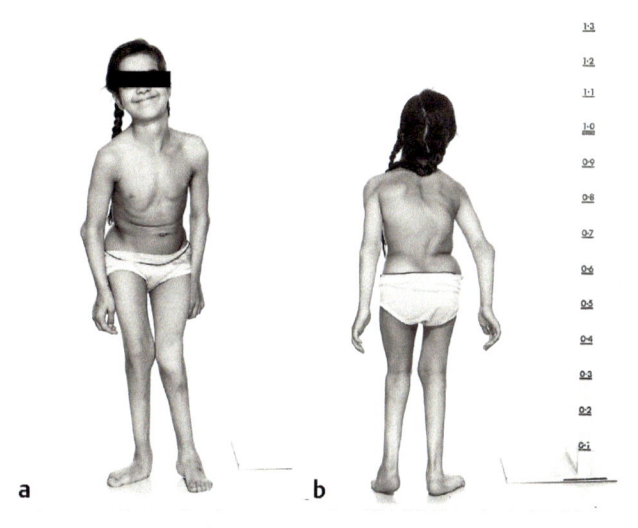

Fig. 6.69 Larsen's syndrome (flattened facies, multiple congenital dislocations, foot deformities).

produced.[181] In Silver's syndrome[182] of congenital hemihypertrophy (shortness of stature and elevated urinary gonadotrophins), a mild scoliosis is common and this is generally related to the characteristic leg length inequality that occurs in these patients.[182] However, Specht also reported curves that were intrinsic to the spine and many of these were associated with congenital vertebral anomalies.[183] The Freeman-Sheldon whistling face syndrome[184] of cranio-carpo-tarsal dystrophy, along with microstomia and enophthalmos, is associated with many musculoskeletal problems, including scoliosis in about 50% of cases. It is difficult to be certain quite what the nature of these deformities is, but platyspondyly and congenital vertebral anomalies can certainly be present, indicating that these curves can be of both congenital and dysplastic varieties. Congenital spinal deformities are also not uncommon in arthrogryposis multiplex congenita[185] but this is categorized now as a neuromuscular disorder.

Lumbar and Sacral Agenesis

This condition was first described in the middle of the 19th century[186] and varies according to the extent of the embryopathological defect. Low lesions have a milder clinical picture than high lesions and are 10 times more common.[187] With mild low lesions there may be no deformity or weakness at all, but with a complete lumbar absence the appearance is that of a sitting Buddha with marked attenuation of the pelvis and buttocks and grossly deformed lower extremities. In more than one-third of cases there are congenital anomalies of the urogenital or alimentary systems, and in complete lumbar lesions with spinopelvic instability the compressive effect of a collapsing spinopelvic kyphosis can compromise these organs. There have been several attempts at classifying these anomalies,[186,188–190] but Renshaw proposed a sensible four-part classification based on 23 patients whom he had carefully evaluated[191] (▶ Fig. 6.70).

Congenital Deformities

1. Type 1 lesions (total or partial unilateral sacral agenesis) were the least common and encountered in only two of his patients. Although both patients had an oblique lumbosacral joint with a mild scoliosis, these did not progress and treatment was not required for their spines. More distally there was only one calcaneovarus foot deformity treated conservatively, and both patients were community ambulators (▶ Fig. 6.70a and ▶ Fig. 6.71a).
2. Type 2 (partial sacral agenesis, with a partial but bilaterally symmetrical defect) was the most common type of defect and 12 patients were so affected (▶ Fig. 6.70b). Two had an unstable spinopelvic junction and two others were myelodysplastic. The other eight patients had levels of motor paralysis corresponding to within one segment of the level of the vertebral deficit, but sensation was intact at least down to S4. A scoliosis developed in six patients, three of which were of the congenital bony variety and three associated with myelodysplasia. Hip dislocation was present in three patients and foot deformities in five. Eight patients in this type 2 group were fully ambulatory.
3. Type 3 (variable lumbar and total sacral agenesis with the ilia articulating with the side of the lowest vertebra present) was present in five patients, but in three the spinopelvic articulations were stable. A progressive kyphosis developed in the other two and a long thoracolumbar paralytic scoliosis was noted in a further two. Four had bilateral hip dislocations, knee contractures, and severe foot deformities (▶ Fig. 6.70c and ▶ Fig. 6.71b).
4. Type 4 (variable lumbar and total sacral agenesis with the lowest vertebra resting above either fused ilia or an iliac amphiarthrosis), the most severe type, occurred in four patients, only one of whom did not have spinopelvic kyphosis or scoliosis (▶ Fig. 6.70d and ▶ Fig. 6.71c). All these patients had bilateral severe hip flexion

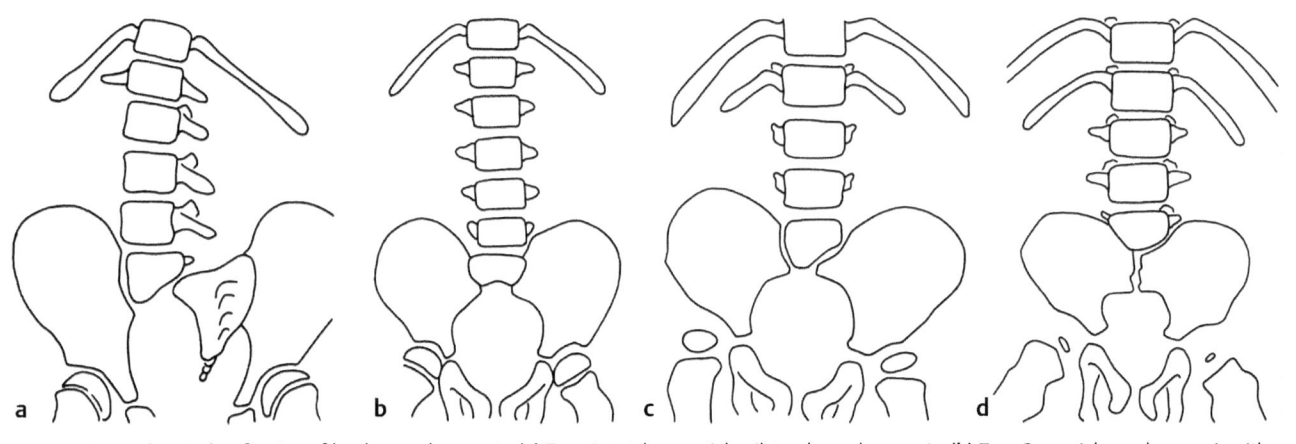

Fig. 6.70 Renshaw's classification of lumbosacral agenesis. (a) Type 1: total or partial unilateral sacral agenesis. (b) Type 2: partial sacral agenesis with a stable spinopelvic junction. (c) Type 3: complete sacral and partial lumbar agenesis with the lowest lumbar vertebra articulating with the ilia. (d) Type 4: complete sacral and partial lumbar agenesis with the lowest lumbar vertebra merely resting on the conjoined ilia.

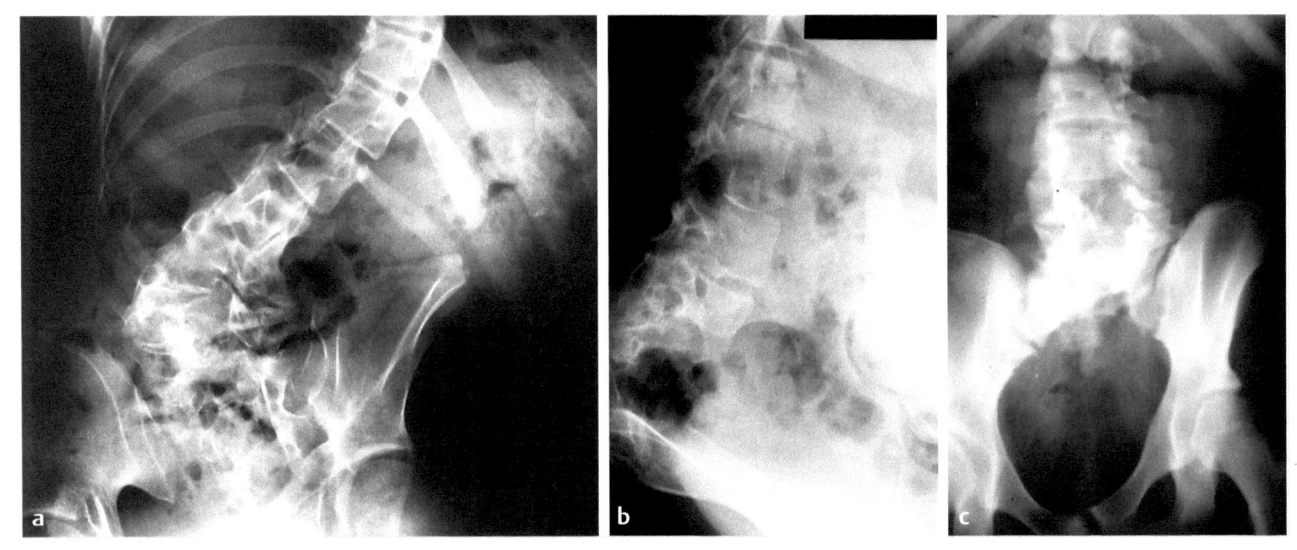

Fig. 6.71 (a) Type 1, (b) type 3, (c) type 4.

contractures, and popliteal webbing. All had severe bilateral foot deformities.

Although these individuals clearly do not tend to reproduce, there is evidence of a familial basis to the condition.[187] However, of greater interest is the observation that in about 20% of cases there is maternal diabetes.[191,192] It is also interesting that when insulin is administered to the very early developing chick lumbosacral agenesis can be induced.[193]

In the management of these patients it is essential to view them holistically with the musculoskeletal system in association with the urogenital and alimentary tracts. As Hensinger and MacEwen rightly state, "it is the responsibility of the orthopaedist to see that the urinary tract is being evaluated."[194] Accordingly, a team approach is necessary. The musculoskeletal consequences for a type 1 patient are minimal with the occasional mild deformity. Most patients encountered would be type 2 and spinal, spinopelvic, hip, knee, and foot deformities may all require surgical treatment. The great majority of type 3 and 4 patients require multiple surgical procedures.

The nonspinal aspects of this condition can be managed in one of two principal ways. For the severe atrophic and fixed lower extremity the limb is not conserved and following subtrochanteric amputation walking is facilitated with a bucket-type prosthesis.[195] This treatment program is only applicable to those with an unsalvageable extremity. On the other hand, there are those who favor limb retention, and so an aggressive surgical treatment program to correct whatever deformities are present is required. In favor of the latter treatment is the fact that sensation is unusually well preserved in comparison with motor power in these patients, and thus protective sensation in the lower extremities militates against pressure ulceration and in favor of the use of orthoses.

There are two areas of surgical consideration for the spine in these patients: spinopelvic instability and scoliosis. Patients with sacral agenesis who lack stability of the spine need surgical stabilization as this allows them to sit with their hands free, permits stretching and/or surgical release of contractures lower down, and protects viscera from compression. Perry has operated two such cases and after a period of halo-femoral traction, performing a posterior thoraco-iliac fusion through a halo-femoral plaster cast.[196] The kyphotic segment in the lower thoracic region was osteotomized to correct the sagittal plane component of the deformity and this was held with a combination of distraction and compression systems. Renshaw reported four cases of spinopelvic fusion for instability and, although operative detail was not reported, demonstrated successful fusion, recommending that this should be performed at an early age.[191] His patients were better sitters, had improved ilial conduits and respiratory reserve and could use their orthoses, or prostheses, more efficiently.

Two types of structural spinal deformity above the pelvis may be encountered in these patients: a congenital bony scoliosis, or a paralytic deformity, not dissimilar to that encountered with myelodysplasia, which may be present also. The indication for surgical treatment of these higher spinal deformities is to improve function when it is the spine, and nothing else, which jeopardizes sitting stability or walking potential. These are treated as for congenital or paralytic scoliosis respectively.

Genetic Considerations

When a congenital lesion presents itself clinically it is not unnatural for the family to enquire about the risks of other or subsequent children in the family being involved and what the future is for the offspring of the child concerned. Wynne-Davies studied the heritable implications in the families of more than 300 children with congenital vertebral anomalies and considered three groups of patients: those with an isolated vertebral anomaly such as a hemivertebra, those with multiple vertebral defects, and those with vertebral anomalies in association with the spina bifida syndrome.[197] She found that the single defects were sporadic and inferred that there was no genetic risk, although Winter puts the chances at about 1 in 100 for first-degree relatives.[198] Those with multiple defects or those in association with the spina bifida syndrome have a very definite risk estimated to be about 5 to 10%. Of the various twin studies that have been reported, most have shown only one twin with a congenital deformity.[198-201] Where both of identical twins have been affected there is evidence of variable expressivity.[202,203] In the uncommon collection of syndromes such as spondylocostal dysplasia where multiple congenital vertebral anomalies occur along with abnormalities elsewhere in the body, both autosomal recessive and dominant modes of inheritance have been described.[204-210]

Congenital Deformities

Case Gallery

Here is the case gallery for the congenital chapter with four more interesting cases. Try and describe each radiograph and then give a thought to surgical options. We suppose that doing nothing is one surgical option.

Case 1: Multiple Hemivertebrae—T1, T8, T11

See ▶ Fig. 6.72.

Comment

Three posterior hemi-vertebrectomies is a lot of surgery to go through not without risk, and so you have to be familiar with the surgical techniques involved and have a full risks-and-rewards discussion with the patient. The patient was very keen to have their unacceptable shape improved and it seemed that either doing three hemi-vertebrectomies or doing none were the only options.

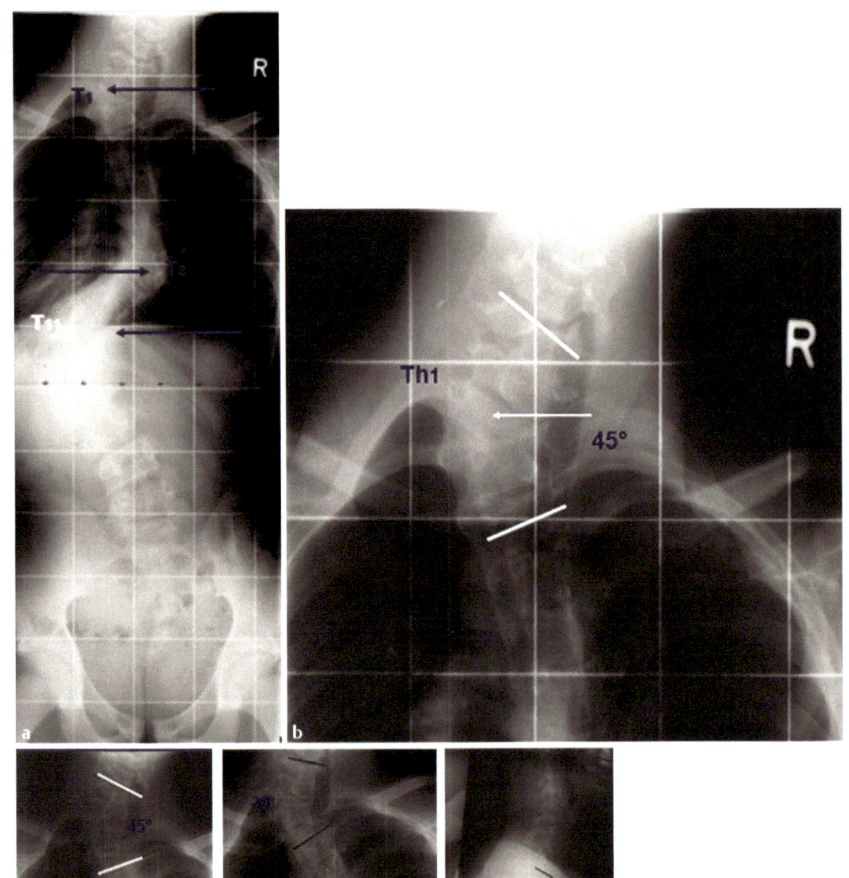

Fig. 6.72 (a) PA radiograph showing multiple hemivertebrae at T1 to the left, T8 to the right, and T11 to the left. (b) Close up tomogram showing several congenital anomalies in the lower neck with a hemivertebra at T1 with its additional rib. (c) PA radiograph showing the size of each component of the deformity. (d,e) PA and lateral radiographs after excision of the T11 hemivertebra and instrumentation.

Congenital Deformities

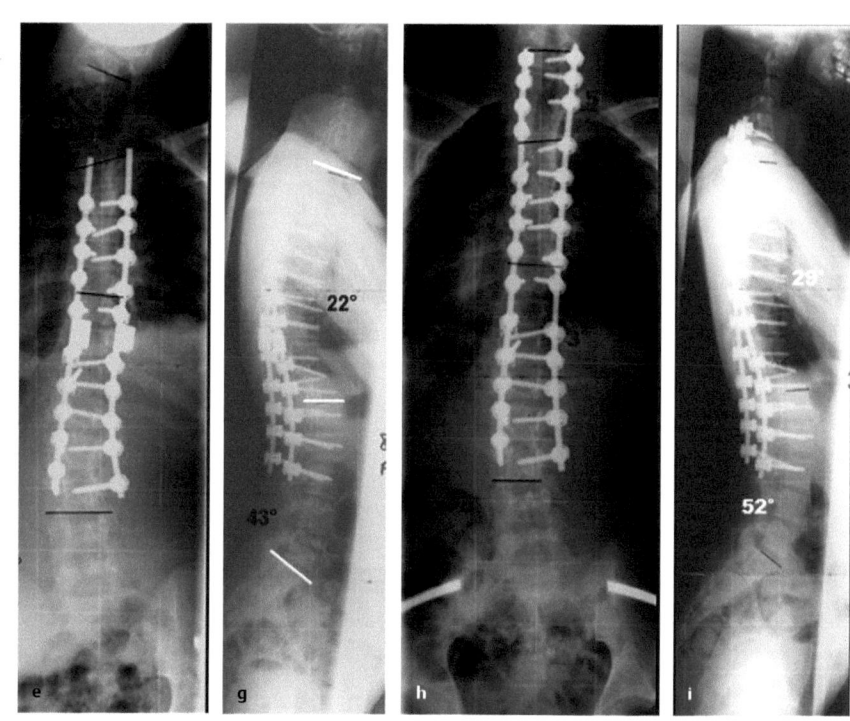

Fig. 6.72 (*continued*) **(f,g)** PA and lateral radiographs after excision of the T8 hemivertebra with extension of the instrumentation upward. **(h,i)** PA and lateral radiographs after excision of the T1 hemivertebra with completion of the instrumentation. There is a straight spine in the frontal plane but rather flat in the sagittal plane. This is a nicely corrected and well-balanced spine.

Congenital Deformities

Case 2: Hemivertebrae Plus Contralateral Bar

See ▶ Fig. 6.73. These high thoracic/cervicothoracic cases are very challenging, but they do produce significant deformities and patients are very pleased with the results. Always check the vertebral artery status before surgery.

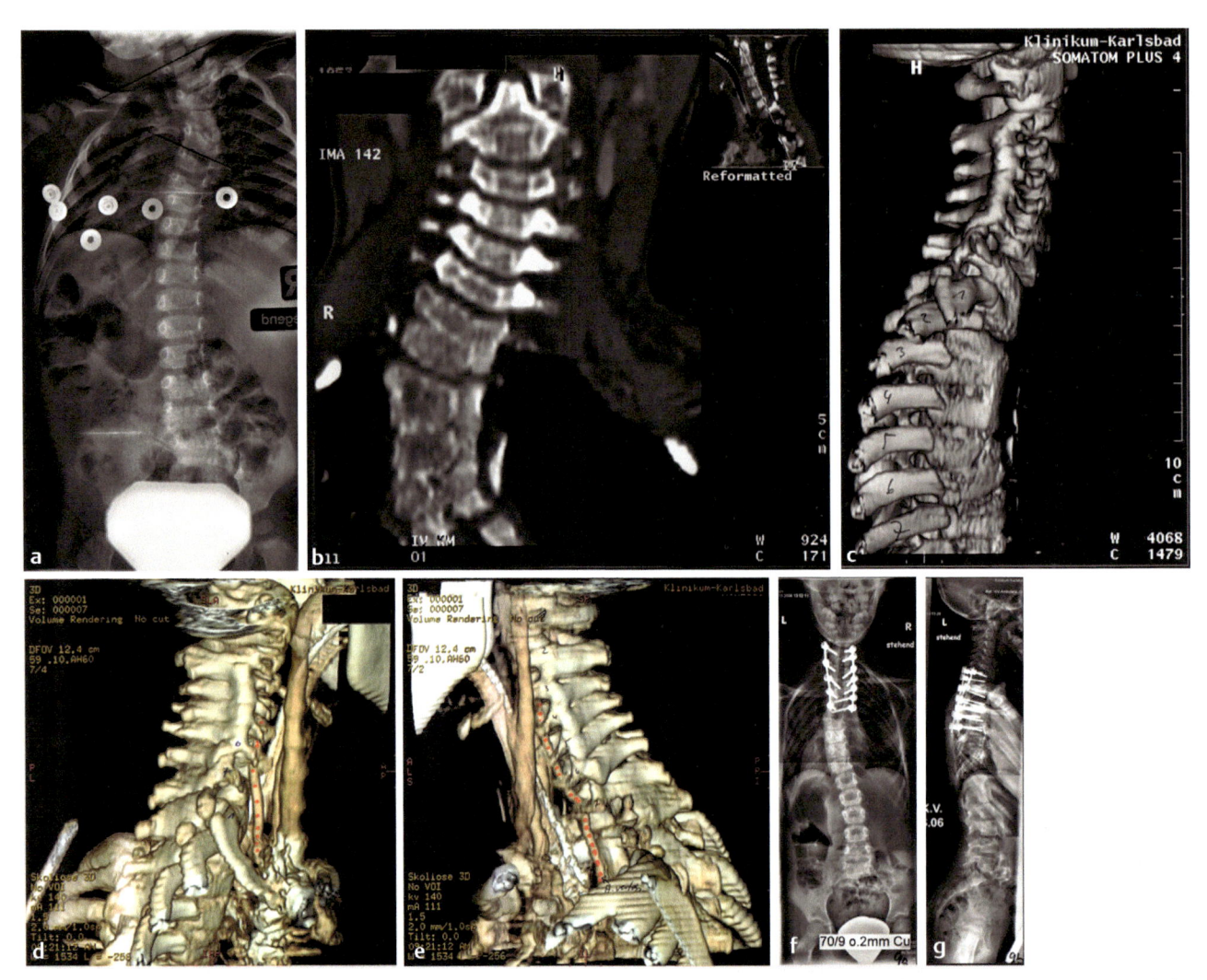

Fig. 6.73 (a) PA radiograph showing several block vertebrae with hemivertebrae at T2 and T4, and a contralateral unilateral bar with its associated rib fusions. (b) PA plain tomogram and (c) lateral 3D CT scan showing that the C7 and T1 are a block vertebra segmented from T2/T3 block vertebra with the hemivertebra at T4 fused to T5. (d,e) 3D CT angiography showing the major neck vessels and in particular that the vertebral arteries are not anomalous. (f,g) PA and lateral radiographs after apical wedge resection through the entire spine including the bar showing an excellent correction at follow-up 2 years later.

Case 3: Lower Lumbar/Lumbosacral Anomalies

See ▶ Fig. 6.74. The key to surgery here is providing a stable square base for the spine above which has been achieved by wedge resection of L4/5 and local instrumentation only.

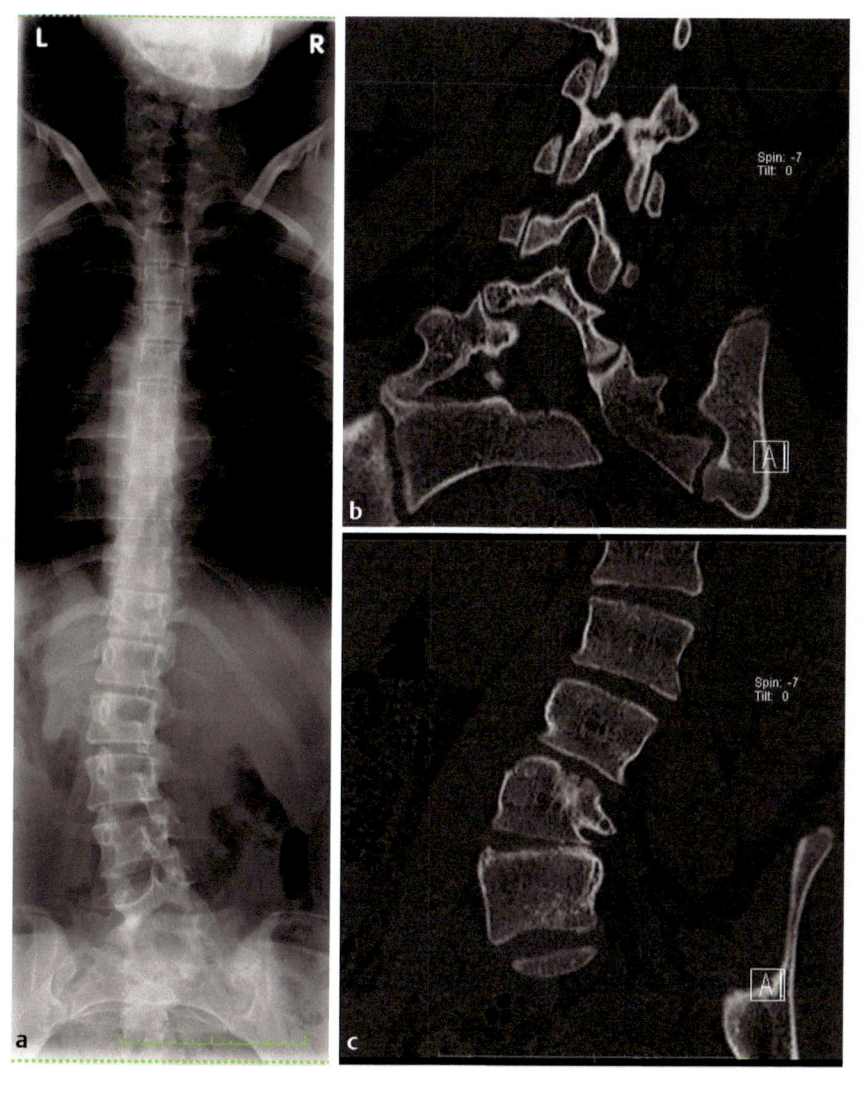

Fig. 6.74 (a) PA full length spine radiograph showing what appears to be unilateral sacralization of L5 tilting the spine above to the left. (b) PA CT scan of the lumbosacral spine showing the asymmetric transverse process/lateral masses of L5 with a fibrous joint to the ala of the sacrum on the right side. This boy was 12 years old in his prepubertal growth phase. (c) PA CT slice through the lower lumbar spine showing deformation of the L4 vertebral body favoring the right side.

Congenital Deformities

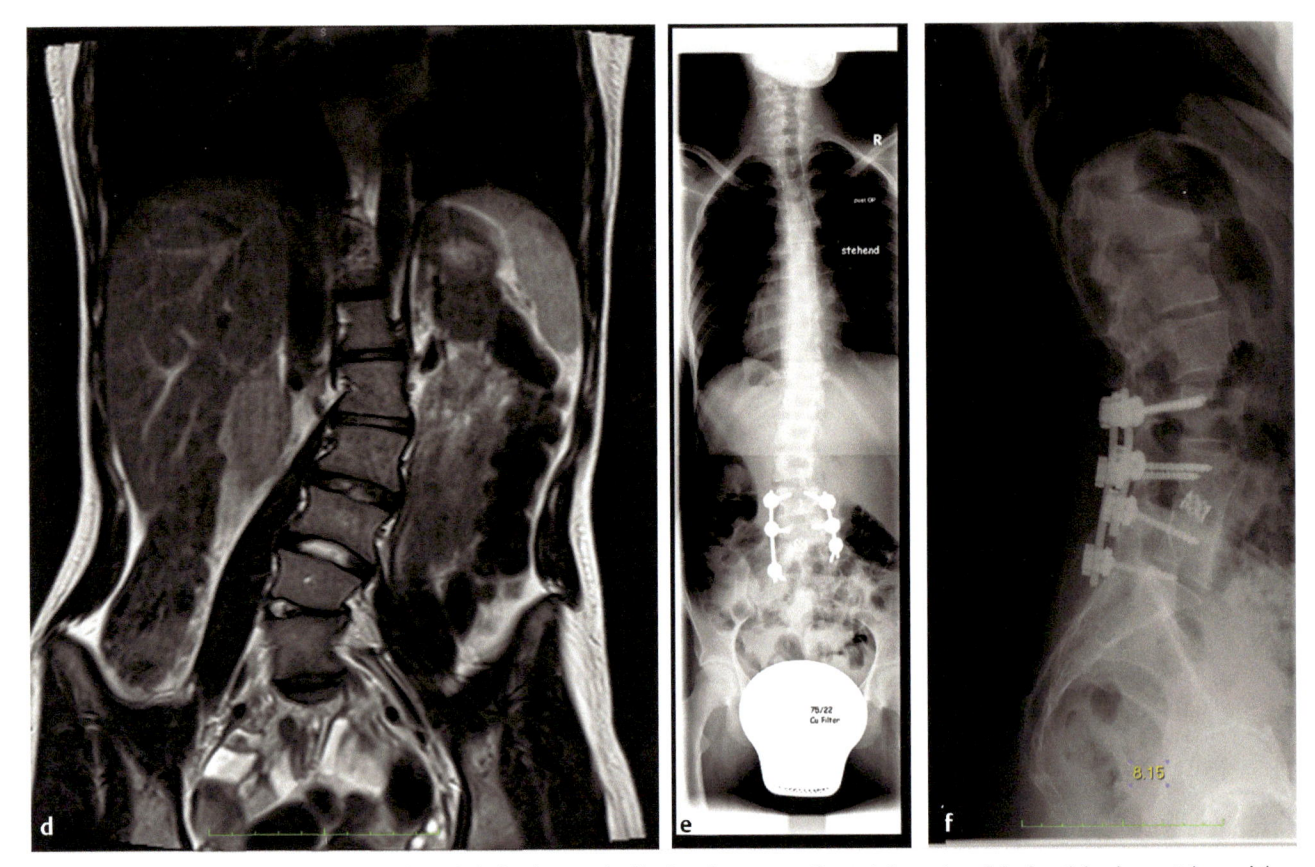

Fig. 6.74 (*continued*) (**d**) Coronal MRI scan through the lumbar vertebral bodies showing significant deformation of the fourth lumbar vertebra and the compensatory curve above. (**e,f**) PA and lateral radiographs after wedge resection at the L4/5 level and short segment instrumentation showing how nicely the spine has re-stacked above.

Case 4: Thoracic Meningocele

See ▶ Fig. 6.75. This is a 9-year-old boy with a thoracic meningocele but no neurological deficit. There is a T1 hemivertebra above the spinal bifida level angulating the head off to the left. Below that is a thoracolumbar scoliosis. Follow-up was possible immediately after surgery but the boy was unable to leave his country for 6 years thereafter.

Comment

Another of these difficult high thoracic deformities and again it is important to check on the local arterial anatomy going upward. T1 hemivertebrectomy left significant deformity lower down and so correction of the thoracolumbar spine was necessary. A deformed spine with the head angulating off to the left was not an acceptable situation for this boy.

Congenital Deformities

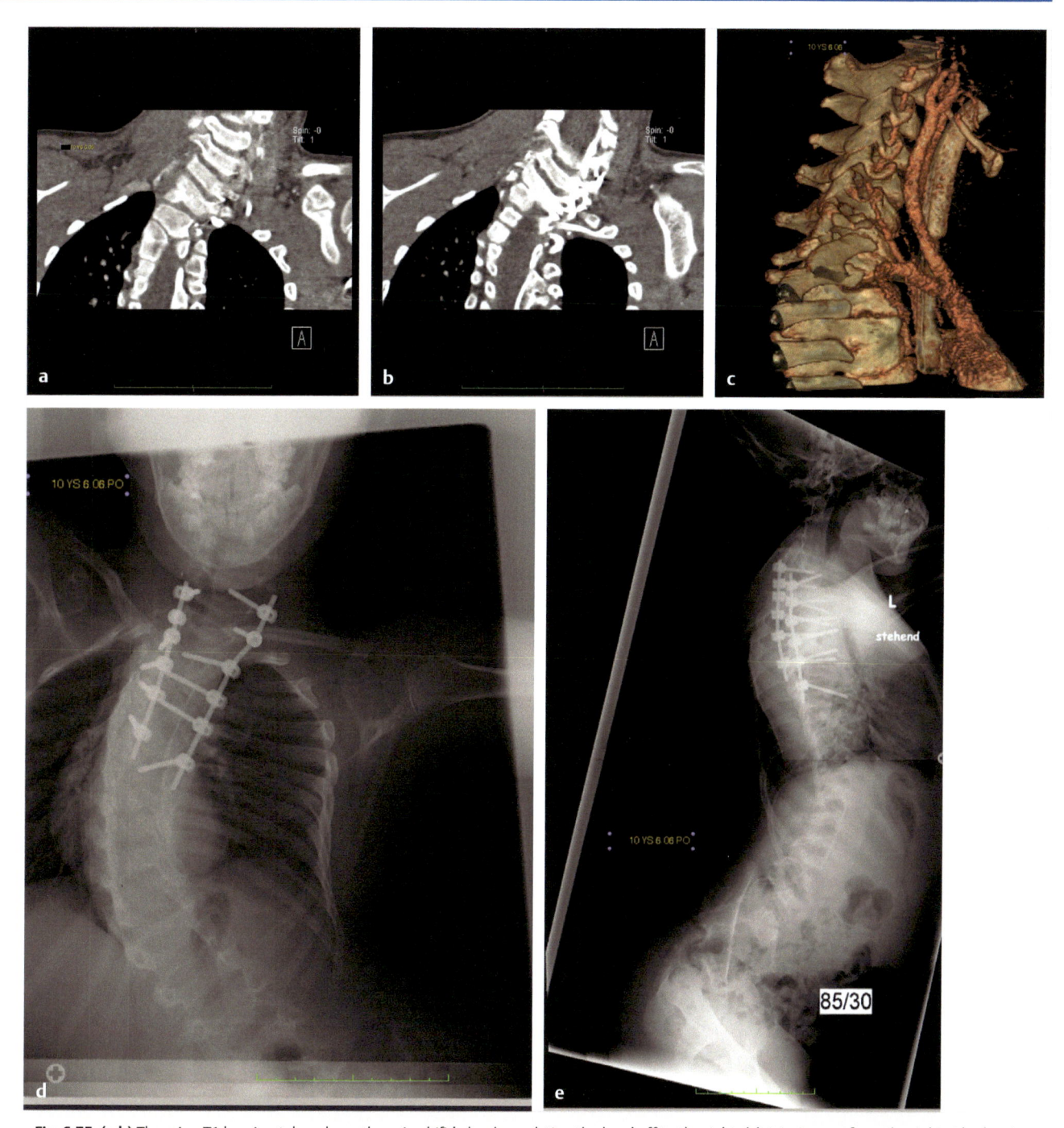

Fig. 6.75 (a,b) There is a T1 hemivertebra above the spina bifida level angulating the head off to the right. (c) Arteriogram from the right side showing the brachiocephalic artery dividing into the common carotid and subclavian which latter gives off the vertebral artery going up into the transverse process foramina. (d,e) PA and lateral radiographs after wedge resection including the hemivertebra and short segment fixation and stabilization.

Congenital Deformities

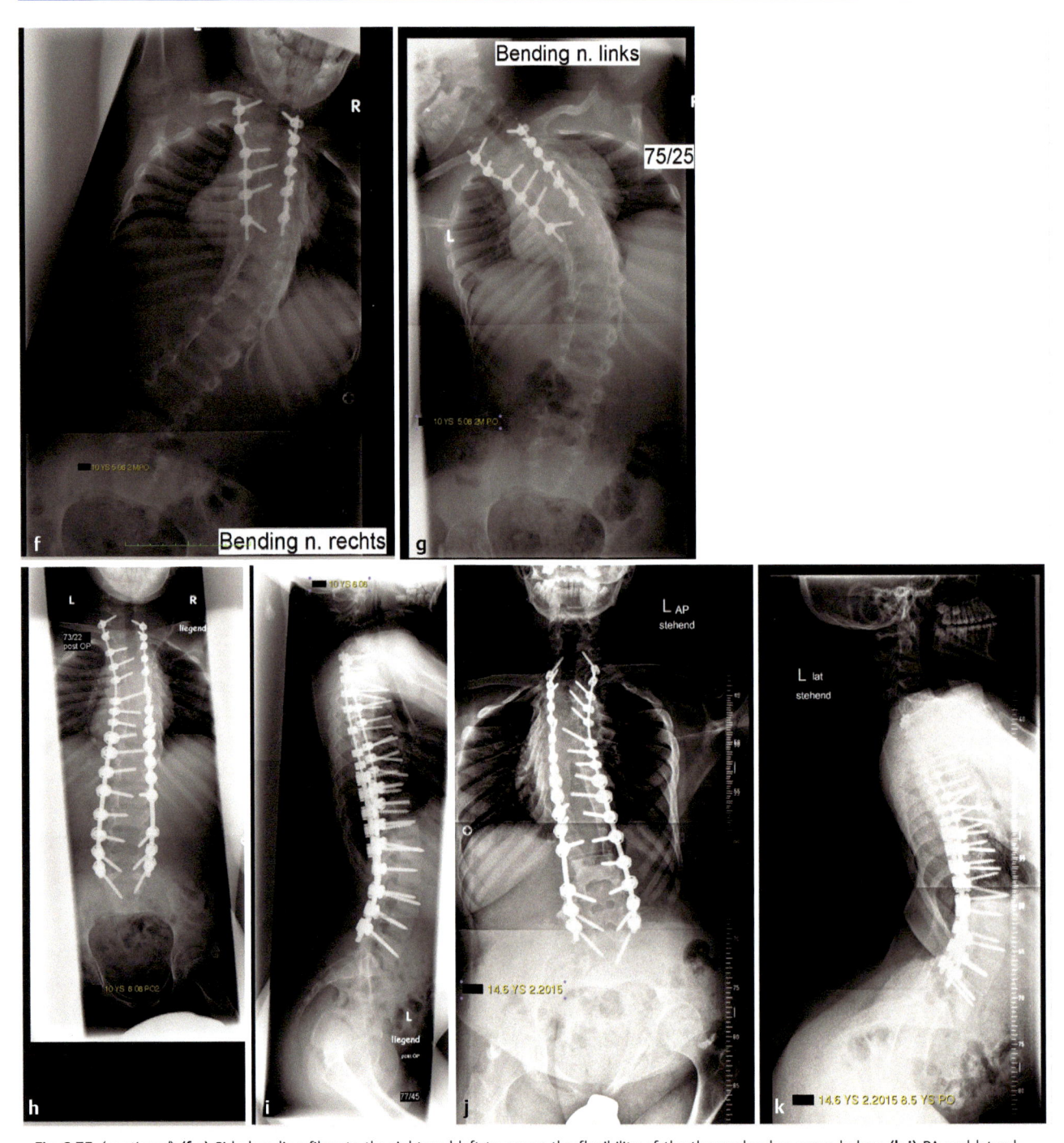

Fig. 6.75 (*continued*) **(f,g)** Side-bending films to the right and left to assess the flexibility of the thoracolumbar curve below. **(h,i)** PA and lateral radiographs post thoracolumbar surgery showing a good balanced correction of the thoracolumbar spine down to L5 and a reasonable sagittal profile. **(j,k)** PA and lateral radiographs 5 years postoperatively showing maintenance of the corrected position.

References

Note: References in **bold** are Key References.

[1] Keen WW, Coplin WML. Sacrococcygal tumour. Surg Gynecol Obstet. 1906; 3:661–671

[2] Bremer JL. Dorsal intestinal fistula; accessory neurenteric canal; diastematomyelia. AMA Arch Pathol. 1952; 54(2):132–138

[3] Fallon M, Gordon ARG, Lendrum AC. Mediastinal cysts of fore-gut origin associated with vertebral abnormalities. Br J Surg. 1954; 41(169):520–533

[4] **Beardmore HE, Wiglesworth FW. Vertebral anomalies and alimentary duplications; clinical and embryological aspects. Pediatr Clin North Am. 1958; 5:457–474**

[5] Bentley JF, Smith JR. Developmental posterior enteric remnants and spinal malformations: the split notochord syndrome. Arch Dis Child. 1960; 35:76–86

[6] Watterson RL, Fowler I, Fowler BJ. The role of the neural tube and notochord in development of the axial skeleton of the chick. Am J Anat. 1954; 95(3):337–399

[7] Sensenig EC. The early development of the human vertebral column. Contrib Embryol. 1949; 33(213-221):21–42

[8] Flint OP. Cell interactions in the developing axial skeleton in normal and mutant mouse embryos. In: Ede DA, et al. (eds). Vertebral Limb and Somite Morphogenesis. Cambridge: Cambridge University Press; 1977:465–484

[9] **Tanaka T, Uhthoff HK. Significance of resegmentation in the pathogenesis of vertebral body malformation. Acta Orthop Scand. 1981; 52(3):331–338**

[10] Dodds GS. Anterior and posterior rhachischisis. Am J Pathol. 1941; 17(6):861–872, 3

[11] Saunders RL. Combined anterior and posterior spina bifida in a living neonatal human female. Anat Rec. 1943; 87:225–278

[12] Prop N, Frensdorf EL, van de Stadt FR. A postvertebral entodermal cyst associated with axial deformities: a case showing the "entodermal-ectodermal adhesion syndrome". Pediatrics. 1967; 39(4):555–562

[13] **Smithells RW, Sheppard S, Schorah CJ, et al. Apparent prevention of neural tube defects by periconceptional vitamin supplementation. Arch Dis Child. 1981; 56(12):911–918**

[14] Feller A, Sternberg H. Zur Kenntnis der Fehlbildungen der Wirbelsäule. Virchows Arch. 1930; 278:566–609

[15] Junghanns H. Die Fehlbildungen der Wirbelkörper. Arch Orthop Unfallchir. 1937; 38:1–24

[16] Bardeen CR. The development of the thoracic vertebrae in man. Am J Anat. 1905; 4:163–174

[17] Wyburn GM. Observations on the development of the human vertebral column. J Anat. 1944; 78(Pt 3):94–102, 2

[18] Peacock A. Observations on the prenatal development of the intervertebral disc in man. J Anat. 1951; 85(3):260–274

[19] Tanaka T, Uhthoff HK. The pathogenesis of congenital vertebral malformations. A study based on observations made in 11 human embryos and fetuses. Acta Orthop Scand. 1981; 52(4):413–425

[20] Valentin B, Putscher W. Dysontogenetische Blockwirbel und Gibbushbildung. Z Orthop Ihre Grenzgeb. 1936; 64:338–369

[21] Ehrenhaft JL. Development of the vertebral column as related to certain congenital and pathological changes. Surg Gynecol Obstet. 1943; 76:282–292

[22] Overgaard K. On Bechterew's disease from the roentgenologic point of view. Acta Radiol. 1945; 26:185–209

[23] Tsou PM. Embryology of congenital kyphosis. Clin Orthop Relat Res. 1977 (128):18–25

[24] **Schmorl G, Junghanns H. The Human Spine in Health and Disease. 2nd ed. New York: Grune and Stratton; 1971**

[25] Lereboullet AC. Recherches sur les monstruosities du brochet observées dans l'oeuf et sur les modes de production. Ann Sci Nat 4 ser. Zoologie. 1863; 20:177

[26] Hertwig O. Urmund und spina bifida. Arch Mikr Anat. 1892; 39:353–504

[27] Bell HH. Anterior spina bifida and its relation to a persistence of the neurenteric canal. J Nerv Ment Dis. 1923; 57:445

[28] Luksch F. Ueber Myeloschisis mit abnormer Darmause Mündung. Z Heilk. 1903; 24:143–156

[29] Gruber GB. Ungewöhnliche neuroenterische Kommunikation bei Rhachischisis anterior und posterior. Virchows Arch. 1923; 247:401: (Pathol Anat)

[30] Johnston TB. Partial duplication of the notochord in a human embryo of 11 mm greatest length. J Anat. 1931; 66(Pt 1):48–49

[31] Fraser JE. Proceedings of the Antatomical Society of Great Britain and Ireland. J Anat. 1931; 66:135

[32] Sparrow DB, Chapman G, Smith AJ, et al. A mechanism for gene-environment interaction in the etiology of congenital scoliosis. Cell. 2012; 149(2):295–306

[33] **Deacon P, Flood BM, Dickson RA. Idiopathic scoliosis in three dimensions. A radiographic and morphometric analysis. J Bone Joint Surg Br. 1984; 66(4):509–512**

[34] **Dickson RA, Lawton JO, Archer IA, Butt WP. The pathogenesis of idiopathic scoliosis. Biplanar spinal asymmetry. J Bone Joint Surg Br. 1984; 66(1):8–15**

[35] **Dickson RA. Idiopathic scoliosis: foundation for physiological treatment. Ann R Coll Surg Engl. 1987; 69(3):89–96**

[36] **Millner PA, Dickson RA. Idiopathic scoliosis: biomechanics and biology. Eur Spine J. 1996; 5(6):362–373**

[37] Winter RB, Moe JH, Eilers VE. Congenital scoliosis, a study of 234 patients treated and untreated. J Bone Joint Surg. 1968; 50A:15–47

[38] Nasca RJ, Stilling FH, III, Stell HH. Progression of congenital scoliosis due to hemivertebrae and hemivertebrae with bars. J Bone Joint Surg Am. 1975; 57(4):456–466

[39] **McMaster MJ, Ohtsuka K. The natural history of congenital scoliosis. A study of two hundred and fifty-one patients. J Bone Joint Surg Am. 1982; 64(8):1128–1147**

[40] **McMaster MJ, David CV. Hemi-vertebra as a cause of scoliosis. J Bone Joint Surg. 1986; 68B:588–595**

[41] Kleinberg p. Scoliosis. Pathology, Etiology and Treatment. Baltimore: Williams and Wilkins; 1951

[42] MacEwen GD, Conway JJ, Miller WT. Congenital scoliosis with a unilateral bar. Radiology. 1968; 90(4):711–715

[43] Kuhns JG, Hormel RS. Management of congenital scoliosis: review of 170 cases. Arch Surg. 1952; 65:250–263

[44] Billing EL. Congenital scoliosis: an analytical study of its natural history. J Bone Joint Surg. 1955; 37A:404–405

[45] Wax JR, Watson WJ, Miller RC, et al. Prenatal sonographic diagnosis of hemivertebrae: associations and outcomes. J Ultrasound Med. 2008; 27(7):1023–1027

[46] Winter RB, Moe JH, MacEwen GD, et al. The Milwaukee Brace in the nonoperative treatment of congenital scoliosis. Spine. 1976; 1:85–96

[47] **Winter RB, Moe JH. The results of spinal arthrodesis for congenital spinal deformity in patients younger than five years old. J Bone Joint Surg Am. 1982; 64(3):419–432**

[48] **Leatherman KD. The management of rigid spinal curves. Clin Orthop Relat Res. 1973(93):215–224**

[49] **Roaf R. The treatment of progressive scoliosis by unilateral growth arrest. J Bone Joint Surg Br. 1963; 45(4):637–651**

[50] Winter RB. Convex anterior and posterior hemiarthrodesis and hemiepiphyseodesis in young children with progressive congenital scoliosis. J Pediatr Orthop. 1981; 1(4):361–366

[51] Winter RB, Lonstein JE, Denis F, Sta-Ana de la Rosa H. Convex growth arrest for progressive congenital scoliosis due to hemivertebrae. J Pediatr Orthop. 1988; 8(6):633–638

[52] Walhout RJ, van Rhijn LW, Pruijs JE. Hemi-epiphysiodesis for unclassified congenital scoliosis: immediate results and mid-term follow-up. Eur Spine J. 2002; 11(6):543–549

[53] **Andrew T, Piggott H. Growth arrest for progressive scoliosis. Combined anterior and posterior fusion of the convexity. J Bone Joint Surg Br. 1985; 67(2):193–197**

[54] **Leatherman KD, Dickson RA. Two-stage corrective surgery for congenital deformities of the spine. J Bone Joint Surg Br. 1979; 61-B(3):324–328**

[55] Royle ND. The operative removal of an accessory vertebra. Med J Aust. 1928; 1:467–468

[56] Compere EL. Excision of hemivertebrae for correction of congenital scoliosis. J Bone Joint Surg. 1932; 14:555–562

[57] Von Lackum HL, Smith A de F. Removal of vertebral bodies in the treatment of scoliosis. Surg Gynecol Obstet. 1933; 57:250–256

[58] Wiles P. Resection of dorsal vertebrae in congenital scoliosis. J Bone Joint Surg Am. 1951; 33 A(1):151–154

[59] **Roaf R. Wedge resection for scoliosis. J Bone Joint Surg Br. 1955; 37-B(1):97–101**

[60] Hodgson AR, Stock FE. Anterior spinal fusion a preliminary communication on the radical treatment of Pott's disease and Pott's paraplegia. Br J Surg. 1956; 44(185):266–275

[61] **Hodgson AR. Correction of fixed spinal curves. J Bone Joint Surg Am. 1965; 47:1221–1227**

[62] Dommisse G, Enslin TB. Hodgson's circumferential osteotomy in the correction of spine deformity. J Bone Joint Surg. 1970; 52B:778

[63] Bradford DS, Boachie-Adjei O. One-stage anterior and posterior hemivertebral resection and arthrodesis for congenital scoliosis. J Bone Joint Surg Am. 1990; 72(4):536–540

[64] Houlte DC, Winter RB, Lonstein JE, Denis F. Excision of hemi-vertebrae and the treatment of congenital scoliosis. J Bone Joint Surg. 1995; 77B:159–171

[65] Zidorn T, Krauspe R, Eulert J. Dorsal hemivertebrae in children's lumbar spines. Spine. 1994; 19(21):2456–2460

[66] **Nakamura H, Matsuda H, Konisishi S, Yamano Y. Single stage excision of hemi-vertebrae via the posterior approach alone for congenital spine deformity: follow-up period longer than ten years. Spine. 2002; 27:110–115**

[67] Shono Y, Abumi K, Kaneda K. One-stage posterior hemivertebra resection and correction using segmental posterior instrumentation. Spine. 2001; 26(7):752–757

[68] **Ruf M, Harms J. Hemivertebra resection by a posterior approach: innovative operative technique and first results. Spine. 2002; 27(10):1116–1123**

[69] **Ruf M, Harms J. Pedicle screws in 1- and 2-year-old children: technique, complications, and effect on further growth. Spine. 2002; 27(21):E460–E466**

[70] Ferree BA. Morphometric characteristics of pedicles of the immature spine. Spine. 1992; 17(8):887–891

[71] Zindrick MR, Knight GW, Sartori MJ, Carnevale TJ, Patwardhan AG, Lorenz MA. Pedicle morphology of the immature thoracolumbar spine. Spine. 2000; 25(21):2726–2735

[72] **Ruf M, Harms J. Posterior hemivertebra resection with transpedicular instrumentation: early correction in children aged 1 to 6 years. Spine. 2003; 28(18):2132–2138**

[73] **Hedequist DJ, Hall JE, Emans JB. Hemivertebra excision in children via simultaneous anterior and posterior exposures. J Pediatr Orthop. 2005; 25(1):60–63**

[74] Xu W, Yang S, Wu X, Claus C. Hemivertebra excision with short-segment spinal fusion through combined anterior and posterior approaches for congenital spinal deformities in children. J Pediatr Orthop B. 2010; 19(6):545–550

[75] Garrido E, Tome-Bermejo F, Tucker SK, Noordeen HN, Morley TR. Short anterior instrumented fusion and posterior convex non-instrumented fusion of hemivertebra for congenital scoliosis in very young children. Eur Spine J. 2008; 17(11):1507–1514

[76] Elsebaie HB, Kaptan W, Elmiligui Y, et al. Anterior instrumentation and correction of congenital spinal deformities under age of 4 without hemivertebrectomy: a new alternative. Spine. 2010; 35:E218–E222

[77] Yu Y, Chen WJ, Qiu Y, et al. [Early outcome of one-stage posterior transpedicular hemi-vertebra resection in the treatment of children with congenital scoliosis]. Zhonghua Wai Ke Za Zhi. 2010; 48(13):985–988

[78] Peng X, Chen L, Zou X. Hemivertebra resection and scoliosis correction by a unilateral posterior approach using single rod and pedicle screw instrumentation in children under 5 years of age. J Pediatr Orthop B. 2011; 20(6):397–403

[79] Lenke LG, O'Leary PT, Bridwell KH, Sides BA, Koester LA, Blanke KM. Posterior vertebral column resection for severe pediatric deformity: minimum two-year follow-up of thirty-five consecutive patients. Spine. 2009; 34(20):2213–2221

[80] Yaszay B, O'Brien M, Shufflebarger HL, et al. Efficacy of hemivertebra resection for congenital scoliosis: a multicenter retrospective comparison of three surgical techniques. Spine. 2011; 36(24):2052–2060

[81] **Ruf M, Jensen R, Letko L, Harms J. Hemivertebra resection and osteotomies in congenital spine deformity. Spine. 2009; 34(17):1791–1799**

[82] Marshall RE, Graham CB, Scott CR, Smith DW. Syndrome of accelerated skeletal maturation and relative failure to thrive: a newly recognized clinical growth disorder. J Pediatr. 1971; 78(1):95–101

[83] Tsou PM, Yau ACMC, Hodgson AR. Congenital spinal deformities: natural history, classification, and the roles of anterior spinal surgery in management. J Bone Joint Surg. 1974; 56A:1767

[84] Greig DM. Congenital kyphosis. Edinburgh Med J. 1916; 16:93–99

[85] **James JIP. Kyphoscoliosis. J Bone Joint Surg Br. 1955; 37-B(3):414–426**

[86] Depalma AF, McKeen WB. Congenital kyphoscoliosis with paraplegia. Clin Orthop Relat Res. 1965; 39(39):190–196

[87] **Winter RB, Moe JH, Wang JF. Congenital kyphosis. Its natural history and treatment as observed in a study of one hundred and thirty patients. J Bone Joint Surg Am. 1973; 55(2):223–256**

[88] James JIP. Proceedings: Paraplegia in congenital kyphoscoliosis. J Bone Joint Surg Br. 1975; 57(2):261

[89] Winter RB. Congenital kyphosis. Clin Orthop Relat Res. 1977(128):26–32

[90] Mayfield JK, Winter RB, Bradford DS, Moe JH. Congenital kyphosis due to defects of anterior segmentation. J Bone Joint Surg Am. 1980; 62(8):1291–1301

[91] **Lonstein JE, Winter RB, Moe JH, et al. Neurologic defects secondary to spinal deformity. A review of the literature and report of 43 cases. Spine. 1980; 5:331–355**

[92] Borkow SE, Kleiger B. Spondylolisthesis in the newborn. A case report. Clin Orthop Relat Res. 1971; 81(81):73–76

[93] Matthäus H. Ein Beitrag zur Behandlung der angeborenen Lumbalkyphose. Z Orthop Ihre Grenzgeb. 1974; 112(6):1312–1314

[94] Finnegan WJ, Chung SMK. Complete spondylolisthesis in an infant. Treatment with decompression and fusion. Am J Dis Child. 1975; 129(8):967–969

[95] von Rokitansky KF. Handbuch der Pathologischen Anatomie. Vol 11. Vienna: Braumuller und Seidel; 1844

[96] von Schrick FG. Die angeborene kyphose. Zeitschrift für orthopädische Chirurgie. 1932; 56:238–259

[97] **McMaster MJ, Singh H. Natural history of congenital kyphosis and kyphoscoliosis. A study of one hundred and twelve patients. J Bone Joint Surg Am. 1999; 81(10):1367–1383**

[98] Kim HW, Weinstein SL. Atypical congenital kyphosis. Report of two cases with long-term follow-up. J Bone Joint Surg Br. 1998; 80(1):25–29

[99] **Tsirikos AI, McMaster MJ. Infantile developmental thoracolumbar kyphosis with segmental subluxation of the spine. J Bone Joint Surg Br. 2010; 92(3):430–435**

[100] Zeller RD, Ghanem I, Dubousset J. The congenital dislocated spine. Spine. 1996; 21(10):1235–1240

[101] Campos MA, Fernandes P, Dolan LA, Weinstein SL. Infantile thoraco-lumbar kyphosis secondary to lumbar hypoplasia. J Bone Joint Surg. 2008; 90(8):1726–1729

[102] Raycroft JF, Curtis BH. Spinal curvature in myelomeningocele. Natural history and etiology. In: American Academy of Orthopaedic Surgeons Symposium on Myelomeningocele. St Louis: C.V. Mosby Co.; 1972

[103] Banta JV, Whiteman S, Dyck PM, et al. Fifteen year review of myelodysplasia. J Bone Joint Surg. 1976; 58A:726

[104] Shurtleff DB, Goiney R, Gordon LH, Livermore N. Myelodysplasia: the natural history of kyphosis and scoliosis. A preliminary report. Dev Med Child Neurol Suppl. 1976; 18 37:126–133

[105] Cheuk DK, Wong V, Wraige E, et al. Surgery for scoliosis in Duchenne muscular dystrophy. Cochrane Database Syst Rev. 2007; 24(1):CD005375

[106] **Allen BL, Jr, Ferguson RL. L-rod instrumentation for scoliosis in cerebral palsy. J Pediatr Orthop. 1982; 2(1):87–96**

[107] Hoppenfield S. Congenital kyphosis in myelomeningocele. J Bone Joint Surg. 1967; 49:276–280

[108] Sriram K, Bobechko WP, Hall JE. Surgical management of spinal deformities in spina bifida. J Bone Joint Surg Br. 1972; 54(4):666–676

[109] Lichenstein BW. 'Spinal dysraphism', spina bifida and myelodysplasia. Arch Neurol Psychiatry. 1940; 44:792–810

[110] Ollivier CP. Triate des maladies de la moelle epiniere. 3rd ed. Paris: Crevot; 1827

[111] Perret gov. Diagnosis and treatment of diastematomyelia. Surg Gynecol Obstet. 1957; 105(1):69–83

[112] James CCM, Lassman LP. Spinal dysraphism. An orthopaedic syndrome in children accompanying occult forms. Arch Dis Child. 1960; 35:315–327

[113] Freeman LW. Late symptoms from diastematomyelis. J Neurosurg. 1961; 18:538–541

[114] Till K. Spinal dysraphism. A study of congenital malformations of the lower back. J Bone Joint Surg Br. 1969; 51(3):415–422

[115] James CCM, Lassman LP. Diastematomyelia and the tight filum terminale. J Neurol Sci. 1970; 10(2):193–196

[116] James CCM, Lassman LP. Spinal dysraphism, spina bifida occulta. London, Butterworth, 1972

[117] Guthkelch AN. Diastematomyelia with median septum. Brain. 1974; 97(4):729–742

[118] Hoffman HJ, Hendrick EB, Humphreys RP. The tethered spinal cord: its protean manifestations, diagnosis and surgical correction. Childs Brain. 1976; 2(3):145–155

[119] Belmont PJ, Jr, Kuklo TR, Taylor KF, Freedman BA, Prahinski JR, Kruse RW. Intraspinal anomalies associated with isolated congenital hemivertebra: the role of routine magnetic resonance imaging. J Bone Joint Surg Am. 2004; 86-A(8):1704–1710

[120] Gillespie R, Faithfull DK, Roth A, Hall JE. Intraspinal anomalies in congenital scoliosis. Clin Orthop Relat Res. 1973(93):103–109

[121] Winter RB, Haven JJ, Moe JH, Lagaard SM. Diastematomyelia and congenital spine deformities. J Bone Joint Surg Am. 1974; 56(1):27–39
[122] McMaster MJ. Occult intraspinal anomalies and congenital scoliosis. J Bone Joint Surg Am. 1984; 66(4):588–601
[123] Tredway TL, Musleh W, Christie SD, Khavkin Y, Fessler RG, Curry DJ. A novel minimally invasive technique for spinal cord untethering. Neurosurgery. 2007; 60(2) Suppl 1:ONS70–ONS74, discussion ONS74
[124] Potts MB, Wu JC, Gupta N, Mummaneni PV. Minimally invasive tethered cord release in adults: a comparison of open and mini-open approaches. Neurosurg Focus. 2010; 29(1):E7
[125] Leatherman KD, Dickson RA. The Management of Spinal Deformities. Chapter 6 : Congenital deformities, Figure 6.28 "arthroscopy" of the dural contents. London: John Wright; 1988
[126] Mehta VA, Gottfried ON, McGirt MJ, Gokaslan ZL, Ahn ES, Jallo GI. Safety and efficacy of concurrent pediatric spinal cord untethering and deformity correction. J Spinal Disord Tech. 2011; 24(6):401–405
[127] Reigel DH, Tchernoukha K, Bazmi B, Kortyna R, Rotenstein D. Change in spinal curvature following release of tethered spinal cord associated with spina bifida. Pediatr Neurosurg. 1994; 20(1):30–42
[128] Arnold J.. Myelocyste, Transposition von Gewebskeimen und Sympodie. Beitr z Path Anat u z Allg Path. 1894; 16:1–28
[129] Chiari H. Ueber die Veränderungen des Kleinhirns, des Pons und der Medulla oblongata in Folge von congenitaler hydrocepholie des Grosshirns. Denkschr d K Akad d wissensch in Vienna. 1895; 63:71–116
[130] Lichtenstein BW. Distant neuroanatomic complications of spinal bifida (spina dysraphism). Hydrocephalus, Arnold-Chiari deformity, stenosis of aqueduct of Sylvius etc; pathogenesis and pathology. Arch Neurol Psychiatry. 1942; 47:195–241
[131] Steele GH. The Arnold-Chiari malformation. Br J Surg. 1947; 34 (135):280–282
[132] Garceau GJ. The filum terminale syndrome (the cord-traction syndrome). J Bone Joint Surg Am. 1953; 35-A(3):711–716
[133] Cornips EM, Vereijken IM, Beuls EA, et al. Clinical characteristics and surgical outcome in 25 cases of childhood tight filum syndrome. Eur J Paediatr Neurol. 2012; 16(2):103–117
[134] Hajnovic L, Trnka J. Tethered spinal cord syndrome—the importance of time for outcomes. Eur J Pediatr Surg. 2007; 17(3):190–193
[135] Colombo LF, Motta F. Consensus conference on Chiari: a malformation or an anomaly? Scoliosis and others orthopaedic deformities related to Chiari 1 malformation. Neurol Sci. 2011; 32 Suppl 3:S341–S343
[136] Hall PV, Lindseth RE, Campbell RL, et al. Myelodysplasia in developmental scoliosis. A manifestation of syringomyelia. Spine. 1976; 1:49–55
[137] Hamilton JJ, Schmidt AC. Scoliosis with spontaneous transposition of the spinal cord. Clinical and autopsy study. J Bone Joint Surg Am. 1975; 57 (4):474–477
[138] Carvell JE, Dickson RA. Spontaneous transposition of the spinal cord. J Bone Joint Surg Br. 1982; 64(4):413–415
[139] Klippel M, Feil A. Un cas d'absence des vertèbres cervicales. Nov iconog Salpêtrière. 1912; 25:223–250
[140] Bertolotti M.. Le anomalie congenite del rachide cervicale. Chir organi movimento. 1920; 4:395–499
[141] Haller von A. Icones Anatomical. A Vandenhoek: Gottingen: 1743. Cited In: Winter RB, Lonstein JE, Leonard AS, eds. Congenital Deformities of the Spine. New York: Thieme; 1983
[142] Sprengel OK. Die angeborene Verschiebung des Schutterblattes nach oben. Archiv für Klinische Chururgie, Berlin. 1891; 42:544–549
[143] Hensinger RN, Lang JE, MacEwen GD. Klippel-Feil syndrome; a constellation of associated anomalies. J Bone Joint Surg Am. 1974; 56(6):1246–1253
[144] Eelen H, Fabry G. Congenital scoliosis. A follow-up study. Acta Orthop Belg. 1977; 43(5):585–597
[145] König F. Eine neue Operation des angeborenen Schulterblatthochstandes. Beitr Klin Chir 1914;94:530–537. Cited in Lange M. Orthopädisch-chirurgische Operationslehre. Munich: JF Bergmann; 1951
[146] Schrock RD. Congenital elevation of the scapula. J Bone Joint Surg. 1926; 8:207–215
[147] Inclan A. Congenital elevation of the scapula or Sprengel's deformity: two clinical cases treated with Ober's operation. Cir ortop traum Habana. 1949; 15:1
[148] Green WT. The surgical correction of congenital elevation of the scapula (Sprengel's deformity). J Bone Joint Surg. 1957; 39A:1439
[149] Jeannopoulos CL. Observations on congenital elevation of the scapula. Clin Orthop. 1961; 20(20):132–138
[150] Woodward JW. Congenital elevation of the scapula: correction by release and transplantation of muscle origins – a preliminary report. J Bone Joint Surg. 1961; 43A:219–228
[151] Robinson RA, Braun RM, Mack P, et al. The surgical importance of the clavicular component of Sprengel's deformity. J Bone Joint Surg. 1967; 49A:1481
[152] Digennaro GL, Fosco M, Spina M, Donzelli I. Surgical treatment of sprengel shoulder: experience of the Rizzoli Orthopaedic Institute 1975-2010. J Bone Joint Surg Br. 2012; 94B:709–712
[153] Erskine CA. An analysis of the Klippel-Feil syndrome. Arch Pathol (Chic). 1946; 41:269–281
[154] Gray SW, Romaine CB, Skandalakis JE. Congenital fusion of the cervical vertebrae. Surg Gynecol Obstet. 1964; 118:373–385
[155] Shoul MI, Ritvo M. Clinical and roentgenologic manifestations of the Klippel-Feil syndrome. AJR Am J Roentgenol. 1972; 68:369–385
[156] Southwell RB, Reynolds AF, Badger VM, Sherman FC. Klippel-Feil syndrome with cervical compression resulting from cervical subluxation in association with an omo-vertebral bone. Spine. 1980; 5(5):480–482
[157] Moore WB, Matthews TJ, Rabinowitz R. Genitourinary anomalies associated with Klippel-Feil syndrome. J Bone Joint Surg Am. 1975; 57(3):355–357
[158] Vitko RJ, Cass AS, Winter RB. Anomalies of the genitourinary tract associated with congenital scoliosis and congenital kyphosis. J Urol. 1972; 108(4):655–659
[159] MacEwen GD, Winter RB, Hardy JH. Evaluation of kidney anomalies in congenital scoliosis. J Bone Joint Surg Am. 1972; 54(7):1451–1454
[160] Owen R. The association of axial skeleton defects with gastrointestinal and genitourinary abnormalities. In: Zorab PA (ed). Scoliosis. Proceedings of a Fifth Symposium held at the Cardiothoracic Institute, Brompton Hospital, London. September 1976. London: Academic Press; 1977:209–214
[161] Shaw-Smith C. Oesophageal atresia, tracheo-oesophageal fistula, and the VACTERL association: review of genetics and epidemiology. J Med Genet. 2006; 43(7):545–554
[162] Nader A, Sedivy R. [Rokitansky's first description of a spondylocostal dysplasia, dysostosis]. Wien Med Wochenschr. 2004; 154(19–20):472–474
[163] Jarcho S, Levin PM. Hereditary malformation of the vertebral bodies. Bull Johns Hopkins Hosp. 1938; 62:216–226
[164] Lavy NW, Palmer CG, Merritt AD. A syndrome of bizarre vertebral anomalies. J Pediatr. 1966; 69(6):1121–1125
[165] Moseley JE, Bonforte RJ. Spondylothoracic dysplasia—a syndrome of congenital anomalies. Am J Roentgenol Radium Ther Nucl Med. 1969; 106 (1):166–169
[166] Ramírez N, Cornier AS, Campbell RM, Jr, Carlo S, Arroyo S, Romeu J. Natural history of thoracic insufficiency syndrome: a spondylothoracic dysplasia perspective. J Bone Joint Surg Am. 2007; 89(12):2663–2675
[167] Campbell RM, Jr, Smith MD, Mayes TC, et al. The effect of opening wedge thoracostomy on thoracic insufficiency syndrome associated with fused ribs and congenital scoliosis. J Bone Joint Surg Am. 2004; 86-A(8):1659–1674
[168] Hell AK, Campbell RM, Hefti F. The vertical expandable prosthetic titanium rib implant for the treatment of thoracic insufficiency syndrome associated with congenital and neuromuscular scoliosis in young children. J Pediatr Orthop B. 2005; 14(4):287–293
[169] Teli M, Hosalkar H, Gill I, Noordeen H. Spondylocostal dysostosis: thirteen new cases treated by conservative and surgical means. Spine. 2004; 29 (13):1447–1451
[170] Emans JB, Caubet JF, Ordonez CL, Lee EY, Ciarlo M. The treatment of spine and chest wall deformities with fused ribs by expansion thoracostomy and insertion of vertical expandable prosthetic titanium rib: growth of thoracic spine and improvement of lung volumes. Spine. 2005; 30(17) Suppl:S58–S68
[171] Fette A, Rokitansky A. Thoracoplasty for treatment of asphyxiating thoracic dysplasia in a newborn. J Pediatr Surg. 2005; 40(8):1345–1348
[172] Groenefeld B, Hell AK. Ossifications after vertical expandable prosthetic titanium rib treatment in children with thoracic insufficiency syndrome and scoliosis. Spine. 2013; 38(13):E819–E823
[173] Campbell RM, Jr. VEPTR: past experience and the future of VEPTR principles. Eur Spine J. 2013; 22 Suppl 2:S106–S117
[174] Aarskog D. Pterygium syndrome. Birth Defects Orig Artic Ser. 1971; 7 (6):232–234
[175] Silver W, Steier M, Schwartz O, Zeichner MB. The Holt-Oram syndrome with previously undescribed associated anomalies. Am J Dis Child. 1972; 124 (6):911–914
[176] Goldenhar M. Associations malformaties de l'oeil et de l'oreille, en particular le syndrome dermoids épibulbaire - appendices avriculaires-fistula avris

[177] congenital et ses relations avec la dysostose mandibulo-faciale. J Genet Hum. 1952; 1:243–282
[177] **Tsirikos AI, McMaster MJ. Goldenhar-associated conditions (hemifacial microsomia) and congenital deformities of the spine. Spine. 2006; 31(13): E400–E407**
[178] Sherk HH, Whitaker LA, Pasquariello PS. Facial malformations and spinal anomalies. A predictable relationship. Spine. 1982; 7(6):526–531
[179] Wall JF, Kane WJ. Scoliosis in Apert's syndrome (acrocephalosyndactyly). J Bone Joint Surg. 1974; 56A:1763
[180] Larsen LJ, Schottstaedt ER, Bost FC. Multiple congenital dislocations associated with characteristic facial abnormality. J Pediatr. 1950; 37(4):574–581
[181] Micheli LJ, Hall JE, Watts HG. Spinal instability in Larsen's syndrome: report of three cases. J Bone Joint Surg Am. 1976; 58(4):562–565
[182] Silver HK, Kiyasu W, George J, Deamer WC. Syndrome of congenital hemihypertrophy, shortness of stature, and elevated urinary gonadotropins. Pediatrics. 1953; 12(4):368–376
[183] **Specht EE, Hazelrig PE. Orthopaedic considerations of Silver's syndrome. J Bone Joint Surg Am. 1973; 55(7):1502–1510**
[184] Rinksy LA, Bleck EE. Freeman-Sheldon ('whistling face') syndrome. J Bone Joint Surg. 1976; 58A:149–150
[185] **Drummond DS, Mackenzie DA. Scoliosis in arthrogryposis multiplex congenita. Spine. 1978; 3(2):146–151**
[186] Banta JV, Nichols O. Sacral agenesis. J Bone Joint Surg Am. 1969; 51(4):693–703
[187] Reeve AW, Mortimer JG. Lumbo-sacral agenesis or rumplessness. N Z Med J. 1971; 73(469):340–345
[188] Mongeau M, Leclaire R. Complete agenesis of the lumbosacral spine: a case report. J Bone Joint Surg Am. 1972; 54(1):161–164
[189] Foix C, Hillemand P. Dystrophie cruro-vésico-fessière par angénésie sacrococcygienne. Rev Neurol. 1924; 40:450–468
[190] Smith ED. Congenital sacral anomalies in children. Aust N Z J Surg. 1959; 29:165–176
[191] **Renshaw TS. Sacral agenesis. J Bone Joint Surg Am. 1978; 60(3):373–383**
[192] Johanna B, Evans EB, Eggers GWN. Partial and complete agenesis or malformation of the sacrum with associated anomalies. J Bone Joint Surg. 1959; 41A:497–518
[193] Duraiswami PK. Experimental causation of congenital skeletal defects and its significance in orthopaedic surgery. J Bone Joint Surg Br. 1952; 34-B(4):646–698

[194] Hensinger RN, MacEwen GD. Congenital anomalies of the spine. In: Rothman RH, Simeone FA (eds). The Spine. Philadelphia: WB Saunders; 1975: 157–270
[195] Frantz CH, Aitken GT. Complete absence of the lumbar spine and sacrum. J Bone Joint Surg Am. 1967; 49(8):1531–1540
[196] **Perry J, Bonnett CA, Hoffer MM. Vertebral pelvic fusions in the rehabilitation of patients with sacral agenesis. J Bone Joint Surg Am. 1970; 52(2):288–294**
[197] Wynne-Davies R. Congenital vertebral anomalies: aetiology and relationship to spina bifida cystica. J Med Genet. 1975; 12(3):280–288
[198] Winter RB. Congenital Deformities of the Spine. New York: Thieme-Stratton Inc; 1983:48
[199] Peterson HA, Peterson LFA. Hemivertebrae in identical twins with dissimilar spinal columns. J Bone Joint Surg Am. 1967; 49(5):938–942
[200] Bonicoli F, Delvecchio E. [Scoliosis in monochorial twins (pathogenetic considerations)]. Chir Organi Mov. 1968; 57:178–186
[201] Hattaway GL. Congenital scoliosis in one of monozygotic twins: a case report. J Bone Joint Surg Am. 1977; 59(6):837–838
[202] McKinley LM, Leatherman KD. Idiopathic and congenital scoliosis in twins. Spine. 1978; 3(3):227–229
[203] Haffner J. Eineiige Zwillinge mit symmetrischer Wirbelsäulendeformität. Keilwirbel. Acta Radiol. 1936; 17:529–541
[204] Akbarnia BA, Moe JH. Familial congenital scoliosis with unilateral unsegemented bar. Case report of two siblings. J Bone Joint Surg Am. 1978; 60(2):259–261
[205] Caffey JP. Paediatric X-ray Diagnosis. 5th ed. Chicago: Year Book Medical Publishers; 1957:1109
[206] Rimoin DL, Fletcher BD, McKusick VA. Spondylocostal dysplasia. A dominantly inherited form of short-trunked dwarfism. Am J Med. 1968; 45(6):948–953
[207] Norum RA. Costovertebral anomalies with apparent recessive inheritance. Birth Defects. 1969; 5:326–329
[208] Cantú JM, Urrusti J, Rosales G, Rojas A. Evidence for autosomal recessive inheritance of costovertebral dysplasia. Clin Genet. 1971; 2(3):149–154
[209] Pérez-Comas A, García-Castro JM. Occipito-facial-cervico-thoracic-abdomino-digital dysplasia; Jarcho-Levin syndrome of vertebral anomalies. Report of six cases and review of the literature. J Pediatr. 1974; 85(3):388–391
[210] Bartsocas CS, Kiossoglou KA, Papas CV, Xanthou-Tsingoglou M, Anagnostakis DE, Daskalopoulou HD. Costovertebral dysplasia. Birth Defects Orig Artic Ser. 1974; 10(9):221–226

Chapter 7

Neuromuscular Deformities

7.1	Introduction	*216*
7.2	Cerebral Palsy	*216*
7.3	Poliomyelitis	*221*
7.4	The True Neuromuscular Diseases of Childhood	*224*
7.5	Peripheral Neuropathies, Friedreich's Ataxia, and Arthrogryposis Multiplex Congenita	*225*
7.6	Scoliosis in the True Neuromuscular Diseases	*228*
7.7	The Other True Neuromuscular Diseases	*229*
7.8	Duchenne Muscular Dystrophy	*229*
Case Gallery		*232*

7 Neuromuscular Deformities

7.1 Introduction

The term neuromuscular disease in childhood refers to those conditions generally hereditary that affect the spinal cord, peripheral nerves, neuromuscular junctions, and muscles.[1] This classification can be seen in ▶ Table 7.1.

It is crucially important for the spinal surgeon to understand the fundamentals of these conditions, their prognosis, and their treatment so that the spine is not isolated from the underlying condition. Although cerebral palsy (CP) and poliomyelitis are not strictly "true" neuromuscular deformities in the child, notwithstanding, these conditions can produce significant spinal deformities and thus it is appropriate to describe them in a section on neuromuscular deformities.

7.2 Cerebral Palsy

This refers to all those conditions in which interference with the control of the motor system arises as a result of lesions within the brain. Despite the significant advances made in obstetric and pediatric practice since Little first described perinatal cerebral palsy (CP),[2] along with a significant reduction in neonatal death rate, the incidence of CP has remained much the same with about 2 per 1,000 affected children.[3] Cerebral palsy is caused by a broad group of developmental, genetic, metabolic, ischemic, infectious disorders and others that result in a common group of neurological phenotypes (▶ Table 7.2). CP can be associated with other abnormalities[4] of speech (25–80%), vision (34–80%), and intellect as well as epilepsy (33%) but many individuals with CP perform intellectually well with no evidence of cognitive dysfunction and 60% achieve gainful employment.[5] CP subtypes have historically been considered as being prenatal, perinatal, and postnatal.[6] There is a mortality rate of 10% in the first year while prenatal and perinatal types are clinically manifest by the age of 3 years; 10% of cerebral palsy cases are postnatal.

The Collaborative Perinatal Project in which just over 50,000 children were regularly monitored from in utero to the age of 7 years showed that most children with CP were born at term following uncomplicated pregnancies and deliveries.[7] Antenatal factors causing abnormal brain development were found in more than three-quarters. Asphyxia during delivery was found in fewer than 10% but exposure to maternal infection in utero was a significant risk factor confirmed by raised levels of inflammatory cytokines. Low birth weight was also a significant factor particularly if less than 1 kg.

Physiologically 50% are spastic, 25% athetoid, 7% rigid, 5% ataxic, and the remainder mixed.[4] There are four principal clinical groups: spastic hemiplegia, spastic quadriplegia, extrapyramidal cerebral palsy, and minimal brain dysfunction (maybe just a clumsy child). All hemiplegics are able to walk independently although contractures can produce a poor base for balance and all have one normal hand allowing them to participate in some type of occupation. While the extrapyramidal group demonstrates the involuntary movements of tension athetosis which hinders effective walking, sitting, and head control throughout life compounded by contractures, these are the most intelligent children in the whole range of cerebral palsies. It is behavioral abnormalities, mental retardation, and epilepsy that are the principal obstacles to competitive performance in adult life. In quadriplegia, however, mental impairment is commonly considerable[5] and it is not often to find normal intelligence. There is a close correlation between intelligence and

Table 7.1 Neuromuscular disorders

Spinal muscular atrophy
- Infantile (Werdnig-Hoffmann)
  - Group 1 – severe
  - Group 2 – intermediate
  - Group 3 – mild
- Juvenile (Kugelberg-Welander)

Peripheral neuropathies
- Peroneal muscular atrophy
  - Charcot-Marie-Tooth
  - Neuronal atrophy variant
  - Roussy-Lévy
- Hypertrophic polyneuritis
  - Dejerine-Sottas
  - Refsum's form
  - Dominant spastic form

Friedreich's ataxia
Arthrogryposis
The muscular dystrophies
- Duchenne
- Becker
- Limb girdle
- Facio-scapulo-humeral
- Congenital muscular dystrophy

Congenital myopathies
Familial dysautonomia
Malignant hyperpyrexia

Table 7.2 Classification of cerebral palsy and major causes

Motor syndrome	Neuropathology	Major causes
Spastic diplegia	Periventricular leukomalacia (PVL)	Prematurity Ischemia Infection Endocrine/metabolic (e.g., thyroid)
Spastic quadriplegia	PVL Multicystic encephalomalacia Malformations	Ischemia, infection Endocrine/metabolic, general developmental
Hemiplegia	Stroke in utero or neonatal	Thrombophilic disorders Infection Genetic/development Periventricular hemorrhagic infarction
Extrapyramidal (athetoid, dyskinetic)	Pathology: putamen, globus pallidus, thalamus, basal ganglia	Asphyxia Kernicterus Mitochondrial Genetic/metabolic

Source: With permission from Johnston MV. Encephalopathies. In: Kliegman RM, Behrman RE, Jenson HB, Stanton BF, eds. Nelson Textbook of Pediatrics. 18th ed. Philadelphia: Saunders Elsevier; 2008:2494.

physical handicap and this is particularly important as regards treatment because patient enthusiasm and drive are essential to a successful rehabilitation program[8] and psychological help is therefore necessary to optimize the program. The role of the educational psychologist is extremely important to assess and advise child, family, and surgeon. As a result of the Warnock report in the United Kingdom (a government report on the Education of Handicapped Children and Young People in 1978) appreciably more children have gone to their local school albeit with appropriate support,[9] demonstrating the essential requirement for good team work. Consequently, a multidisciplinary approach including social as well as physical and academic development is necessary to address treatment for these patients in a holistic fashion. At the same time, it is important to appreciate that 25% of patients can attend ordinary schools while a further 25% are so retarded that permanent sheltered residential conditions are required. Minimal brain dysfunction may be the lesion in a substantial number of mentally retarded children. It is very important for the orthopaedic surgeon to appreciate that at least 50% of all children with CP have a significant sensory impairment and so surgeons should not be under the illusion that the problem is essentially a motor one.[10]

Computed tomography (CT) or magnetic resonance imaging (MRI) may show an atrophic cerebral hemisphere with a dilated lateral ventricle contralateral to the side of the affected extremities in diplegia although MRI is far more sensitive than CT for most lesions in CP.[11]

7.2.1 General Orthopaedic Principles

The basic underlying principles governing the orthopaedic management of neuromuscular conditions are probably known to all orthopaedic surgeons but a more comprehensive knowledge (although not detailed) is required to set the scene for spinal deformities. Getting this additional knowledge (and understanding it) is not easy and, for example, James Robb's chapter in *Children's Orthopaedics and Fractures*[12] is a must-read providing us with so much important information in such a short and readable text. (There will be many more chapters in pediatric orthopaedic textbooks that you can look at but this one is particularly good.) Deformities may be mobile or fixed due to disorganized posture, balance, and movement. Delay in acquiring motor skills means that these appear late and maybe fewer than normal. If equilibrium is poor, then movement may not be able to be initiated even though voluntary motion is possible. Postural control of the trunk and head are crucial matters for the orthopaedic spine surgeon because, for surgery with a collapsing CP spine in the sitter, it must be the spine that is causing loss of sitting stability and balance and not retarded postural mechanisms. Normal postures develop as muscles shorten or by a compensatory mechanism to maintain equilibrium. To stand erect may require spasticity as a compensation. It is not isolated muscle groups that are spastic but an imbalance between agonists and antagonists with the effect that the weaker antagonist produces deformity that can be well seen at the hip.

Gait is particularly important to understand in the ambulatory CP patient which is very difficult with multiple lower limb joint deformities. Robb recommends physiotherapy records with the use of gait scores, such as the Edinburgh Gait Score.[13]

In addition to gait analysis, it is particularly important to examine gait in detail and a comprehensive evaluation would include kinematics, kinetics, energy consumption, and dynamic electromyography. Interestingly gait analysis was first used clinically to optimize management in CP children.[14] This is the area that is really important for the orthopaedic spine surgeon. Assessment of sitting stability prior to surgery is relatively straightforward but which walkers merit correction and fusion of their scoliosis is much more difficult to define particularly in those with already difficult walking ability.

Surgery in such cases can render the ambulatory patient unable to walk which was pointed out in the very responsible article by Lonstein from Minneapolis.[15] Understanding more about the complexities of gait by way of this comprehensive gait evaluation would be very important here before surgery as for the walker it would be easy to do more harm than good. A preoperative trial in a brace or cast to see the effect on ambulation would seem a rather simplistic notion but may be very useful in doubtful cases.

"The aim of clinical examination and gait analysis is to define a list of biomechanical problems apart from the neurological disorder"[12] and therefore an important aim in the management of patients with CP involves control of posture and daily activities during which the available range of joint movement and muscle length should be used. "Compromises may have to be made between in the balance of benefit from intervention and the disadvantages, for example, standing with the knees bent places a load on the quadriceps which is tiring while straightening the knees can solve this stance phase problem for the patient but may cause difficulties in the swing phase of gait."[12] Orthopaedic procedures for the lower limbs may involve muscle or tendon lengthening, tendon transfers, tenotomy, and bony operations to improve rotational problems, to relocate joints, and neurectomy. Treatment for hip dislocation is indicated for instability, reduced motion, and pain although whether the cerebral palsy hip is really painful is uncertain.[16] Passive physiotherapy stretching and intramuscular Botulinum toxin A, in conjunction with functional and positional orthoses, are part of the therapeutic armamentarium for the appendicular skeleton. As regards the lower limb, adductor tenotomy and obturator neurectomy are important to try and keep the adducted internally rotated and flexed hip in joint with or without additional femoral or acetabular osteotomy and this is certainly going to be very important in trying to maintain walking ability.

The windswept deformity, where there is significant adduction at one hip and abduction at the other (▶ Fig. 7.1), is a typical finding in the nonwalker and necessarily contributes to pelvic obliquity. It is extremely difficult to treat. Graham, one of the real experts in cerebral palsy orthopaedic treatment, found that abduction, bracing, and Botulinum toxin injections were not effective in a comparative trial.[17] However "one hip in and one hip out" is not a satisfactory endpoint. Treatment for this situation is very difficult but left untreated does lead to pelvic obliquity which is a very undesirable platform for the spinal deformity above and can cause great difficulty with perineal hygiene. In this regard the complex lumbopelvic movements required for ambulation can be markedly disrupted by making the thoracolumbar spine straight but absolutely stiff with surgery.[15]

Of course while the orthopaedic spine surgeon may well be consulted when the child is at an early age if the degree of

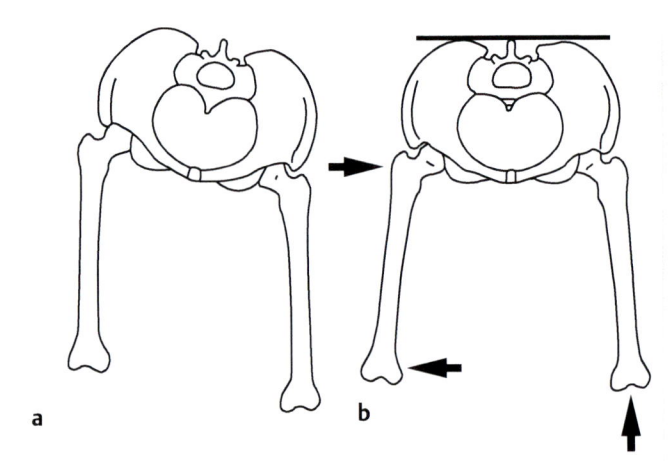

Fig. 7.1 Windswept deformity in cerebral palsy. (a) One hip adducted the other abducted, a common cause of pelvic obliquity. (b) The treatment aim would be to surgically get the hip on the high side abducted and contained to try and square the pelvis. (Reproduced with the permission from Springer Publishing, Children's Orthopaedics and Fractures, 3rd Ed, Eds Benson M, Fixsen J, Macnicol M, Parsch K, Chapter 3, Fig 3.6.)

cerebral palsy is severe, most often it is the adverse effect of growth that leads to presentation to the scoliosis surgeon and by this time the patient will have been seen and treated perhaps on many occasions by his pediatric orthopaedic surgical colleague in which case it will be imperative to review the overall aims and objectives for that particular patient so that the scoliosis surgery fits into a sensible and comprehensive treatment schedule. Of course those with minimal brain dysfunction and a spinal deformity that will not trouble function should not be ignored as such individuals surely deserve the same sort of attention to the psychosocial aspects of deformity and their effect on personal dignity as the patient with idiopathic scoliosis.

7.2.2 The Spine in Cerebral Palsy

Robson looked at the prevalence rate of scoliosis in adolescents and young adults with CP and examined 152 diplegics and athetoids.[18] There were 73 deformities of which half were structural and the remainder related to pelvic obliquity.

Males and females were equally represented. Balmer and McKeown looked at 100 children with CP and found 21 with a scoliosis measuring 10 degrees or more, only 2 of which were larger than 60 degrees.[19] The biggest group of children with CP was studied by Samilson and Bechard and of 906 children 232 had a spinal deformity, of which 193 were spastic quadriplegics.[20] The most severe curves were in the thoracolumbar region, compounded in the majority of cases by either a fixed pelvic obliquity or a hip contracture or dislocation (▶ Fig. 7.2). One New York group found the prevalence rate of scoliosis with CP to be of the order of 40%, with only one case greater than 40 degrees.[21]

Early experience of surgery for CP scoliosis focused on posterior fusion with Harrington instrumentation.[22] However, whereas the polio thoracolumbar C-shaped collapsing scoliosis does remain flexible for a longish period of time, the same cannot be said for the much more rigid cerebral palsy curve. Accordingly, there is a trend for the more severe curves to be dealt with by a preliminary anterior instrumentation stage. Dwyer invented the anterior instrumentation that bears his name[23] and indeed it was first designed for the treatment of thoracolumbar and lumbar idiopathic curves but many scoliosis surgeons were concerned about going anteriorly for idiopathic cases and so it gained popularity as an initial anterior instrumentation and fusion worldwide for neuromuscular curves, including CP. The principle behind this was that with secure fixation and fusion down to L5 then this favorably corrected pelvic obliquity because of the attachment of L5 to S1 by the immensely strong iliolumbar and lumbosacral ligaments. Then in the second stage segmental spinal instrumentation posteriorly allowed the back of the spine to be stacked up above this solid base (▶ Fig. 6.50g and ▶ Fig. 7.3).

In the early 1980s Lonstein and Akbarnia reported the Minneapolis experience of 109 scolioses in CP and mental retardation.[15] They noted the important difference between balanced and unbalanced curve configurations which comprised 44 and 63, respectively, of the 107 CP patients with a scoliosis. Traction was of no benefit, not surprisingly. For balanced curves not involving the sacrum a posterior approach alone sufficed and of course these were ambulatory patients toward the mild end of the CP spectrum. For unbalanced curves involving the pelvis, both anterior and posterior approaches were necessary but complications occurred in more than 80% of patients making scoliosis surgery for CP scoliosis a very important risks and rewards equation. Some who were walkers were rendered wheelchair bound by stiffening the lumbar spine in an area where the somewhat bizarre lumbopelvic spinal movements are required for ambulation. They emphasized that the best indication for surgery in CP was the patient with the unbalanced curve down to the pelvis who was a permanent sitter and was losing sitting stability and, of course, to aid perineal hygiene. With the advent of segmental wiring to posterior L rods[24] it was thought that perhaps this more rigid posterior procedure would suffice but of the 27 patients so treated 10 required an additional anterior procedure.[15]

Then in the early 1980s Zielke in Germany brought out an updated anterior metalwork system[25] which gradually replaced the Dwyer. So it came to be that surgery for balanced curves not involving the pelvis treatment was by single-stage posterior segmental instrumentation while for the unbalanced collapsing C-shaped thoracolumbar curves anterior and posterior instrumentation and fusion became the norm in all but the most moderate and flexible cases (▶ Fig. 6.50g and ▶ Fig. 7.3). It is however the *very devil* to obtain a lumbosacral fusion in paralytic scoliosis and, indeed, the excellent John Hall in Boston told us that that he didn't think he had ever managed to achieve an L5/S1 fusion in such cases.

Neuromuscular Deformities

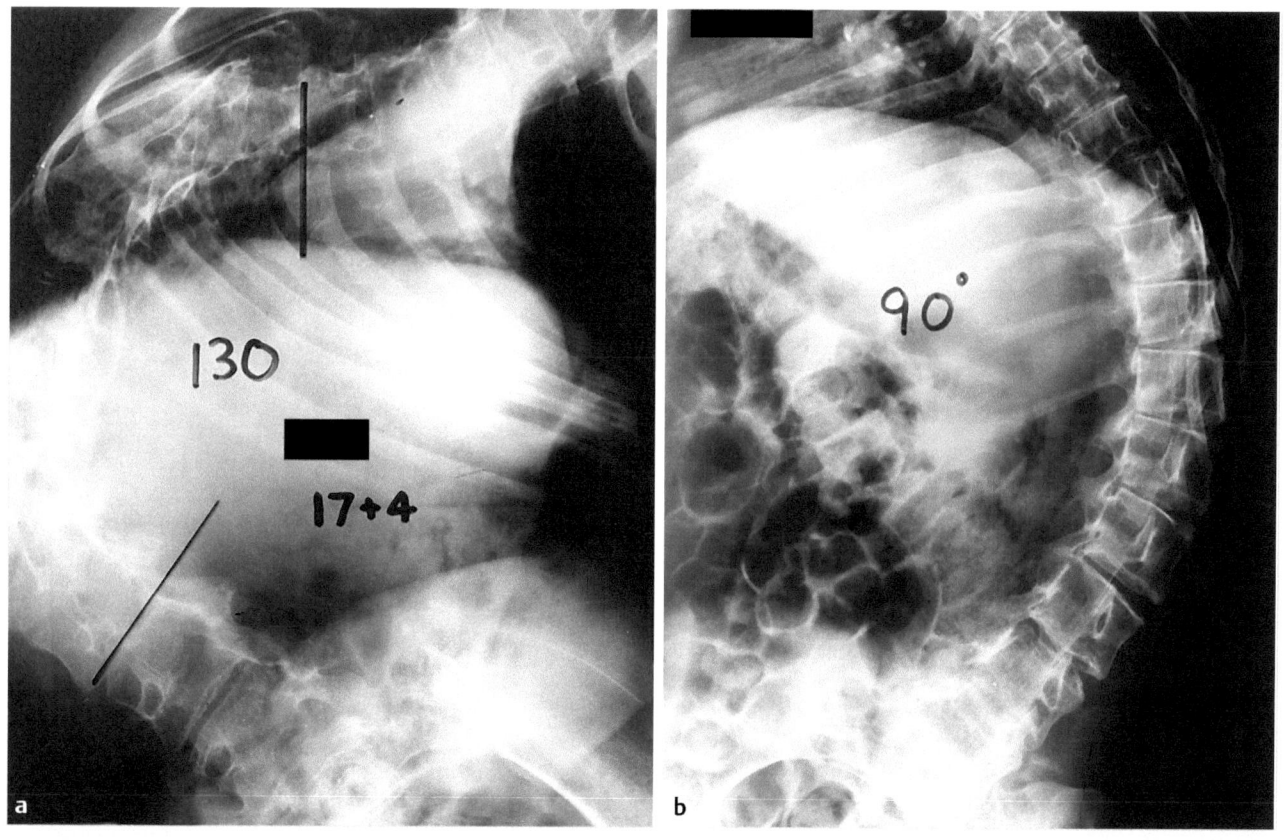

Fig. 7.2 (a,b) Two severe thoracolumbar collapsing C-shaped curves down to fixed pelvic obliquity. These two teenagers had always been bed-ridden. They were pain free. Surgery was neither indicated nor prescribed.

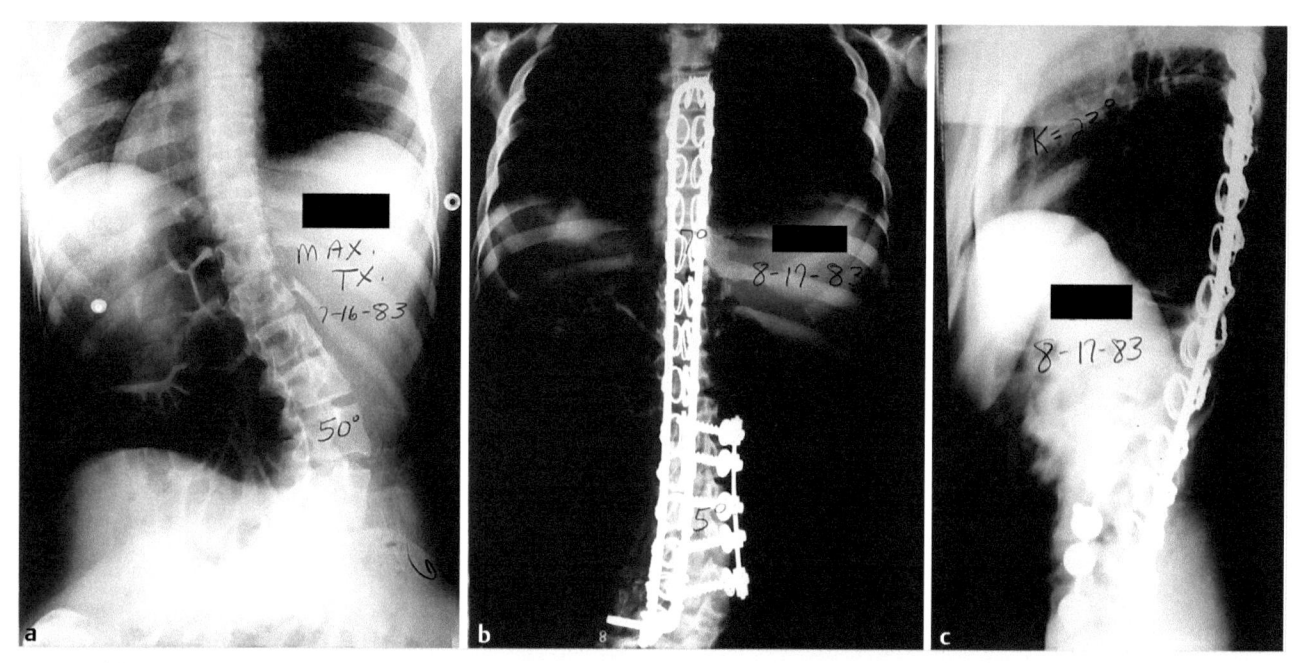

Fig. 7.3 (a) Maximum traction PA X-ray of a C-shaped thoracolumbar curve with pelvic obliquity showing better than expected flexibility. **(b,c)** PA and lateral X-rays after anterior Zielke instrumentation and fusion and posterior unit rod fixation to the sacrum. Anterior and posterior instrumentation and fusion ensured this excellent correction was maintained.

Neuromuscular Deformities

Debate continued however about fixation to the sacrum as it became quite clear that sacral bone did not appear to be strong enough and the L5/S1 joint was very difficult to fuse in neuromuscular cases. Alan and Ferguson addressed this by developing transiliac metalwork extension into the pelvis, referred to as the Galveston technique, and focused particularly on CP and poliomyelitis cases[26] (▶ Fig. 7.4). They demonstrated improved results in having a more securely instrumented base for the construct and fusion above.

In 1991 the Minneapolis experience was published of 68 cases of neuromuscular scoliosis and pelvic obliquity corrected by the Luque-Galveston procedure.[27] Thirty-four had CP and the other 34 had other neuromuscular diseases. The average age at surgery was 14 years and 20 patients had an anterior fusion without instrumentation. The scoliosis averaged 73 degrees before surgery and 33 degrees at a minimum 4-year follow-up. Those having their preliminary anterior diskectomy had a more severe scoliosis and greater pelvic obliquity but the percentage correction was similar. There were instrumentation problems in just over 20% but only four had broken rods and there were no broken wires. Seven had pseudarthroses. Three patients had minor transient neurological problems. They concluded by saying that the Luque-Galveston procedure was the most effective available method of treatment for neuromuscular spine deformities requiring fusion to the sacrum. In addition, anterior fusion from T10 to the sacrum reduces the pseudarthrosis rate and improves the correction of scoliosis and pelvic obliquity. So that was the state of play in the 1990s—but, in scoliosis surgery, the status quo never lasts for long.

When the Luque construct was introduced there were two L rods with the shorter L angulated down into the ilium. Separate, unlinked rods could however swivel or translate with respect to one another, leading to a loss of curve correction and pelvic obliquity and so a one piece "unit rod" construct was developed.[28] This one piece unit rod comprised two L rods with a U connection at the top to provide greater stability and maintenance of correction of both the spinal curvature and the pelvic obliquity (▶ Fig. 7.3). Then came a report of a comparative study of 15 patients treated with a unit rod construct versus 15 treated with two L rods.[29] The correction of both Cobb angle and pelvic obliquity was much greater in those treated with the unit rod construct. This second generation segmental instrumentation technique, whether two rods or one-unit rod, continued to dominate the scene. Meanwhile in France a third generation instrumentation system was being developed by Cotrel and Dubousset whereby with the use of two rods and hooks distraction and compression could be applied on the same rod at different sites.[30] This is the prototype for all subsequent third generation systems albeit now with much greater use of transpedicular fixation particularly in the lower spine. In 2006 the Milan Group published the results of 60 patients with CP treated with CD instrumentation with a mean follow-up of 6.5 years.[31] There were 34 posterior only and 26 anterior and posterior procedures. Scoliosis correction and pelvic obliquity correction were 60% and 40%, respectively. They claimed to have a lower pseudarthrosis rate than with second generation systems. As usual, complications in CP patients were considerable.

The Seoul Group, in a retrospective study of 55 cases, showed that the amount of pelvic obliquity preoperatively mattered as regards the need for and success of pelvic fixation. If pelvic obliquity was greater than 15 degrees, then pelvic fixation was necessary but not if preoperative pelvic obliquity was less than 15 degrees.[32] The results were poor, however, if pelvic obliquity exceeded 15 degrees and there was no pelvic fixation.

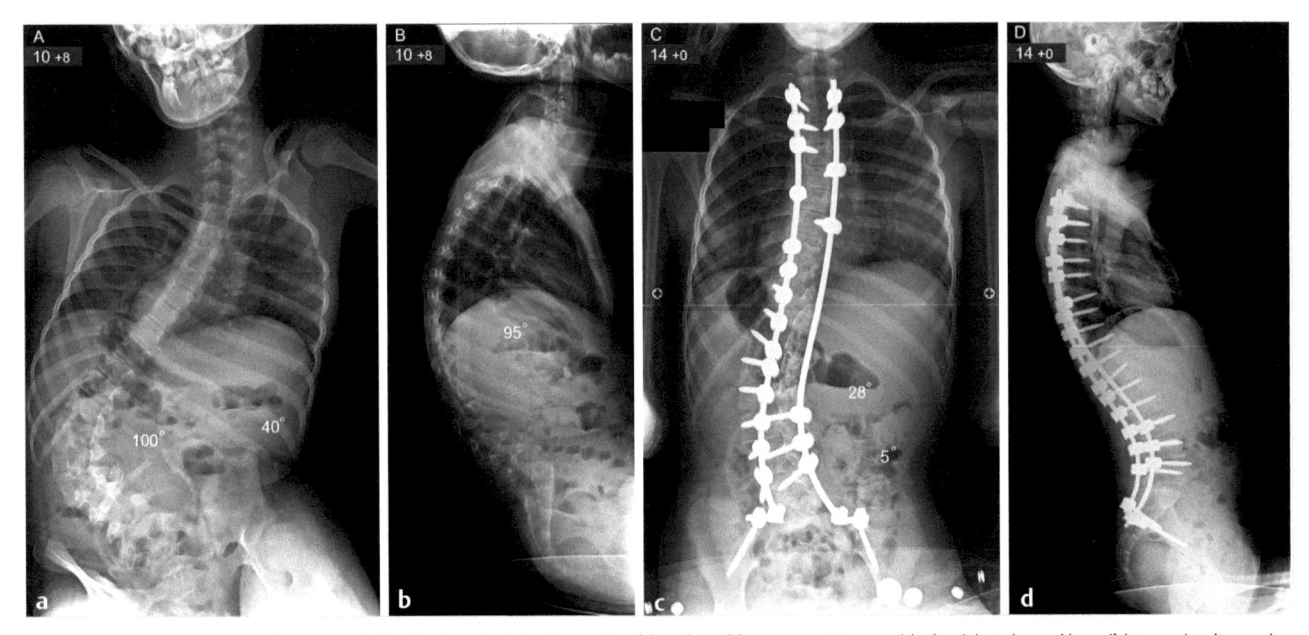

Fig. 7.4 (a) Typical severe collapsing C-shaped lordoscoliosis with considerable pelvic obliquity in a 10-year-old wheelchair-bound boy. (b) Lateral radiograph showing the characteristic pseudokyphotic appearance when lateral X-rays of the patient and not the deformity are taken. (c) PA radiograph at follow-up more than 3 years after long transpedicular fixation down to the pelvis where Galveston-type fixation has been used. There is a superb correction of the scoliosis underpinned by almost complete correction of the pelvic obliquity. (d) Lateral radiograph postoperatively showing a very nice re-creation of a natural sagittal profile. Once the scoliosis is corrected the spine is brought toward the midline and so the lateral X-ray of the patient more closely resembles a true lateral X-ray of the deformity. (We are most grateful to our colleague and friend Professor Thanos Tsrikos for the case shown in Fig. 7.4.)

In a recent review of 52 scoliosis patients with CP who underwent posterior only pedicle screw fixation the Cobb angle was improved from 77 degrees to 32 degrees and the overall pelvic obliquity from 9 degrees to 4 degrees. Interestingly, the mean age of these patients was all of 22 years, very much older than the usual age of 14 years or thereabouts at the time of surgery, and there were two perioperative deaths and one temporary neurological problem! The amount of pelvic obliquity going in being less than 10 degrees certainly wasn't substantial.[33] Others reported good results with transpedicular instrumentation.[34]

Posterior multilevel vertebral osteotomy (average number of osteotomies four) in seven CP patients achieved improvement in Cobb angles and pelvic obliquity from 118 degrees and 17 degrees to 49 degrees and 8 degrees, respectively, without any neurological or vascular injuries and with no postoperative ventilatory support required.[35] The mean age was all of 21 years and follow-up only 2 years.

In a retrospective study of 61 patients with CP, 19 had a unit rod correction with anterior release compared with 42 without an anterior release. Not surprisingly those who underwent an anterior release had larger curves averaging 91 degrees versus 72 degrees for the posterior only construct. Similarly, pelvic obliquity was 26 degrees in the anterior release and 19 in the posterior only group. Percentage corrections were similar but of course these groups were not really comparable.[36] In a recent study of how beneficial surgery is in spastic CP, 84 patients/families of spastic CP patients responded to a questionnaire and although the overall satisfaction rate was more than 90% functional improvements were much less.[37]

In one study 26 patients underwent posterior only surgery compared with 26 who underwent anterior and posterior surgery; no benefit was claimed for a preliminary anterior release. All patients underwent halo-femoral traction preoperatively.[38] No anterior instrumentation was however used and so unless the anterior tension side is closed down after diskectomies, and therefore shortened with instrumentation, it may be that the maximum benefit of an anterior procedure wasn't achieved.

In 2011 Lonstein published the results of 93 patients instrumented with the Luque-Galveston technique who had CP or encephalopathy with a preoperative scoliosis Cobb angle of 72 degrees corrected down to 33 degrees but there were complications in more than half the patients.[39] However, there were no deaths or neurological complications and only one wound infection. There was a pseudarthrosis rate of 7.5% but most of the complications were relatively minor.

The Edinburgh Group recently published their results of 45 consecutive patients with quadriplegia who underwent pedicle screw instrumentation.[40] All were wheelchair bound with a collapsing thoracolumbar scoliosis and pelvic obliquity. The mean age was 13 years and the scoliosis was corrected from 83 degrees to 21 degrees and the pelvic obliquity from 24 degrees to 4 degrees. These are excellent results (▶ Fig. 7.4). There was no neurological deficit but one deep infection and one reoperation for prominent implants. Very good parent satisfaction was reported. The Swiss Group who looked at health-related quality of life after spinal fusion for patients with CP noted high levels of satisfaction but these did not correlate with objective radiographic improvements.[41]

The Dallas Group reported 53 patients with significant infection after instrumentation for scoliosis—10 had CP while 21 had idiopathic scoliosis.[42] In this group of patients there was a 50% chance that the infection would remain if all the instrumentation was not removed. Coagulase-negative *Staphylococcus* was the organism in nearly 50% of cases and they recommended that prophylactic antibiotic coverage for this organism must be used at the time of the initial spinal fusion.[41]

There is no doubt that when properly indicated and prescribed spinal deformity surgery can be hugely beneficial in terms of quality of life in these unfortunate CP patients.

7.3 Poliomyelitis

Poliomyelitis is an acute infectious disease caused by a neurotropic group of viruses spread as direct person to person contact with infected mucus, phlegm, or feces. Entry is through the mouth and nose and into the intestinal and respiratory tracts and then to the blood and lymph channels to the central nervous system. Both the anterior horn cells of the spinal cord and centers in the brain stem nuclei are involved in the infectious process and it was shown 60 years ago that infected nerve cells undergo chromatolysis and that the pathogenesis was not simply due to inflammatory edema. Bodian also pointed out that as a result the nerve cells are either destroyed or not and only in the latter event was recovery possible.[43] Outbreaks occurred in both the UK and United States in the early 19th century. Major epidemics occurred 100 years later in the 1940s. Routine vaccination has seen very few cases in the Western hemisphere but outbreaks still occur in underdeveloped or developing countries but a huge worldwide vaccination program has left polio cases in only a few places in Africa and South Asia, with a 95% reduction in cases over the past 30 years.[44]

The condition can be subclinical (95%), nonparalytic, or paralytic and there are three traditional phases: the acute phase, the convalescent phase, and the residual phase. During the stage of paralysis that extends from the end of the acute phase through the convalescent phase, musculoskeletal management lies principally in the prevention of deformity. The convalescent phase—when recovery can occur—lasts up to 2 years although most of this recovery occurs in the first 3 to 6 months. It is in the residual phase of paralytic poliomyelitis where orthopaedic deformities may require reconstructive surgery.[45]

Deformities can be fixed or mobile and for mobile deformities physiotherapy and splintage, dynamic or static, are the basis of treatment. Splintage is required to keep the joint in the overcorrected position to prevent recurrence. Although previous generations of consultant orthopaedic surgeons were very often "brought up," so to speak, on the array of conservative and surgical treatment required for poliomyelitis, younger generations have missed this unique experience and would do well with familiarizing themselves about the principles of surgical treatment in poliomyelitis as a background to learning and understanding surgical treatment for the polio spine. A good summary can be found in Chow.[45] Clearly as regards scoliosis the status of the lower extremities is particularly important and again the spine should not be isolated from the other affected joints. These may contribute to or cause pelvic obliquity.

Table 7.3 Pelvic obliquity

Type	Cause
Infrapelvic	Leg length inequality
Transpelvic	Unequal contraction/contracture of iliopsoas
Suprapelvic	Collapsing thoracolumbar paralytic scoliosis

Yount described the abduction deformity due to iliotibial band tightness and indeed recommended division of this band in such circumstances.[46] However, Kaplan did not believe it was a significant deforming force.[47] The hip joint itself dislocating as a result of paralysis with progressive coxa valga is a major factor in producing pelvic obliquity and may require soft tissue or bony surgery according to the stage of the dislocation process.[48] Where pelvic obliquity is really important is in its true causation[49–51] (▶ Table 7.3). There are three types of pelvic obliquity—infrapelvic, transpelvic, and suprapelvic—and more often than not while the hip may contribute to an unstable pelvis the chief deforming force lies with the collapsing spinal deformity above (suprapelvic pelvic obliquity). Suprapelvic pelvic obliquity is the unstable paralytic C-shaped thoracolumbar scoliosis that goes down to the pelvis and causes the pelvic obliquity (down on the convex side) (▶ Fig. 7.4). All too often trying to treat transpelvic pelvic obliquity, such as, the Sharrard transfer of iliopsoas posterior and lateral to the hip joint through a large hole in the ilium,[52] necessarily fails when the real cause of the pelvic obliquity is the collapsing paralytic scoliosis above.

7.3.1 The Spine in Poliomyelitis

It is difficult to determine the prevalence rate of spinal deformity in poliomyelitis but in the 1920s a third of cases of scoliosis were due to poliomyelitis.[53] Fifty years ago in Oxford only 19 of the 321 cases of scoliosis were due to poliomyelitis.[54] There have been several attempts to relate muscle paralysis to curve characteristics.[55–60] The most detailed study was performed by James in 193 patients with polio scoliosis and he compared their muscle function with 280 patients with polio but with no spinal deformity.[57] A total of 118 of his cases were thoracic curves and those with a high thoracic apex had the worst prognosis—the majority going on to develop curves measuring 100 degrees or more by maturity. He noted the high prevalence rate of intercostal muscle paralysis on the convex side. This combined with the characteristic convex rib drooping and crowding clearly differentiated the thoracic polio scoliosis from the idiopathic one and put James very much against the concept that there was a subclinical neuromuscular problem at the heart of idiopathic scoliosis, another nail in the coffin of the neuromuscular advocates. A total of 47 of his curves were thoracolumbar and he incriminated weakness of the lateral abdominal flexor muscles while quadratus lumborum weakness specifically was responsible for his 17 lumbar cases. Only 13 were double structural thoracic and lumbar curves. He noted that the function of the midline muscles (erector spinae and the anterior abdominals) only influenced spinal shape in the sagittal plane. Then in the same journal Roaf reported his experience and considered four types of deformity: the thoracolumbar C-shaped curve, the collapsing combined thoracic and lumbar curve, the primary lumbar curve, and the primary thoracic curve.[58] He observed that the thoracolumbar C curve was mild, not usually rotated, and was due to gravity shifting the trunk toward the weak side. He noted this curve to be a very flexible one and responded well to surgical correction. He also noted that some mild C-shaped curves did go on to the collapsing combined type for which treatment was much more difficult and had to involve an extensive fusion. Interestingly for the primary thoracic curve he felt that closing wedge osteotomy provided a better correction than posterior fusion. Garrett reduced these different types to two groups: those as a result of asymmetric paralysis that produced higher curves and those due to symmetric collapsing paralysis that involved the sacrum with pelvic obliquity and required a fusion to the pelvis.[59] Garrett's two subgroups are probably the best and simplest way of looking at the polio scoliosis spine. Pavon and Manning noted a leg length inequality to be present in at least half of all patients which contributed an infrapelvic mechanism to the suprapelvic pelvic obliquity.[61]

For polio curves not extending down to the pelvis, Milwaukee brace treatment was popular years ago in the hope that the necessary surgical stabilization could be delayed but there is no evidence that this form of treatment was effective and indeed the brace was specifically designed to support the polio spine after surgery and not as a conservative treatment option.[62] Before the era of Harrington instrumentation surgical treatment was a difficult matter, correction being obtained by cast techniques. Then through a window in the back of the cast a posterior fusion was performed with whatever bone could be found, pelvic or tibial.[63] This was then followed by a period of prolonged recumbency followed by mobilization with a spinal support. Not surprisingly the pseudarthrosis rate was high and curve correction disappointing.[64] When Harrington instrumentation began to be used[65] this heralded the era of poliomyelitis distraction instrumentation for the spine and then the Milwaukee brace to support the paralytic spine postoperatively. While the period of recumbency was only of the order of 3 weeks for the instrumented cases, the pseudarthrosis rate was unfortunately unchanged.[66] Meanwhile Dwyer in Australia produced his anterior instrumentation (albeit for idiopathic scoliosis) which appeared to be eminently suitable for the paralytic deformity in polio.[23] Then the Hong Kong Group revolutionized the treatment of the collapsing paralytic polio curve by establishing that both anterior and posterior instrumentation and fusion were necessary with first stage anterior Dwyer instrumentation down to the fifth lumbar vertebra and second stage Harrington instrumentation.[67] Fixation down to the fifth lumbar vertebra influenced the obliquity of the first sacral segment because of the attachment of the immensely strong iliolumbar and lumbosacral ligaments. Thus arose the concept that it was the obliquity of the pelvis which was the primary target for surgical treatment although of course the scoliosis was corrected pari passu. In the second stage there was a long posterior fusion to the sacrum using Harrington instrumentation.[68] In due course the Zielke system was introduced providing more anterior rigidity.[69] Then the segmental instrumentation system devised by Luque in Mexico was developed whereby the generally early flexible polio curve could be managed by one posterior operation.[70] Not surprisingly there was a higher correction rate with a lower complication rate including pseudarthrosis and loss of correction. For cases with particularly severe pelvic obliquity Alan and Ferguson introduced the concept of passing the short arm of the L rod into the pelvis (the Galveston technique).[26]

Two important series of patients with poliomyelitis and scoliosis were published one involving the Hong Kong patients[71] and the other the patients in Taiwan.[72] Leong and colleagues reviewed 110 patients with paralytic scoliosis who were operated upon, 58 had lumbar curves, 26 thoracic curves, 14 long C-shaped curves, 8 had thoracolumbar curves, and 4 had double major curves. These patients had developed polio before the age of 3 years. The average age of surgery was in the early teens. The earliest surgical experience involved Harrington instrumentation only but much better results were achieved with preliminary anterior Dwyer instrumentation followed by posterior fusion at a second stage (▶ Fig. 7.5). Percentage correction of Cobb angle varied from 50% to almost 100% and this related strongly to initial curve angle (53 degrees to 105 degrees). They used traction for bigger rigid curves which of course makes biomechanical sense (the bigger a curve is the more it requires a pull from top and bottom while milder curves require a push from the side) (▶ Fig. 7.6). Posterior fusions alone had a 25% pseudarthrosis rate while with combined anterior and posterior fusions the pseudarthrosis rate was reduced to 7% with none in thoracic curves and 12% in the long C-shaped curves.[71]

The Taiwan Group reported on 118 consecutive patients with post-poliomyelitis paralytic scoliosis.[72] Ninety-two of the cases were double thoracic and lumbar curves and 20 were thoracic and thoracolumbar double structural curves. They looked at

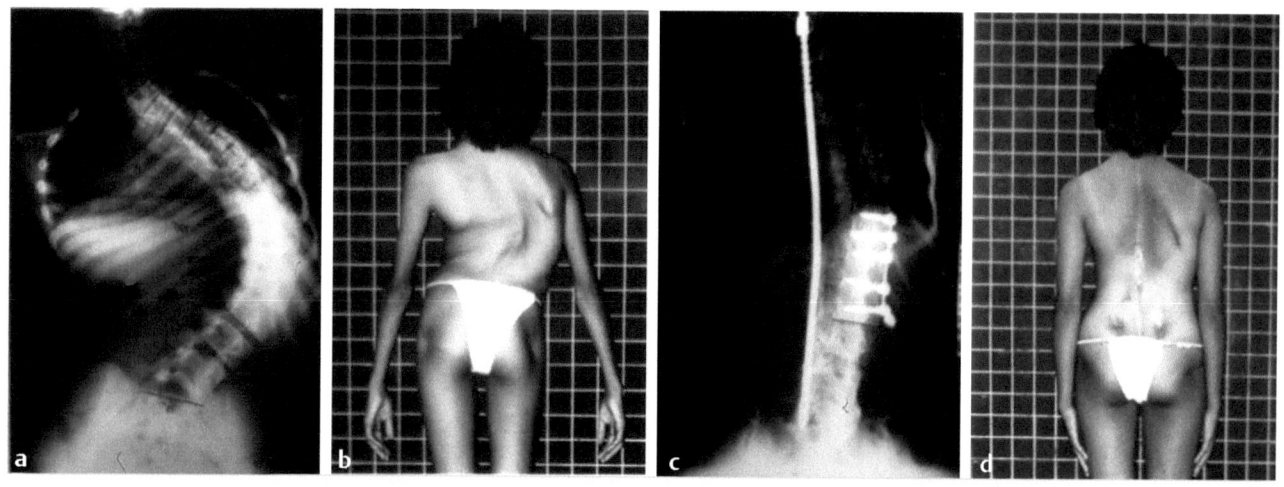

Fig. 7.5 (a) PA radiograph of a low thoracic polio curve in a girl of 14. (b) Clinical view of this significant deformity. (c) After anterior apical Dwyer instrumentation and a long Harrington rod showing an excellent correction and a solid spinal fusion. (d) Clinical appearance 2 years after surgery showing an excellent correction and a well-balanced spine. (We are most grateful to our colleagues Professors John Leong and Ken Cheung for the cases shown in ▶ Fig. 7.5 and ▶ Fig. 7.6.)

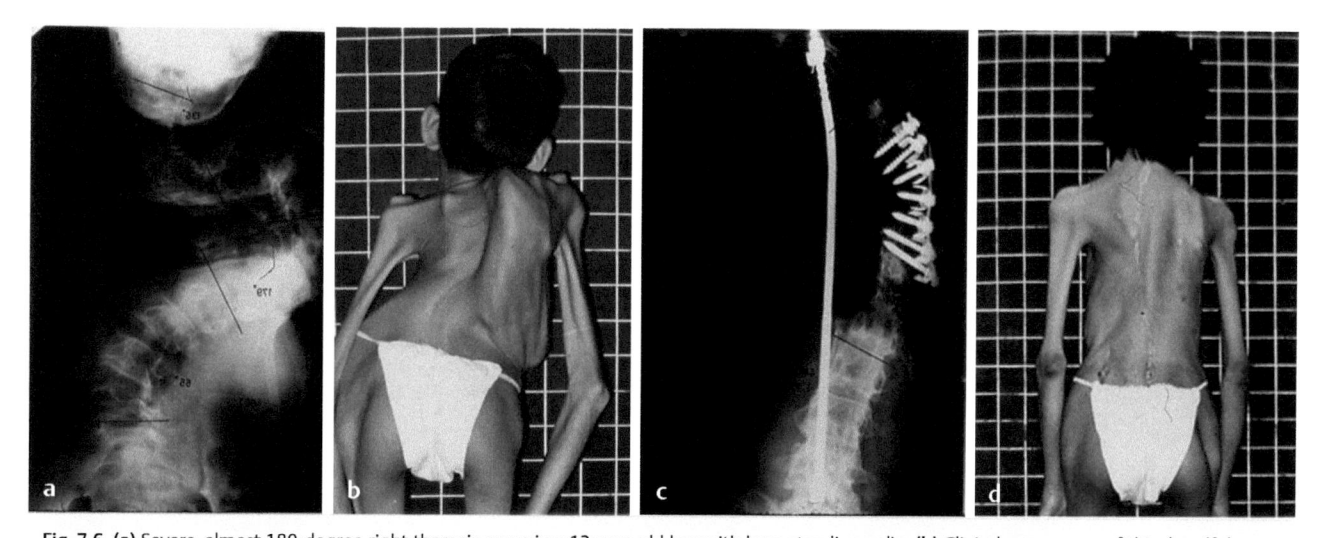

Fig. 7.6 (a) Severe, almost 180-degree right thoracic curve in a 13-year-old boy with long-standing polio. (b) Clinical appearance of this dreadful curve with a rib hump so bad as to warrant the term ridge-back. (c) After interval halo-pelvic traction a PA radiograph after anterior Dwyer instrumentation and a long posterior Harrington rod showing an excellent correction and a solid fusion. (d) Clinical photograph showing an excellent correction and a well-balanced spine. This was 40 years ago and you could hardly get a better correction using modern instrumentation.

those who had a posterior spine fusion with Harrington instrumentation and those who had two-stage anterior spine fusion with Dwyer instrumentation followed by posterior fusion with Harrington instrumentation. The 19 patients who had posterior procedures only had a 44% correction of pelvic obliquity from 28 to 14 degrees. The 82 patients who underwent two-stage anterior and posterior instrumentation and fusion had a correction of pelvic obliquity from 37 degrees to 17 degrees (55%). You cannot compare these sorts of curves with different severities of pelvic obliquity. The upper and lower curves were much greater in those who underwent a two-stage procedure and correction of both pelvic obliquity and Cobb angle were accordingly much better. There was one posterior death and five wound infections. There were three dislodged hooks and two pseudarthroses while there were two vertebral fractures and two pulled out staples as a result of the anterior Dwyer instrumentation.

We probably shall not see polio surgery series anywhere near these numbers in the future bearing in mind the success of the vaccination program.

7.4 The True Neuromuscular Diseases of Childhood

These neuromuscular diseases are a wide variety of disorders depending upon which part of the neuromuscular chain is involved. Thus the anterior horn cell is the site of muscular atrophies, the peripheral nerve for peripheral neuropathies, the neuromuscular junction for myasthenic syndromes, and skeletal muscle for the myopathies and muscular dystrophies. However, more than one area can be involved—for instance, learning difficulties with Duchenne muscular dystrophy.

There is an array of investigative techniques available to help differentiate these various conditions including muscle biopsy, neurophysiology, biochemistry, and muscle imaging, such as, MRI. In addition, some neuromuscular diseases are diagnosable with modern, very sensitive DNA tests. Clinical assessment is invaluable with, for instance, fasciculation, atrophy, and reduced tendon reflexes typical of anterior horn cell disease while absent tendon reflexes and muscle atrophy without fasciculation are typical of peripheral neuropathies. Weakness with preserved tendon reflexes is typical of the myopathies and muscular dystrophies.

7.4.1 Spinal Muscular Atrophy

When Werdnig and Hoffmann described the condition of infantile muscular atrophy at the end of the last century[73,74] they referred to a very serious muscular atrophy occurring within a few months of birth leading to death within 2 years. Fifty years later it became apparent that there was a later onset variety with a much better prognosis now referred to as the Kugelberg-Welander variety[75] and that the early onset Werdnig-Hoffman disease can have a variable course with one in five children having a prolonged survival.[76] The condition is now regarded as being one continuum with age at diagnosis and the extent of clinical involvement being the most important factors determining the prognosis.[77] Spinal muscular atrophy (SMA) is the result of anterior horn cell disease. The most common type of SMA is caused by deletions in the *SMN1* gene while others are much less common.[78] This is in effect a pathological continuation of the process of apoptosis (programmed cell death) that is normal in embryonic life.

Classification is clinical and based on age of onset and motor function while lifespan depends on respiratory and bulbar function. The common pathological denominator is degeneration of the anterior horn cells of the spinal cord resulting in symmetrical muscle weakness of the trunk and proximal muscles including those of the shoulder and pelvic girdle. The intercostal muscles are affected but the diaphragm is spared.[79]

There is a positive family history in 60% and it is thought to be both autosomal and recessively inherited with an equal gender distribution. In addition, an autosomal dominant inheritance has been described as a rare form. Clinically there is objective evidence of muscle weakness, hypotonia, areflexia, finger tremor, tongue fasciculation, and preserved sensation. The legs are weaker than the arms and proximal muscle groups are weaker than distally.[80] ▶ Table 7.4 summarizes the key clinical features of the different types.

SMA type 1 has severe hypotonia, thin muscle mass, respiratory distress, and inability to feed and they lie flaccid with no head control with more than three quarters dying within the first 2 years. In type 2 the ability to suck, swallow, and breathe is adequate in early infancy but there is progressive weakness. If they survive into school years or beyond they are confined to an electric wheelchair and are severely handicapped. Type 3 Kugelberg-Welander disease is the mildest form of SMA and these patients may well survive into middle adult life. Fasciculations of many muscles proximally are a specific clinical feature as well as the tongue. Intelligence is normal and importantly, unlike Duchenne dystrophy, the heart is not involved. Diagnosis is a combination of clinical history, physical examination, and three investigations—serum enzyme studies, electrophysiology, and nerve and muscle biopsy.[79] Creatine phosphokinase and aldolase are usually elevated mildly but may be normal in contradistinction to the great rises found in Duchenne dystrophy. Electromyography (EMG) is positive for neurogenic dysfunction while muscle biopsy shows group atrophy of both type 1 and type 2 fibers with persisting groups of hypertrophic fibers.[80] These are useful to differentiate the condition from Becker and limb girdle muscular dystrophies. However, the simplest and most definitive diagnostic test is a molecular genetic marker in blood for the *SMN* gene detected by DNA probes in blood samples or in muscle biopsy.[81] Testing chorionic villi tissues is available for prenatal diagnosis. Unfortunately, no medical treatment is able to delay the progression of this condition. Previous names such as myotonia, amyotonia congenita, and congenital hypotonia are better not used.[80]

Table 7.4 SMA; clinical spectrum

Type	Age of onset	Motor skills	Life expectancy
Werdnig-Hoffmann	<6 months	Never sits alone	80% die by 2 years
Intermediate	6–18 months	Sits alone, unable to walk	Variable
Kugelberg-Welander	>18 months	Walks more than four steps alone	Normal

General Orthopaedic Problems

Just as there is a spectrum of disease severity so there is a spectrum of function and disability. All patients who live long enough end up in a wheelchair and those with milder forms may walk for several years while others are always wheelchair-sitters. It is important to assess these children frequently as they would appear to be often neglected such that contractures develop secondarily which can render a potential walker wheelchair bound. Contractures do not appear to affect non-walkers in terms of sitting stability or discomfort. There are two main areas for orthopaedic concern: the hips and the spine. There is a tendency for coxa valga to develop into frank dislocation which may affect the stability of the pelvis and thus compound a scoliosis above. While Shapiro felt there was a definite role for varus derotation femoral osteotomy in this condition,[1] others feel that this attempt to avoid hip dislocation does not have good results to the point where surgery is not justified.[82] It has been suggested that such hips should merely be observed rather than undergoing surgical treatment.[83]

7.5 Peripheral Neuropathies, Friedreich's Ataxia, and Arthrogryposis Multiplex Congenita

Although it is convenient to group these conditions together because of their common involvement of the nervous system, their heritable pattern and their high incidence of orthopaedic problems,[80,84] there are important differences between them.[85] For instance, the absence of cerebellar disease distinguishes the peripheral neuropathies from Friedreich's ataxia while arthrogryposis poses an additional problem of severe and stiff joint deformity.

7.5.1 The Peripheral Neuropathies

Peroneal Muscular Atrophy

In 1886 Tooth reported on five children with distal limb weakness and wasting suggesting that the primary pathology was in nerve.[85] The same year Charcot and Marie reported five further cases.[86] Their three names became eponymously associated with the peripheral neuropathies. The classification of Charcot-Marie-Tooth (CMT) disease is based on electrophysiological criteria. Type 1 represents demyelinating neuropathies while type 2 axonal neuropathies. Type 1 shows a median nerve motor conduction velocity of less than 38 milliseconds while the axonal group has a higher velocity, more than 38 milliseconds. The diagnosis is a combination of the clinical picture of motor difficulties of some sort—developmental delay, hypotonia, pes cavus, and clawing of the toes—along with abnormal peripheral neurophysiology. CMT is the most common form caused by a duplication of the chromosome 17p11.2.[87] It is autosomal dominant and accounts for 70% of cases of peripheral neuropathy.

There is a neuronal atrophy variant with electromyographic findings very similar to the spinal muscular atrophies. Reflexes are present and there is no evidence of demyelination. The third variety, referred to as Roussy-Lévy disease, is similar to the classic form of CMT disease but is associated with hand tremor.

Hypertrophic Polyneuritis

In the Déjérine-Sottas form of this condition there is marked fibrosis of nerves with segmental demyelination. The condition is recessively inherited and presents in infancy. Children affected walk late and are often wheelchair bound in their teens.

In the Refsum's form of the disease there is peripheral neuropathy in association with eye, ear, and heart problems and this has been referred to as a lipid storage disease because of the greatly elevated levels of phytanic acid. There is a rare dominant form with spastic paraplegia.

Friedreich's Ataxia

This is an autosomal recessive spinocerebellar degenerative condition presenting in late childhood or teenage years. This has a prevalence rate of 1 in 48,000. The gene is mapped to 9q13 and laboratory diagnosis is by determining the number of GAA repeats in a child with progressive ataxia.[88] The clinical presentation is usually in the form of pes cavus with an awkward gait but the prognosis is very much more serious than with the peripheral neuropathies, the majority soon becoming wheelchair bound (▶ Fig. 7.7). Death occurs as a result of cardiomyopathy generally before the age of 40 years. The cerebellar signs are ataxia, nystagmus, dysphasia, and loss of dorsal column function which are all clinically obvious.

In the peripheral neuropathies and Friedreich's ataxia cavus feet are the rule and it is important to try and avoid a rigid deformity.[89,90] Girdlestone flexor to extensor transfer is successful for the passively correctable deformity[90] but if the deformity is rigid then a plantigrade foot is best achieved by triple arthrodesis.

Arthrogryposis

This is a strange but interesting condition of multiple joint contractures at birth often associated with a neuropathic or myopathic process that was first described by Otto in the middle of the last century.[91] Sheldon in 1932 referred to the condition as amyoplasia congenita because of the lack of muscle development.[92] The incidence is thought to be of the order of 1 in 10,000 births and Hall describes the condition in detail.[93] The cause is thought to be due to unfavorable uterine factors in early pregnancy such as oligohydramnios.[94] The diagnosis is assisted by the following investigations: radiographs of the whole spine and CT of the head, chromosome analysis, collagen biochemistry, biochemical investigations to exclude myopathic disorders, electrophysiology, and muscle and nerve biopsy. The diagnosis can be made on clinical grounds at birth but the necessary neuromuscular biopsy investigation should be delayed for 3 months.[95] Because of the neuromuscular association the diagnosis of congenital muscular dystrophy is often added to that of arthrogryposis.

Because of joint deformities that are stiff, conservative treatment by way of physiotherapy and splinting should be started early and can be very successful. Limb deformities are more severe distally with the feet and hands nearly always involved. Hip splintage should be avoided because of the risk of avascular necrosis. Because of the general health problems of feeding, swallowing, sucking, weight gain, and recurrent chest infections early on in life corrective surgery should be delayed until

Neuromuscular Deformities

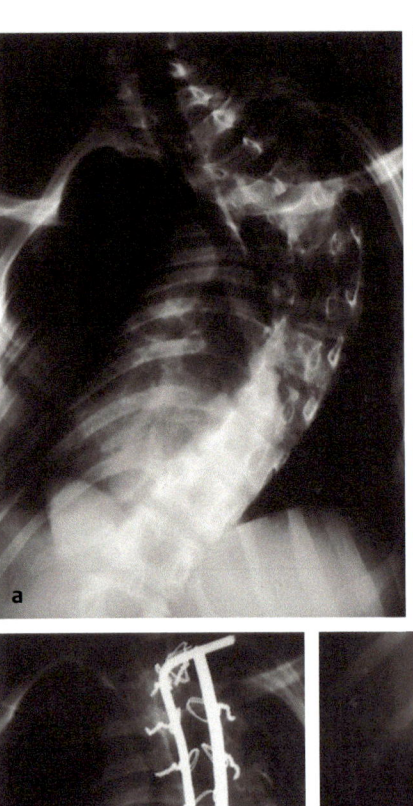

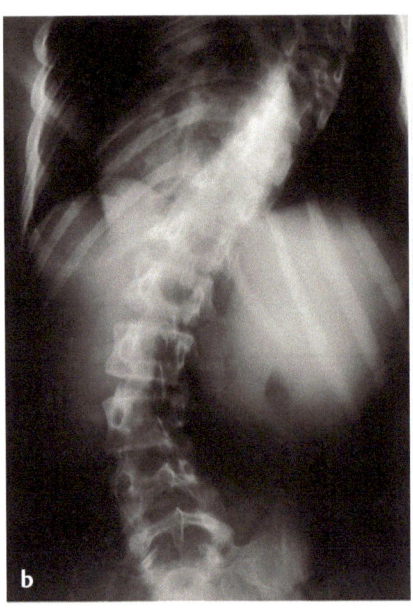

Fig. 7.7 Frontal radiographs of the (**a**) top and (**b**) bottom half of the spine of a teenage boy with Friedreich's ataxia who was falling out of his wheelchair. Frontal radiographs of the (**c**) top and (**d**) bottom half of the spine after full-length spinal instrumentation. This led to restoration of sitting stability and markedly improved function.

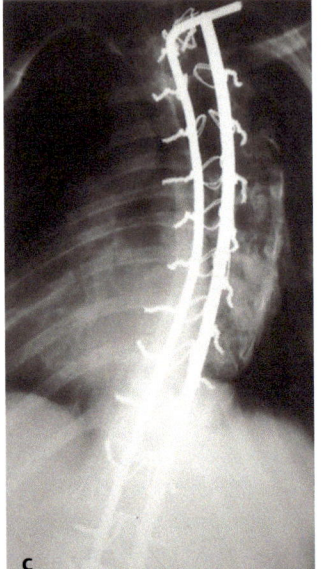

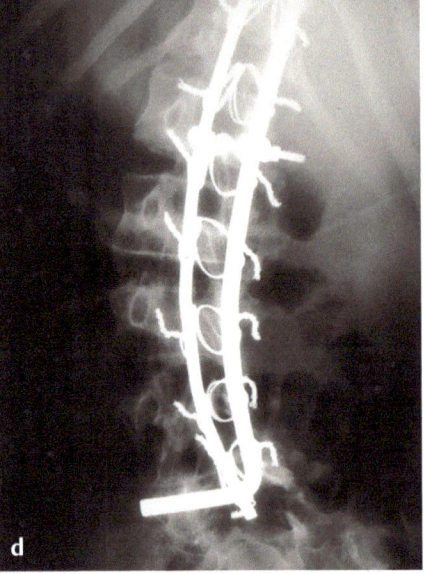

the child is thriving.[96] Virtually all joints in the appendicular skeleton can be involved and the rigid club foot occurs in more than three quarters, hip dislocation in half, and significant involvement of the upper extremity in a quarter.[97] If stiffness is not correctable by physiotherapy and splintage then surgery is necessary but not before the age of 4 to 5. Rigid foot deformities are amenable to talectomy while success has been demonstrated using the Ilizarov technique. One or both hips may be dislocated and if both are then it is advisable that they be left alone. Locating the hips often leads to more stiffness but good results can be obtained.[98] For the upper limbs children can develop remarkable trick movements and surgery should be considered very carefully and this is why surgery should be delayed until the age of 4. Surgical treatment should be considered only with the careful assessment of a skilled physiotherapist and an occupational therapist.

7.5.2 The Muscular Dystrophies

There are a number of muscular dystrophies with the common pathological denominator of dystrophic muscle changes, differences in fiber size, necrosis, and splitting of fibers, along with excess fatty and fibrous tissue. DNA analysis identifies the specific types but there are also important clinical differences.

Duchenne and Becker Muscular Dystrophy

These are referred to as dystrophinopathies and are the most common types of muscular dystrophy with a prevalence rate of about 3 per 100,000. They are X-linked recessive. Duchenne muscular dystrophy (DMD) and Becker muscular dystrophy (BMD) are now considered to be part of a spectrum in boys, with Duchenne having absence of dystrophinism while in Becker there is only partial absence.[99] Loss of walking ability before the age of 13 occurs with Duchenne, while ability to walk

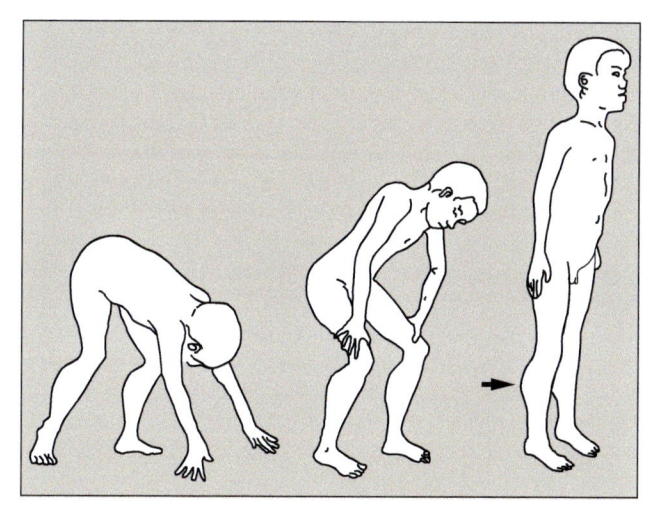

Fig. 7.8 Gower's sign in DMD. When Duchenne children get up, they literally "climb up their legs." (Reproduced with the permission from Springer Publishing, Children's Orthopaedics and Fractures, 3rd Ed, Eds Benson M, Fixsen J, Macnicol M, Parsch K, Chapter 16, Fig 16.7.)

beyond 16 occurs with Becker although loss of walking ability can occur any time in between. Boys start by climbing up their legs (Gower's sign) (▶ Fig. 7.8). Dystrophine is a 427kDa protein which is part of the muscle cell plasma membrane.[100] It is located on the X chromosome and apparently is the largest human gene so far cloned. With translocation involving the X chromosome rare female cases can occur while the female carriers may have obvious muscle weakness.[101] Creatine phosphokinase and aldolase are very elevated. The average age at diagnosis is about 4.5 years with wheelchair dependency averaging 10 years and death at 20–25 years. Ventilatory support can improve longevity and quality of life. Some degree of learning disability occurs in more than a third.

It is important that preoperative cardiac and pulmonary assessments are performed before surgery because of the associated respiratory problems and cardiomyopathy. As regards the legs in nonwalkers, there is no indication to release the hip and knee contractures but the equinus deformity at the ankle and foot can be treated by tendo Achillis and tibialis posterior lengthening.[102] This is particularly indicated as regards shoe fitting or pressure symptoms on the foot plate of a wheelchair but the period of walking is brief anyway as energy consumption is too great. Death from progressive respiratory failure occurs in the late teens to early twenties. Improvements in survival can be attributed to correction of the scoliosis and management of the chest infections.

Limb Girdle Muscular Dystrophy

This dystrophy is characterized by proximal limb weakness and can have as severe a phenotype as in DMD or a very mild one. Limb girdle muscular dystrophy (LGMD) is now classified as to whether it is autosomal dominant or autosomal recessive.

Facioscapulohumeral Myopathy

As its name would suggest this dystrophy is characterized by facial and scapular muscle weakness with winging of the scapulae and weak proximal upper limb muscles. High frequency hearing loss is very common; cardiac involvement is rare.

Congenital Muscular Dystrophy

Again this is where Dubowitz has made such important advances.[80] These are heterogeneous conditions genetically but a common denominator is muscle weakness and hypotonia. There may be raised creatine phosphokinase levels and dystrophic changes on biopsy. All are autosomal recessive. There may be learning difficulty and a number of eye abnormalities such as myopia and cataract.

7.5.3 Congenital Myopathies

Dubowitz did much pioneering work on the congenital myopathies and an important matter here is that they are generally nonprogressive.[80] They usually present in infancy with hypotonia and delayed motor development. There are a number of different varieties according to the genetic defect and these are myotubular, nemaline rod, central core, and minicore myopathies. The same morphological changes and clinical features can be seen in genetically heterogeneous conditions, particularly nemaline myopathy. Determination of the genotype in a child with a congenital myopathy allows more informative genetic counseling and the possibility of antenatal diagnosis.

There are a number of other areas affected such as gallstones and renal stones but because of vitamin K responsive coagulopathy it is important that prior to scoliosis surgery such patients should be appropriately assessed hematologically. Important clinical features in most of these congenital myopathies are respiratory insufficiency and cardiomyopathy. It is of note that in central core myopathy developmental hip dysplasia may occur.

7.5.4 Familial Dysautonomia

This is an interesting syndrome where in association with defective lacrimation there is reduced appreciation of pain.[103] It only occurs in individuals of Ashkenazi Jewish origin. There is muscular incoordination, stumbling gait, fractures, and osteochondritis but the most common musculoskeletal manifestation is a scoliosis.[104] With general anesthesia hypotension, cardiac arrest, and temperature irregularity are serious threats. In eight cases of general anesthesia in these patients there were six episodes of severe hypotension and two deaths.[105] In one of two operated cases there was a concerning period of hyperpyrexia 2 weeks after surgery with temperatures in excess of 40 degrees. It would appear that there is a basic inability to release catecholamines and thus intravenous epinephrine is an important therapeutic agent. The main lesson to be learned from this condition, as with malignant hyperpyrexia, is the presentation by way of scoliosis and evidence of myopathy of unclear etiology that demands particularly careful assessment. It would appear that with these relatively modest curve sizes surgery need not be considered.

7.5.5 Malignant Hyperpyrexia

This is an inherited disorder of skeletal muscle in which affected individuals can develop a rapid rise in body temperature and a severe metabolic disturbance in response to a triggering stimulus which may be stress related to trauma or one of a number of anesthetic drugs, notably inhalational agents and depolarizing muscle relaxants.[106] During such episodes there is marked muscular rigidity, the body core temperature can rise by 6°C per hour and there is cyanosis, acidosis, hypercalcemia, and myoglobinemia. Such episodes have a mortality in excess of 50%. Musculoskeletal abnormalities include a mild myopathy, ligamentous laxity, recurrent joint dislocation, and club foot. In one series 40% of cases presented initially to an orthopaedic surgeon.[107] In addition, hernia, strabismus, and ptosis are common. The syndrome was first accurately described by Denborough and Lovell in 1960 and this led to worldwide recognition and awareness of the condition.[108] There is an autosomal dominant mode of inheritance with variable penetration and expressivity. The prevalence rate in the UK is around 1 in 50,000 although much less in the United States. There is a clinically detectable myopathy but most appear to lead a normal active life. Involvement of the spinal musculature may produce a scoliosis or deformities in the sagittal plane with an increased thoracic kyphosis and lumbar lordosis. There would also appear to be an increased prevalence rate of congenital spinal deformities. An investigation by the internationally renowned Leeds Malignant Hyperpyrexia Investigation Unit with vast numbers of patients[109] revealed a mild scoliosis in about 20% but these would appear to have only limited progression potential.[110] The risk of serious anesthetic complications during operative treatment should ward off any consideration of surgical intervention.

7.6 Scoliosis in the True Neuromuscular Diseases

7.6.1 Spinal Muscular Atrophy

Clearly respiratory problems are the limiting factor in spinal surgery in this condition but, unlike DMD, the heart is not affected. As with all neuromuscular conditions the function of the patient is the critical factor. There is no reason why mildly affected Kugelberg-Welander cases should not have their appearance just as respected as those with idiopathic scoliosis. These will be thoracic curves and can be managed by a posterior approach. Clearly it is better to avoid a transthoracic procedure.

At the other end of the spectrum is the severely affected younger patient with a collapsing paralytic curve with pelvic obliquity whose sitting stability is being jeopardized. In these cases, a long posterior procedure down to the pelvis is generally recommended. In the middle of course there are those who are still ambulatory with thoracolumbar curves and, again, it is extremely important to watch their gait pattern, and perhaps immobilize the torso in a brace, to really see if correcting and thereby making their deformity rigid is in their best functional interest. Of course in rapidly progressive curves this status may be fairly short-lived before they naturally go into a wheelchair but for those with better expectations a good risks and rewards analysis is essential.

However, with more severe cases there comes less good pulmonary function. Postoperative atelectasis or a chest infection occurs in virtually all patients and some may require continued endotracheal intubation while others may require a preoperative tracheostomy followed postoperatively by vigorous respiratory and physical therapy. In addition, mortality is not insignificant with 2 out of 14 patients reported in 1976[105] and 1 out of 16 cases in 1982,[111] both series from distinguished centers. However, going back to these early series it is quite remarkable what can be done with a simple posterior fusion with Harrington instrumentation, the illustrations enhancing Hensinger and MacEwen's paper being quite remarkable.[105] We may get less complications nowadays; there were three pseudarthroses in 14 patients in one series[105] but our correctability will not be much better. In one series treated with Luque type instrumentation the decline in lung function seen preoperatively was actually reversed with a significant improvement at follow-up averaging 13 years.[112] The Cobb angle correction was only 40% but that isn't the reason for carrying out surgery in wheelchair-bound patients with spinal muscular atrophy (SMA) or indeed any other neuromuscular disease; rather, it is to provide a stable spine and to free the hands for prehensile function (▶ Fig. 6.50g). So probably Cobb angle doesn't matter although it seems imperative to measure and report it. This review did at least confine itself to patients with spinal muscular atrophy, and there were all of 43 of them.[112] Most reports about scoliosis treatment in neuromuscular diseases contained a wide variety of diagnoses and in some it is not possible to readily subdivide them according to diagnosis or there may be three with one diagnosis and four or five with another brought into the grand total.[113,114]

One group tried to treat patients with intermediate SMA with a telescopic growing rod but, in collapsing neuromuscular conditions, without concomitant fusions this was destined to fail and indeed did so in 15 patients.[115] Recently Sucato provided an overview of spine deformity in SMA and he described the condition and its surgical treatment admirably.[116] He did not recommend anterior surgery alone but did recommend posterior spinal fusion with segmental pedicular instrumentation from T2 to the pelvis in all patients who are not ambulatory. Although frontal plane correction was between a third and a half this is really irrelevant because what is required is a stable spine in the sitting position with release of the upper extremities for prehensile function and not to be used to hold themselves up with a collapsing spine in a wheelchair. In most reported series parents were satisfied with the result but in one series[117] two ambulatory patients lost the ability to walk following surgery while six patients who had previously been able to sit independently could not maintain a sitting position without support postoperatively. This again, like cerebral palsy, indicates the problem of doing long spinal fusions in ambulatory patients while the six patients who previously had been able to sit independently in the Granata et al series probably shouldn't have had surgery in the first place because the indication for surgery in nonwalkers is being unable to sit independently in the wheelchair. It is critically important in neuromuscular spinal deformity to address the functional needs of the patient only. Then came four papers from the Guro Hospital in Korea[118-122] and there seems to be a fair amount of salami slicing here. The first paper talks about 24 patients, 9 with DMD and 5 with SMA, and describes correction of apical axial rotation with pedicle screws but Cobb angle and pelvic obliquity were also reported upon.[118] The next paper talks about 26 patients, 10 with DMD and 5 with SMA (i.e., one additional

DMD patient; there was also one more cerebral palsy patient) making up the total of 26.[119] Then, more importantly, the same group a year later report upon 36 patients with DMD.[120] Then in 2010 the same group reported upon 27 patients, 18 with DMD and 9 with SMA.[121] Clearly the numbers don't add up here and there is a mix of neuromuscular disorders but the Cobb angle correction was 70% and the pelvic obliquity was corrected from 16 degrees to 9 degrees on average. These cases were instrumented with posterior-only pedicle screw fixation. Another group in Korea compared outcomes between muscular dystrophy and SMA.[122] Corrections of both Cobb angle and pelvic obliquity were significantly better in the SMA group than the DMD group. There did not seem to be a difference in pulmonary outcomes. Patients tended to have a vital capacity less than 30%.

Then, in 2008, from various centers in Holland, a Dutch guideline for the treatment of scoliosis in neuromuscular disorders was published.[123] They looked at a number of neuromuscular conditions including SMA and their guidelines as regards SMA refer to delay in surgery until 7 to 9 years of age and then carrying out a spinal fusion with multiple pedicle screws but putting screws around the curve apex to reduce crank shafting with growth.

Now we come to another paper from the Guro hospital in Korea again lumping together different causes of neuromuscular scoliosis in 55 patients but the message from them is that if the pelvic obliquity is more than 15 degrees pelvic fixation is required but not if the obliquity angle is less than 15 degrees.[32]

A paper from Baltimore looked at SMA cases and indicated that there were several potential therapeutic compounds being studied in clinical trials aiming to increase the amount of SMN protein.[124]

Then another paper from the Guro hospital group in Korea reported on surgical complications in neuromuscular scoliosis operated on by posterior pedicle screw fixation and the complications were considerable—most of them pulmonary in nature—but there were two deaths, one due to cardiac arrest and the other due to hypovolemic shock.[125] They also talked about intraoperative blood loss of more than 3.5 L. There was also one complete spinal cord injury.

In 2011 the St Louis Group published on the outcome of surgery for scoliosis in SMA focusing on major curve progression. This was a 5-year radiographic study on 22 SMA patients focusing on Cobb angles from T5 to T12 and T12 to the sacrum. Postoperative curve progression tended to occur in younger patients, not surprisingly with bigger Cobb angles and shorter fusions.[126]

However, a group from Johns Hopkins reported on good results with growing rods for scoliosis in SMA. The correction of Cobb angle was from 90 to 55 degrees and pelvic obliquity from 31 to 11 degrees. These were 15 patients with SMA and they were treated with growing rods for 3 years. There was also improvement in space-available-for-lung ratio but rib collapse was not halted.[127]

7.7 The Other True Neuromuscular Diseases

Back in 1985 there was a paper from the Minneapolis group about 19 patients with Friedreich's ataxia.[128] There were 12 boys and 7 girls and the age of onset averaged 9 years with the earliest being 3 years of age. The average loss of ambulation date was 20 years of age and 12 had cardiac problems. There were six thoracic curves and six thoracolumbar curves. Double thoracic and thoracolumbar/lumbar curves were present in seven. Like with all scoliosis deformities brace treatment was unsuccessful. Twelve patients had surgery, 10 with Harrington instrumentation and 2 with Luque instrumentation. The preoperative Cobb angle averaged 49 degrees and postoperatively 26 degrees. The only significant complication was one case of cardiomyopathy successfully treated.

Labelle et al in 1986 questioned whether the spinal deformity in Friedreich's ataxia behaved like an idiopathic curve or a typical neuromuscular scoliosis.[129] Fifty-six patients with Friedreich's ataxia were studied with an average follow-up of 9 years. Scoliosis of more than 10 degrees was found in all patients. They also mentioned significant hyperkyphosis, which of course doesn't exist, the lateral view of the patient appearing to show kyphosis which is just a reflection of the scoliosis with a significant amount of apical rotation (see Chapter 3). There was an equal gender distribution and most curves were single thoracolumbar. Twenty progressed to be more than 60 degrees. In a study of the variability of somatosensory cortical evoked potential monitoring during spinal surgery it was noted that with those with neuromuscular problems, particularly with ataxia, had high variability and weak amplitudes of responses.[130] This confirms that it is essential when contemplating surgery for a neuromuscular scoliosis that somatosensory evoked potentials should be carried out preoperatively as this will provide very important information.

The Dallas group in 2007 reported on 298 patients with CMT and looked at them epidemiologically finding 45 patients with scoliosis with an average age at diagnosis of 13 years and an average curve magnitude at diagnosis of 28 degrees. One third were left thoracic. The majority progressed and surgery was performed with long posterior spinal fusions. Intraoperative neurological monitoring was possible in only a small minority. There were no significant neurological complications.[131]

7.8 Duchenne Muscular Dystrophy

As with SMA there is much recent information about scoliosis in DMD. In 2002 a prospective cohort study of 44 DMD subjects was examined six monthly to assess ambulation.[132] Various measures were recorded including ambulatory status, anthropometric data, muscle strength, functional status, and use of standing and walking aids. Those with impaired hip extension and ankle dorsiflexion strength were more than 10 times more likely to stop ambulating within 2 years. These are very important primary predictors of loss of ambulation in DMD. In 2002 the Nottingham and Oswestry Scoliosis Groups looked at the need for pelvic or lumbar fixation in the surgical management of DMD. Essentially lumbar fixation to L5 was adequate if the surgery was performed early,[133] soon after becoming wheelchair bound, and these were smaller curves with minimal pelvic obliquity. By contrast older children with bigger curves and established pelvic obliquity should have pelvic fixation.

The Royal National Orthopaedic Hospital in London in 2003 reported on 30 patients with scoliosis and DMD, 17 with predicted forced vital capacities more than 30% and 13 with less than 30%.[134] There were no significant risk differences between the groups. One in each group required temporary tracheostomy.

Then in 2004 the Manchester, UK, group led by our colleague Charles Galasko who has vast experience of DMD reported on 85 consecutive patients who underwent spinal fusion over a period of 16 years as regards postoperative progression of the scoliosis and pelvic obliquity.[135] A total of 55 were instrumented using the Luque unit rod system and 19 with pedicle screws; 15 were instrumented down to L5 and 15 to S1 with 7 instrumented above to the L3/4 level. The postoperative follow-up was 4 years on average. There was only one perioperative death and three cases of metalwork failure. A fusion to S1 did not provide any benefit over a more proximal fusion. The Newcastle, UK, Scoliosis Unit reported on the correction of DMD in patients with preexisting respiratory failure.[136] The mean age at surgery was 12 years and the mean follow-up 4 years and eight patients were studied. The mean preoperative Cobb angle was 70 degrees and this was improved to 30 degrees on average by surgery. The mean vital capacity at the time of surgery was only 20%. There were no major cardiac or pulmonary complications and this confirmed the important view that these patients can be operated upon safely.

The famous Dubowitz neuromuscular center at Hammersmith Hospital, London, UK, looked at their huge 10-year experience of scoliosis management in 123 patients with DMD; 10% did not have a scoliosis. They were at least 17 years old at the time of the study. Surgery was considered in 70 cases and eventually performed in 40%. They found that in 17 years there was no difference in survival, respiratory impairment, or sitting comfort in all patients managed conservatively or with surgery. They confirmed that it was important to understand the natural history of scoliosis in DMD in helping families and clinicians making risks and rewards decisions.[137]

In 2007 the Hong Kong Group carried out a systematic review of DMD and scoliosis and interrogated several databases including the Cochrane Neuromuscular Disease Group and Cochrane Back Group, the Centre Register for Control Trials, Medline etc.[137] A total of 402 studies were identified and 36 met the inclusion criteria of controlled clinical trials using random or quasi-random allocation of treatment. They concluded that there were no randomized controlled trials to evaluate effectiveness of scoliosis in DMD and therefore no evidence-based recommendations could be made for clinical practice. They concluded that patients should be informed of the uncertainty of benefits and potential risks of surgery for scoliosis and that clearly randomized controlled trials were needed. No sensible person would ignore these results. Scoliosis surgeons experienced with the condition of DMD particularly from national centers that attract large numbers of cases have already shown that, while there are obvious risks, there are also ample rewards. In the 1970s and 1980s when surgery for DMD was first carried out there was a high mortality rate of 10%.

Leatherman's group in Louisville reported on their first five patients with DMD treated with segmental spinal instrumentation and noted a 50% correction but there was one death 48 hours after surgery due to pulmonary failure.[138] At that time it would appear that 40 degrees was the critical threshold beyond which curve progression with functional loss was the rule[139] and that is why Leatherman stressed the need to tackle the early flexible curve before it threatens sitting stability,[138] a message that has been regularly repeated since. Not surprisingly, with more modern posterior techniques and considerable further experience in these National Regional Scoliosis Centres the complication rate has diminished and of course the quality of intensive care has greatly increased. One of the problems with DMD is the relatively small number of cases and thus randomized controlled trials may not be the way forward and perhaps this reinforces the need to measure all the relevant variables in these cases so that as much reliable information as possible can be gathered.

The Boston Group in 2007 showed that carrying out a posterior spinal fusion for scoliosis in DMD actually diminished the subsequent rate of respiratory decline compared to a nonoperated control group. Here we now have confirmed organic benefit of scoliosis surgery in DMD.[140] Now we can therefore add considerable respiratory benefit to functional outcome in cases of DMD. The report from the Hospital for Sick Children in Toronto demonstrated that surgery for scoliosis did improve quality of life in DMD. Quality of life is assessed on a 10-point scale: 0 (death) to 10 (perfect health). This has been used to demonstrate the efficacy of hip replacements with significant economic benefit to the UK Health Service.[141]

The Balgrist Clinic in Zurich, Switzerland, reported on 20 consecutive patients with scoliosis in DMD who were operated upon down to the pelvis.[142] The average scoliosis was quite rightly not severe and improved on average from 44 degrees to 10 degrees while the pelvic obliquity improved from 14 to 3 degrees. There were no metalwork complications or respiratory complications but unfortunately one patient died postoperatively due to known cardiomyopathy. The same sort of good results have been reported from Japan particularly on those with a very low FVC.[143] Another report from Japan compared autogenous iliac crest bone graft versus allograft bone in scoliosis surgery in DMD patients.[144] There was no difference in the outcome as regards the scoliosis and pelvic obliquity correction but half of the autogenous iliac crest bone graft group had significant donor site pain which severely limited their physical function causing difficulties in wheelchair sitting.

Hassan Dashti is now a lead clinician in the Manchester neuromuscular scoliosis center where there is a multidisciplinary team approach to the treatment of DMD so essential to obtaining optimal outcomes in these challenging cases. He very kindly let us have some of his cases to illustrate in this chapter (▶ Fig. 7.9, ▶ Fig. 7.10, and ▶ Fig. 7.11) and the case gallery.

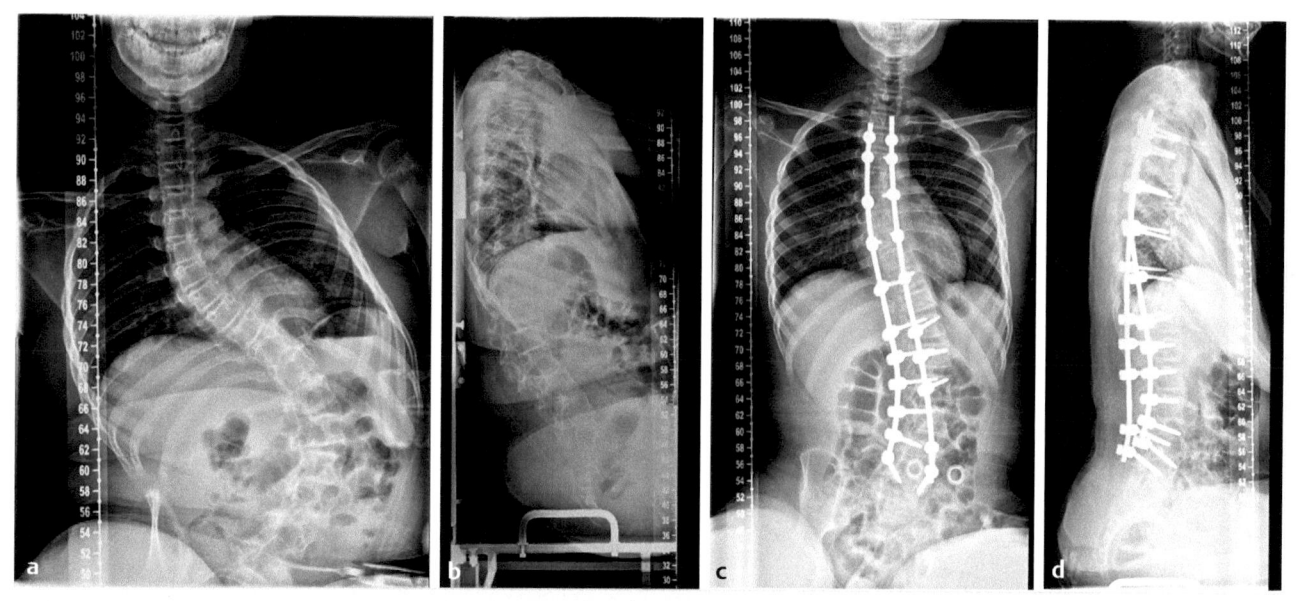

Fig. 7.9 **(a,b)** PA and lateral radiographs before surgery showing a 90-degree collapsing neuromuscular lordoscoliosis with 45 degrees of pelvic obliquity in a boy with DMD. **(c,d)** PA and lateral radiographs postoperatively showing an excellent correction of the scoliosis and the pelvic obliquity reduced to less than 20 degrees. The use of transpedicular fixation has certainly enhanced the correctability and maintenance of that correction in these difficult cases. The second and third cases (▶ Fig. 7.10 and ▶ Fig. 7.11) were DMD brothers both with some learning difficulties. Case 2 was aged 15 with mainly pain on sitting.

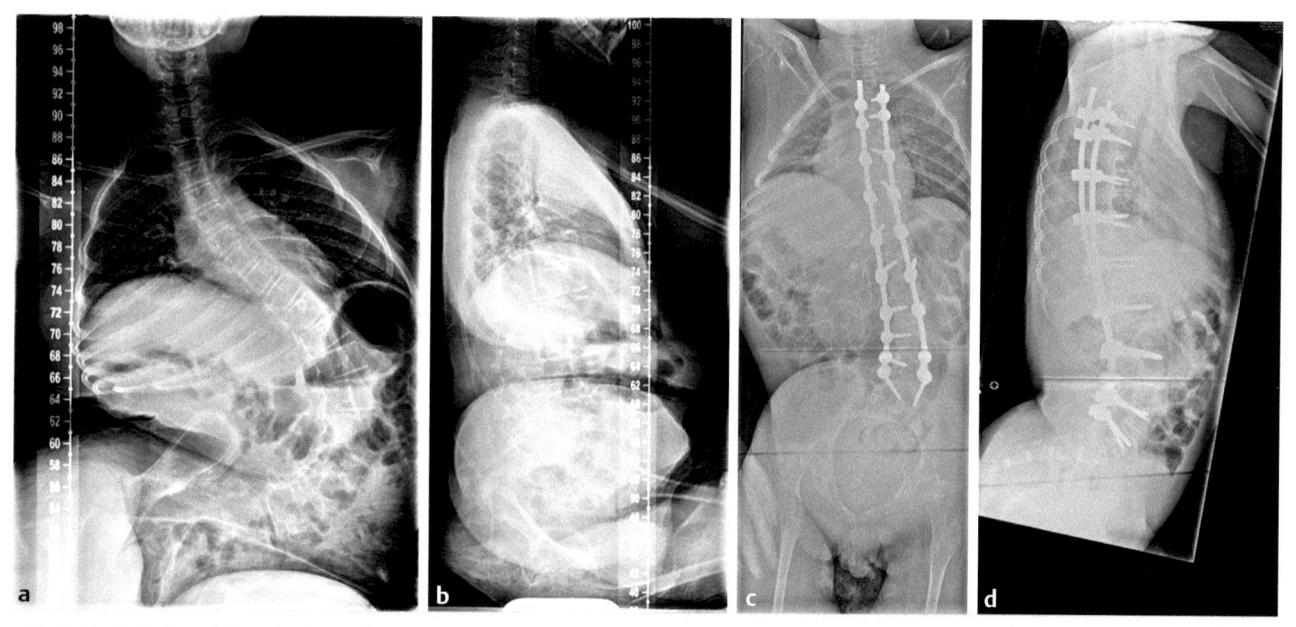

Fig. 7.10 **(a,b)** PA and lateral radiographs preoperatively showing a gross collapsing neuromuscular lordoscoliosis and all of 90 degrees of pelvic obliquity typical of DMD. **(c,d)** PA and lateral radiographs after surgical correction showing excellent correction of the scoliosis but more importantly the pelvic obliquity was reduced down to less than 10 degrees.

Neuromuscular Deformities

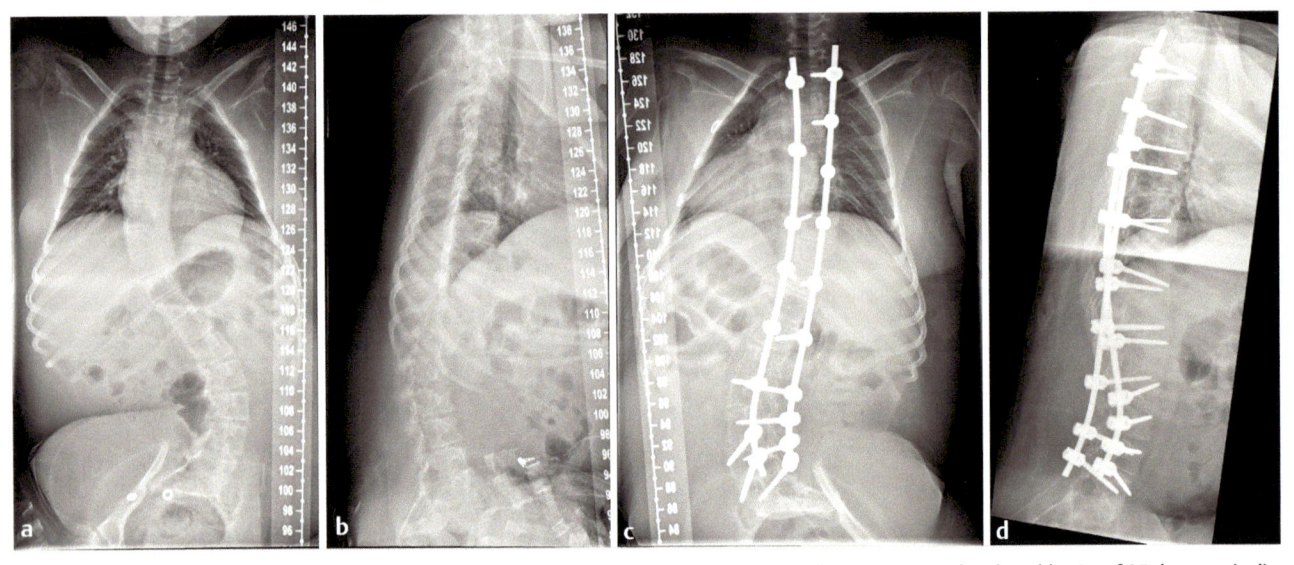

Fig. 7.11 DMD case. (a,b) PA and lateral radiographs preoperatively with the usual C-shaped collapsing curve with pelvic obliquity of 25 degrees. (c,d) are PA and lateral radiographs postoperatively showing excellent correction of the scoliosis and the pelvic obliquity down to 15 degrees. Earlier surgery was planned but due to low weight issues a feeding gastrostomy for hyperalimentation was required to improve his nutritional status and surgery had to be delayed by a period of about a year. It is now recognized that the earlier surgery is carried out, the better the functional result.

Case Gallery

Case 1

Comment

A boy of 17 with DMD and a typical collapsing lordoscoliosis and pelvic obliquity. He had problems with pain and seating with costopelvic skin breakdown. He also had severe nutritional deficiency and required a feeding gastrostomy preoperatively to hyperaliment him to become fit for surgery. See ▶ Fig. 7.12a–c.

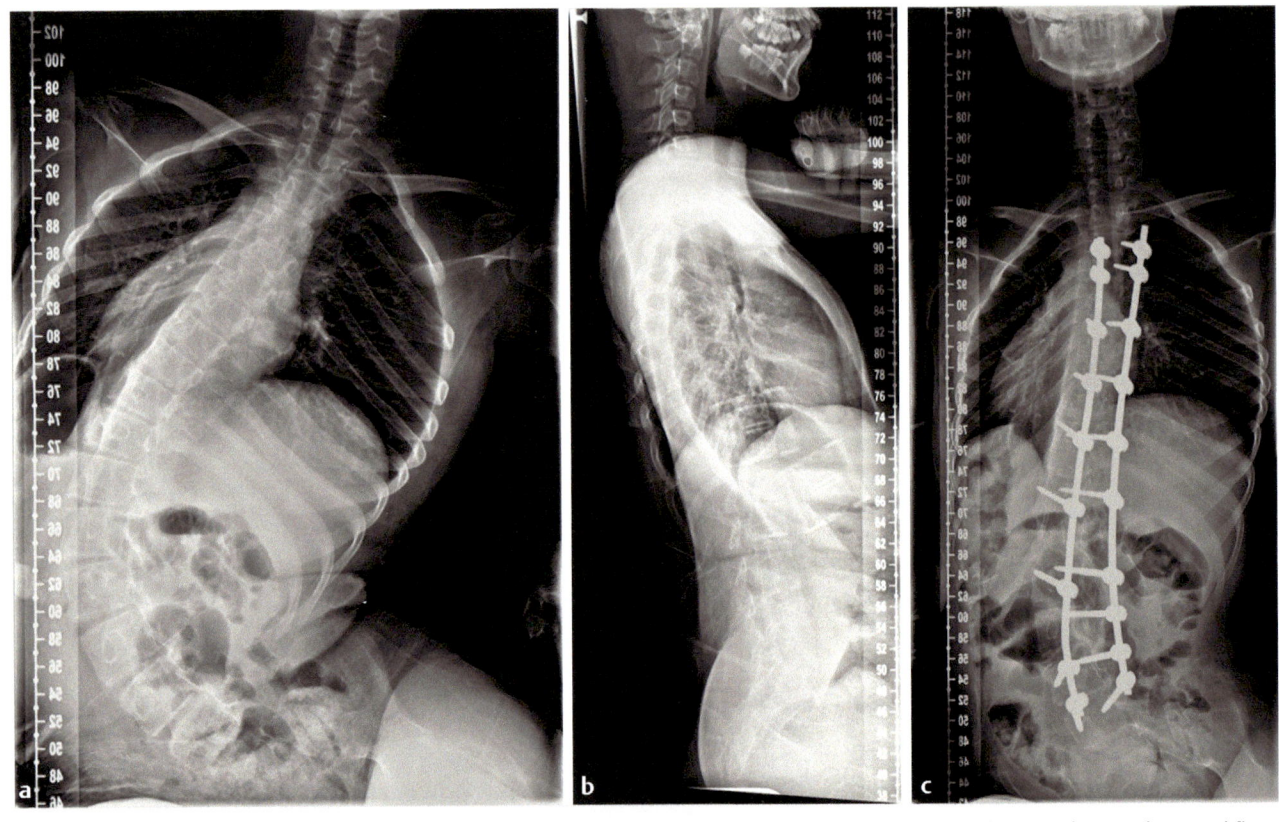

Fig. 7.12 (a) Typical collapsing lordoscoliosis with significant pelvic obliquity measuring 60 degrees. (b) Lateral radiograph showing the typical flat back. (c) PA radiograph after surgery with transpedicular fixation. The pelvic obliquity has been reduced to less than 20 degrees.

This is an excellent case for teaching purposes and for personal reflection. First of all, there is still a trend for having to deal with these difficult DMD cases at this sort of age (17) and not earlier in the natural history of this dreadful condition. The boy had pain over the concavity where there was painful costopelvic skin breakdown which of course would not have occurred with a lesser Cobb angle in a younger patient. Then he had problems with painful seating in that he simply could not get comfortable in any position which is a very severe disability when, of course, you spend nearly all your day in the wheelchair. It is becoming more and more common to have to hyperaliment in these patients whose nutritional status descends into danger territory for major spinal surgery. Another great case from our technically skilled colleague Hasan Dashti in Manchester.

References

Note: References in **bold** are Key References.

[1] **Shapiro F, Bresnan MJ. Orthopaedic management of childhood neuromuscular disease. Part I: Spinal muscular atrophy. J Bone Joint Surg Am. 1982; 64(5):785–789**

[2] Little WJ. On the influence of abnormal parturition, labour, premature birth and asphyxia neonatorum on the mental and physical condition of the child especially in relation to deformities. Transactions of the Obstetric Society of London. 1862; 3:243–344

[3] Stanley FJ, Blair E, Alberman E. How common are the cerebral palsies? In: Stanley F, Blair E, Alberman E (eds). Cerebral palsies: epidemiology and causal pathways. London: Mac Keith Press/Cambridge University Press; 2000:22–39

[4] Brown JK, Minns RA. Mechanisms of deformity in children with cerebral palsy. Sem Orthop. 1989; 4:236–255

[5] Pollock GA, Stark G. Long-term results in the management of 67 children with cerebral palsy. Dev Med Child Neurol. 1969; 11(1):17–34

[6] Courville CB. Cerebral Palsy. Los Angeles: San Lucas Press; 1954

[7] Nelson KB, Ellenberg JH. Antecedents of cerebral palsy. Multivariate analysis of risk. N Engl J Med. 1986; 315(2):81–86

[8] Miller E, Rosenfeld GB. Psychological evaluation of children with cerebral palsy and its implications in treatment. AMA Am J Dis Child. 1952; 84(4):504–505

[9] Warnock HM. Special Educational Needs: Report of the Committee of Enquiry into the Education of Handicapped Children and Young People. London: HMSO; 1978

[10] Tizard JP, Paine RS, Crothers B. Disturbances of sensation in children with hemiplegia. J Am Med Assoc. 1954; 155(7):628–632

[11] Krägeloh-Mann I, Hagberg B, Petersen D, Riethmüller J, Gut E, Michaelis R. Bilateral spastic cerebral palsy—pathogenetic aspects from MRI. Neuropediatrics. 1992; 23(1):46–48

[12] **Robb JE, Brunner R. Orthopaedic management of cerebral palsy. In: Benson M, Fixsen J, Macnicol M, Parsch K (eds). Children's Orthopaedics and Fractures. 3rd ed. London: Springer; 2010:307–325**

[13] Read HS, Hazlewood ME, Hillman SJ, Prescott RJ, Robb JE. Edinburgh visual gait score for use in cerebral palsy. J Pediatr Orthop. 2003; 23(3):296–301

[14] **Graham HK, Harvey A. Assessment of mobility after multi-level surgery for cerebral palsy. J Bone Joint Surg Br. 2007; 89(8):993–994**

[15] **Lonstein JE, Akbarnia A. Operative treatment of spinal deformities in patients with cerebral palsy or mental retardation. An analysis of one hundred and seven cases. J Bone Joint Surg Am. 1983; 65(1):43–55**

[16] Cooperman DR, Bartucci E, Dietrick E, Millar EA. Hip dislocation in spastic cerebral palsy: long-term consequences. J Pediatr Orthop. 1987; 7(3):268–276

[17] Graham HK, Boyd R, Carlin JB, et al. Does botulinum toxin a combined with bracing prevent hip displacement in children with cerebral palsy and "hips at risk"? A randomized, controlled trial. J Bone Joint Surg Am. 2008; 90(1):23–33

[18] Robson P. The prevalence of scoliosis in adolescents and young adults with cerebral palsy. Dev Med Child Neurol. 1968; 10(4):447–452

[19] Balmer GA, MacEwen GD. The incidence and treatment of scoliosis in cerebral palsy. J Bone Joint Surg Br. 1970; 52(1):134–137

[20] Samilson R, Bechard R. Scoliosis in cerebral palsy; incidence, distribution of curve patterns, natural history and thoughts on etiology. Curr Pract Orthop Surg. 1973; 5:183–205

[21] Rosenthal RK, Levine DB, McCarver CL. The occurrence of scoliosis in cerebral palsy. Dev Med Child Neurol. 1974; 16(5):664–667

[22] **MacEwen GD. Operative treatment of scoliosis in cerebral palsy. Reconstr Surg Traumatol. 1972; 13:58–67**

[23] Dwyer AF, Newton NC, Sherwood AA. An anterior approach to scoliosis. A preliminary report. Clin Orthop Relat Res. 1969; 62(62):192–202

[24] Luque ER. Segmental spinal instrumentation for correction of scoliosis. Clin Orthop Relat Res. 1982(163):192–198

[25] Zielke K. [Ventral derotation spondylodesis. Results of treatment of cases of idiopathic lumbar scoliosis (author's (author's transl)]. Z Orthop Ihre Grenzgeb. 1982; 120:320–329

[26] Allen BL, Jr, Ferguson RL. L-rod instrumentation for scoliosis in cerebral palsy. J Pediatr Orthop. 1982; 2(1):87–96

[27] Gau Y-L, Lonstein JE, Winter RB, Koop S, Denis F. Luque-Galveston procedure for correction and stabilization of neuromuscular scoliosis and pelvic obliquity: a review of 68 patients. J Spinal Disord. 1991; 4(4):399–410

[28] Bell DF, Moseley CF, Koreska J. Unit rod segmental spinal instrumentation in the management of patients with progressive neuromuscular spinal deformity. Spine. 1989; 14(12):1301–1307

[29] Bulman WA, Dormans JP, Ecker ML, Drummond DS. Posterior spinal fusion for scoliosis in patients with cerebral palsy: a comparison of Luque rod and Unit Rod instrumentation. J Pediatr Orthop. 1996; 16(3):314–323

[30] Dubousset J, Graf H, Miladi L, et al. Spinal and thoracic derotation with CD instrumentation. Orthop Trans. 1986; 10:36

[31] Teli MG, Cinnella P, Vincitorio F, Lovi A, Grava G, Brayda-Bruno M. Spinal fusion with Cotrel-Dubousset instrumentation for neuropathic scoliosis in patients with cerebral palsy. Spine. 2006; 31(14):E441–E447

[32] Modi HN, Suh SW, Song HR, Yang JH, Jajodia N. Evaluation of pelvic fixation in neuromuscular scoliosis: a retrospective study in 55 patients. Int Orthop. 2010; 34(1):89–96

[33] Modi HN, Hong JY, Mehta SS, et al. Surgical correction and fusion using posterior-only pedicle screw construct for neuropathic scoliosis in patients with cerebral palsy: a three-year follow-up study. Spine. 2009; 34(11):1167–1175

[34] Whitaker C, Burton DC, Asher M. Treatment of selected neuromuscular patients with posterior instrumentation and arthrodesis ending with lumbar pedicle screw anchorage. Spine. 2000; 25(18):2312–2318

[35] Suh SW, Modi HN, Yang J, Song HR, Jang KM. Posterior multilevel vertebral osteotomy for correction of severe and rigid neuromuscular scoliosis: a preliminary study. Spine. 2009; 34(12):1315–1320

[36] Auerbach JD, Spiegel DA, Zgonis MH, et al. The correction of pelvic obliquity in patients with cerebral palsy and neuromuscular scoliosis: is there a benefit of anterior release prior to posterior spinal arthrodesis? Spine. 2009; 34(21):E766–E774

[37] Watanabe K, Lenke LG, Daubs MD, et al. Is spine deformity surgery in patients with spastic cerebral palsy truly beneficial?: a patient/parent evaluation. Spine. 2009; 34(20):2222–2232

[38] Keeler KA, Lenke LG, Good CR, Bridwell KH, Sides B, Luhmann SJ. Spinal fusion for spastic neuromuscular scoliosis: is anterior releasing necessary when intraoperative halo-femoral traction is used? Spine. 2010; 35(10):E427–E433

[39] **Lonstein JE, Koop SE, Novachek TF, Perra JH. Results and complications after spinal fusion for neuromuscular scoliosis in cerebral palsy and static encephalopathy using luque galveston instrumentation: experience in 93 patients. Spine. 2012; 37(7):583–591**

[40] Tsirikos AI, Mains E. Surgical correction of spinal deformity in patients with cerebral palsy using pedicle screw instrumentation. J Spinal Disord Tech. 2012; 25(7):401–408

[41] Bohtz C, Meyer-Heim A, Min K. Changes in health-related quality of life after spinal fusion and scoliosis correction in patients with cerebral palsy. J Pediatr Orthop. 2011; 31(6):668–673

[42] **Ho C, Skaggs DL, Weiss JM, Tolo VT. Management of infection after instrumented posterior spine fusion in pediatric scoliosis. Spine. 2007; 32(24):2739–2744**

[43] Bodian D. A reconsideration of the pathogenesis of poliomyelitis. Am J Hyg. 1952; 55(3):414–438

[44] Hull HF, Aylward RB. Progress towards global polio eradication. Vaccine. 2001; 19(31):4378–4384

[45] Chow W, Li YH, Leong CYJ. Poliomyelitis. In Benson M, Fixsen J, Macnicol M, Parsch K (eds). Children's Orthopaedics and Fractures. 3rd ed. London: Springer; 2010:287–305

[46] Yount CC. The role of the tensor fasciae femoris in certain deformities of the lower extremities. J Bone Joint Surg. 1926; 8:171–193

[47] Kaplan EB. The iliotibial tract; clinical and morphological significance. J Bone Joint Surg Am. 1958; 40-A(4):817–832

[48] Somerville EW. Paralytic dislocation of the hip. J Bone Joint Surg Br. 1959; 41-B(2):279–288

[49] Raycroft JF, Curtis BH. Spinal curvature in myelomeningocele. Natural history and etiology. In: American Academy of Orthopaedic Surgeons Symposium on Myelomeningocele. St Louis: C.V. Mosby Co.: 1972

[50] Mayer L. Further studies of fixed paralytic pelvic obliquity. J Bone Joint Surg. 1936; 18:87–100

[51] Irwin CE. Subtrochanteric osteotomy in poliomyelitis. J Am Med Assoc. 1947; 133(4):231–235

[52] Sharrard WJW. The distribution of the permanent paralysis in the lower limb in poliomyelitis; a clinical and pathological study. J Bone Joint Surg Br. 1955; 37-B(4):540–558

[53] Steindler A. Diseases and deformities of spine and thorax. St Louis: CV Mosby; 1929

[54] Scott JC. Scoliosis: Lecture delivered at the Royal College of Surgeons of England on 7th October, 1949. Ann R Coll Surg Engl. 1950; 6(2):73–98

[55] Colonna PC, Vom Saal F. A study of paralytic scoliosis based on 500 cases of poliomyelitis. J Bone Joint Surg. 1941; 23:335–353

[56] Lowman CL. The relation of the abdominal muscles to paralytic scoliosis. J Bone Joint Surg. 1932; 14:763–772

[57] **James JIP. Paralytic scoliosis. J Bone Joint Surg Br. 1956; 38-B(3):660–685**

[58] **Roaf R. Paralytic scoliosis. J Bone Joint Surg Br. 1956; 38-B(3):640–659**

[59] Garrett AL, Perry J, Nickel VL. Stabilisation of the collapsing spine. J Bone Joint Surg Am. 1961; 43:474–484

[60] Hamel AL, Moe JH. The collapsing spine. Surgery. 1964; 56:364–373

[61] Pavon SJ, Manning C. Posterior spinal fusion for scoliosis due to anterior poliomyelitis. J Bone Joint Surg Br. 1970; 52(3):420–431

[62] Blount WP, Moe JH. The Milwaukee Brace. Baltimore: Williams & Wilkins; 1973

[63] Risser JC. Scoliosis: the application of body casts for the correction of scoliosis. Instructional Course Lecture. Am Acad Orthop Surg. 1955; 12:255–259

[64] Gucker T, III. Experiences with poliomyelitic scoliosis after fusion and correction. J Bone Joint Surg Am. 1956; 38-A(6):1281–1300

[65] Harrington PR. Surgical instrumentation for management of scoliosis. J Bone Joint Surg Am. 1960; 42:1448

[66] Bonnett C, Brown JC, Perry J, et al. Evolution of treatment of paralytic scoliosis at Rancho Los Amigos Hospital. J Bone Joint Surg Am. 1975; 57(2):206–215

[67] O'Brien JP, Yau ACMC. Anterior and posterior correction and fusion for paralytic scoliosis. Clin Orthop Relat Res. 1972; 86(86):151–153

[68] **O'Brien JP, Dwyer AP, Hodgson AR. Paralytic pelvic obliquity. Its prognosis and management and the development of a technique for full correction of the deformity. J Bone Joint Surg Am. 1975; 57(5):626–631**

[69] Griss P, Harms J, Zielke K. Ventral derotation spondylodesis (VDS). In: Dickson RA, Bradford DS (eds). Management of Spinal Deformities. London: Butterworths International Medical Reviews; 1984:193–236

[70] Luque ER. Paralytic scoliosis in growing children. Clin Orthop Relat Res. 1982 (163):202–209

[71] **Leong JC, Wilding K, Mok CK, Ma A, Chow SP, Yau AC. Surgical treatment of scoliosis following poliomyelitis. A review of one hundred and ten cases. J Bone Joint Surg Am. 1981; 63(5):726–740**

[72] Mayer PJ, Dove J, Ditmanson M, Shen YS. Post-poliomyelitis paralytic scoliosis. A review of curve patterns and results of surgical treatments in 118 consecutive patients. Spine. 1981; 6(6):573–582

[73] Werdnig G. Zwei frühinfantile hereditäre Fälle von progressiver Muskelatrophie unter dem Bilde der Dystrophie, aber auf neuritischer Grundlage. Arch Psychiatr Nervenkr. 1891; 22:437–481

[74] Hoffmann J. Ueber chronische spinale Muskelatrophie in Kindesalter, auf familiärer Basis. Dtsch Z Nervenheilkd. 1893; 3:427–470

[75] Kugelberg E, Welander L. Heredofamilial juvenile muscular atrophy simulating muscular dystrophy. AMA Arch Neurol Psychiatry. 1956; 75(5):500–509

[76] **Dubowitz V. Benign infantile spinal muscular atrophy. Dev Med Child Neurol. 1974; 16(5):672–675**

[77] Munsat TL, Woods R, Fowler W, Pearson CM. Neurogenic muscular atrophy of infancy with prolonged survival. The variable course of Werdnig-Hoffmann Disease. Brain. 1969; 92(1):9–24

[78] Lefebvre S, Bürglen L, Reboullet S, et al. Identification and characterization of a spinal muscular atrophy-determining gene. Cell. 1995; 80(1):155–165

[79] Bunch WH. Muscular dystrophy. In: Hardy JH (ed). Spinal deformity in Neurological and Muscular Disorders. St Louis: CV Mosby; 1974

[80] **Dubowitz V. Muscle Disorders in Childhood. Philadelphia: WB Saunders; 1978**

[81] Hardart MKM, Truog RD. Spinal muscular atrophy—type I. Arch Dis Child. 2003; 88(10):848–850

[82] Zenios M, Sampath J, Cole C, Khan T, Galasko CS. Operative treatment for hip subluxation in spinal muscular atrophy. J Bone Joint Surg Br. 2005; 87(11):1541–1544

[83] Sporer SM, Smith BG. Hip dislocation in patients with spinal muscular atrophy. J Pediatr Orthop. 2003; 23(1):10–14

[84] Forgan L, Munsat TL. Spinocerebellar degenerative disease. In: Hardy JH (ed). Spinal Deformity in Neurological Muscular Disorders. St Louis: CV Mosby; 1974

[85] Tooth HH. The peroneal type of muscular atrophy. London: HK Lewis; 1886

[86] Charcot JM, Marie P. Su rune forme particuliére d'atrophie musculaire progressive souvent familial, debutante par les pieds et les jambs, et atteignant plus tard les mains. Rev Medicale Fr. 1886; 6:97–138

[87] Timmerman V, Nelis E, Van Hul W, et al. The peripheral myelin protein gene PMP-22 is contained within the Charcot-Marie-Tooth disease type 1A duplication. Nat Genet. 1992; 1(3):171–175

[88] Morrison PJ. The spinocerebellar ataxias: molecular progress and newly recognized paediatric phenotypes. Eur J Paediatr Neurol. 2000; 4(1):9–15

[89] Makin M. The surgical management of Friedreich's ataxia. J Bone Joint Surg Am. 1953; 35-A(2):425–436

[90] Taylor RG. The treatment of claw toes by multiple transfers of flexor into extensor tendons. J Bone Joint Surg Br. 1951; 33-B(4):539–542

[91] Otto AG. Monstorum Sexentorum Descriptio Anatomica. Vratislavial: Museum Anatomica Pathologieum; 1847:323

[92] Sheldon W. Amyoplasia Congenita: (Multiple congenital articular rigidity: Arthrogryposis multiplex congenita). Arch Dis Child. 1932; 7(39):117–136

[93] Hall JG. Overview of arthrogryposis. In: Staheli LT, Hall JG, Jaffe KM, Pahoike DE (eds). Arthrogryposis: A Text Atlas. Cambridge: Cambridge University Press; 1998:1–25

[94] **Wynne-Davies R, Williams PF, O'Connor JCB. The 1960s epidemic of arthrogryposis multiplex congenita: a survey from the United Kingdom, Australia and the United States of America. J Bone Joint Surg Br. 1981; 63-B(1):76–82**

[95] **Shapiro F, Bresnan MJ. Orthopaedic management of childhood neuromuscular disease. Part II: peripheral neuropathies, Friedreich's ataxia, and arthrogryposis multiplex congenita. J Bone Joint Surg Am. 1982; 64(6):949–953**

[96] Robinson RO. Arthrogryposis multiplex congenita; feeding, language and other health problems. Neuropediatrics. 1990; 21(4):177–178

[97] **Gibson DA, Urs ND. Arthrogryposis multiplex congenita. J Bone Joint Surg Br. 1970; 52(3):483–493**

[98] Akazawa H, Oda K, Mitani S, Yoshitaka T, Asaumi K, Inoue H. Surgical management of hip dislocation in children with arthrogryposis multiplex congenita. J Bone Joint Surg Br. 1998; 80(4):636–640

[99] Arahata K, Ishiura S, Ishiguro T, et al. Immunostaining of skeletal and cardiac muscle surface membrane with antibody against Duchenne muscular dystrophy peptide. Nature. 1988; 333(6176):861–863

[100] Bonilla E, Samitt CE, Miranda AF, et al. Duchenne muscular dystrophy: deficiency of dystrophin at the muscle cell surface. Cell. 1988; 54(4):447–452

[101] Greenstein RM, Reardon MP, Chan TS. An X-autosome translocation in a girl with Duchenne muscular dystrophy – evidence for DMD gene localisation. Pediatr Res. 1977; 11:457

[102] Siegel IM, Miller JE, Ray RD. Subcutaneous lower limb tenotomy in the treatment of pseudohypertrophic muscular dystrophy. Description of technique and presentation of twenty-one cases. J Bone Joint Surg Am. 1968; 50(7):1437–1443

[103] Riley CM, Day RL, et al. Central autonomic dysfunction with defective lacrimation; report of five cases. Pediatrics. 1949; 3(4):468–478

[104] Riley CM, Moore RH. Familial dysautonomia differentiated from related disorders. Case reports and discussions of current concepts. Pediatrics. 1966; 37(3):435–446

[105] **Hensinger RN, MacEwen GD. Spinal deformity associated with heritable neurological conditions: spinal muscular atrophy, Friedreich's ataxia, familial dysautonomia, and Charcot-Marie-Tooth disease. J Bone Joint Surg Am. 1976; 58(1):13–24**

[106] Gronert GA. Malignant hyperthermia. Anesthesiology. 1980; 53(5):395–423

[107] Britt BA, Kalow W. Malignant hyperthermia: a statistical review. Can Anaesth Soc J. 1970; 17(4):293–315
[108] Denborough MA, Forster JF, Lovell RR, Maplestone PA, Villiers JD. Anaesthetic deaths in a family. Br J Anaesth. 1962; 34:395–396
[109] Ellis FR, Harriman DGF. A new screening test for susceptibility to malignant hyperpyrexia. Br J Anaesth. 1973; 45(6):638
[110] Deacon P, Dickson RA. Unpublished data.
[111] **Riddick MF, Winter RB, Lutter LD. Spinal deformities in patients with spinal muscle atrophy: a review of 36 patients. Spine. 1982; 7(5):476–483**
[112] **Robinson D, Galasko CS, Delaney C, Williamson JB, Barrie JL. Scoliosis and lung function in spinal muscular atrophy. Eur Spine J. 1995; 4 (5):268–273**
[113] Thacker M, Hui JH, Wong HK, Chatterjee A, Lee EH. Spinal fusion and instrumentation for paediatric neuromuscular scoliosis: retrospective review. J Orthop Surg (Hong Kong). 2002; 10(2):144–151
[114] Takeshita K, Lenke LG, Bridwell KH, Kim YJ, Sides B, Hensley M. Analysis of patients with nonambulatory neuromuscular scoliosis surgically treated to the pelvis with intraoperative halo-femoral traction. Spine. 2006; 31 (20):2381–2385
[115] Fujak A, Ingenhorst A, Heuser K, Forst R, Forst J. Treatment of scoliosis in intermediate spinal muscular atrophy (SMA type II) in childhood. Ortop Traumatol Rehabil. 2005; 7(2):175–179
[116] **Sucato DJ. Spine deformity in spinal muscular atrophy. J Bone Joint Surg Am. 2007; 89 Suppl 1:148–154**
[117] Granata C, Cervellati S, Ballestrazzi A, Corbascio M, Merlini L. Spine surgery in spinal muscular atrophy: long-term results. Neuromuscul Disord. 1993; 3 (3):207–215
[118] Modi HN, Suh SW, Song HR, Lee SH, Yang JH. Correction of apical axial rotation with pedicular screws in neuromuscular scoliosis. J Spinal Disord Tech. 2008; 21(8):606–613
[119] Modi HN, Suh SW, Song HR, Fernandez HM, Yang JH. Treatment of neuromuscular scoliosis with posterior-only pedicle screw fixation. J Orthop Surg. 2008; 3(3):23
[120] Mehta SS, Modi HN, Srinivasalu S, et al. Pedicle screw-only constructs with lumbar or pelvic fixation for spinal stabilization in patients with Duchenne muscular dystrophy. J Spinal Disord Tech. 2009; 22(6):428–433
[121] Modi HN, Suh S-W, Hong J-Y, Cho J-W, Park J-H, Yang J-H. Treatment and complications in flaccid neuromuscular scoliosis (Duchenne muscular dystrophy and spinal muscular atrophy) with posterior-only pedicle screw instrumentation. Eur Spine J. 2010; 19(3):384–393
[122] Chong HS, Moon ES, Kim HS, et al. Comparison between operated muscular dystrophy and spinal muscular atrophy patients in terms of radiological, pulmonary and functional outcomes. Asian Spine J. 2010; 4(2):82–88
[123] Mullender M, Blom N, De Kleuver M, et al. A Dutch guideline for the treatment of scoliosis in neuromuscular disorders. Scoliosis. 2008; 3:14
[124] Burnett BG, Crawford TO, Sumner CJ. Emerging treatment options for spinal muscular atrophy. Curr Treat Options Neurol. 2009; 11(2):90–101
[125] Modi HN, Suh SW, Yang JH, et al. Surgical complications in neuromuscular scoliosis operated with posterior- only approach using pedicle screw fixation. Scoliosis. 2009; 4:11
[126] Zebala LP, Bridwell KH, Baldus C, et al. Minimum 5-year radiographic results of long scoliosis fusion in juvenile spinal muscular atrophy patients: major curve progression after instrumented fusion. J Pediatr Orthop. 2011; 31 (5):480–488
[127] McElroy MJ, Shaner AC, Crawford TO, et al. Growing rods for scoliosis in spinal muscular atrophy: structural effects, complications, and hospital stays. Spine. 2011; 36(16):1305–1311
[128] **Daher YH, Lonstein JE, Winter RB, Bradford DS. Spinal deformities in patients with Friedreich ataxia: a review of 19 patients. J Pediatr Orthop. 1985; 5(5):553–557**
[129] Labelle H, Tohmé S, Duhaime M, Allard P. Natural history of scoliosis in Friedreich's ataxia. J Bone Joint Surg Am. 1986; 68(4):564–572
[130] Lubicky JP, Spadaro JA, Yuan HA, Fredrickson BE, Henderson N. Variability of somatosensory cortical evoked potential monitoring during spinal surgery. Spine. 1989; 14(8):790–798
[131] Karol LA, Elerson E. Scoliosis in patients with Charcot-Marie-Tooth disease. J Bone Joint Surg Am. 2007; 89(7):1504–1510
[132] Bakker JP, De Groot IJ, Beelen A, Lankhorst GJ. Predictive factors of cessation of ambulation in patients with Duchenne muscular dystrophy. Am J Phys Med Rehabil. 2002; 81(12):906–912
[133] Sengupta DK, Mehdian SH, McConnell JR, Eisenstein SM, Webb JK. Pelvic or lumbar fixation for the surgical management of scoliosis in duchenne muscular dystrophy. Spine. 2002; 27(18):2072–2079
[134] Marsh A, Edge G, Lehovsky J. Spinal fusion in patients with Duchenne's muscular dystrophy and a low forced vital capacity. Eur Spine J. 2003; 12 (5):507–512
[135] Gaine WJ, Lim J, Stephenson W, Galasko CS. Progression of scoliosis after spinal fusion in Duchenne's muscular dystrophy. J Bone Joint Surg Br. 2004; 86 (4):550–555
[136] Gill I, Eagle M, Mehta JS, Gibson MJ, Bushby K, Bullock R. Correction of neuromuscular scoliosis in patients with preexisting respiratory failure. Spine. 2006; 31(21):2478–2483
[137] **Kinali M, Messina S, Mercuri E, et al. Management of scoliosis in Duchenne muscular dystrophy: a large 10-year retrospective study. Dev Med Child Neurol. 2006; 48(6):513–518**
[138] Leatherman KD, Johnson J, Holt R, et al. A clinical assessment of 357 cases of segmental spinal instrumentation. In: Luque ER (ed). Segmental Spinal Instrumentation. Thorofare: Slack Inc.; 1984:165–184
[139] Cheuk DK, Wong V, Wraige E, et al. Surgery for scoliosis in Duchenne muscular dystrophy. Cochrane Database Syst Rev. 2007; 24(1):CD005375
[140] Velasco MV, Colin AA, Zurakowski D, Darras BT, Shapiro F. Posterior spinal fusion for scoliosis in duchenne muscular dystrophy diminishes the rate of respiratory decline. Spine. 2007; 32(4):459–465
[141] Mercado E, Alman B, Wright JG. Does spinal fusion influence quality of life in neuromuscular scoliosis? Spine. 2007; 32(19) Suppl:S120–S125
[142] Hahn F, Hauser D, Espinosa N, Blumenthal S, Min K. Scoliosis correction with pedicle screws in Duchenne muscular dystrophy. Eur Spine J. 2008; 17 (2):255–261
[143] **Takaso M, Nakazawa T, Imura T, et al. Surgical management of severe scoliosis with high-risk pulmonary dysfunction in Duchenne muscular dystrophy. Int Orthop. 2010; 34(3):401–406**
[144] Nakazawa T, Takaso M, Imura T, et al. Autogenous iliac crest bone graft versus banked allograft bone in scoliosis surgery in patients with Duchenne muscular dystrophy. Int Orthop. 2010; 34(6):855–861

Chapter 8

Deformities Associated with Neurofibromatosis

8.1	Introduction	238
8.2	Axial Skeletal Lesions in Neurofibromatosis	239
8.3	Spinal Deformities in Neurofibromatosis	239
8.4	Management of Spinal Deformities in Neurofibromatosis	242
8.5	Cervical and Cervicothoracic Spine Deformities	247
Case Gallery		249

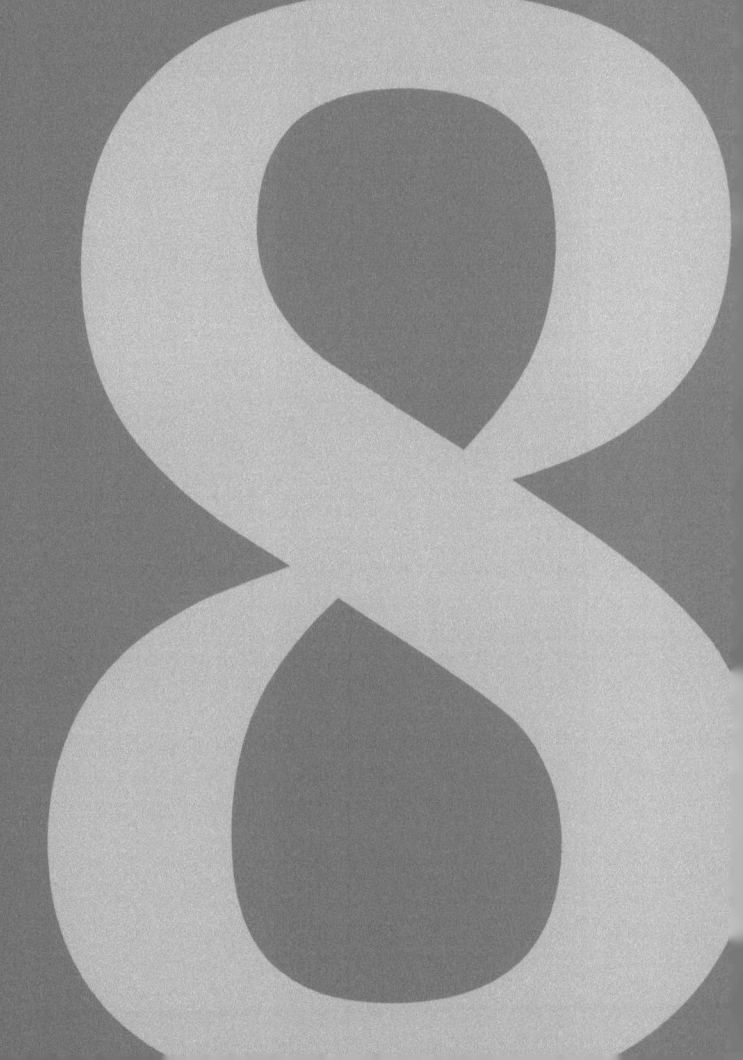

8 Deformities Associated with Neurofibromatosis

8.1 Introduction

Von Recklinghausen's disease of the nervous system (neurofibromatosis [NF1]) is to be differentiated from von Recklinghausen's disease of bone (hyperparathyroidism). It is a common autosomal dominant disorder (▶ Fig. 8.1). NF1 arises from an abnormality of neural crest differentiation and migration during early embryogenesis.

There are two discrete forms: NF1 and NF2. NF1 is the most common with an incidence rate of 1 in 4,000 live births. NF1 is caused by a defect in the gene for the protein neurofibromin which is a tumor suppressor gene. It was NF1 that was described by von Recklinghausen but like so many medical conditions that are referred to eponymously it was originally described about a century before von Recklinghausen's description.[1] Early work by Smith recorded both the clinical and postmortem findings and he thought that the tumors were connected to minute nerve branches.[2] Interestingly he did not mention involvement of the skeleton. Then Virchow[3] studied carefully the pathology of the nodules and determined that these were true neoplasms and not neuromata. Von Recklinghausen himself demonstrated nerve elements in the fibrous tissue tumors and correlated the nerve and skin lesions.[4] Chauffard then demonstrated that the pigmented skin lesions were characteristic of the disease as were the tumors.[5] The diagnostic value of these café-au-lait spots (melanin deposits in the basal skin layers) was reaffirmed by Thannhauser who recommended a careful search elsewhere for other lesions when the characteristic skin lesions were noted.[6] Whitehouse increased the diagnostic value of café-au-lait spots by recommending that at least six should be present[7] and the axilla is a favorite location. NF1 may involve virtually every system and organ in the body and so clinical manifestation may vary considerably. It is rather like scoliosis itself, not so much being a matter of having the condition but rather how much of it you have.

That the condition can affect all components of the musculoskeletal system supports the opinion that the pathogenesis involves embryological or developmental failure of both ectodermal and mesodermal tissues.[8–10]

NF1 is diagnosed when two of the seven signs listed in ▶ Table 8.1 are present.

There should be six café-au-lait spots measuring 1.5 cm in the adolescent and 0.5 cm in the young confirming that the activity of these areas of pigmentation and indeed the tumors are further related to sex hormone status[11] (▶ Fig. 8.2).

Lisch nodules are hamartomata in the iris present in three-quarters of cases of NF1 with an increasing prevalence rate with age so that all adults have them.

There should be two or more neurofibromata or one plexiform neurofibroma and, interestingly, these can involve the nerves and blood vessels of the gut as well as the musculoskeletal system.

All orthopaedic surgeons have known about the osseous changes in von Recklinghausen's disease with long bone pseudarthroses being common along with dystrophic scoliosis although the latter, perhaps surprisingly, is not sufficiently specific enough to be a diagnostic criterion.

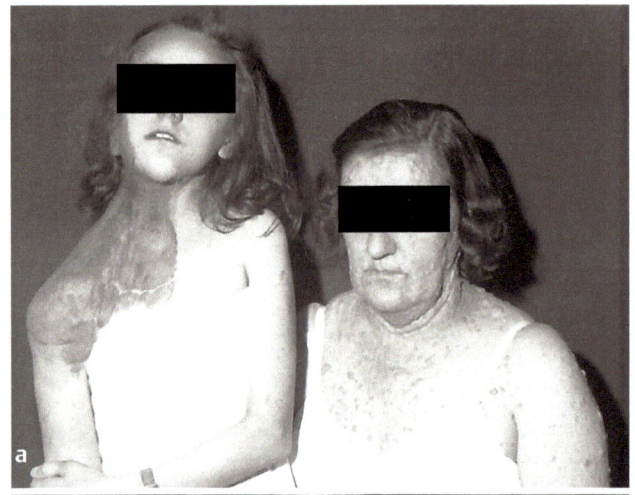

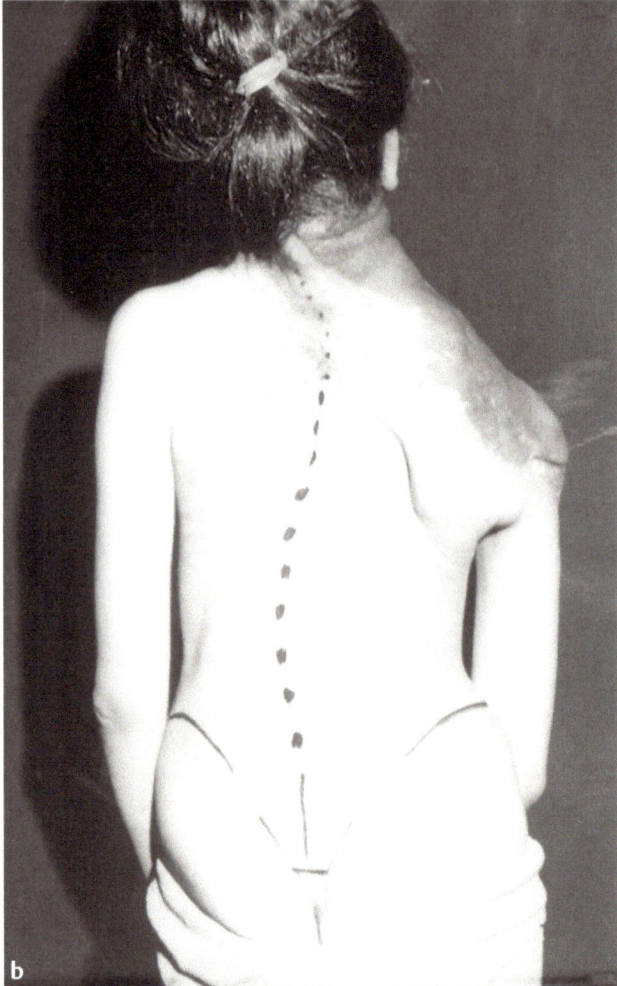

Fig. 8.1 (a) Mother and daughter with NF1, the former with multiple cutaneous nodules (fibroma molluscum) and the latter with a cutaneous plexiform neurofibroma (elephantiasis neuromatosa). (b) Back view of the daughter showing a high thoracic curve.

Deformities Associated with Neurofibromatosis

Table 8.1 Diagnostic signs in NF1

- Café au lait spots
- Axillary/inguinal freckling
- Lisch nodules in the iris
- Neurofibromata
- A distinctive bony lesion
- Optic gliomas
- An affected first degree relative

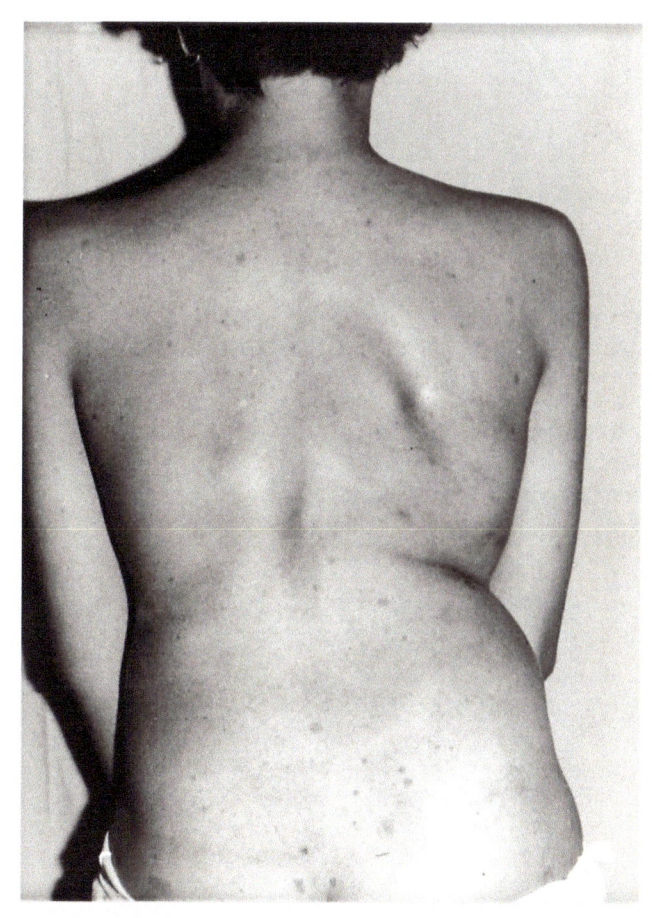

Fig. 8.2 Multiple cutaneous café-au-lait spots. Note also the surface appearance of a short angular thoracolumbar scoliosis with a lot of rotation.

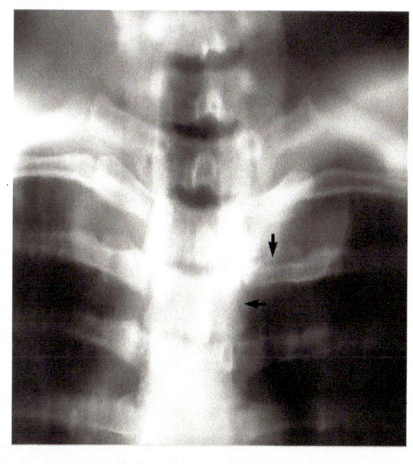

Fig. 8.3 PA tomogram of the upper thoracic spine showing the rib pencilling (*vertical arrow*) and the vertebral scalloping (*horizontal arrow*) typical of neurofibromatosis.

Sphenoid dysplasia is also distinctive.

An affected first degree relative is also diagnostic but there is a high rate of mutation approaching 50%.[12]

There is a definite risk of the tumors becoming malignant and changing into the highly lethal neurofibrosarcoma, variably estimated at between 5% and 10%.

8.2 Axial Skeletal Lesions in Neurofibromatosis

With the passage of time more attention was naturally focused on skeletal radiology in NF1. Prevalence rates of skeletal involvement in less than 30% of cases[13] soon rose to more than 50%[14] as the importance of spinal involvement became recognized. Hunt and Pugh,[15] in documenting the skeletal lesions in NF1, put much weight on spinal involvement. In addition to describing these spinal deformities, tibial pseudarthroses, and orbital defects, they stressed the importance of attenuated pencilled ribs, enlarged intervertebral foramina, and in particular the scalloped appearances of the vertebrae themselves (▶ Fig. 8.3). An early single case report of scalloping due to pressure from an adjacent neurofibroma[16] led to the initial view that dysplastic bodies and enlarged foramina were due to pressure from local tumor involvement but this was soon repudiated by the observation that scalloping occurred most commonly without any local tumor tissue.[17] Meanwhile, operatively and radiographically it had been demonstrated that these characteristic skeletal lesions often occurred in association with local meningoceles and dural enlargements (ectasia) such that these were incriminated in the pathological process.[15,18–22] There is undoubtedly an association, but the relative paucity of such radiological findings in the great majority of cases lends support to the view of Heard and Payne[17] that these dystrophic changes are primary, and therefore in some way associated with the underlying condition, while the meningeal dilatations are merely filling the greater available space. There is certainly no evidence of neurofibromatous tissue as a causative factor at the apex of spinal deformities.[23]

8.3 Spinal Deformities in Neurofibromatosis

8.3.1 Pattern of Deformity

Once again the chief confusing factor as regards the description of the deformity has been an analysis of anteroposterior (AP) and lateral radiographs of the patient and not the deformity (see Chapter 3). In this respect kyphoscoliosis comes through as the main spinal deformity, but it is not possible, as with other causes of scoliosis,[24] for the condition of kyphoscoliosis to really exist. Roaf in his classic text[25] likened the curve pattern in NF1 to that in idiopathic scoliosis, namely a lordoscoliosis, although also recognizing a common shorter and more angular curve

(▶ Fig. 8.4). He further pointed out[26] "if kyphosis means an increase in length of the posterior elements of the vertebral column relative to the anterior elements the use of the term is certainly erroneous" in relation to kyphoscoliosis. When Weiss, in attributing recognition of the high incidence of scoliosis in von Recklinghausen's disease to another dermatologist Engman, described spinal curvatures,[27] he wisely did not go much further.

Subsequent studies of the pattern of deformity showed that it can be divided into two groups of cases: patients with a diagnosis of NF1 who have been examined for the presence of a spinal deformity, and patients presenting as the result of a spinal deformity in the clinic in association with NF1. It is only possible to look at the prevalence rate of spinal deformity in the first group, but as Scott pointed out[28] even this group are selected to a degree by presenting to hospital as a result of one or more components of their condition. Nonetheless, in these studies of patients with NF1, the prevalence rate of spinal deformity ranges from 20 to 40%.[22,28–31] Most of these studies could find no particular pattern of deformity,[22,28,29] although the thoracic curve was the most common site encountered. Chaglassian[31] looked at 141 cases and found 37 cases of scoliosis (26%), the majority having long idiopathic-type curves with only 16 short, sharp angular ones. Although he could detect no particular curve pattern it is interesting that the average age of presentation of the 21 long curves was 7 years, while that of the 16 short curves was surprisingly 10 years. These 141 cases were all diagnosed according to the criteria of Crowe et al[32] and therefore this series did not contain any formes frustes of neurofibromatosis. Laws and Pallis looked at 18 unselected cases of NF1 and found a spinal deformity in seven (39%), but none were short angular curves.[22] Scott[28] could find no uniformity in length or direction of thoracic curves. However, in seven cases he observed evidence of a congenital bony anomaly in the form of fused ribs or hemivertebrae.

Meanwhile, Cobb had clearly stated that there were two types of scoliosis in neurofibromatosis: a milder idiopathic type and a particularly progressive short angular dystrophic type.[33] Moreover, he stated that the diagnosis could be made radiographically on the basis of this very characteristic short angular curve. He also pointed out that later in childhood some curves did appear congenital but there were always earlier films that showed normal vertebrae. Apart from prevalence rate all that can be said from these studies is that the thoracic curve is the most commonly encountered and it is more often of a long idiopathic type than a short angular dystrophic type.

Other studies of spinal deformity in NF1 concern patients who have presented as a result of a spinal deformity.[34–44] These therefore represent an extremely selected group from which it would be quite incorrect to infer anything about prevalence rates and patterns of deformity. Quite naturally in this selected group the most common curve encountered is the short angular dystrophic curve. This situation is analogous with studies of idiopathic scoliosis in which data derived from scoliosis clinics describe the thoracic curve site as the most common with a significant female preponderance, whereas data from community screening studies reveal a more even gender ratio and the lumbar spine is now found to be preponderant.[45]

Thus it is the short sharp angular dystrophic curve that attracts the attention of the scoliosis surgeon.[34–44] Veliskakis looked at 55 patients with a spinal deformity and found 43 patients with short angular curves with wedging that often looked like a hemivertebra.[37] There was an equal gender distribution but there were more left-sided curves. In contradistinction to Chaglassian et al,[31] he found that the short curves appeared, as expected, at an early age and progressed more rapidly. Kyphosis was noted to be common and the severity of the kyphosis was proportional to the severity of the lateral spinal curvature. This implies that AP and lateral views of the patient were assessed, which gave the spurious appearance of a kyphosis. (If you're not with us go back and read Chapter 3 again). Dawson et al looked at 41 cases and followed them for 5 years.[38] Twenty-one were sharp angular curves, nine were pseudo-idiopathic, and the appearance of a kyphosis was seen in 14 patients. The 14 cases that progressed only did so by 30 degrees in 5 years. Moe et al reported 100 dystrophic curves out of a total of 112 cases of spinal deformity in neurofibromatosis.[42] They noted that all dystrophic curves progressed but only seven were lordotic. Winter et al then reviewed 102 patients, 80 of whom had dystrophic changes.[43] They described 31 as having kyphoscoliosis, 49 as scoliosis only, with no kyphotic component (he accepted 49 degrees of kyphosis as normal), and only 5 lordoscoliotic curves.

These reports demonstrate clearly that it is not possible to accurately define curve pattern from AP and lateral views of the patient. We have already seen (see Chapters 2 and 3) the spurious appearance of spinal deformities when inappropriate views of them are taken, but there is still much that can be learned about a spinal deformity from an AP view of the patient. Roaf[25,26] clearly understood the spine in three dimensions; he stressed the simple geometrical point that if there is rotation of a scoliosis with

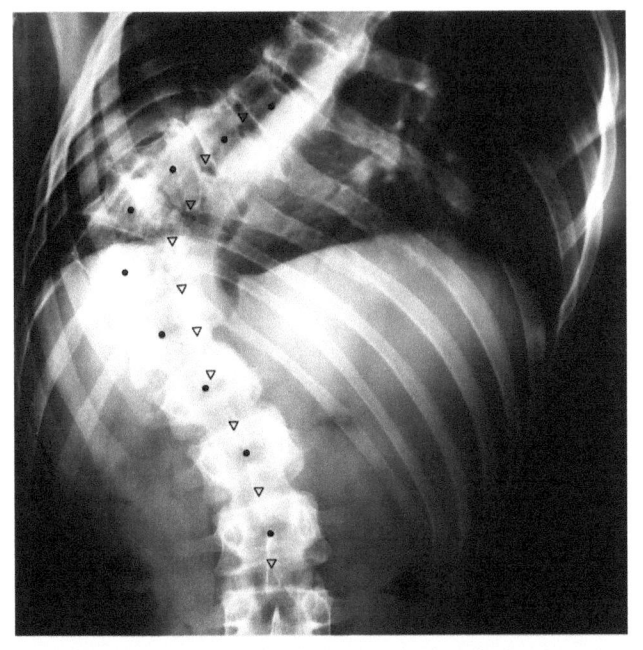

Fig. 8.4 PA view of the short sharp angular curve typical of von Recklinghausen's disease. There are black dots over the middle of the bodies and triangles over the spinous processes confirming lordosis. Note that there are only four really angulated and rotated vertebrae in this curve.

the vertebral bodies toward the convexity and the spinous processes toward the concavity then the line of the vertebral bodies is longer than the line of the posterior elements which, in conjunction with the direction of rotation, implies that the front of the spine is longer than the back and therefore these curves are *all* lordoscolioses. Moreover, in these studies of patients with neurofibromatosis and a spinal deformity,[34–44] all the AP radiographic illustrations confirm the presence of a lordoscoliosis. Vlok, however, recognized these radiographic features, and in his report of 21 cases[44] noted a short sharp angular dystrophic curve in 9 cases, all of which had a lordosis. Furthermore, the average curve magnitude of the lordoscolioses was significantly greater at 74 degrees than those who had a true kyphosis in which average curve magnitude was only 25 degrees (there being no buckling or "spinning" potential with a kyphotic spine).

Although by far the most common deformity in NF1 is the lordoscoliosis, this does not imply that these spines cannot be kyphotic. However, it does indicate that the area of kyphosis exists alone or lies above or below the scoliosis, where the vertebrae are not rotated. We therefore have the elementary principle that the pattern of spinal deformity in NF1 is similar to idiopathic spinal deformities. The thoracic lordoscoliosis seen in the NF1 patient is comparable to the idiopathic scoliotic deformity, while the thoracic kyphosis, with rotated lordoscoliosis below, is comparable to the Scheuermann's deformity albeit more angular.[46] The prevalence rate of clinically significant deformities in neurofibromatosis is however 150 times greater than in otherwise normal children (30% and 0.2%, respectively), and this is entirely attributable to the dystrophic nature of the vertebrae. The forces acting on the spine, which 98% of normal children can resist, cannot be resisted by the dystrophic vertebrae of any more than 70% of patients with von Recklinghausen's disease. Moreover, if the dystrophic process is particularly obvious,[34–44] then the short sharp angular curve is produced, whereas with little or no dystrophic change the longer idiopathic-type curve is produced.[22,28–31] In the former situation the spine fails locally, whereas in the latter the spine fails over a greater area.

It is far better to be less prescriptive about scoliosis in NF1 and not simply try to divide the curves into angular dystrophic and long idiopathic type curves because there is clearly a spectrum from one to the other; the more evidence of systemic von Recklinghausen's disease, the more dystrophic features there are whereas the less the evidence of NF1, the more the patient resembles a normal child with the more prevalent long idiopathic type deformity. In von Recklinghausen's disease dystrophic curves always require an anterior spinal fusion in addition to a posterior one to try and mitigate a strong tendency for curve progression after surgery. In addition, knowing the unpredictability of the von Recklinghausen's scoliosis, you should always carry out a front and back fusion regardless of whether you think the curve is dystrophic or not. If you don't do this, then the von Recklinghausen scoliosis will make you regret that you had not done so. Do not forget the aphorism of the philosopher Santayana* "those who cannot remember history are condemned to repeat it."

Moreover, in an excellent review from the Royal National Orthopaedic Hospital in London,[47] they pointed out that modulation from initially idiopathic type curves to dystrophic ones occurs commonly and in the 91 cases they reported 80% of children under the age of 7 modulated and 25% of those over the age of 7. There are two particularly important discriminating factors, one obviously being patient age, and the other the presence of rib pencilling. All the more reason therefore for assuming dystrophism in all NF1 spinal deformity cases.

While the otherwise normal child who develops an idiopathic spinal deformity does not do so in the cervical region, the dystrophic vertebral situation in the patient with von Recklinghausen's disease facilitates the production of cervical spine deformities.[48,49] Yong-Hing[49] from Dean MacEwen's center in Wilmington noted that of 56 patients, 17 had cervical deformities and 15 of these occurred in association with significant deformities lower down in the spine. The majority of these were angular kyphoses, although lordoses were not uncommon. These deformities so high in the spine tend to resist rotation, but in the cervicothoracic junction serious rotational abnormalities can be produced in the presence of an underlying lordosis.

There are therefore four patterns of spinal deformity which can be encountered in the patient with neurofibromatosis:
1. An inconsequential nonstructural lumbar curve consequent upon leg-length inequality caused by local hemihypertrophy.
2. The idiopathic-type long lordoscoliosis.
3. The dystrophic short angular lordoscoliosis.
4. An angular thoracic or cervical kyphosis that can occur alone, or above a compensatory lordosis that has rotated to the side.

8.3.2 Neurological Involvement

Neurological deficits secondary to a spinal deformity are very prevalent in association with NF1, second only to congenital spine deformities.[50] In a superb report by Curtis et al of 8 cases, with a review of the literature,[51] they found 32 cases of NF1 with paraplegia from the end of the 19th century.[52–71] Analysis of these cases demonstrated two clear patterns of spontaneous neurological involvement affecting the spine in von Recklinghausen's disease. The most common situation is a low cervical or high thoracic paraplegia in association with a local angular kyphosis for which laminectomy is disastrous. In other words, the last thing angular dystrophic kyphosis in the growing child wants is removal of the posterior spinal column which of course is the only local tension member and if removed rapidly leads to accelerated progression of the deformity. If a laminectomy is required for removal of an intradural lesion, then it is mandatory to carry out a concomitant spinal fusion procedure. This clearly cannot be a posterior fusion because there are no posterior elements left and so anterior or lateral intertransverse fusion is necessary, and preferably both. Cobb stated so succinctly[33] "the spinal deformity resulting from neurofibromatosis may be horrible, but laminectomy without stabilization will make it a nightmare." The second type of neurological problem is that associated with local tumor formation, is much less

---

*Jorge Agustín Nicolás Ruiz de Santayana (1863–1952), Spanish-born American philosopher, poet, and humanist.

common than in association with a spinal deformity itself, and can arise anywhere in the spine. It is only in this group that laminectomy, followed by tumor removal, is of benefit. Again there should be no hesitation in carrying out a concomitant spinal fusion.

8.4 Management of Spinal Deformities in Neurofibromatosis

8.4.1 Scoliosis

Retrospective analyses of the treatment of these spinal deformities have produced interesting but in no way surprising information that tells more about the natural history of these deformities than the efficacy of treatments prescribed. Conservative treatment has been in the form of traditional Milwaukee bracing and, of course, the different "responses to treatment" are attributable solely to whether the curve was more of the mild idiopathic type or tended toward the more progressive angular dystrophic variety. Even now, when it has been confirmed that there is no evidence base in support of orthotic treatment for any kind of scoliosis[72] except perhaps a circumferential torso support device for the collapsing neuromuscular curve, the Milwaukee or one of its underarm forms still has its proponents. Of course the most recent brace trial[73] had a number of serious flaws—no randomization, more of the progressive thoracic curves in the control group than the treated group biasing natural history, and stopping before the attainment of spinal maturity to mention but a few. Even forgetting about these discrepancies the results were extraordinary. Using an increase in Cobb angle by 6 degrees as failure the control group was significantly worse than the brace group with the electrical stimulation (LESS[74]) group worst. Not only should orthotic treatment for idiopathic scoliosis be binned or kicked into the long grass but we are talking about scoliosis in NF1 and it is positively harmful in those children whose curves are known to have significant progression potential. Fiddling about with bracing for a number of months or years simply delays surgical treatment for a condition that most definitely requires it. Not surprisingly it was the short angular dystrophic curve that responded "less well" to brace treatment.

Cobb[33] stated that it was better to fuse earlier than to wait and accordingly most of these reports favored early surgical intervention in the nature of posterior fusion with or without instrumentation. Rapp and Glock, however, disagreed with those that said the scoliosis always needed early fusion and emphasized that age played a major part in determining treatment.[75] They were essentially emphasizing that growth velocity was the final common denominator and that fusion would be all the more definitive the closer to the end of adolescent growth. Consequently early results of posterior fusion were not encouraging and in Dawson's series of 27 operations, the average correction was only 23 degrees, 6 of whom subsequently lost correction and a further 6 developed pseudarthroses.[38] In Stagnara's series of 37 cases there was little difference in postoperative progression between posterior fusion and posterior fusion along with metalwork which averaged about 23 degrees.[39] He did however perform some extensive anterior and posterior fusions but the numbers were not sufficient to attribute benefit. In Winter's series of 102 patients[43] he tried to divide kyphosis into two groups, above or below 50 degrees. For those with a kyphosis of less than 50 degrees a posterior fusion alone was satisfactory but for those more than 50 degrees there was a two-thirds incidence of pseudarthrosis and in such cases he recommended quite rightly an additional anterior fusion. However, in Professor Tanner's wonderful book *Growth at Adolescence*,[76] he nicely describes the growth velocity curve of normal children along with standard centile charts to record serial measurements,[77] and not those with notoriously progressive deformities such as von Recklinghausen's disease. These unfortunate children do not behave according to Tanner's normal child and that is why aggressive curves such as neurofibromatosis, early onset idiopathic, and congenital present earlier with a much worse progression potential than their idiopathic counterpart. Although George Rapp from Indianapolis meant well by telling us to pay attention to adolescent growth[75]—the simple fact is that you have to step in surgically as and when the patient tells you, which is sooner rather than later regardless of precise chronological age. Moreover, 90% of height gain during adolescence occurs in the legs and not much in the spine, so concern about stunting spinal growth is not really justified.

Have we made much progress since these earlier reports mainly in the 1970s? Reviewing now the last 20 or so years of publications concerning spinal deformities in association with NF1 one sees the same sort of results replicated. There is also the same tendency to divide curves into the dystrophic and non-dystrophic varieties when there is no clear discriminatory point between them. We can certainly all recognize the very dystrophic curve (short, sharp, angular, considerable apical wedging, rib pencilling, large foramina, lots of rotation) but it is much more difficult to fix a point down the pathway to dystrophism to confirm two discrete categories. Our basic message to all young and aspiring scoliosis surgeons is to assume they are all of the dystrophic variety (which they may well be) and treat them in the same aggressive surgical manner—anterior and posterior.

Surprisingly, at the height of the French revolution, CD instrumentation was regarded as being the universal panacea for all scolioses and was used as the first segmental instrumentation for neurofibromatosis. In Miami, Harry Shufflebarger reported on 11 NF1 patients, 10 with idiopathic-like curves and 1 dysplastic. Correction in all three planes was very satisfactory but the dysplastic NF1 patient required further anterior surgery.[78] Then Holt and Johnson from the Leatherman centra in Louisville in 1989 reported five dystrophic NF1 patients treated with CD instrumentation with only one posterior and the rest front and back procedures. Despite this, three patients showed significant progression that required further surgery and they quite rightly talked about the "tendency to extraordinary progression with growth."[79]

In 1999 the spine surgeons from the Rizzoli Institute in Bologna reported on 56 cases of dystrophic curves divided, as Winter had originally suggested, into those with a kyphosis less (group 1) or more than 50 degrees[80] (group 2). Despite stating that they had previously recommended anterior and posterior surgery[81] they carried out posterior surgery alone in 19 cases and only combined anterior and posterior in the remaining 6! The average age of the children was 13 years but did go down in range to 4 years. Only 10 of these posterior fusion patients achieved stabilisation, the initial Cobb angle being 71 degrees with 33 degrees of kyphosis going down to 45 degrees and 25 degrees, respectively, at surgery, deteriorating with time to 54 degrees and 31 degrees. Even in group 2 children they still did 11 posteriorly and 20 anteriorly and posteriorly. Failure to stabilize the curve occurred in more than 50% of those who underwent posterior fusion alone and less than 25% in those who had anterior and posterior fusions. They warned again that the severe dystrophic curve always requires combined anterior and posterior stabilization, particularly in younger patients, "even if the sagittal curves do not become pathologic by the time of presentation."

In 2005 a review of neurofibromatosis in terms of diagnosis and treatment was published from London and again categorized the curves into dystrophic and nondystrophic types although emphasized that that should be based on a meticulous assessment of the spine with both plain films and magnetic resonance imaging (MRI) to highlight radiologically undetectable dysplastic features that would determine prognosis and surgical planning[47] (▶ Table 8.2). When MRI scanning of the whole spine is carried out to identify vertebral dysplasia then in one-third of cases of NF1 initially classified on plain films as having nondystrophic curves did have typical vertebral dysplasia and hence were therefore dystrophic curves. Nondystrophic curves could be managed as for idiopathic scoliosis whereas dystrophic curves required anterior and posterior fusion of the entire structural curve with abundant autologous bone graft. Assessing carefully these MRI scan features indicating dystrophic change markedly assists in the division between dystrophic and nondystrophic curves and indicate that when there were three or more dysplastic features present the risk of curve progression was significantly increased in 85% of patients, with rib pencilling being the most important single factor.

From the above it doesn't look as though there are many scolioses in von Recklinghausen's disease that are not dystrophic (15% or less) in which case the message—treat them all as dystrophic anyway—sounds like even better advice (no apologies for telling you again).

China seems to have become an important source of scoliosis literature in recent years and in 2009 the Changhai Orthopaedic Department[82] reported on 19 patients with NF1 noting that posterior instrumented fusion alone was not adequate to correct scoliosis. They say because of weak bone structure but while this is true (dystrophic change) time allows spinal growth to significantly alter vertebral shape, particularly at the apex of the curve where the vertebrae can look like hemivertebrae, and so accelerates and potentiates early and progressive deformity.

Table 8.2 Typical dysplastic changes evident on plain radiographs in patients with NF1[22,26,37,43]

- Vertebral scalloping (considered to be present when the depth of scalloping is more than 3 mm in the thoracic spine or more than 4 mm in the lumbar spine)—this is either associated with dural ectasia or neural tumor
- Rib pencilling (considered to be present when the width of the rib is smaller than that of the narrowest portion of the second rib)
- Transverse process spindling
- Paravertebral soft tissue mass
- Short curve with a lot of apical rotation
- Intervertebral foraminal enlargement
- Widened interpediculate distances
- Dysplastic pedicles
- Vertebral dysplasia is best shown up on MRI scanning

They looked at whether extension of the fusion beyond the usual neutral to neutral vertebrae would enable posterior instrumented fusion to be effective. Their patients were aged more than 10 years and their scolioses were less than 90 degrees. There were 16 dystrophic and 3 nondystrophic curves. In the dystrophic curves the initial Cobb angle was 68 degrees with 30 degrees of kyphosis and this was reduced to 27 and 30 degrees at a minimum of 2 years' follow-up. A pseudarthrosis only occurred in one patient.

This goes back to the old notion of end-to-end posterior fusion (parallelism), rather than neutral to neutral, for younger idiopathic curves.[83] Although this seemed to be successful in their series the Cobb angle or degree of kyphosis did not seem excessive whereas with aggressive dystrophic curves both measures are usually considerably greater. The power of transpedicular instrumentation seems to result in a well corrected and stable curve, at least in Li's series,[82] but the real message of having to go end-to-end should be to mandate an anterior and posterior fusion.

Then the Cairo Group reported 32 cases of dystrophic NF1 again divided into two groups according to the angle of pseudokyphosis, less than and more than 45 degrees.[84] All underwent what they describe as aggressive anterior and posterior surgery with an average of four apical disks removed. When the deformity is as angular as can occur in NF1 then the spine above and below the apex angulates away from the surgeon but it is usually possible to remove at least four intervertebral disks including the growth plates. Taking out first the apical three disks usually allows a degree of curve improvement bringing the disks above and below more accessible. Then posterior transpedicular instrumentation with some sublaminar wires was the basis of the second stage. Their results were perhaps surprisingly good with a preoperative Cobb angle of 100 degrees being reduced to 40 degrees in both groups and with no significant loss of correction over a 3-year follow-up.[84]

In 2010 16 patients with dystrophic NF1 deformities were reported having undergone corpectomy and circumferential spinal fusion alleging that vertebral body resection had not previously been investigated[85] although we reported on vertebral body resection for severe dystrophic curves from the Leatherman spine center back in 1988.[86] Leatherman's closing wedge resection (▶ Fig. 6.19) has become the model for all subsequent techniques.[87,88] There was a correction of Cobb angle in the frontal and lateral planes of 90 degrees and 70 degrees respectively down to 50 degrees each with just a few degrees lost in the frontal plane and 13 degrees in the lateral plane at 7-year follow-up.[85]

Rib head protrusion into the central canal in NFI cases has been described several times with or without spinal cord dysfunction since the first description in 1986[89,90] (▶ Fig. 8.5) Clearly if this occurs then rib resection and spinal canal decompression is required as part of the surgical strategy.

Recommended Treatment for Scoliosis in Association with Neurofibromatosis

While the so-called dystrophic curve is readily recognizable even by plain X-rays (▶ Fig. 8.4, ▶ Table 8.2), MRI scanning is mandatory as part of the assessment of these children[47] and adds a considerable degree of precision as regards recognition of dystrophic curves to the plain films and thus to diagnosis.

Deformities Associated with Neurofibromatosis

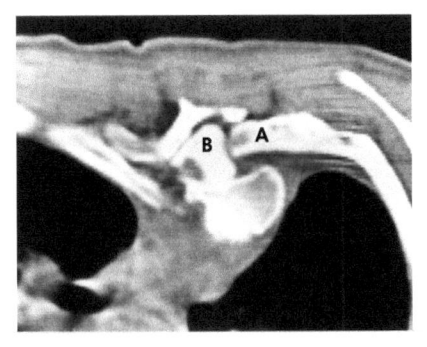

Fig. 8.5 The rib head (A) has dislocated through the enlarged foramen and is compressing the cord (B).

It is not possible nevertheless to absolutely differentiate dystrophic from so-called nondystrophic curves and to all intents and purposes it is essential to regard all scolioses in NFI as dystrophic and therefore carry out both anterior and posterior fusion. With the less severe deformity good results can be achieved by anterior soft tissue release (multiple apical diskectomy with removal of all growth plate cartilage) followed by posterior fusion of the entire structural curve with transpedicular instrumentation. For more severe angular deformities apical wedge resection is required in addition to multiple diskectomies and thereby excellent and reliable results can be achieved. It is far better to do what is necessary to start with, that is, anterior and posterior fusion, rather than posterior surgery alone and then have to perform more complex revision rescue surgery later on (▶ Fig. 8.6 and ▶ Fig. 8.7).

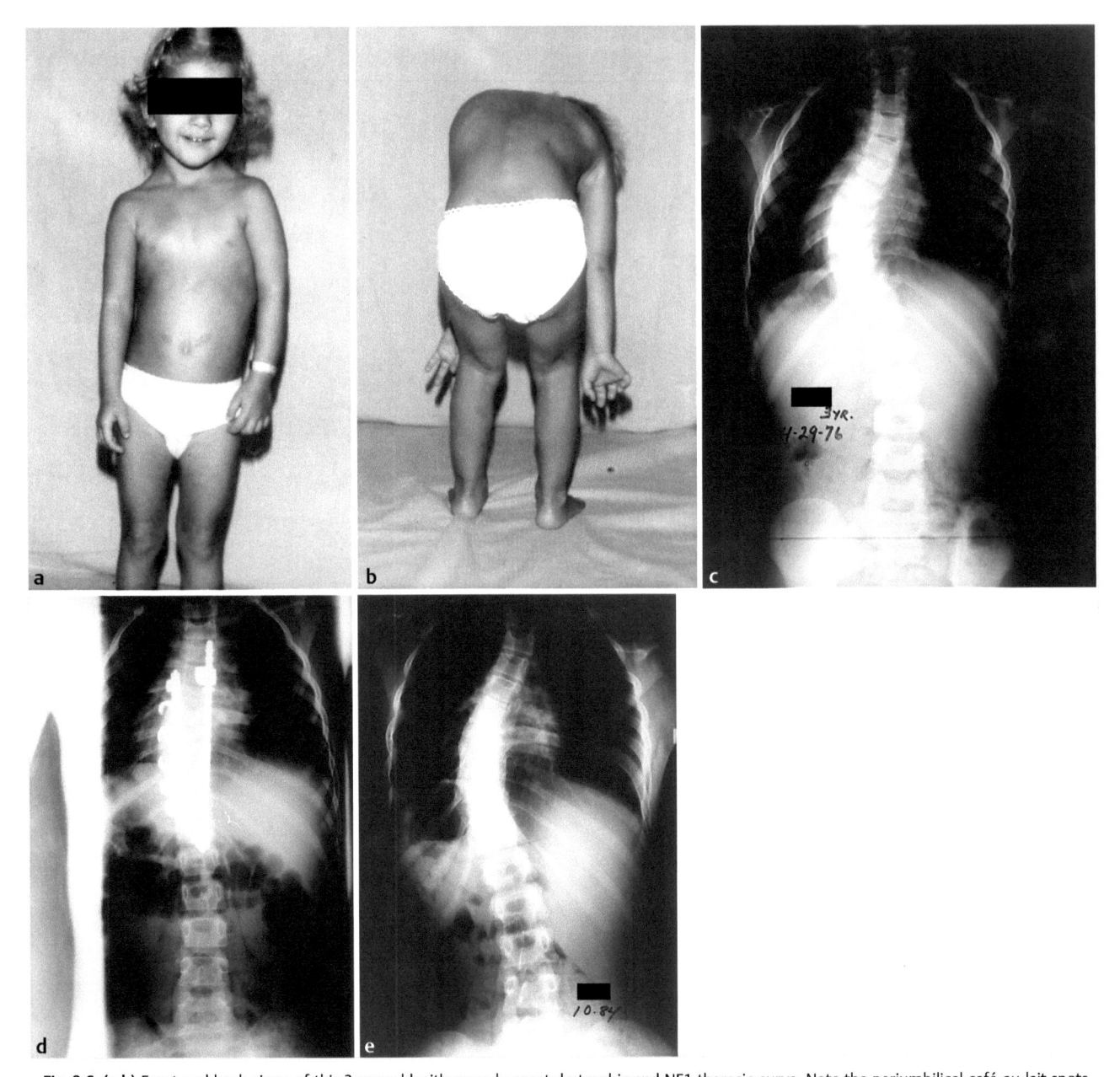

Fig. 8.6 (a,b) Front and back views of this 3-year-old with an early onset dystrophic and NF1 thoracic curve. Note the periumbilical café-au-lait spots plus a considerable amount of rotation (one of Leatherman's own cases). **(c)** PA radiograph of this particularly dystrophic thoracic curve. **(d)** After two-stage anterior multiple diskectomy and growth plate removal and posterior fusion with instrumentation. We felt that the adverse biology had been adequately countered. **(e)** After 11 years, at the end of growth and metalwork removal, the good correction has been sustained.

8.4.2 Kyphosis

When true planar views of spinal deformities in von Recklinghausen's disease are obtained it will be observed that the great majority are lordoscolioses, despite the clinical appearance and the AP and lateral views of the patient. The management strategy for these deformities is similar to those of congenital origin (see Chapter 6). The strong likelihood of neurological problems developing as the cord is bow-strong across the back of the kyphosis indicates that treatment is required whenever these deformities are encountered. Conservative therapy is useless. Do not fall into the trap of carrying out a posterior

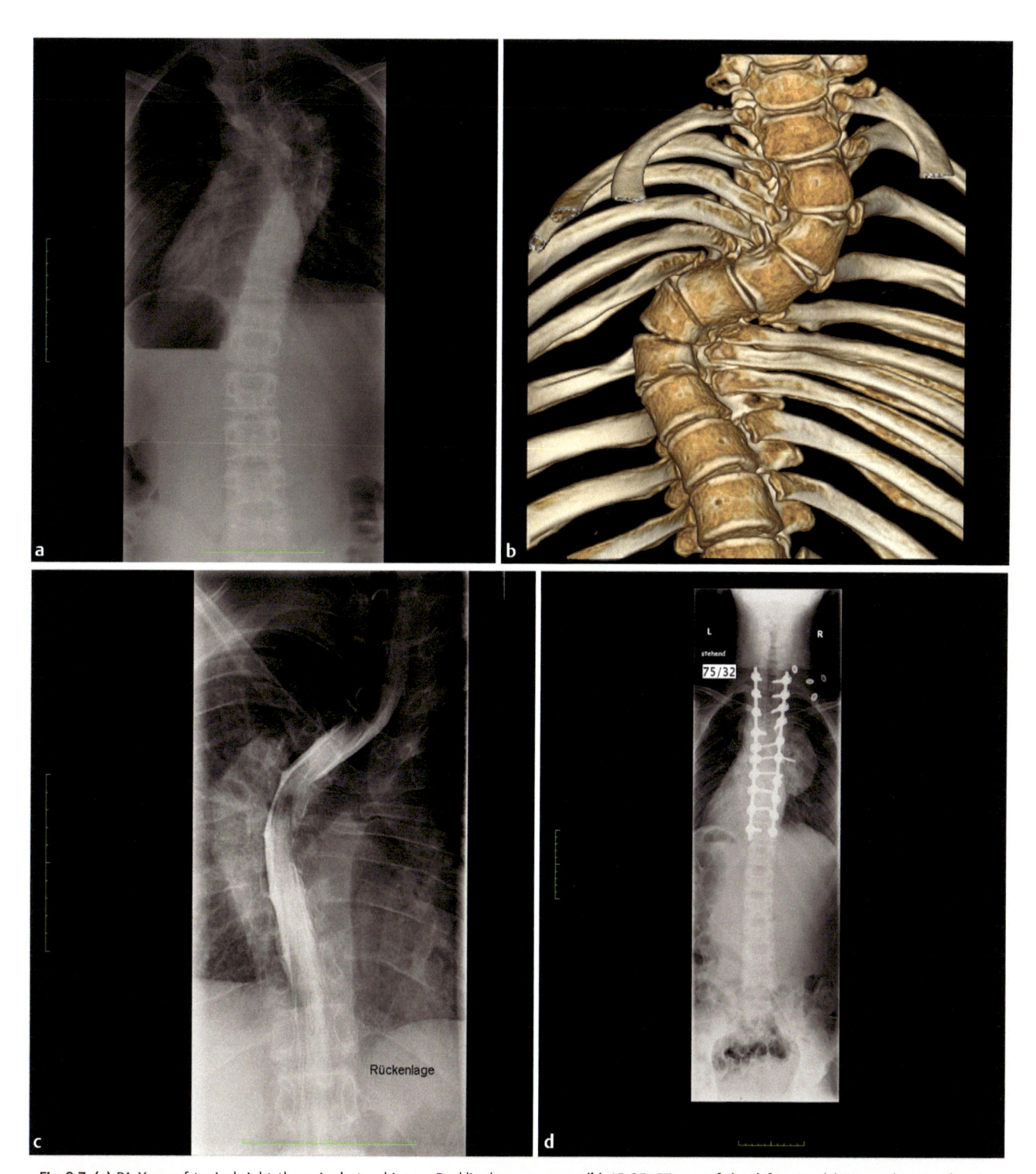

Fig. 8.7 (a) PA X-ray of typical right thoracic dystrophic von Recklinghausen curve. (b) AP 3D CT scan of the deformity. (c) PA myelogram showing thinning of the dye column over the apex of the deformity. (d) PA radiograph after apical wedge resection and posterior transpedicular instrumentation.

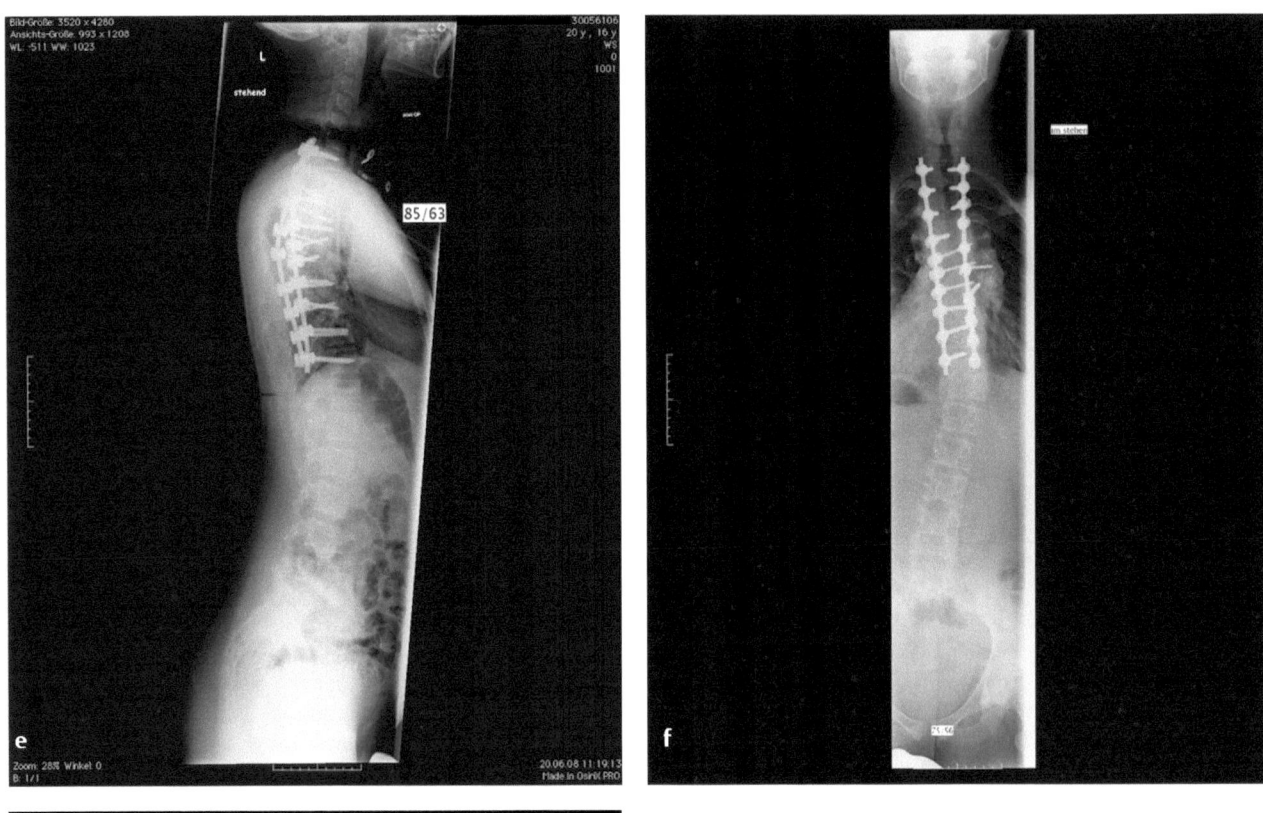

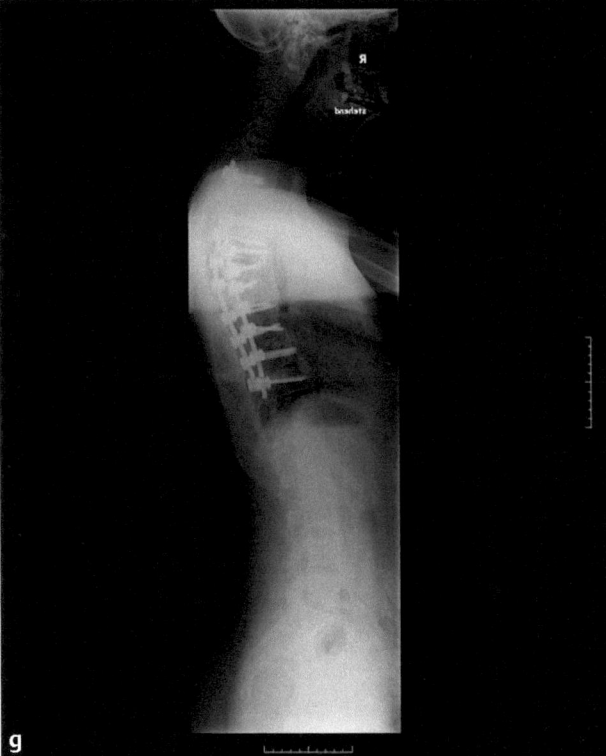

Fig. 8.7 (*continued*) (**e**) Lateral radiograph showing restoration of the normal thoracic kyphosis. (**f**) PA radiograph at the end of growth showing some "adding on" of the right thoracic curve but a well-balanced spine. (**g**) Lateral radiograph showing maintenance of the same thoracic kyphosis.

instrumented fusion alone for the relatively mild deformity, always carry out anterior and posterior surgery. The first stage involves removal of the apical disks and growth plates, the insertion of autogenous iliac crest interbody graft material, and a strong anterior strut graft of either iliac crest or fibular bone[71,91] (▶ Fig. 5.11d). Stagnara taught us how to raise an osteoperiosteal flap[92] which forms a rich vascular cancellous bed for the anterior construct such that failure of fusion is virtually unheard of. Then the entire deformity is neutralized posteriorly by metalwork. Thereby a correction of the kyphotic deformity of the order of 50% can be expected by this two-stage procedure.[93]

If the kyphotic deformity is both severe, and accompanied by neurological signs, then anterior cord decompression is the only treatment of choice (▶ Fig. 8.8). Merely obtaining some correction of the kyphotic deformity without vertebral body resection at the curve apex cannot be relied upon to rid the patient of neurological signs. Accordingly, the anterior aspect of the spinal cord must be seen to be completely decompressed and this implies the same apical wedge resection procedure that should be performed for the congenital kyphosis associated with neurological signs and after adequate anterior decompression, intervertebral graft material, and a strong anterior strut graft/cage completes the anterior stage.

8.5 Cervical and Cervicothoracic Spine Deformities

Deformities in the cervical spine are either angularly kyphotic or hyperlordotic. For the kyphotic deformity, anterior strut grafting/cage is again necessary but if this is accompanied by neurological signs then anterior vertebral body resection at the curve apex is necessary both to correct the deformity and to be certain that the anterior aspect of the cord is adequately decompressed. Again the posterior aspect of the spine is neutralized using posterior metalwork. It may be helpful to consider halo immobilization to support the potentially unstable spine and to fix to it a jacket to allow the patient to be ambulatory.

The rotated lordoscoliosis in the cervicothoracic region is a very difficult deformity to treat in the patient with dystrophic NF1. It is also difficult to evaluate radiologically and three-dimensional computed tomography (CT) is required. Furthermore, the scoliotic deformity may be double structural with a low cervical curve in one direction and a high thoracic curve in the other. Fortunately, these deformities are not commonly encountered but the anterior surgical procedures for those who do need treatment can be particularly exacting. In general treatment should be reserved for the kyphotic deformity that is associated with a neurological deficit. For this anterior vertebral body resection, spinal cord decompression, or diskectomy, the removal of the growth plates and both strut and cancellous bone grafting are necessary.

The cervicothoracic junction can be awkward to get at anteriorly and there are a number of ways in which this can be achieved.

The deformity may have to be approached with a sternal splitting exposure originally described by Cauchoix et al[94] and popularized by Fang et al for spinal tuberculosis.[95] These descriptions of the anterior approach to the cervicothoracic region have tended to focus on gaining access to short spinal segments. However, Tredwell's group in Vancouver recently described patients who were managed with a combined anterior neck and sternal splitting approach[96] (▶ Fig. 8.9) particularly useful for accessing multilevel spine deformities in children. Two of the six patients who were described had deformities secondary to NF1. It is very well worthwhile looking at this paper, the diagrams are excellent. Clearly a spinal surgeon has to involve their cardiothoracic colleague to display and mobilize the anatomy in the front of the upper thoracic spine. The upper part of the incision is a straightforward longitudinal one down the medial border of sternomastoid muscle, which is later retracted laterally along with the neurovascular sheath. After division of omohyoid, sternohyoid, and sternothyroid muscles the incision is extended downward as a midline sternotomy approach. After removal of the thymus gland the brachiocephalic trunk is mobilized with a vessel loop and then it can be seen that the lower anterior cervical spine and the upper thoracic spine are exposed contiguously. The trachea and esophagus are then retracted from the midline and the innominate artery displaced forward and downward. Access down to T4 should thus be facilitated although it has to be said that, after safe exposure with your cardiovascular colleague, in the presence of angular kyphosis, the orthopaedic part of the procedure (i.e., multiple diskectomies and body resection) is by no means straightforward. Then the deformity should be supported posteriorly using posterior metalwork. Again it is doubtful whether posterior fusion is required on the tension side of a kyphosis as sufficient biological support should have been provided by the anterior interbody and strut grafting part of the procedure.

There is no doubt that this sort of approach for more lengthy exposures anteriorly over the cervicothoracic junction is very useful. However, we have found that approaching the front of the upper thoracic spine so as to resect and replace vertebral bodies can be carried out more easily by the costo-transversectomy approach, removing the transverse processes and posterior portions of the first three ribs (▶ Fig. 6.47).

In patients with dystrophic NF1 with thoracolumbar spinal deformities, cervical spine problems have been noted in a quarter to a half.[97] It is not uncommon for the orthopaedic spine surgeon to be referred a patient after having had previous cervical spine surgery, generally because of a progressive kyphosis when the back of the cervical spine has been destabilized. In this respect laminectomy without concomitant stabilization of the neck is disastrous. There can however be neurofibromas themselves in the neck and atlantoaxial subluxation/dislocation has been reported.[98] Because of the more generous dimensions of the cervical canal and cervical cord (3:1), some pathologies may remain asymptomatic but clearly symptomatic mass lesions causing symptoms may require to be removed and, if performed by posterior laminectomy, posterior instrumentation and lateral mass fusion of the particular area must be carried out—hence the critical importance of full MRI in the evaluation of the NF1 patient. Again halo immobilization may be invaluable particularly when the bone to support metalwork is in itself dystrophic.

Deformities Associated with Neurofibromatosis

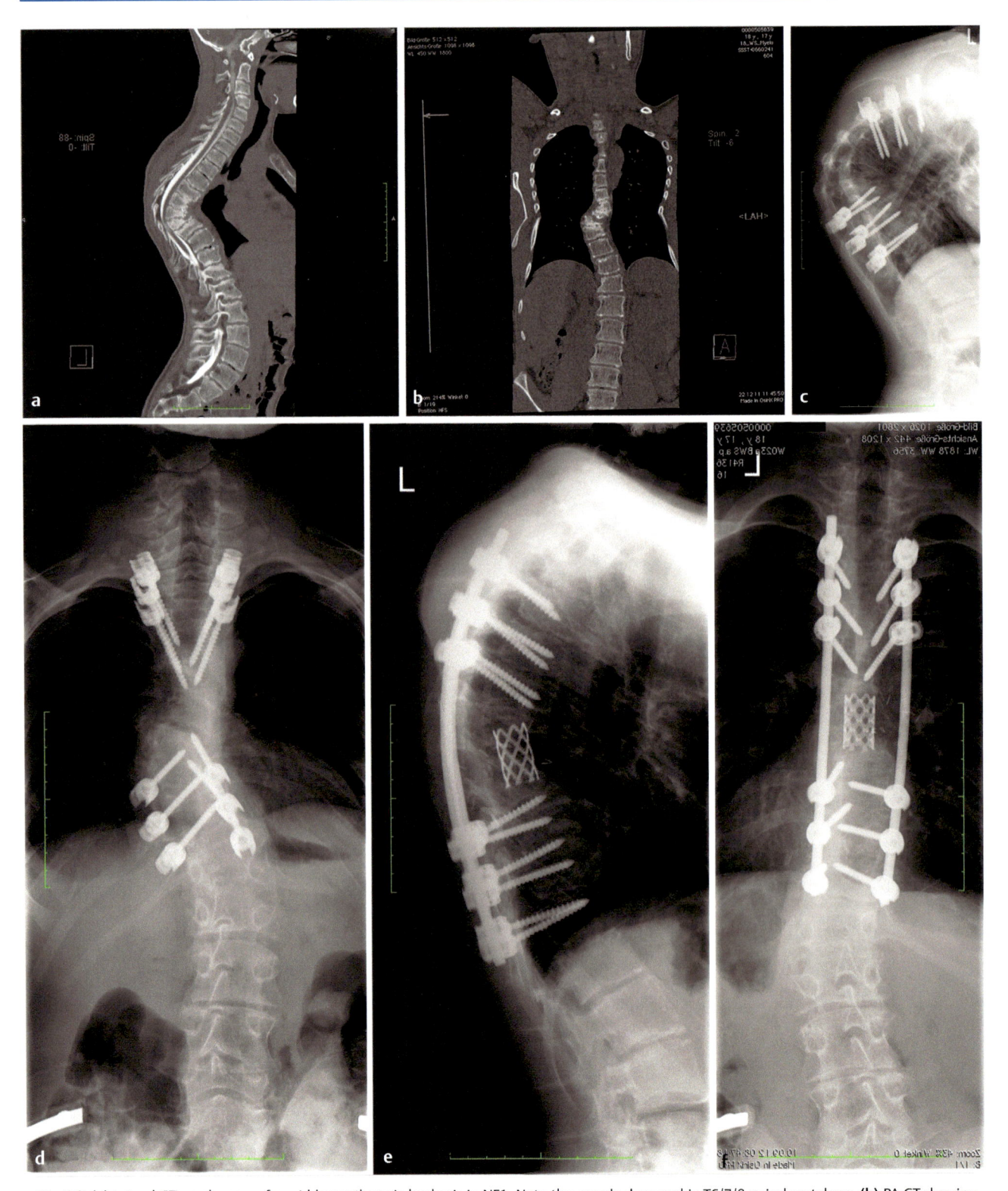

Fig. 8.8 (a) Lateral CT myelogram of a mid-lower thoracic kyphosis in NF1. Note the grossly dysmorphic T6/7/8 apical vertebrae. (b) PA CT showing that, as is often the case, there is some deformation in the frontal plane. Why should the kyphotic process be symmetrical? (c) Lateral radiograph showing that prior to surgical resection pedicular screws have been placed three above and three below. It is much easier and safer to do this before the spine becomes unstable. (d) PA view of the pre-AVR metalwork. (e) Lateral radiograph after apical resection of most of the three dystrophic apical vertebrae and replacement with a bone graft–filled cage. (f) PA radiograph showing the frontal appearance of a very solid construct.

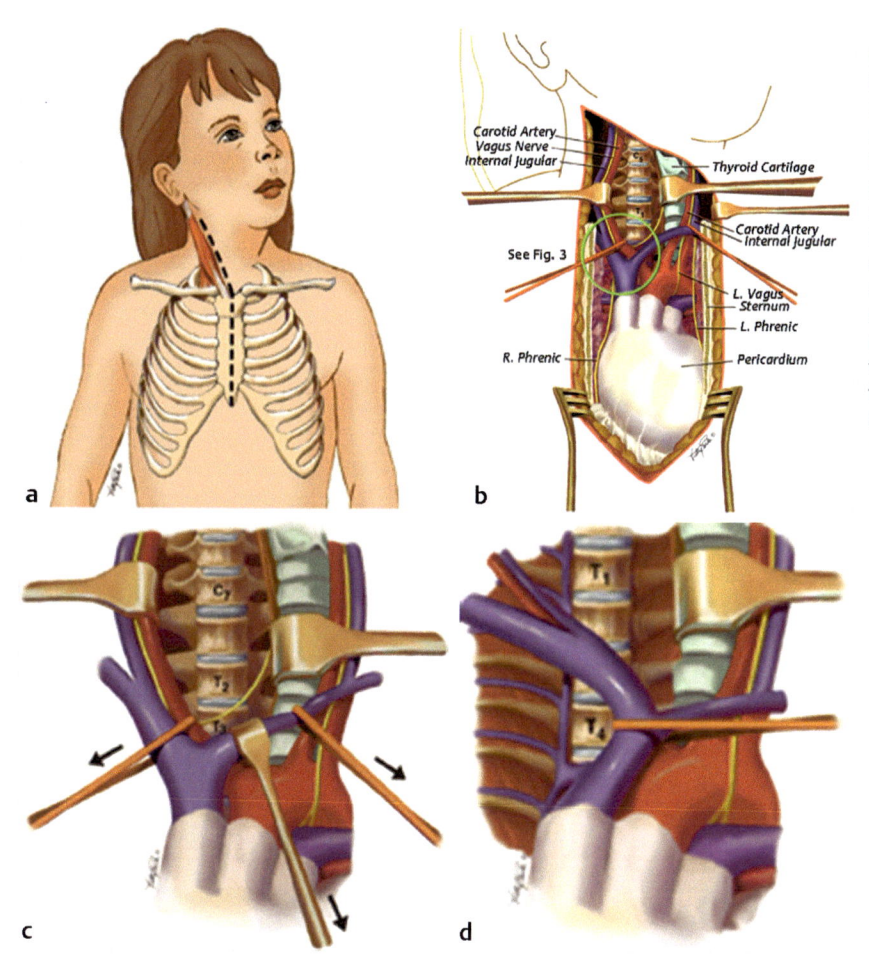

Deformities Associated with Neurofibromatosis

Fig. 8.9 (a) The patient is placed on the operating table in a supine position and the neck is hyperextended and turned to the left, allowing a right-sided approach. (b) The sternum is opened, the thymus gland resected, and the brachiocephalic trunk is mobilized to allow contiguous access to the anterior cervical spine and upper thoracic spine. (c) Retraction of the trachea, esophagus, and innominate artery provides access to the lower cervical and upper thoracic spine. (d) Medial displacement of the brachiocephalic trunk allows more distal access to the thoracic spine. (Reproduced with permission from Lippincott WW, Spine 2005, Vol 30 (11), pp. E305-310, figs 1–4.)

Case Gallery

Case 1: Thoracolumbar Kyphosis

Refer to ▶ Fig. 8.10a–c. Can you accurately describe the MRI scan appearances in ▶ Fig. 8.10a? There were upper motor neurone symptoms but no signs. What should you do in this premenarchal girl?

Comment

Spinal cord compression symptoms are much easier to resolve than physical signs and so anterior cord decompression is required with appropriate reconstruction as in ▶ Fig. 8.10b, c.

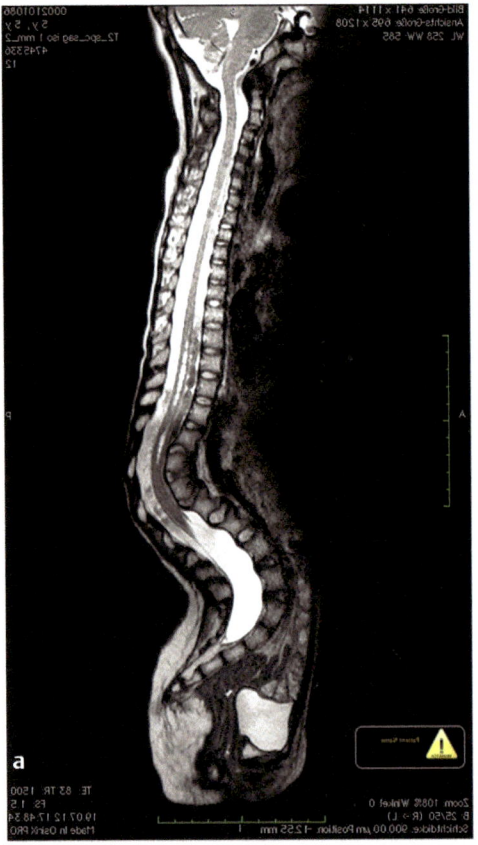

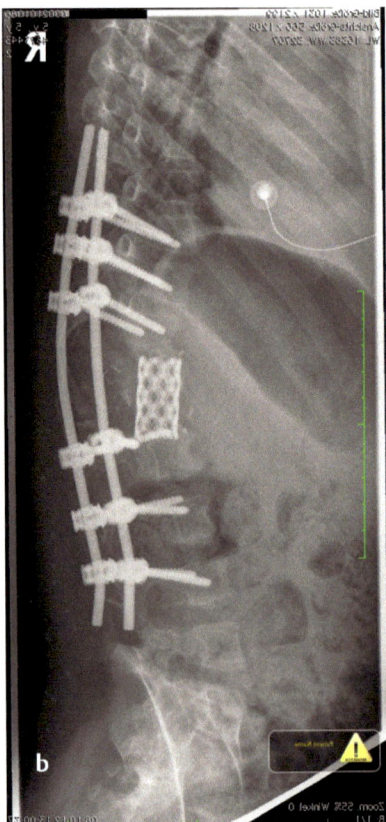

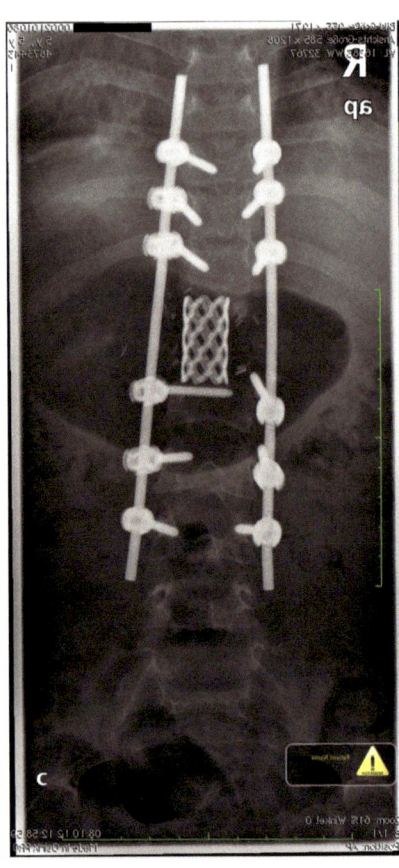

Fig. 8.10 (a) T2 sagittal MRI scan of a von Recklinghausen thoracolumbar kyphosis with two anteriorly wedged vertebrae which could be described as bullet-shaped. These bullet-shaped vertebrae are more characteristic of skeletal dysplasias and mucopolysaccharidoses. This appearance can occur with NF1 giving a resultant significant kyphosis. Note the dural ectasia lower down. This is not primarily ectasia of the dura but rather a very much enlarged extradural space, particularly in the lumbar region, which has to be obligatorily filled with dura. (b) Lateral radiograph after three above and three below transpedicular fixation and then vertebral body resection with cage replacement. (c) PA X-ray showing again a solid metalwork construct. There were symptoms but no neurological signs in this growing child, and there certainly won't be any now.

References

Note: References in **bold** are Key References.

[1] Tilesius Von Tilenau WG. Historia Pathologica Singularis Cutis Turpitudinus. Leipzig: SL. Crussius; 1793
[2] Smith RW. A Treatise on the Pathology, Diagnosis and Treatment of Neuroma. Dublin: Hodges and Smith; 1849
[3] Virchow R. Die Krankhaften Geschwütsle. Vol 3. Berlin: A Hirschwald; 1863: 233
[4] von Recklinghausen FD. Ueber die Multiplen Fibrome der Haut und ihre Beziehung zu den Multiplen Neuromen. Berlin: A Hirschwald; 1882
[5] Chauffard A. Dermo-fibromatose pigmentaire (ou neuro-fibromatose généralisée). Mort par adénoma des capusules surréndes et du pancréas. Bulletins et Mémoires de la Société Medicale des Hôpitaux de Paris. Trolsième Série. 1896; 13:777
[6] Thannhauser SJ. Neurofibromatosis (von Recklinghausen) and osteitis fibrosa cystica localisata et disseminata (von Recklinghausen). Medicine. 1944; 23:105
[7] Whitehouse D. Diagnostic value of the café-au-lait spot in children. Arch Dis Child. 1966; 41(217):316–319
[8] Payne JF. Multiple neuro-fibromata in connection with molluscum fibrosum. Trans Pathol Soc Lond. 1887; 38:69
[9] Inglis K. The influence of intrinsic factors in the causation of disease in man: illustrated by neurofibromatosis and lesions with which it is sometimes associated. Med J Aust. 1956; 43(11):429–434
[10] Meszaros WT, Guzzo F, Schorsch H. Neurofibromatosis. Am J Roentgenol Radium Ther Nucl Med. 1966; 98(3):557–569
[11] Penfield W, Young AW. The nature of von Recklinghausen's disease and the tumors associated with it. Arch Neur Psych. 1930; 23(2):320–344
[12] Fienman NL, Yakovac WC. Neurofibromatosis in childhood. J Pediatr. 1970; 76 (3):339–346
[13] **Holt JF, Wright EM. The radiologic features of neurofibromatosis. Radiology. 1948; 51(5):647–664**
[14] Allibone EC, Illingworth RS, Wright T. Neurosis fibromatosis (von Recklinghausen's disease) of the vertebral column. Arch Dis Child. 1960; 35:153–158
[15] **Hunt JC, Pugh DG. Skeletal lesions in neurofibromatosis. Radiology. 1961; 76:1–20**
[16] Levene LJ. Bone changes in neurofibromatosis; report of a case with coincidental osteitis deformans and review of the literature. AMA Arch Intern Med. 1959; 103(4):570–580
[17] Heard G, Payne EE. Scolloping of the vertebral bodies in von Recklinghausen's disease of the nervous system (neurofibromatosis). J Neurol Neurosurg Psychiatry. 1962; 25(4):345–351
[18] Pohl R. Meningokele im Brustraum unter dem Bilde eines intrathorakalen Rundschattens. Röntgenpraxix. 1933; 5:747–749
[19] Nanson EM. Thoracic meningocele associated with neurofibromatosis. J Thorac Surg. 1957; 33(5):650–662
[20] Sammons BP, Thomas DF. Extensive lumbar meningocele associated with neurofibromatosis. Am J Roentgenol Radium Ther Nucl Med. 1959; 81 (6):1021–1025
[21] Zacks A. Atlanto-occipital fusion, basilar impression, and block vertebrae associated with intraspinal neurofibroma, meningocele, and von Recklinghausen's disease. Radiology. 1960; 75:223–231
[22] **Laws JW, Pallis C. Spinal deformities in neurofibromatosis. J Bone Joint Surg Br. 1963; 45(4):674–682**

[23] Inglis K. The nature of neurofibromatosis and related lesions, with special reference to certain lesions of bones: Illustrating the influence of intrinsic factors in disease when development of the body is abnormal. J Pathol Bacteriol. 1950; 62(4):519–530

[24] Carrière G, Huriez AC, Gervois M, Dupret R. La Gliofibromatose de Recklinghausen. Paris: Doin et Cie; 1938

[25] Roaf R. Scoliosis. Edinburgh. ES Livingstone; 1966

[26] **Roaf R. The basic anatomy of scoliosis. J Bone Joint Surg Br. 1966; 48 (4):786–792**

[27] Weiss RS, . (A) von Recklinghausen's disease in the Negro. (B) Curvature of the spine in von Recklinghausen's disease. Arch Derm Syphilol. 1921; 3:144–151

[28] Scott JC. Scoliosis and neurofibromatosis. J Bone Joint Surg Br. 1965; 47:240–246

[29] Hagelstam L. On the deformities of the spine in multiple neurofibromatosis (von Recklinghausen). Acta Chir Scand. 1946; 93(2–5):169–193

[30] Simmons EH, Thomas AF. Neurofibromatosis associated with scoliosis. J Bone Joint Surg. 1976; 58A:155

[31] **Chaglassian JH, Riseborough EJ, Hall JE. Neurofibromatous scoliosis. Natural history and results of treatment in thirty-seven cases. J Bone Joint Surg Am. 1976; 58(5):695–702**

[32] Crowe FW, Schull WJ, Neel JVA. Clinical, Pathological and Genetic Study of Multiple Neurofibromatosis. Springfield, MO: CC Thomas; 1956

[33] Cobb JR. Discussion. J Bone Joint Surg. 1950; 32A:617, 626

[34] James JIP. Scoliosis. Edinburgh: E & S Livingstone; 1967

[35] Marchetti PG. Le Scoliosi. Rome: A Gaggi; 1968

[36] James JIP. The etiology of scoliosis. J Bone Joint Surg Br. 1970; 52(3):410–419

[37] Veliskakis KP, Wilson PD, Levine DB. Neurofibromatosis and scoliosis. Significance of the short angular spinal curve. J Bone Joint Surg. 1970; 52A:833

[38] **Dawson EG, Moe JH, Pedras CCV. Spinal deformity in neurofibromatosis – natural history, classification and treatment. J Bone Joint Surg. 1973; 55A:1321–1322**

[39] Stagnara P, Biot B, Fauchet R. Évaluation critique du traitement chirurgical des lésions vertébrales de la neurofibromatose. Rev Chir Orthop Repar Appar Mot. 1975; 61:17–38

[40] Savini R, Vicenzi G. Deformities of the spine in neurofibromatosis. Clinical and radiographic study of 46 cases. Ital J Orthop Traumatol. 1976; 2(1):37–50

[41] Simmons EH, Thomas AF. Scoliosis associated with neurofibromatosis. J Bone Joint Surg. 1976; 58B:141

[42] Moe JH, Winter RB, Bradford DS, et al. Scoliosis and Other Spinal Deformities. Philadelphia: W B Saunders; 1978

[43] Winter RB, Moe JH, Bradford DS, Lonstein JE, Pedras CV, Weber AH. Spine deformity in neurofibromatosis. A review of 102 patients. J Bone Joint Surg. 1979; 61A:677–694

[44] Vlok GJ. Neurofibromatous scoliosis. J Bone Joint Surg. 1979; 61B:258

[45] Stirling AJ, Howel D, Millner PA, Sadiq S, Sharples D, Dickson RA. Late-onset idiopathic scoliosis in children six to fourteen years old. A cross-sectional prevalence study. J Bone Joint Surg Am 1996; 78:1330–1336

[46] Deacon P, Berkin CR, Dickson RA. Combined idiopathic kyphosis and scoliosis. An analysis of the lateral spinal curvatures associated with Scheuermann's disease. J Bone Joint Surg Br. 1985; 67(2):189–192

[47] Tsirikos AI, Saifuddin A, Noordeen MH. Spinal deformity in neurofibromatosis type-1: diagnosis and treatment. Eur Spine J. 2005; 14(5):427–439

[48] Klose. Recklinghausensche Neurofibromatose mit schwerer Deformierung de Halswirbelsäule. Klin Wochenschr. 1926; 5:817

[49] Yong-Hing K, Kalamchi A, MacEwen GD. Cervical spine abnormalities in neurofibromatosis. J Bone Joint Surg Am. 1979; 61(5):695–699

[50] **Lonstein JE, Winter RB, Moe JH, Bradford DS, Chou SN, Pinto WC. Neurologic deficits secondary to spinal deformity. A review of the literature and report of 43 cases. Spine. 1980; 5(4):331–355**

[51] Curtis BH, Fisher RL, Butterfield WL, Saunders FP. Neurofibromatosis with paraplegia. Report of eight cases. J Bone Joint Surg Am. 1969; 51(5):843–861

[52] Meslet PAF. Contribution à l'Étude des Névromes Plèxiformes, These de Bordeaux No 6, 1892. Cited by Curtis, Fisher, Butterfield et al; 1969

[53] Sieveking H. Kompression des Cervikalmarkes durch ein im Wirbelkanal liegendes Neurofibrom bei einem Fall von multiplen Nevromen. In: Jahrbucher der Hamburgischen Stattskranken-Stalten. Bd IV Jahrung 1893–94. Hamburg and Leipzig: Leopold Voss; 1896:260

[54] Berggün E. Ein Fall von allgemeiner Neurofibromatose Bei Einem 11 jährigen Knaben. Arch Kinderheilkd. 1896; 21:89–113

[55] Hirsch E. Fall von Querschnittsläsion des Rückenmarks bei Morbus Recklinghausen in Abhängigkeit von Schwangerschaft. Med Klin. 1927; 23:983–984

[56] Euziere Lamarque P, Viallefont H, et al. Un cas de maladie de Recklinghausen avec cyphoscoliose et paraplegie. Arch Soc Sci Med Biol Montpellier. 1929; 10:340–348

[57] Draganescu S, Dumitriu F, Vasiliu DO. Paraplegia in course of scoliosis co-existent with Recklinghausen's disease. Spitatul. 1929; 49:160–162. Cited by Curtis et al 1969

[58] Gorlitzer V. Neurofibromatosis Recklinghausen excessive und Skelettmissbldung. Arch Derm Syphilol. 1930; 159:510–522

[59] Michaëlis L. Uber Wirbelsäulenveränderungen Bei Neurofibromatose. Bruns's Beitr Klin Chir. 1930; 150:574–587

[60] Miller A. Neurofibromatosis with reference to skeletal changes, compression myelitis and malignant degeneration. Arch Surg. 1936; 32(1):109–122

[61] Ruhlin CW, Albert S. Scoliosis complicated by spinal-cord involvement. J Bone Joint Surg Am. 1941; 23(4):877–886

[62] Heuyer G, e Feld M. Paraplégie par cyphoscoliose au cours d'une maladie de Recklinghausen. Rev Neurol. 1944; 76:257–260

[63] Ford FR. Paraplegia due to severe scoliosis. In: Disease of the Nervous System in Infancy. Childhood and Adolescence. 3rd ed. Springfield. CC Thomas; 1952:1007–1008

[64] Kerr JG. Scoliosis with paraplegia. J Bone Joint Surg Am. 1953; 35-A(3):769–773

[65] Semat P, Damasio GR, Niviere J, Chenillet G. Neurofibromatosis de Recklinghausen et Paraplègic Spinale Aiguë. J Radiol. 1956; 37:468–470

[66] David M, Hecaen H, Bonis A. Tumeurs du syteme nerveux central et maladie de Recklinghausen. Ann Chir. 1956; 32:335–354

[67] Schulte-Brinkmann W, Von Mallinckroot H. Wirbelsäulenveränderungen Bei der Neurofibromatose von Recklinghausen unter Einschluss der intrathorakelen Meningozele. Beitr Klin Chir. 1960; 200:257–273

[68] Heard GE, Holt JF, Naylor B. Cervical vertebral deformity in von Recklinghausen's disease of the nervous system. A review of necropsy findings. J Bone Joint Surg. 1962; 44B:880–885

[69] Juncos RA, Abdala J. [CERVICAL SPINAL CORD COMPRESSION IN A CASE OF VON RECKLINGHAUSEN'S NEUROFIBROMATOSIS]. Rev Med Cordoba. 1963; 51:59–64

[70] Curtis BH, Butterfield WL, Saunders FP. Neurofibromatosis of the spine with paralysis. J Bone Joint Surg. 1966; 48A:1023

[71] **Johnson JTH, Robinson RA. Anterior strut grafts for severe kyphosis. Results of 3 cases with a preceding progressive paraplegia. Clin Orthop Relat Res. 1968; 56(56):25–36**

[72] Dickson RA, Weinstein SL. Review article – bracing (and screening) – Yes or No. J Bone Joint Surg (Br). 1999; 81B(2):193–198

[73] Nachemson AL, Peterson LE. Effectiveness of treatment with a brace in girls who have adolescent idiopathic scoliosis. A prospective, controlled study based on data from the Brace Study of the Scoliosis Research Society. J Bone Joint Surg Am. 1995; 77(6):815–822

[74] Axelgaard J, Brown JC. Lateral electrical surface stimulation for the treatment of progressive idiopathic scoliosis. Spine. 1983; 8(3):242–260

[75] Rapp GF. Glock p. Scoliosis in neurofibromatosis. J Bone Joint Surg. 1969; 51A:203

[76] Tanner JM. Growth at Adolescence. 2nd ed. Oxford: Blackwell Scientific; 1962

[77] Tanner JM, Whitehouse RH, Takaishi M. Standards from birth to maturity for height, weight, height velocity, and weight velocity: British children, 1965. II. Arch Dis Child. 1966; 41(220):613–635

[78] **Shufflebarger HL. Cotrel-Dubousset instrumentation in neurofibromatosis spinal problems. Clin Orthop Relat Res. 1989(245):24–28**

[79] Holt RT, Johnson JR. Cotrel-Dubousset instrumentation in neurofibromatosis spine curves. A preliminary report. Clin Orthop Relat Res. 1989(245):19–23

[80] Parisini P, Di Silvestre M, Greggi T, Paderni S, Cervellati S, Savini R. Surgical correction of dystrophic spinal curves in neurofibromatosis. A review of 56 patients. Spine. 1999; 24(21):2247–2253

[81] Savini R, Parisini P, Cervellati S, Gualdrini G. Surgical treatment of vertebral deformities in neurofibromatosis. Ital J Orthop Traumatol. 1983; 9(1):13–24

[82] Li M, Fang X, Li Y, Ni J, Gu S, Zhu X. Successful use of posterior instrumented spinal fusion alone for scoliosis in 19 patients with neurofibromatosis type-1 followed up for at least 25 months. Arch Orthop Trauma Surg. 2009; 129 (7):915–921

[83] Brown LP, Stelling FH. Parallelism in scoliosis. J Bone Joint Surg. 1974; 56A:444

[84] Koptan W, ElMiligui Y. Surgical correction of severe dystrophic neurofibromatosis scoliosis: an experience of 32 cases. Eur Spine J. 2010; 19(9):1569–1575

[85] Shahcheraghi GH, Tavakoli AR. Corpectomy and circumferential spinal fusion in dystrophic neurofibromatous curves. J Child Orthop. 2010; 4(3):203–210

[86] Leatherman KD, Dickson RA. The Management of Spinal Deformities. Wright; 1988:243
[87] Suk SI, Chung ER, Kim JH, Kim SS, Lee JS, Choi WK. Posterior vertebral column resection for severe rigid scoliosis. Spine. 2005; 30(14):1682–1687
[88] Letko L, Jenson RG, Harms J. The treatment of rigid adolescent idiopathic scoliosis: releases, osteotomies, and apical vertebral column resection. In: Newton, O'Brien, Shufflebarger, Betz, Dickson, Harms, eds. Idiopathic Scoliosis – The Harms Study Group Treatment Centre. Stuttgart: Thieme; 2010:188–199
[89] **Flood BM, Butt WP, Dickson RA. Rib penetration of the intervertebral foraminae in neurofibromatosis. Spine. 1986; 11(2):172–174**
[90] Kishen TJ, Mohapatra B, Diwan AD, Etherington G. Post-traumatic thoracic scoliosis with rib head dislocation and intrusion into the spinal canal: a case report and review of literature. Eur Spine J. 2010; 19(12) Suppl 2:S183–S186
[91] Leatherman KD, Dickson RA. The Management of Spinal Deformities. Stoneham, MA: Wright; 1988:246
[92] Stagnara P, Gounot J, Fauchet R, Jouvinroux P. Les greffes antérieures par voie thoracique dans le traitement des déformations et dislocations vertébrales en cyphose et cyphoscoliose. Rev Chir Orthop Repar Appar Mot. 1974; 60:39–56
[93] **Leatherman KD, Dickson RA. Two-stage corrective surgery for congenital surgery for congenital spine deformities. J Bone Joint Surg. 1977; 59B:497**
[94] Cauchoix J, Binet JP. Anterior surgical approaches to the spine. Ann R Coll Surg Engl. 1957; 21(4):237–243
[95] Fang HSY, Ong GB, Hodgson AR. Anterior spinal fusion: The operative approaches. Clin Orthop Relat Res. 1964; 35(35):16–33
[96] Mulpuri K, LeBlanc JG, Reilly CW, et al. Sternal split approach to the cervicothoracic junction in children. Spine. 2005; 30(11):E305–E310
[97] Atkins JC, Ratvich MD. Children's Hospital of Pittsburgh. The Operative Management of Von Recklinghausens NF1 in Children, with special reference to regions of the head and neck. Surgery. 1977; 82:343
[98] Toiohido I, Miyasak K, Hiroshi A. Atlanto-axial dislocation with NF1. J Neurosurg. 1983; 68:451

Chapter 9

Spinal Deformity due to Tumors

9.1	Intradural Tumors	*254*
9.2	Syringomyelia	*256*
9.3	Extradural Tumors	*260*
9.4	Tumor-like Lesions	*266*

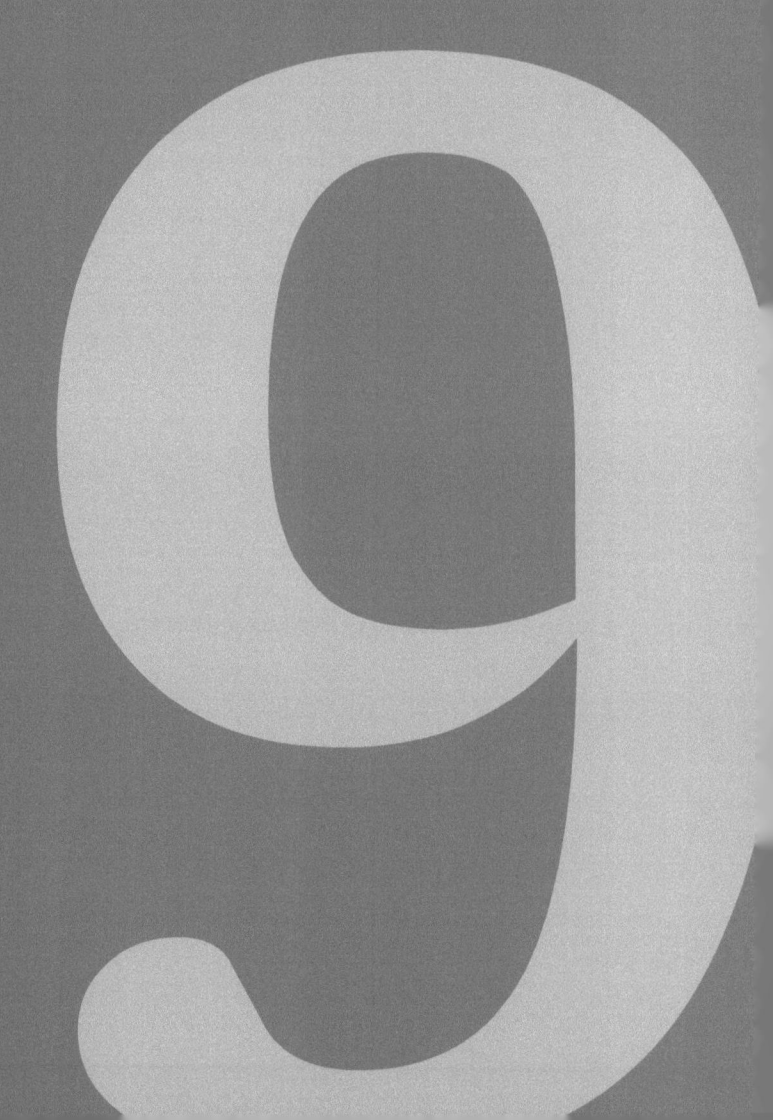

9 Spinal Deformity due to Tumors

There is a wide variety of tumors, tumor-like processes, and cysts that can give rise to a deformity of the growing spine (Fig. 9.1), either by the physical presence of the lesion, or as a result of the necessary treatment in dealing with it. A number of different effects can thereby by produced, which include loss of physical support to the spine, paralysis, and the asymmetric growth effect of radiation therapy, and these effects are frequently present in combination. It is helpful in describing these effects to consider these tumors according to their site. Spinal tumors can be intradural or extradural, the former being the initial management province of the neurosurgeon, while the latter more frequently present to the orthopaedic surgeon. Importantly, quite a different range of pathological tumor types are encountered in children from that found in adults.

Spinal cord tumors in children can be extradural or intradural and if intradural can be either intramedullary or extramedullary (▶ Fig. 9.1). Nowadays in major hospitals there are "spinal teams" comprising both orthopaedic and neurosurgical spine surgeons which markedly helps to look after these combined cases.

9.1 Intradural Tumors

9.1.1 Clinical Features

When spinal cord dysfunction in the child occurs in a subacute or chronic manner, it is most often due to tumor.[1] While meningiomas and neurofibromas are common in adults they are rare in children, in whom the most common intradural spinal neoplasms are gliomas, including astrocytomas and ependymomas (▶ Table 9.1). Neuroblastomas are the second most common neoplasm, but the most common cause of spinal cord compression in the infant.[1] Then come lymphomas, which can be of the Hodgkin's variety, or the non-Hodgkin's lymphosarcoma (lymphocytic or lymphoblastic lymphoma) or reticulum cell sarcoma (histiocytic variety of lymphoma). Developmental lesions such as teratomas and cysts account for most of the remainder.

Tachdjian and Matson have written the most informative orthopaedic article on the subject of intraspinal tumors in children, which should be compulsory reading for all learning spine surgeons.[1] They reported on 30 years' experience in Boston. Spinal intradural tumors were found to be one-fifth as common as intracranial neoplasms. As regards intraspinal tumors, boys were affected twice as commonly as girls, and 50% occurred in the first 4 years of life. Slightly more lesions were benign than malignant, and intramedullary gliomas were the most common, followed by neuroblastomas, and then a collection of developmental tumors, the latter usually encountered in the very young. Lymphosarcomas were found in children of all ages. These tumors occurred throughout the length of the spine, but the thoracic and cervical regions were relatively overrepresented. Limp and leg weakness were the chief presenting features in more than 50% of cases (▶ Table 9.2). Back pain was present in one-third and torticollis in one-fifth. The most important physical findings in order of frequency were pathological reflexes, spastic paralysis, flaccid paralysis, a sensory level, a scoliosis in one-third, and muscle spasm. Tachdjian and Matson also found an incredibly high rate of wrong initial diagnosis, with these tumors commonly masquerading as poliomyelitis, brachial plexus lesions, muscular dystrophy,

Table 9.1 Intradural tumors

Gliomas	Astrocytomas
	Ependymomas
Neuroblastomas	
Lymphomas	Hodgkin's
	Non-Hodgkin's
Reticulum cell sarcomas	
Developmental lesions	Teratomas
	Cysts

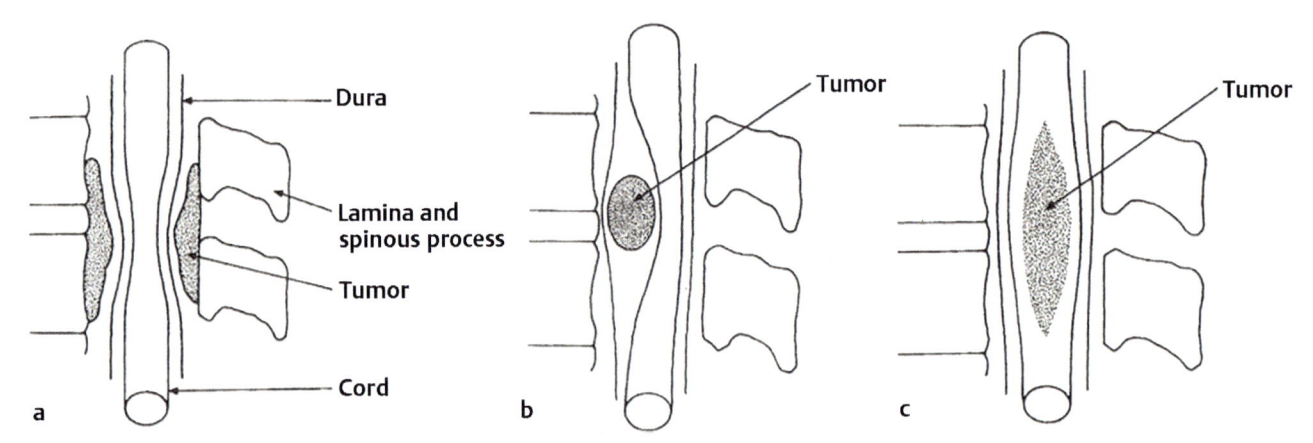

Fig. 9.1 Different categories of spinal cord tumors. (a) Extradural tumor lying outside the thecal sac but within the bony confines of the spinal canal. (b) Intradural extramedullary tumor lying within the thecal sac but outside the spinal cord. (c) Intramedullary tumor entirely in the substance of the spinal cord, causing cord widening. Reproduced with permission by Pediatric Spine, Ed S Weinstein, 2nd Ed, Lippincott PA 2001, Fig 1, p. 710.

Table 9.2 Clinical physical findings (in order of frequency)

General	Neurological
Limp	Pathological reflexes
Gait ataxia	Spastic paralysis
Leg weakness	Flaccid paralysis
Back pain	Sphincter disturbance
Scoliosis	Sensory level
Torticollis	Gait ataxia
Muscle spasm	Leg weakness

Table 9.3 Tachdjian and Matson's principles

- Repeat careful neurological + sphincter exam
- Whole spine radiographs
- MRI in any suspicious case

and postural torticollis. Repeat clinical examination was very important (▶ Table 9.3).

Fraser et al, while reporting on only 15 intradural tumors, again found limp, with limb weakness and back pain, to be the common presenting features, but also noted a sphincter disturbance in one-fifth.[2] Of those children presenting under the age of 6 years, 75% of lesions were malignant, whereas this figure was only 30% for those presenting after the age of 6 years. They also stressed a worrying delay between clinical presentation and diagnosis of spinal tumor. In the infant who has not yet walked the diagnosis is not easy and Balakrishnan et al reported a case of constipation until it was realized that the infant girl was, in fact, paralyzed.[3]

When back pain is the predominant presenting feature it tends to be characteristic. It is continuous, not episodic as with mechanical problems, and steadily worsens with time. It is increased by walking and any jolting increases the severity of the pain. In the older child and adolescent inactivity characteristically increases the pain, such that patients tend to "pace the room" at night in an effort to achieve symptomatic relief.[4] Tumors involving the cord tend to have upper motor neuron features and a gradually progressing sensory disturbance, while those involving the cauda equina have a predominance of lower motor neuron features with painless leg wasting. With intramedullary lesions there is the characteristic suspended disassociated sensory loss with a reduction in pain and temperature but normal appreciation of touch, and this physical sign is common also in syringomyelia. This is caused by dilatation of the central canal by tumor/syrinx causing an interruption of the pain and temperature fibers crossing in the anterior commissure. The vertebral column signs of reduced straight-leg raising, reduced lumbar lordosis, a scoliosis—usually of the nonstructural variety—and local tenderness are all variable and not necessarily present. The scoliosis associated with spinal tumors is atypical and quite different from an idiopathic curve (▶ Fig. 9.2). They may be in the "wrong" direction (e.g., left thoracic). They can be very stiff with muscle spasm, and can be very painful (constant pain worse at night). These are all red flags that should ring alarm bells in the mind of the clinician.

9.1.2 Investigations

Plain radiographs may reveal an increased interpedicular distance which, if more than 3 mm bigger than the adjacent vertebra, is very suggestive of tumor. There is also scalloping of the vertebral margins and pedicular flattening (▶ Fig. 9.3). Foraminal widening occurs with neurofibromas. Magnetic resonance imaging (MRI) has become the imaging modality of choice, has largely replaced computed tomography (CT) myelography (which, however, may be required for the patient who cannot undergo or tolerate MRI), and has revolutionized diagnosis and assessment of spinal cord tumors as well as management and follow-up. Then MRI with gadolinium enhancement aids both identification and vascularity as well as likely pathology.[5] On MRI there tends to be a smooth, curved margin to any filling defect or block and the extent of this may be considerable. If the intradural tumor is intramedullary, then there is expansion of the cord with gradual obliteration of the surrounding subarachnoid space, allowing a thin layer of dye to surround the cord (▶ Fig. 9.1). However, if the tumor is extramedullary, there is widening of the subarachnoid space due to cord displacement, and a concave filling defect.[6] Multiple filling defects are sometimes seen in metastases from medulloblastomas of the central nervous system which have seeded via the cerebrospinal fluid. MRI provides more information about the extent of the tumor and if a vascular tumor is expected then spinal MR angiography may be helpful in assessing the tumor vascularity.

9.1.3 Treatment of Intramedullary Tumors

Laminectomy, with tumor excision, even if subtotal for those that are malignant, has always been the treatment of choice.[1-6] Indeed, operation is always necessary unless there are proven metastases elsewhere. Microsurgical techniques are essential and a wide and deep laminectomy, often with removal of the pedicles, may be required.[6] It is increasingly common to respect the integrity of the spinal column and not remove the entirety of the facet joints bilaterally and then use an ultrasonic aspirator to debulk the tumor.[7] Many malignant tumors cannot be totally removed by surgery and, if the lesion is in the region of the conus, then sphincter preservation implies incomplete excision. Clearly as much tumor as possible should be removed and this may require a surgical revisit. Whereas radiotherapy or chemotherapy was routinely prescribed postoperatively[8] this is now less commonly indicated and it would appear that the host's body defense mechanisms come into play to minimize the deleterious effect of residual tumor. Nonetheless, particularly with the ependymoma, the prognosis is not appreciably reduced by incomplete excision. Of Tachdjian and Matson's 115 cases, 47 died up to 8 years from treatment, but 24 developed full neurological function postoperatively. The 5-year survival from malignant astrocytomas is of the order of 60%.

If the facet joints have to be removed in the cervical or thoracic regions then a local angular kyphosis commonly develops. Nevertheless, even if the integrity of the facet joints is preserved, a progressive gentle kyphosis can occur postoperatively. As a consequence, strategies to prevent these postoperative and essentially iatrogenic deformities have developed. Instead of doing a laminectomy to gain entrance to the canal the

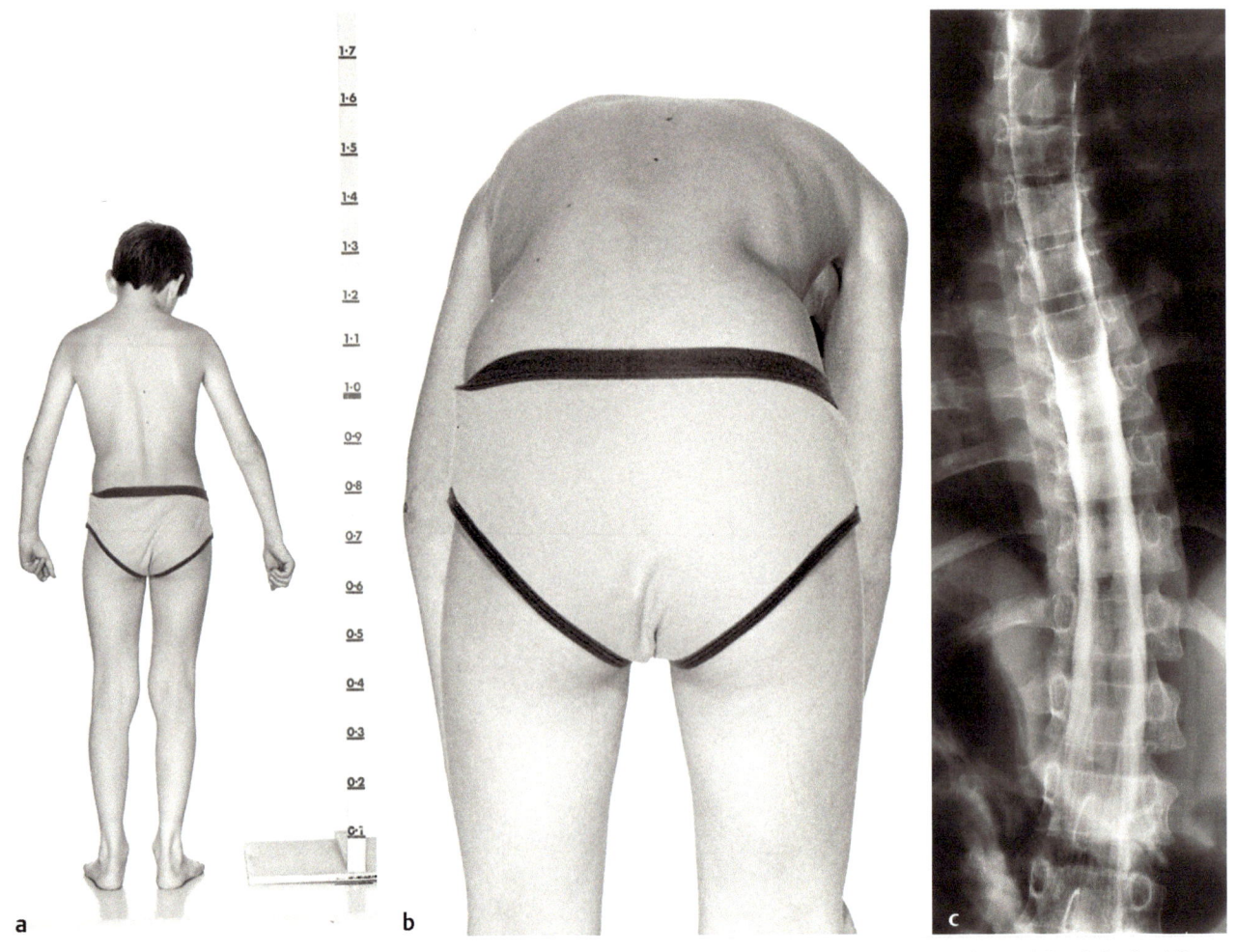

Fig. 9.2 This boy had an intradural astrocytoma and it can be seen that he stands stiffly with muscle spasm and his scoliosis is left-sided—all red flags. (a) Back view erect. (b) Forward bending views of a 10-year-old boy who presented with a mild and stiff idiopathic type deformity but left-sided with not much rotation and with pathological reflexes in association with an intradural astrocytoma. (c) PA myelogram of this boy's spine showing a typical intramedullary tumor (▶ Fig. 9.1c) and a mild scoliosis.

technique of laminoplasty is now more commonly been used. There are various techniques for this including osteotomizing the lateral edge of the lamina on each side and removing the roof of the canal and then reattaching this after the tumor has been removed. A popular alternative is the hinge laminoplasty whereby the laminar osteotomy is only carried out on one side but the other side is tenderized to provide a hinge whereby the spinal canal is hinged open with closure of the hinge at the end of tumor removal. It seems that none of these particular posterior column preservation techniques are immune to the development of a significant postoperative spinal deformity whereas a concomitant spinal fusion procedure posterolaterally with instrumentation protects the great majority of cases from postoperative progressive deformity.[9,10] Particular risk factors for progressive deformity after resection of intramedullary spinal tumors are an age of less than 13 years, a preoperative scoliotic deformity, an increasing number of resections, a tumor-associated syrinx, and surgery spanning the thoracolumbar junction. That was the conclusion of a review of 161 consecutive cases.[11] To this can be added the removal of more than four laminae. We have considerable experience of spinal cord tumors in children in the neurosurgical department in Leeds with whom we work closely in a number of areas. ▶ Fig. 9.4 is an 8-year-old with an intradural intramedullary glioma who presented with a rather mild but painful thoracic scoliosis. The lesion was resected using a laminoplasty approach and a syringoperitoneal shunt inserted to drain the syrinx. This was followed by chemotherapy and radiotherapy to the residual tumor. The scoliosis progressed and so initially growing rod instrumentation was inserted and after several lengthening procedures, the spine was definitively instrumented and fused.

It is worth reiterating that the diagnosis of these lesions can be difficult, and tumor is frequently overlooked, and so it is important to observe Tachdjian and Matson's principles[1] (▶ Table 9.3).

9.2 Syringomyelia

It is useful at this stage to review the condition of syringomyelia, as this intradural problem has some similarities with

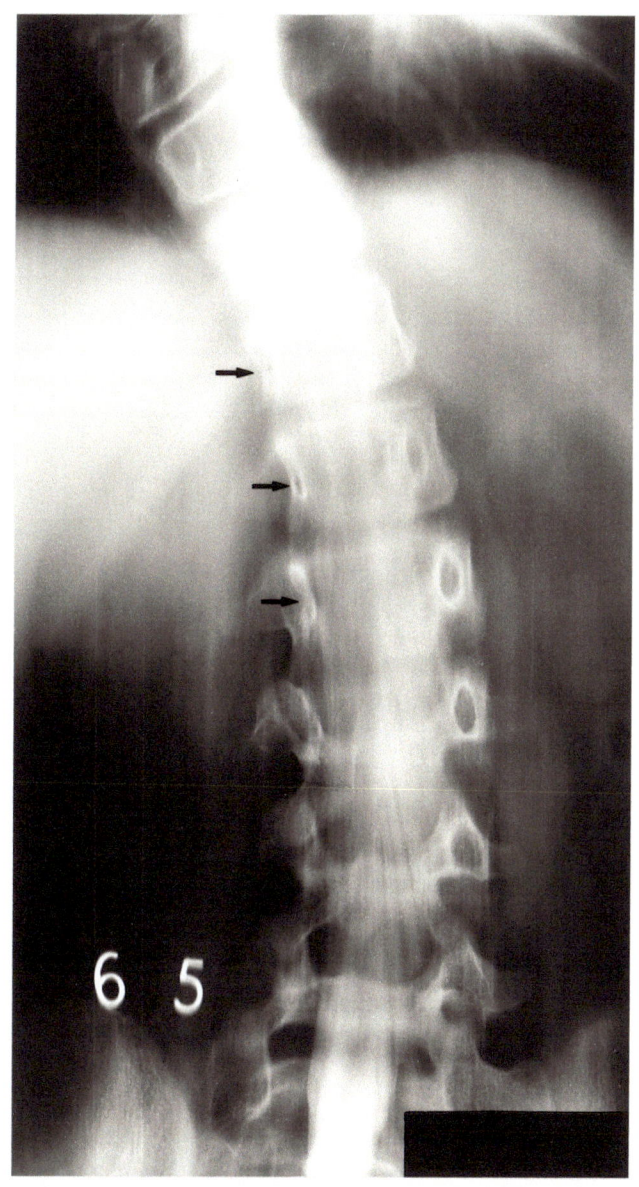

Fig. 9.3 PA myelotomography showing the pedicular flattening (*arrows*) typical of an intradural tumor with a mild nonstructural scoliosis.

normal variant referred to as cerebellar ectopia. In Chiari I the volume of the posterior fossa can be too small for its contents although a tethered cord can also produce the same foramen magnum cerebrospinal fluid (CSF) blockage. Chiari II malformations are all associated with a myelomeningocele.[16]

Williams refers to two pathological types of syringomyelia: the communicating and the noncommunicating varieties.[17,18] In the former there is a communication between the cavity and the posterior fossa, while in the latter fluid has another origin, usually tumor or traumatic paralysis. The orthopaedic features of syringomyelia are also commonly encountered in diastematomyelia and myelomeningocele which has suggested a common origin,[12,19,20] although spina bifida occulta does not occur in syringomyelia any more commonly than in normal people.[20]

Classically there is sensory dissociation with pain and temperature sensation involved but not touch, at the level of the lesion, and weakness and wasting of the muscles of the involved segments. Altered pain and temperature sensation is attributed to the central location of the cavitation in the cord such that the decussating pain and temperature fibers are involved while interference with the local medial nuclear cells, which innervate the trunk muscles, gives rise to the characteristic muscle wasting, particularly of the scapular region.

The most common presenting symptom is pain, felt in the head, neck, trunk, or limbs, which is particularly increased by straining. A history of birth injury or a family history of spina bifida are both important. The cervical spine is the area most often affected, but these cystic lesions may extend up to the medulla and down to the lumbosacral area. In advanced cases the characteristic dissociated sensory loss combined with loss of tendon reflexes makes recognition easy but diagnosis in the earlier stages depends upon a combination of clinical, radiographic, and operative findings. In this respect MRI demonstrates the dilatation while CSF protein determination reveals a moderately elevated level. Plain spinal radiographs may show interpedicular widening and erosion of both neural arches and vertebral bodies locally. Williams has determined that at the C5 level if the size of the canal exceeds that of the vertebral body by 6 mm in the adult then pathological dilatation is present.[17]

Hydrocephalus can be detected in 15% of patients and basilar impression in 55%, with the Klippel-Feil syndrome and spina bifida often being associated.[21] The presence of cervical ribs is also more common and indeed may be associated with signs of peripheral nerve involvement in the upper limb before the true nature of the underlying syringomyelia is discovered.[22] Other limb abnormalities include intrinsic muscle wasting and clawing of the hands, pes cavus, and Charcot's joints, which have been observed in 25% of patients with syringomyelia, 80% of which involve the upper extremity.[23]

9.2.1 Spinal Deformity in Association with Intradural Neoplasms and Syringomyelia

The high prevalence rate of spinal deformities in association with intradural problems is well known.[1–3,19,20,24,25] In many of these reports the issue is clouded by the performance of some sort of surgical intervention, often diagnostic laminectomy, so that there is an iatrogenic component to the deformity.

intradural neoplasms, and both can present with a spinal deformity by similar neurological mechanisms. Syringomyelia is a chronic slowly progressive degeneration of the spinal cord and medulla with cavitation and gliosis within the substance of the cord.[12] This pathological cavitation was first termed syringomyelia by Ollivier in 1827,[13] but Duchenne is attributed with the first clinical description although he called the condition progressive muscular atrophy.[14] It was not until 1882, when Schultze correlated the pathology of syringomyelia with the clinical picture, that the true nature of the syndrome became obvious.[15]

It is important to understand Chiari malformations. Types I and II account for nearly all clinical cases. A Chiari I malformation refers to the descent of the cerebellar tonsils below the plane of the foramen magnum. However, the cerebellar tonsils can be a few millimeters below the foramen magnum as a

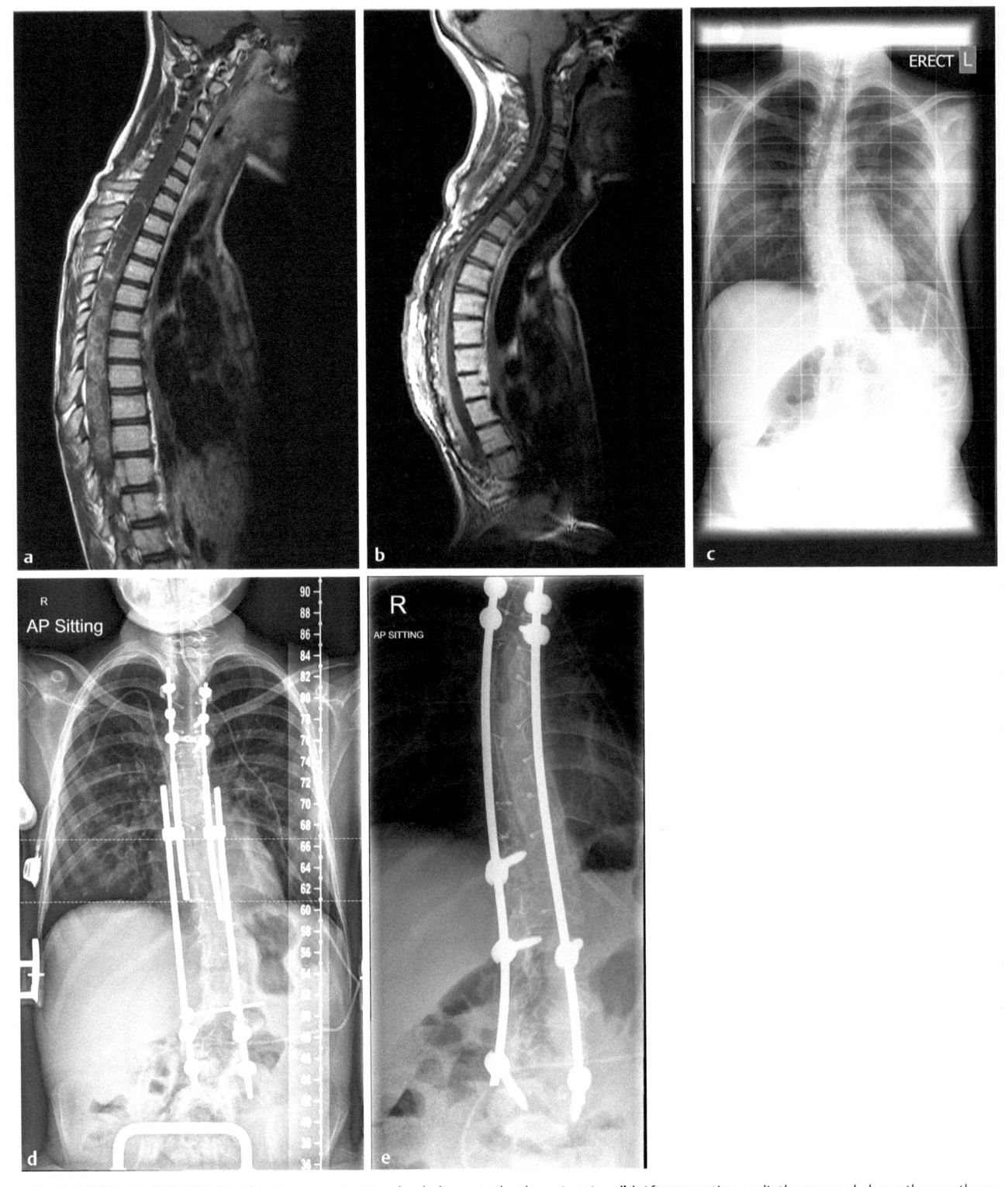

Fig. 9.4 (a) Sagittal T1 MRI slice showing extensive intradural glioma in the thoracic spine. (b) After resection, radiotherapy and chemotherapy there was an increase in the amount of thoracic kyphosis. (c) After surgery and despite laminoplasty, a scoliosis also developed. (d) Because there was a lot of growth to go special instrumentation was in the form of growing dual rods. (e) At the end of growth this was exchanged for definitive metalwork and fusion. (With thanks to Mr. Atul Tyagi, Leeds Teaching Hospitals NHS Trust.)

Nonetheless, there is plenty of evidence that the virgin intradural condition commonly presents in the form of a spinal deformity (▶ Fig. 9.2). Tachdjian and Matson, reporting on 115 intraspinal tumors in children, noted at presentation that 27% had a scoliosis, 15% had a kyphosis, 18% had a torticollis, and that these were often combined.[1,26] There was clearly some confusion between kyphosis and lordosis, as lateral views of the patient and not the deformity were obtained, but it would appear that about 50% of such children do present with a spinal deformity.

They reported on an 11-year-old girl, allegedly presenting with a progressive scoliosis of 5 years' duration, but inspection of the anteroposterior radiograph shows a very mild thoracolumbar curve with little, if any, rotation, and thus the term progressive scoliosis is scarcely applicable. It is also clear that true progressive structural scoliosis is uncommon in association with intraspinal tumors, but the situation, as will be seen, is quite different after these tumors have been dealt with therapeutically. There are several mechanisms by which these mild nonstructural curves can develop. Tachdjian and Matson reported that two-thirds of their patients had either spastic or flaccid paralysis and a quarter had paravertebral muscle spasm,[1] and thus asymmetric muscle action is one mechanism and this is shared with syringomyelia.

Approximately 45% of cases of syringomyelia have a spinal deformity of clinical significance, but if the threshold is lowered to a Cobb angle in excess of 5 degrees then 70% of patients can be shown to have a scoliosis[20] (seven times the normal prevalence rate). This is rather akin to the situation derived from scoliosis screening where the more thorough the search, the higher the prevalence rate of the condition being sought. Indeed, Perret reported that there was always a scoliosis in association with syringomyelia.[27] While the essential lesion of syringomyelia is thought to be overdistension of the embryonic neural tube (hydrocephalomyelia), with associated atresia of the fourth ventricle, the mechanism of production of a scoliosis is thought to be the same as that occurring in poliomyelitis with the lower motor neuron incriminated. As Alexander and Season showed, involvement on the sensory side leads to anterior horn cell chromatolysis, further implicating the efferent pathway.[28] Pincott et al have produced some recent evidence that involvement on the sensory side alone is sufficient to produce a scoliosis,[29] but only of the nonstructural variety. A mild scoliosis is thus a frequent and early finding in syringomyelia and will eventually occur in all cases.

If the diagnosis of syringomyelia is made in the immature individual then as many as 90% will have a scoliosis, whereas only about 50% of mature patients have a spinal deformity.[12,30] These mild curves have a Cobb angle of less than 25 degrees. The great majority are in the thoracic region, the remainder being thoracolumbar, and there is a good correlation between the site of the cord lesion, and thus the level of neurological involvement, and the site of the deformity.[25]

9.2.2 Management of the Scoliosis Associated with Intradural Neoplasms and Syringomyelia

There is necessarily a considerable difference in management, according to whether the underlying problem is a neoplasm or syringomyelia. In the former situation it is extirpation of the growth that is the essential treatment consideration, whereas in syringomyelia there may be a real need to correct the rare severe structural curve. If that is the situation, there is one serious problem and that is the high incidence of paraplegia associated with corrective surgery in syringomyelia scoliosis. This is due to the altered tension on the spinal cord in which there is a significant lesion, which has already rendered local neurological function extremely precarious. Huebert and Mackinnon's two operated cases became paraplegic and died albeit following old-fashioned posterior Harrington distraction instrumentation.[12] MRI would therefore be essential in these cases in order to determine the exact extent of the cavitation and any associated cord tether (▶ Fig. 9.4). Moreover, consultation with an experienced radiologist and neurosurgeon is important in estimating the extent of the underlying lesion before embarking upon spinal surgery. As there is such a high risk of causing neurological damage, then the spine must be shortened at the same time as being straightened, and so anterior and posterior surgery is required. For the moderate deformity this can be achieved by way of anterior multiple diskectomy, followed by posterior transpedicular instrumentation, as with the idiopathic curve. For the more severe deformity, however, the only safe procedure would appear to be wedge resection, thus ensuring that the deformity has been really shortened.[31]

9.2.3 Deformities Associated with the Treatment of Intradural Tumors

The necessary management of intradural malignant neoplasms of childhood unfortunately produces a high prevalence rate of subsequent serious spinal deformity because of the destabilizing effect that laminectomy has on the growing spine. Loss of posterior column support is a serious matter at any age, but the tendency to produce a progressive deformity is magnified during the growth period. Over the past 20 years orthopaedic surgeons have increasingly focused on these problem, but neurosurgeons have been aware of the harmful effects of laminectomy for much longer. In the 1950s Ingraham and Matson warned against laminectomy producing a deformity, particularly when the posterior bone removal was extensive.[32] They noted increased lordosis occurring in the cervical and lumbar regions (▶ Fig. 9.5) and increasing kyphoses in the thoracic region. However, the center of gravity of the body passes in front of the entire spine, just coming in contact with the anterior border of L4, and thus loss of posterior support tends to produce a progressive kyphosis anywhere in the spine. They also noted that the thoracic kyphosis could be asymmetrical thus producing a mild scoliotic component. This coronal plane asymmetry was also noted by Haft et al in 10 out of 17 children who survived following the treatment of spinal tumors.[33] Experienced neurosurgeons repeated the warnings and reported serious spinal deformities in more than 80% of children who underwent laminectomies while stressing the need for orthopaedic assistance.[34,35]

While increasing kyphosis is produced by laminectomy, a collapsing lordoscoliosis is produced by paralysis and the two may coexist with an area of paralytic lordoscoliosis below an area of progressive kyphosis. Moreover, these deformities can occur anywhere in the spine according to the site of the intradural lesion. Cattell and Clark[36] reported on three early adolescents who had undergone laminectomy for meningioma or Schwannoma and subsequently developed significant cervical kyphoses with local instability. The degree of rapidity with which these deformities developed was of considerable importance, as they were established by 3 months following posterior surgery. Wearing a cervical collar gave no protection and anterior strut

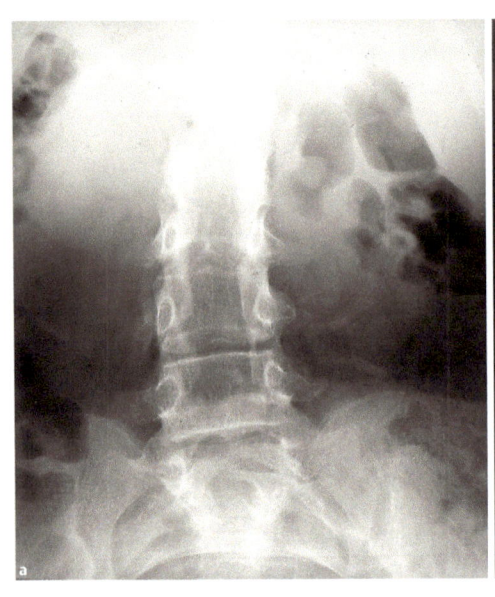

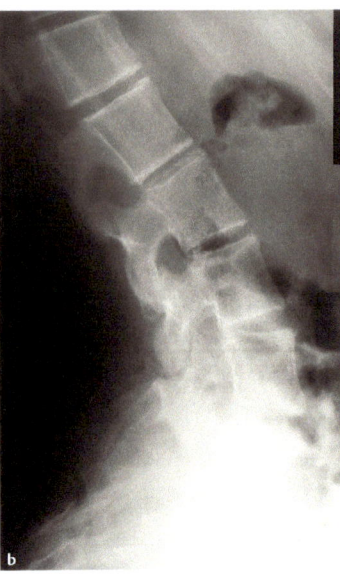

Fig. 9.5 Post-laminectomy lumbar hyperlordosis. **(a)** PA radiograph 4 years after extensive lumbar laminectomy for intradural tumor removal at age 15. **(b)** Lateral radiograph showing the development of a hyperlordosis with growth.

graft fusion throughout the length of the posterior instability was recommended. Sim et al reported on 21 patients (the lower age range of this group included adolescents) and Frank Sim observed a swan-neck combination of lordosis and kyphosis in the cervical region following extensive laminectomy.[37] Early bracing was recommended in any case of extensive laminectomy, but if progression was noted, early anterior fusion was required extending the entire length of the laminectomy.

Lonstein,[38] in reviewing this subject of post-laminectomy kyphosis, described 32 of his own cases and noted that increasing kyphosis was by far the most common deformity with an average Cobb angle of 80 degrees. He described two types of kyphosis: a sharp angular variety if the facet joints were removed, or a longer and more rounded variety if the posterior joints were left intact in which case scoliosis was much less commonly encountered, as would be entirely expected. He also observed that a mild scoliosis could exist referable to the tumor before laminectomy and that, in the presence of paralysis, a collapsing lordoscoliosis could occur below an area of kyphosis associated with laminectomy. By assessing lateral radiographs of the patient and not the deformity there is again confusion between what is kyphosis and lordosis, but it was observed that these deformities progress most during the adolescent growth spurt and that increasing kyphosis can produce its own neurological signs that were not present before. Winter[39] also observed laminectomy producing paraplegia after an interval of 3 years in a child with an intradural astrocytoma and, by the time the patient was 25 years old, the kyphosis had reached 170 degrees.

9.2.4 Treatment of the Postlaminectomy Kyphosis in Association with Intradural Tumors

As neurosurgeons have repeatedly stressed the need for orthopaedic assistance at an early stage then it is clearly advisable for the two disciplines to join forces in the management of these difficult cases. If, the laminectomy has been extensive with posterior joint loss then a serious deformity is much more common, and often of the sinister angular variety (▶ Fig. 9.6). Unless life expectancy is thought to be seriously curtailed by the nature of the underlying tumor, anterior spine stabilization is also essential.[37,38] Posterior fusion is futile, not because there is no transverse process bone to receive grafts, but because this is the tension side of the spine and such a fusion will fail. Lonstein reported a 57% pseudarthrosis rate with posterior fusion only.[38]

In the established kyphosis (▶ Fig. 2.36), particularly if this is threatening the neurological fitness of the patient, then there is no substitute for apical vertebral resection.[31,40] Just as is the case for the congenital kyphosis producing neurological signs, the offending vertebral body or bodies are removed until the dura is totally decompressed. A strong strut graft of corticocancellous bone or nowadays a bone graft filled cage, is keyed into the deficit and then the spine should be stabilized by transpedicular metalwork posteriorly (▶ Fig. 9.6).

9.3 Extradural Tumors

While primary malignant bone tumors affecting the spine are very rare, there are a number of benign tumors or tumor-like conditions that the spinal surgeon will come across from time to time in their practice.

9.3.1 Osteoid Osteoma and Osteoblastoma

Osteoid osteomas are the most common benign tumors of bone and most frequently occur in the lower extremity of children and young adults with a male to female predominance of 3:1. A total of 10% of osteoid osteomas, however, occur in the spine and they usually involve the posterior elements around the pedicle/transverse process junction (▶ Fig. 9.7). Lesions are cortical or subcortical and are commonly surrounded by an area of sclerotic bone. There is a small nidus of vascularized osteoid tissue less than 1 cm in diameter. This nidus is radiolucent. Osteoblastomas are pathologically similar but are only distinguished from osteoid osteomas by size having a diameter

Spinal Deformity due to Tumors

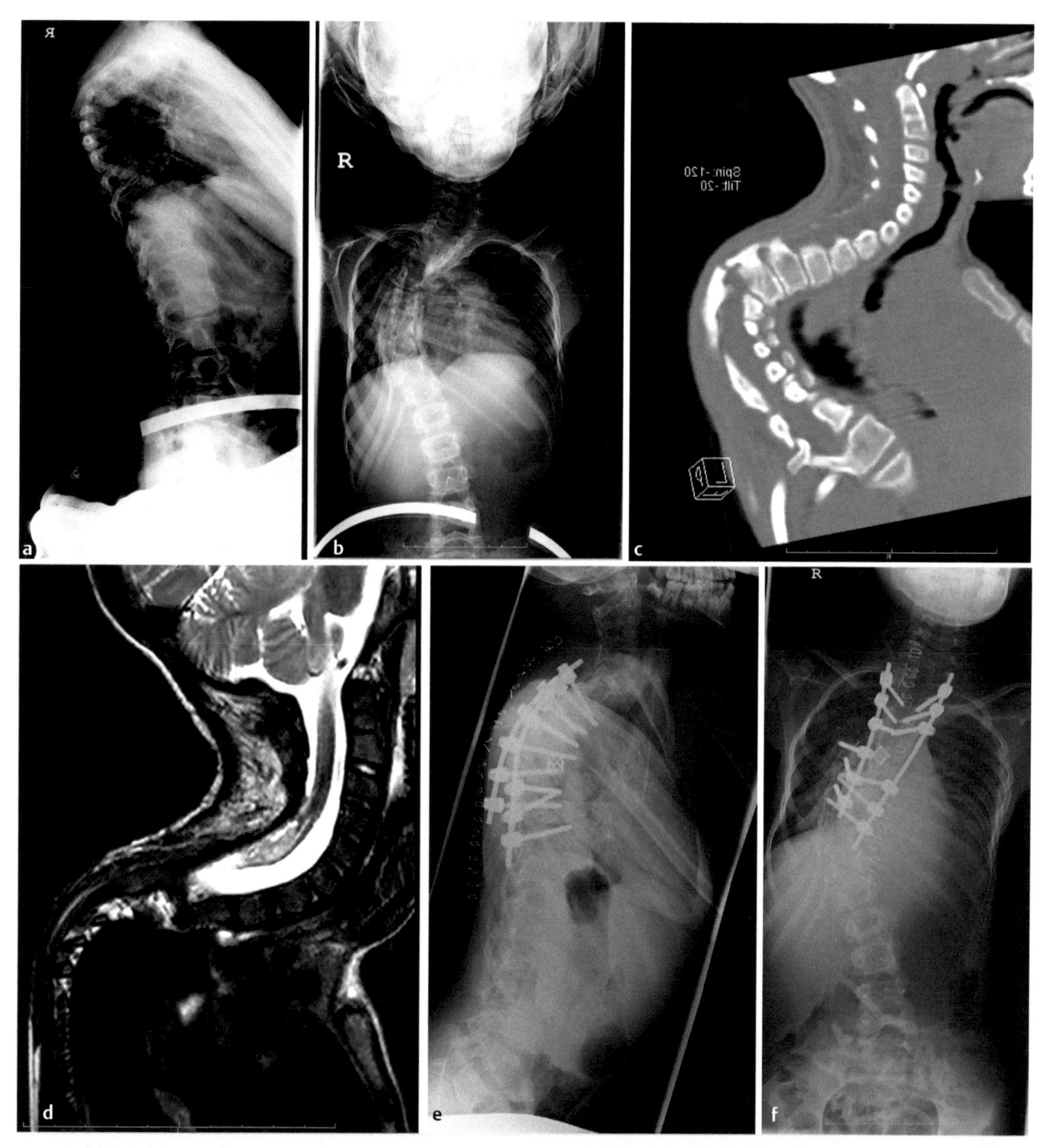

Fig. 9.6 (a) Lateral radiograph showing a severe upper thoracic kyphosis following surgical intervention twice to remove an intradural glioma in a 10-year-old girl. (b) PA radiograph showing a degree of scoliosis due to this asymmetric kyphosis. (c) Lateral tomogram showing the extent of the deformity with the vertebral body bone loss over the apex. (d) Sagittal T2 MRI scan showing a capacious canal above but narrowing over the back of the kyphosis. It is difficult in the presence of kyphosis and a scoliosis to get all of the canal on one slice. (e) Lateral radiograph showing the excellent correction following anterior vertebral body resections over the apex and cage and graft replacement followed by posterior transpedicular metalwork. It was thought that the kyphosis should be addressed surgically first. (f) PA radiograph showing the scoliosis below the corrected kyphosis.

▶

Spinal Deformity due to Tumors

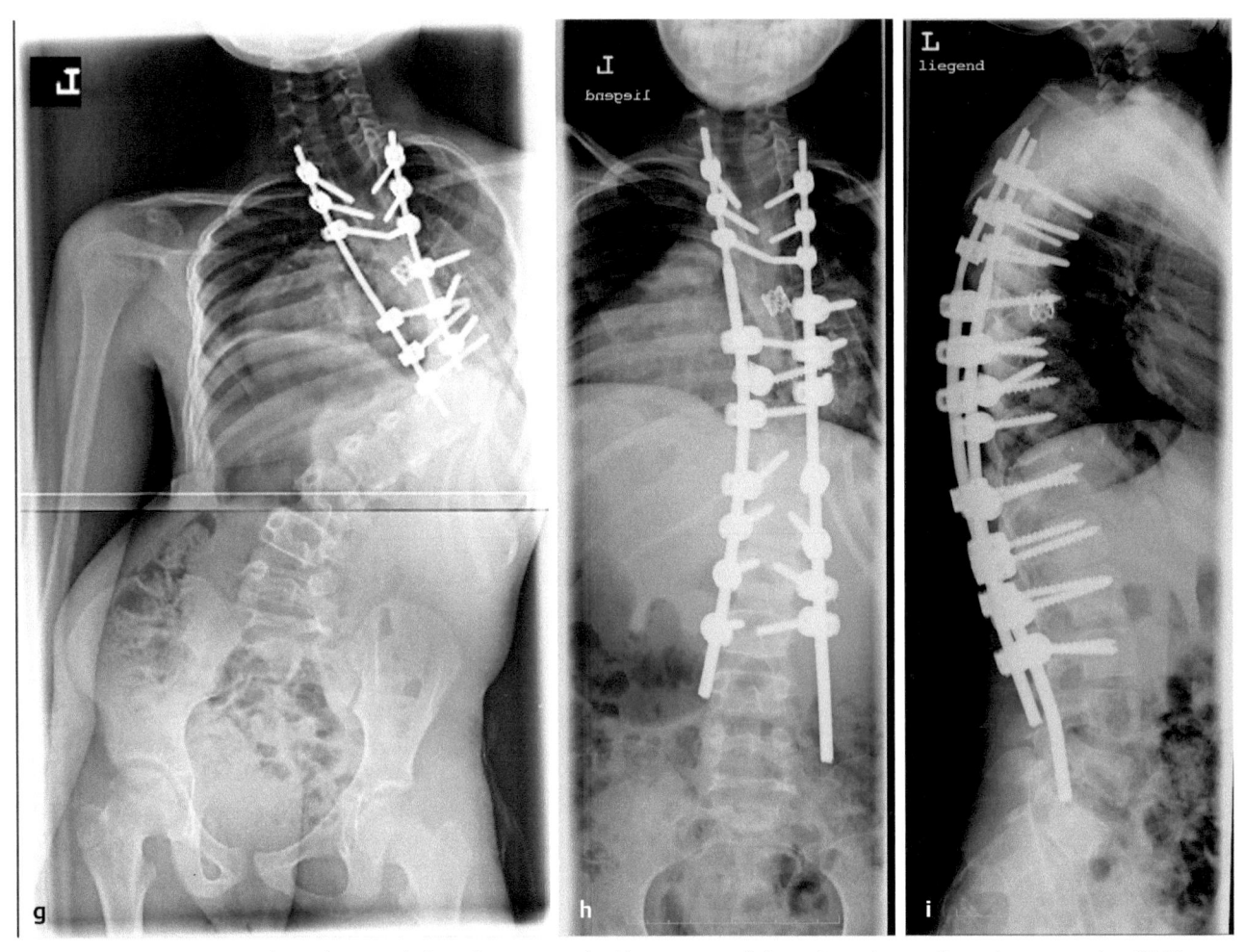

Fig. 9.6 (*continued*) **(g)** PA radiograph 6 months later showing considerable worsening of the scoliosis plus significant decompensation. **(h)** PA radiograph following surgical instrumentation of the scoliosis using dual rods (with a narrow bore for the small upper part of the spine and a wider bore for the scoliosis) with an excellent correction of the deformity. **(i)** Lateral radiograph post-scoliosis surgery showing a reasonable lateral profile.

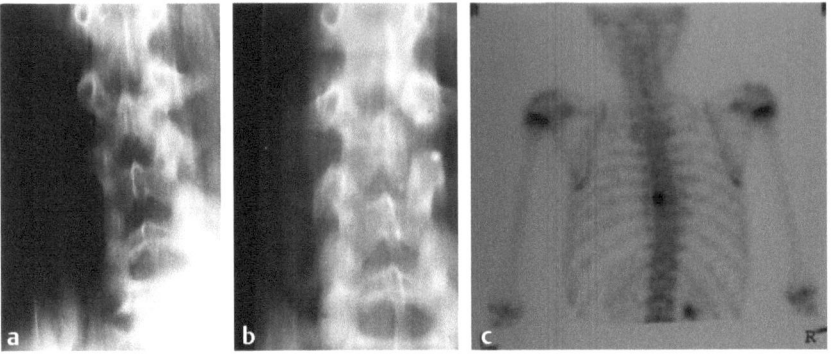

Fig. 9.7 Osteoid osteoma. **(a)** AP tomogram showing a classical osteoid osteoma with a central nidus with surrounding sclerosis. **(b)** PA radiograph after complete removal of the lesion. It is said that neoplastic cells only occupy the central nidus and can therefore be curetted but unless some of the surrounding sclerotic reactionary new bone is also removed then recurrence can occur and is much more difficult to treat. **(c)** Hot spot on the left side at the pedicle transverse process junction of T8 with a scoliosis concave to the side of the lesion. (© With thanks to Dr. James Rankine, Leeds Teaching Hospitals NHS Trust.)

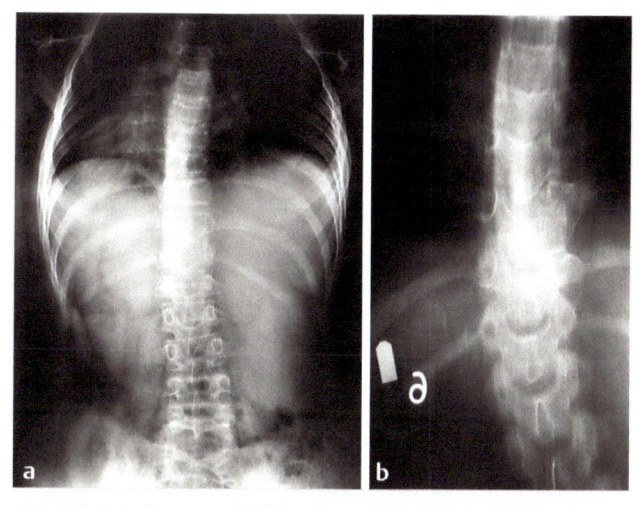

Fig. 9.8 Osteoblastoma. (a) PA radiograph showing a much bigger lesion with absence of left T10 pedicle. (b) AP tomogram showing the full extent of the lesion.

greater than 1.5 cm but there are other distinct radiological features distinguishing the two (▶ Fig. 9.8). Osteoblastomas less frequently produce reactive bone sclerosis and can extend from bone to involve the adjacent soft tissues. They also frequently involve the posterior elements of the spine.

Two cases of osteoid osteoma were described by Bergstrand[41] and then by Jaffe and Mayer.[42] The name osteoid osteoma was not coined until 1935 when Jaffe described five cases.[43] Benign osteoblastomas were described 20 years later.[43–47] In descriptions of natural history, delay in diagnosis is characteristic and the average time from presentation to diagnosis in the 25 cases of Marsh et al was almost 18 months.[48] Moberg[49] pointed out that the natural history of these tumors can be to spontaneously regress but this may take considerable time. The central nidus classically produces prostaglandins, hence the considerable therapeutic response to aspirin or other nonsteroidal anti-inflammatory drugs (NSAIDs) and this in fact can be a useful diagnostic test. Occasionally osteoid osteomas occur in an intra-articular situation and so may produce synovitis with a nonspecific arthropathy again resulting in a delay in diagnosis. In the spine there is a predilection for the thoracolumbar region and their ability to produce a scoliosis in association with pain and marked stiffness bring them to the attention of the scoliosis surgeon.[50] Scolioses are concave to the side of the lesion being sited particularly in the posterior part of the pedicle (▶ Fig. 9.7). These are nonstructural curves produced by local muscle spasm, progression becoming autonomous—not occurring unless surgical treatment has produced a posterior tether.

Radiologically most are visible on plain films as enlargement of the pedicle/transverse process junction but a central radiolucent nidus may not be identified. Radioisotope bone scans are almost invariably positive and the characteristic appearance is an intense area of uptake representing the nidus surrounded by a less intense halo which is the hyperostosis. A positive isotope scan helps to target X-ray/CT examination that, in most cases, will show such specific appearances that pathological confirmation is not required before treatment. As the nidus can be very small, thin 1-mm sections are required so the CT has to be targeted to a specific area guided by the plain radiograph or the isotope bone scan. The increased availability of MRI scanning means that many patients with bone and joint pains are having MRI as the first line of investigation. MRI shows intense edema that can involve the adjacent soft tissues; although the nidus is frequently seen on MRI it may not always be apparent, depending on the thickness of the slices, the obliquity of the sections through the nidus, and partial volume effects. Bone and soft tissue edema can be nonspecific and suggest infection or stress fracture and the radiologist must always consider the diagnosis of osteoid osteoma and perform a CT when necessary.

Whereas excision of the central osteoid tissue within the surrounding reactive bone sclerosis was the treatment of choice in the appendicular skeleton, radiofrequency thermal ablation has taken over with a similar 90% cure rate. The ablation necroses a 1-cm diameter volume of tissue so this form of treatment can only be used in the spine in sites more remote so as to not to produce neurological damage. It would be suitable only for lesions in the vertebral body or the spinous process but at its usual pedicle/transverse process junction or nearby this mandates surgical excision.

Pain disappears immediately after excision as does the secondary nonstructural scoliosis along with its muscle spasm.

Osteoblastomas, the bigger brother of osteoid osteomas, present very similarly clinically but the lesion is much bigger than 1.5 cm and there is no obvious nidus. In this 12-year-old girl there is a missing pedicle on the right side at T10 (▶ Fig. 9.8). Night pain was concerning, however, and her condition improved rapidly with NSAIDs. This area was intensely positive on technetium scanning. Posteroanterior (PA) tomography showed the extent of the lesion, which, on removal, relieved all the symptoms.

9.3.2 Giant Cell Tumor

Although these tumors are rare they are referred to the spinal surgeon as cases of atypical spinal pain and to make a diagnosis.

Sir Astley Cooper[51] first described this tumor in 1818 but it was a century later before the term giant cell tumor was applied.[52] This neoplasm arising from the nonosteogenic supporting connective tissue of the marrow involves the epiphyseal end of long bones and there has been some confusion with aneurysmal bone cysts, although the latter occur in younger patients and in the metaphyseal area of the appendicular

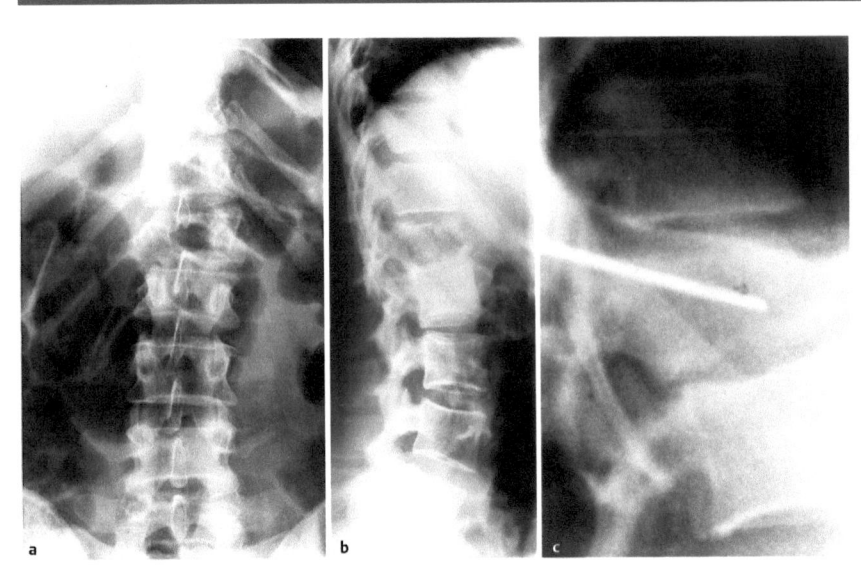

Fig. 9.9 Osteoclastoma. **(a,b)** PA and lateral X-rays showing an osteoclastoma of the L1 vertebral body with cystic dilatation and a fracture of the superior end plate. **(c)** The diagnosis was confirmed by needle biopsy.

skeleton. They do occur in the spine, however; although what were originally thought to be giant cell tumors of the spine were found on reinspection to be nearly all aneurysmal bone cysts and thus spinal giant cell tumors are rare and occasionally occur in the sacrum. Verbiest described five giant cell tumors, three of which involved the cervical spine and two the lumbar spine, all of which were associated with paralysis or signs thereof.[53] Three were in the posterior elements and two in the vertebral bodies. Giant cell tumors have a richly vascular stroma and radiographically appear as a lucent area with expansion and thinning of the surrounding cortex (▶ Fig. 9.9). Aneurysmal cyst in contrast produces a blowout appearance with intracystic soap bubble trabeculation[53] (▶ Fig. 9.10).

Goldenberg,[54] in an analysis of 218 cases of giant cell tumor, observed that all patients were skeletally mature when the diagnosis was made but their age range of 13 to 29 would not appear to go along with this. Nonetheless these tumors must be only exceptionally encountered in the immature and descriptions of the surgical removal all refer to mature patients. The tendency for this tumor to involve both the anterior and posterior elements at the same level indicates that a complete surgical vertebral removal is desirable with appropriate reconstruction.

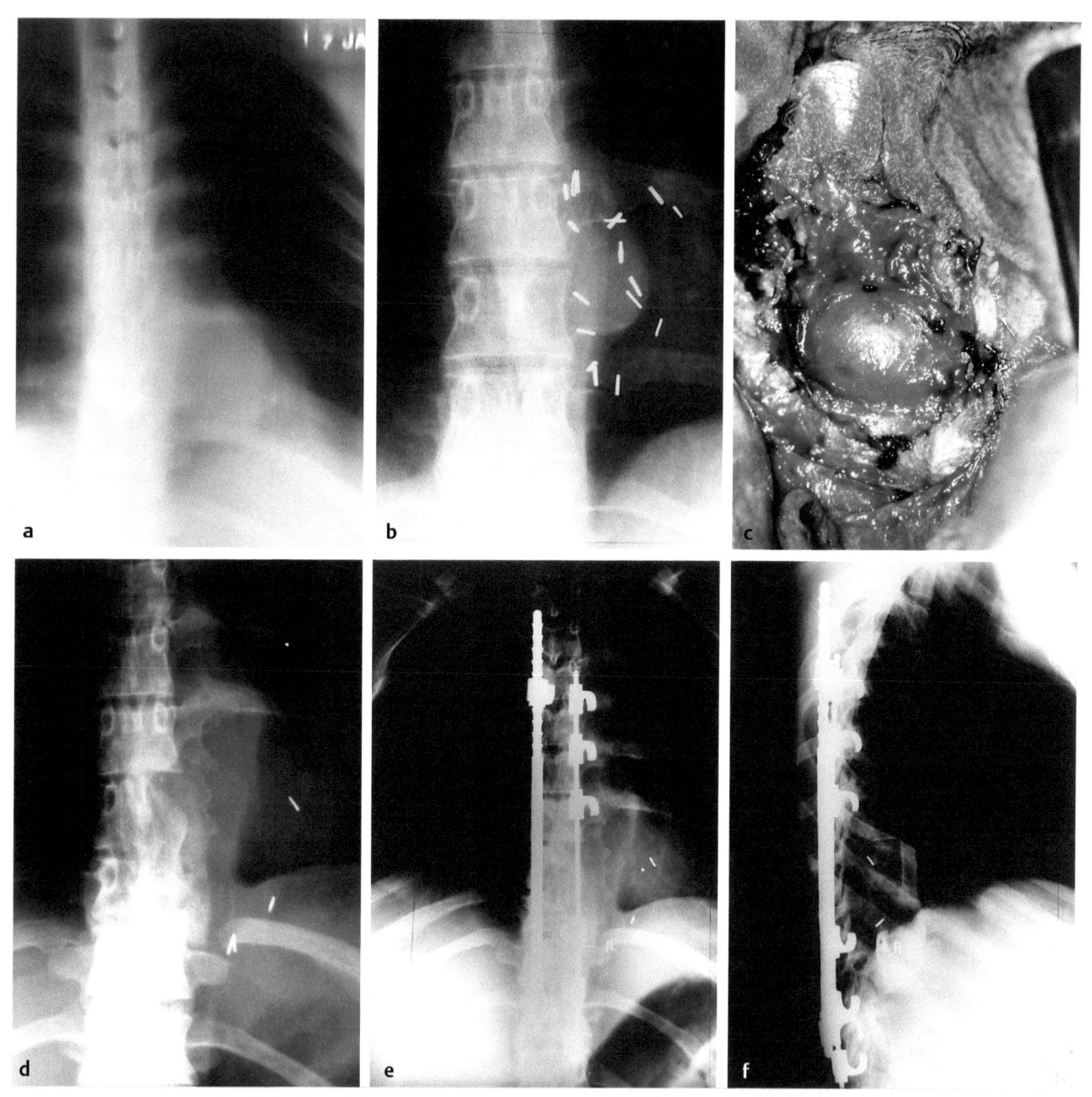

Fig. 9.10 (a) PA radiograph of the thoracic spine of a 15-year-old girl who had previously undergone an unsuccessful attempt to remove an aneurysmal bone cyst by way of costo-tranversectomy. Excessive hemorrhage had been encountered. (b) PA tomogram revealing a much bigger lesion. (c) At thoracotomy this large aneurysmal cyst was encountered and it along with its parent body were excised. Hemorrhage was not excessive. (d) PA radiograph after anterior first stage showing the extent of tumor and bone removal. (e,f) PA and lateral radiographs 1 year after second stage removal of the posterior elements involved with tumor and posterior stabilization and fusion. The anterior strut graft has been well incorporated. The patient had been followed for 12 years without evidence of recurrence.

9.4 Tumor-like Lesions

9.4.1 Aneurysmal Bone Cyst

This lesion, of unknown pathogenesis, is thought to be a vascular disturbance that gives rise to large blood-filled spaces separated by fibrous septa, which contain both osteoid and osteoclasts. Thought formerly to be a variant of the giant cell tumor, Jaffe[55] and Lichtenstein[56] recognized it as a separate entity. It is a lesion of adolescents and young adults and occurs in the metaphyseal region of long bones and in the spine.[53,54] Any spinal lesion that looks as if it might be a giant cell tumor is almost always an aneurysmal cyst and 9 out of 10 of MacCarty's cases in the spine were between the ages of 10 and 15 years.[57] Radiologically these have a blowout appearance with soap bubble trabeculation and while the growth of these cysts might be so rapid as to imply malignancy they are benign and recurrence is not common. One-fifth of all aneurysmal cysts are in the vertebral column (▶ Fig. 9.10) and the lumbar region is most often affected. Not only is this lesion sometimes confused with giant cell tumor but also with benign osteoblastoma also occurs most commonly in the lumbar region.[57]

Although radiation therapy was popular, the current preferred treatment is complete excision of the lesion which requires total vertebrectomy and thorough dural decompression if it is accompanied by unfavorable neurological signs. Verbiest reported two cases of aneurysmal cyst in association with paralysis and thus this danger must be mitigated by thorough surgical extirpation.[53] Strong anterior strut grafting or cage is essential for all cases and as the posterior elements are not uncommonly affected, total vertebrectomy is indicated with additional posterior transpedicular metalwork.

9.4.2 Eosinophilic Granuloma

This is an interesting lesion, most commonly encountered during adolescence and more often single than multiple. The condition was described by Calvé in 1925 and the important differential diagnosis in those days was Pott's disease.[58] The patient had back pain with muscle spasm, tenderness, local spinal rigidity, and a mild kyphos but Calvé's suggested diagnosis of vertebral osteochondritis was based on similar radiographic appearances to Perthes' and Kohler's diseases. It was not until 1953 that Lichtenstein[59] gave the lesion the name histiocytosis X and integrated eosinophilic granuloma of bone with Letterer-Siwe disease and Hand-Schüller-Christian disease as similar lesions with a common histological pattern.

The affected sites in order of frequency are the jaws, the long bones of the lower limbs, vertebral bodies, ribs, and skull.[60] Radiographically long bone lesions appear as sharply defined central lucencies, surrounded by an expanded cortex, often with layers of periosteal calcification resembling osteomyelitis or Ewing's tumor.[61] Lesions of the vertebral bodies, however, go through stages of first a lytic appearance followed by collapse and then increased sclerosis before recovery to a normal height, which may take 1 to 3 years. The findings of a raised erythrocyte sedimentation rate or reduced hemoglobin concentration indicate the disseminated varieties of histiocytosis X with extraskeletal manifestations which may be in liver, lymph nodes, and lungs.[62]

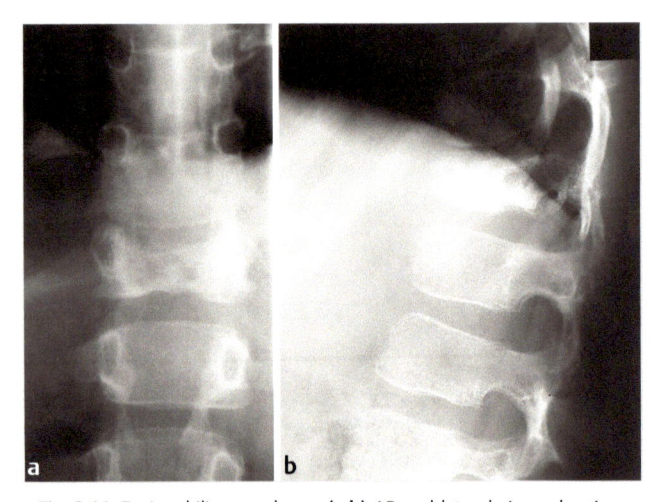

Fig. 9.11 Eosinophilic granuloma. (a,b) AP and lateral views showing the typical appearances of an eosinophilic granuloma on its way to becoming a flatter silver dollar on its edge appearance.

The vertebral bodies can be affected at any age but the implications are different between adolescents and adults. In the latter the vertebral body changes with compression can lead to paralysis.[60,61] In contradistinction, the clinical course is very much more insidious in adolescents, which eventually produces the typical vertebra plana appearance of a silver dollar on its edge (▶ Fig. 9.11) or, on the eastern side of the Atlantic, a biscuit-like appearance, with no such neurological complications and then restitution to normal vertebral height and shape. Treatment is therefore not indicated but biopsy may be required in order to distinguish it from osteomyelitis, Ewing's tumor, or other malignancies.

References

Note: References in **bold** are Key References.

[1] Tachdjian MO, Matson DD. **Orthopaedic aspects of intraspinal Tumors in infants and children.** J Bone Joint Surg Am. 1965; 47:223–248
[2] Fraser RD, Paterson DC, Simpson DA. **Orthopaedic aspects of spinal tumors in children.** J Bone Joint Surg Br. 1977; 59(2):143–151
[3] Balakrishnan V, Rice MS, Simpson DA. Spinal neuroblastomas. Diagnosis, treatment, and prognosis. J Neurosurg. 1974; 40(5):631–638
[4] Fearnside MR, Adams CBT. Tumours of the cauda equina. J Neurol Neurosurg Psychiatry. 1978; 41(1):24–31
[5] McComb JG, Liker MA, Levy ML. In: Weinstein SL, ed. The Pediatric Spine: Principles and Practice. 2nd ed. Lippincott, Williams and Wilkins; 2001:739
[6] Hendrick EB. Spinal cord tumours in children. In: Youmans JR, ed. Neurological Surgery, Vol 5. Philadelphia: WB Saunders; 1982:3215–3221
[7] McComb JG, Liker MA, Levy ML. In: Weinstein SL, ed. The Pediatric Spine: Principles and Practice. 2nd ed. Lippincott, Williams and Wilkins; 2001:713
[8] Wara WM, Sheline GE. Radiation therapy of tumours of the spinal cord. In: Youmans JR, ed. Neurological Surgery, Vol 5. Philadelphia: WB Saunders; 1982:3222–3226
[9] Shikata J, Yamamuro T, Shimizu K, Saito T. Combined laminoplasty and posterolateral fusion for spinal canal surgery in children and adolescents. Clin Orthop Relat Res. 1990(259):92–99
[10] Simon SL, Auerbach JD, Garg S, Sutton LN, Telfeian AE, Dormans JP. Efficacy of spinal instrumentation and fusion in the prevention of postlaminectomy spinal deformity in children with intramedullary spinal cord tumors. J Pediatr Orthop. 2008; 28(2):244–249
[11] Yao KC, McGirt MJ, Chaichana KL, Constantini S, Jallo GI. Risk factors for progressive spinal deformity following resection of intramedullary spinal cord tumors in children: an analysis of 161 consecutive cases. J Neurosurg. 2007; 107(6) Suppl:463–468

[12] Huebert HT, MacKinnon WB. Syringomyelia and scoliosis. J Bone Joint Surg Br. 1969; 51(2):338–343

[13] Ollivier CP. Triate des maladies de la moelle epiniere 3rd Ed. Paris: Crevot; 1827

[14] Duchenne GBA. De l'Electrisation Localisée, 3rd ed. Paris: JB Bailliere et Fils; 1872: 493

[15] Schultze F. Ueber Spalt-. Höhlen-, und Gliombildung im Rückenmarke und in der Medulla Oblongata. Arch Patholo Anatomie Physiol. 1882; 87:510

[16] Chiari H. Uber veranderungen dis kleinhirns denk. 1896, 63: 71–116

[17] Williams B. The distending force in the production of "communicating syringomyelia". Lancet. 1969; 2(7613):189–193

[18] **Williams B. Current concepts of syringomyelia. Br J Hosp Med. 1970; 4:331–342**

[19] Gardner JW, Collis JS. Skeletal anomalies associated with syringomyelia, diastematomyelia, and myelomeningocele. J Bone Joint Surg. 1960; 42-A:1265

[20] **Williams B. Orthopaedic features in the presentation of syringomyelia. J Bone Joint Surg Br. 1979; 61-B(3):314–323**

[21] Finlayson AI. Syringomyelia and related conditions. In: Baker AB, ed. Clinical Neruology. 2nd ed. New York: Harper and Brothers; 1962:1571–1582

[22] Potter JM. Syringomyelia temporarily relieved after scalenotomy. Lancet. 1948; 2(6516):98–99

[23] Meyer GA, Stein J, Poppel MH. Rapid osseous changes in syringomyelia. Radiology. 1957; 69(3):415–418

[24] Woods WW, Pimenta AM. Intramedullary lesions of the spinal cord: Study of sixty-eight consecutive cases. Arch Neurol Psych. 1944; 52:383–399

[25] Simmons EH. The association of scoliosis with syringomyelia and spinal-cord tumours. J Bone Joint Surg. 1973; 55A:440

[26] **Matson DD, Tachdjian MO. Intraspinal tumors in infants and children. Postgrad Med. 1963; 34:279–285**

[27] Perret G. Congenital and developmental anomalies. Skeletal and clinical manifestations of anomalies and defects of the neuraxis. Clin Orthop Relat Res. 1963; 27(27):9–28

[28] Alexander MA, Season EH. Idiopathic scoliosis: an electromyographic study. Arch Phys Med Rehabil. 1978; 59(7):314–315

[29] Pincott JR, Davies JS, Taffs LF. Scoliosis caused by section of dorsal spinal nerve roots. J Bone Joint Surg Br. 1984; 66(1):27–29

[30] McRae DL, Standen J. Roentgenologic findings in syringomyelia and hydromyelia. Am J Roentgenol Radium Ther Nucl Med. 1966; 98(3):695–703

[31] **Leatherman KD, Dickson RA. Two-stage corrective surgery for congenital deformities of the spine. J Bone Joint Surg Br. 1979; 61-B(3):324–328**

[32] Ingraham FD, Matson DD. Neurosurgery of Infancy and Childhood. Springfield, IL Charles C Thomas; 1954

[33] Haft H, Ransohoff J, Carter S. Spinal cord tumors in children. Pediatrics. 1959; 23(6):1152–1159

[34] Gerlach J, Jensen HP, Koss W, et al. Paediatrische Neurochirurgie. Stuttgart: Georg Thieme Verlag; 1967

[35] Matson DD. Neurosurgery of Infancy and Childhood. 2nd ed. Springfield, IL: Charles C Thomas; 1969

[36] **Cattell HS, Clark GL, Jr. Cervical kyphosis and instability following multiple laminectomies in children. J Bone Joint Surg Am. 1967; 49(4):713–720**

[37] Sim FH, Svien HJ, Bickel WH, et al. Swan-neck deformity following multiple laminectomies in children. J Bone Joint Surg. 1967; 49A:713–720

[38] **Lonstein JE. Post-laminectomy kyphosis. Clin Orthop Relat Res. 1977 (128):93–100**

[39] Winter RB, McBride GG. Severe postlaminectomy kyphosis treatment by total vertebrectomy (plus late recurrence of childhood spinal cord astrocytoma). Spine. 1984; 9(7):690–694

[40] Letko L, Jensen RG, Harms J. The treatment of rigid adolescent idiopathic scoliosis: Releases, osteotomies and apical vertebral column resection. In: Newton PO, O'Brien MF, Shfufflebarger HL, Betz RR, Dickson RA, Harms J, eds. Idiopathic Scoliosis. The Harms Study Group Treatment Guide. New York: Thieme; 2010:188–199

[41] Bergstrand H. Uuber eine Eigenartige, Wahrscheinlich Bisher Nicht Beschriebene Osteoblastische Krankheit in Den Langen Knochen der Hand und Des Fusses. Acta Radiologica. 1930; 11(6):596–613

[42] Jaffe HL, Mayer L. An osteoblastic osteoid tissue-forming tumor of a metacarpal bone. Arch Surg. 1932; 24(4):550–564

[43] Jaffe HL. "Osteoid-Osteoma" A Benign Osteoblastic Tumor Composed of Osteoid and Atypical Bone. Arch Surg. 1935; 31:709–728

[44] **Dahlin DC, Johnson EW, Jr. Giant osteoid osteoma. J Bone Joint Surg Am. 1954; 36-A(3):559–572**

[45] Lichtenstein L. Benign osteoblastoma; a category of osteoid-and bone-forming tumors other than classical osteoid osteoma, which may be mistaken for giant-cell tumor or osteogenic sarcoma. Cancer. 1956; 9(5):1044–1052

[46] Jaffe HL. Benign osteoblastoma. Bull Hosp Jt Dis. 1956; 17(2):141–151

[47] **Lichtenstein L, Sawyer WR. Benign osteoblastoma. J Bone Joint Surg Am. 1964; 46:755–765**

[48] Marsh BW, Bonfiglio M, Brady LP, Enneking WF. Benign osteoblastoma: range of manifestations. J Bone Joint Surg Am. 1975; 57(1):1–9

[49] Moberg E. The natural course of osteoid osteoma. J Bone Joint Surg Am. 1951; 33 A(1):166–170

[50] Nemoto O, Moser RP, Jr, Van Dam BE, Aoki J, Gilkey FW. Osteoblastoma of the spine. A review of 75 cases. Spine. 1990; 15(12):1272–1280

[51] Cooper A, Travers B. Surgical Essays. Philadelphia: James Webster; 1818

[52] Bloodgood JC. Bone tumours. Central (medullary) giant-cell tumour (sarcoma) of the lower end of ulna, with evidence that complete destruction of the bony shell or perforation of the bony shell is not a sign of increased malignancy. Ann Surg. 1919; 69(4):345–359

[53] **Verbiest H. Giant-cell tumours and aneurysmal bone cysts of the spine. With special reference to the problems related to the removal of a vertebral body. J Bone Joint Surg Br. 1965; 47(4):699–713**

[54] **Goldenberg RR, Campbell CJ, Bonfiglio M. Giant-cell tumor of bone. An analysis of two hundred and eighteen cases. J Bone Joint Surg Am. 1970; 52 (4):619–664**

[55] Jaffe HL. Aneurysmal bone cyst. Bull Hosp Jt Dis. 1950; 11(1):3–13

[56] Lichtenstein L. Aneurysmal bone cyst. A pathological entity commonly mistaken for giant-cell tumor and occasionally for hemangioma and osteogenic sarcoma. Cancer. 1950; 3:279–289

[57] MacCarty CS, Dahlin DC, Doyle JB, Jr, Lipscomb PR, Pugh DG. Aneurysmal bone cysts of the neural axis. J Neurosurg. 1961; 18:671–677

[58] Calvé J. A localized affection of the spine suggesting osteochondritis of the vertebral body, with the clinical aspect of Pott's disease. J Bone Joint Surg Am. 1925; 7(1):41–46

[59] Lichtenstein L. Histiocytosis X; integration of eosinophilic granuloma of bone, Letterer-Siwe disease, and Schüller-Christian disease as related manifestations of a single nosologic entity. AMA Arch Pathol. 1953; 56(1):84–102

[60] Fitton JM. Cysts and tumours of the musculoskeletal system; clinical aspects of management. In: Harris NH, ed. Postgraduate Textbook of Clinical Orthopaedics. Bristol: Wright; 1983:640–696

[61] Oberman HA. A clinicopathologic study of 40 cases and review of the literature on eosinophilic granuloma of bone. Hand-Schuller-Christian disease and Letterer-Siwe disease. Pediatrics. 1961; 28:307–327

[62] **Lichtenstein L. Histiocystosis X (eosinophilic granuloma of bone, Letterer-Siwe disease, and Schüller-Christian disease). J Bone Joint Surg Am. 1964; 46:76–90**

Chapter 10

Miscellaneous Conditions Associated with Spine Deformities

10.1 Heritable Disorders of Connective Tissue — *270*

10.2 Skeletal Dysplasias — *280*

10 Miscellaneous Conditions Associated with Spine Deformities

In this chapter we have gathered together a number of different conditions, some much more prevalent than others, with the common denominator that they may well present to the scoliosis surgeon with a spinal problem and in some, such as Marfan syndrome, the scoliosis surgeon may be the first clinical port of call while others are also of clinical interest. In many of these it is not a question of surgery for a spinal deformity but rather the scoliosis surgeon may be part of a multidisciplinary team to provide the best holistic management of these children. This is not an unnecessarily exhaustive list, rather it comprises some of the more important conditions with spinal problems.

10.1 Heritable Disorders of Connective Tissue

These disorders of bone matrix are proven or presumed errors of metabolism affecting either the collagenous or noncollagenous components of the matrix. The connective tissue disorders are problems of collagen formation whereas the mucopolysaccharidoses are problems of break down. In osteogenesis imperfecta the features are principally skeletal whereas in the other connective tissue disorders, such as Marfan syndrome and Ehlers-Danlos syndrome, most are extraskeletal.

10.1.1 Osteogenesis Imperfecta: Brittle Bone Syndrome

This is a group of disorders that arise from primary inherited defects in collagen synthesis and have the common feature of bone fragility. Although the condition dates from antiquity—a 3,000-year-old Egyptian specimen resides in the British Museum[1]—the first clinical description was attributed to Ekman.[2] Early classifications of the brittle bone syndrome recognized a severe and lethal sporadic form (osteogenesis imperfecta [OI] congenita) with intrauterine fractures and an early death and a milder dominantly inherited form (OI tarda) which was further subdivided into gravis or levis types according to whether fractures present within the first year of life or thereafter.[3,4] Others favored subdivision into the mild and severe types based upon the presence of long bone deformity (▶ Fig. 10.1 and ▶ Fig. 10.2) and this appears to correlate better with clinical features.[5,6]

The incidence of the condition is 1 in 20,000 at birth with about 80% of cases caused by autosomal dominant mutations of the type I collagen genes, type I collagen being the principal collagen of bone, dentine, and sclera and so these are the tissues most commonly affected in OI.[7] These mutations produce two different protein defects, the first in activating one allele with a 50% reduction in type I collagen in bone while the other has a reduced amount of normal collagen in addition to type I collagen molecules containing mutant collagen genes.[8] As a result the first type produces the mild type I OI form of the disease while the more severe category produces the worst types.

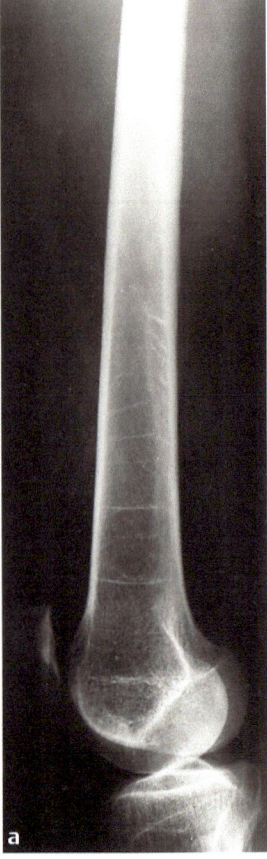

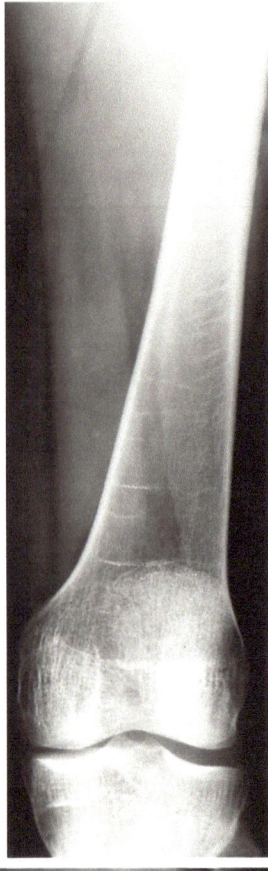

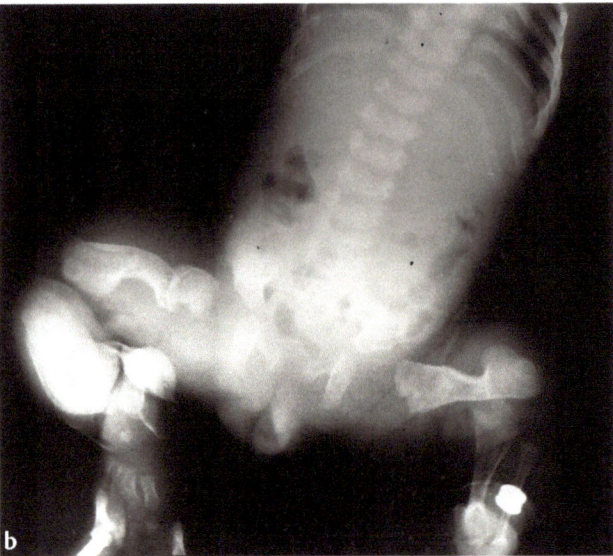

Fig. 10.1 The radiological classification of osteogenesis imperfecta. **(a)** Mild disease showing osteoporosis and Harris' lines. **(b)** Severe disease with multiple fracturing and gross long bone deformity.

There are now some eight types of OI in up-to-date classifications.[7] Type I, with bone fragility but with blue sclerae and autosomal dominant inheritance, is the most common and

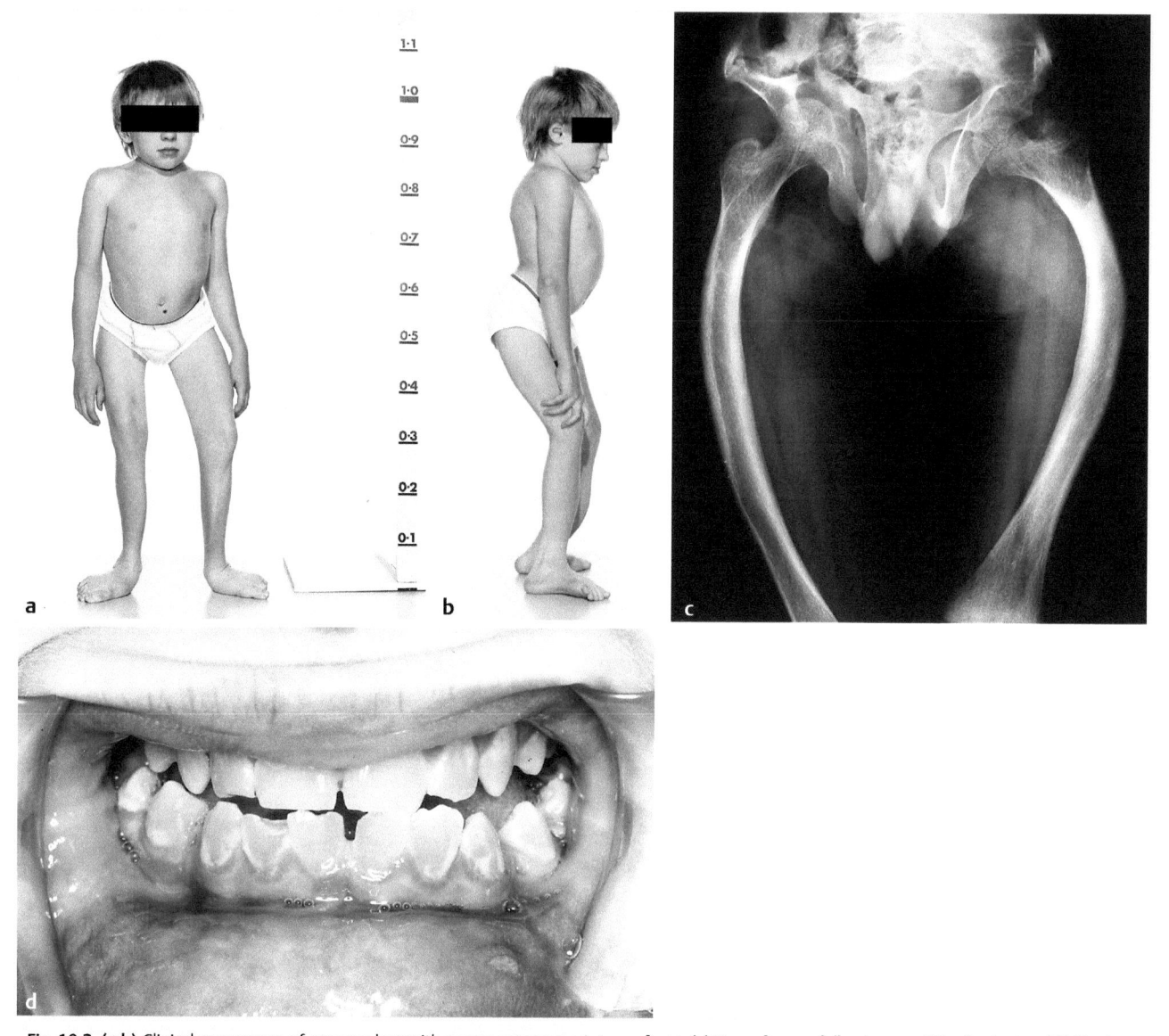

Fig. 10.2 (a,b) Clinical appearance of a young boy with severe osteogenesis imperfecta. **(c)** Varus femurs following repetitive fracturing. **(d)** The boy also had dentinogenesis imperfecta.

mildest form. Fracturing starts to occur when the child starts to walk and the fracture types are similar to those seen in normal children but of course they fracture more easily. The most common biochemical abnormality is defective synthesis of sufficient type I collagen, particularly the alpha 1 (1 chain), which obviously will affect the skeleton as bone contains type I collagen only.[6]

As regards the spine the radiographic changes are indistinguishable from those in juvenile osteoporosis, with multiple compression fractures of the vertebrae that are biconcave[9,10] (▶ Fig. 10.3). About 70% of patients with OI can be shown to have a scoliosis[11,12] (▶ Fig. 10.4) and a similar majority can be shown to have anterior chest deformities in the nature of pectus carinatum, excavatum, or an increased sagittal chest diameter.[12] In a multicenter study of OI in North America involving 544 OI subjects it would seem that type III cases had a higher prevalence rate of severe scoliosis and long bone deformities than types I and IV.[13] Meanwhile in a study of spinal curvature during growth in 316 OI patients scoliosis had a prevalence rate of 50% overall but type III had the highest prevalence rate of 68% with a mean progression rate of 6% per year, while with type IV cases the prevalence rate was 54% and the progression rate 4% per year. The lowest prevalence rate was seen in type I OI with a 39% prevalence rate with progression of 1% per year. For type III patients treatment with bisphosphonates significantly decreased the progression rate.[14]

With so many other dysmorphic problems, altering spinal shape is clearly not a priority and Cobb angle would not be an important variable determining the need for surgery. In addition the history of surgical treatment for scoliosis has demonstrated just the sort of problems that one would anticipate. The earliest report of substantial numbers was by the Scoliosis Research Society.[15] Posterior stabilization was the method of choice, 39 of 55 having Harrington instrumentation with only 4 anterior fusions and 1 combined two-stage procedure. Cobb angle correction was a mere 36 degrees with significant

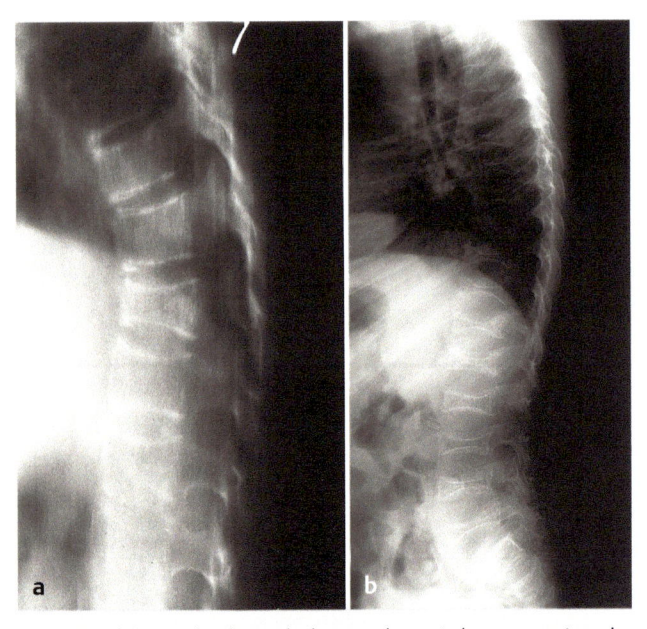

Fig. 10.3 (a) Lateral radiograph showing the typical osteoporosis and biconcave compression fractures of osteogenesis imperfecta. (b) Lateral radiograph of severe spinal disease indistinguishable from idiopathic juvenile osteoporosis.

complications in one-third of cases with loss of instrument attachment to bone and pseudarthrosis being the major culprits.[15] Waugh[16] suggested the use of methyl-methacrylate cement to strengthen hook sites and this has been used in patients with OI.[17] However, with cement augmented pedicle screw instrumentation for the surgical treatment of a scoliosis in OI quite promising results have been reported by Yilmaz et al.[18] There were 10 operated patients, 7 of whom had cement augmented screw insertion at the proximal and distal foundations. The mean Cobb angles to start with were 84 degrees and at follow-up 40 degrees with no instrumentation failures.

10.1.2 Marfan Syndrome

Marfan syndrome is an autosomal dominant disorder in which there is an abnormality in the Fibrillin-1 gene so that this is found in soft tissues.[7] The fibroblast-produced collagen appears unusually soluble. The typical patient is tall and thin with arachnodactyly (hands and feet) and pectus carinatum or excavatum. The tall stature is disproportionate with a reduced upper to lower segment ratio. There is a long narrow face with a high arched palate and eye problems are common including dislocated lenses and retinal detachment (▶ Fig. 10.5). Joints are hypermobile but the most significant problems affect the

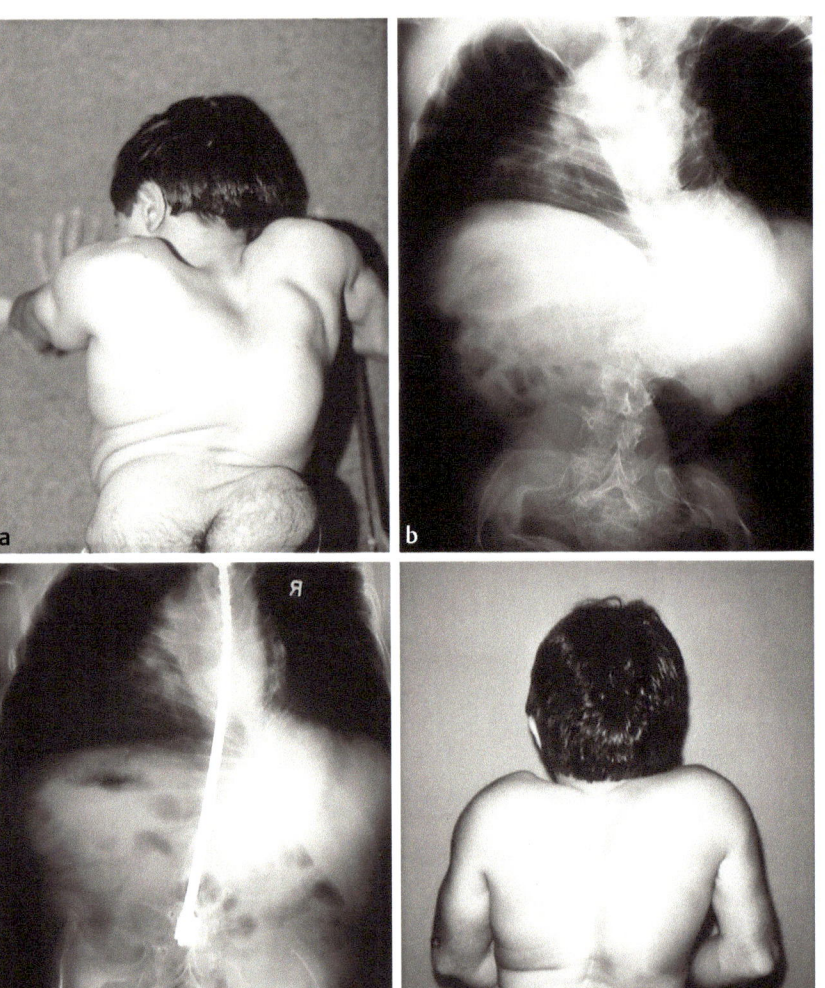

Fig. 10.4 (a) Scoliosis in association with severe osteogenesis imperfecta O.I. with painful costovertebral impingement. (b) PA radiograph showing the severe deformity. (c) After Harrington rod fixation with cementation of the upper and lower hooks. (d) Five years later this correction was sustained and his symptoms remained relieved.

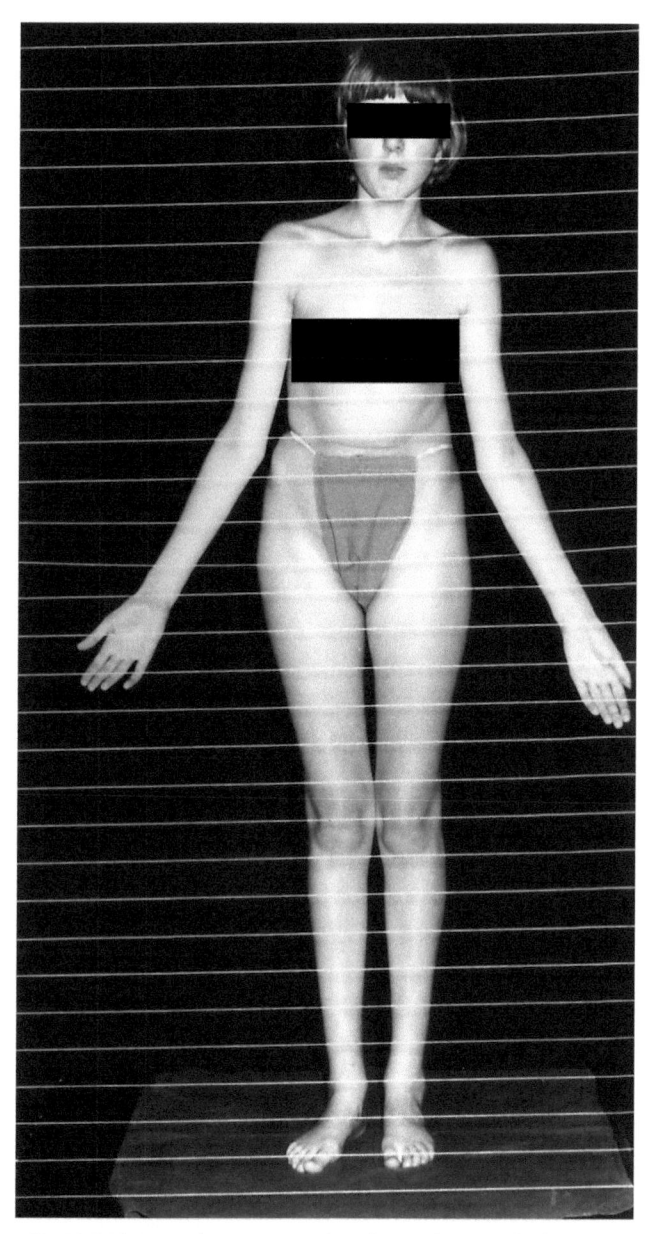

Miscellaneous Conditions Associated with Spine Deformities

Fig. 10.5 The typical appearance of Marfan syndrome: tall, disproportionately long slim limbs, arachnodactyly, and an increased upper to lower segment ratio.

cardiovascular system with aortic incompetence and dissecting aneurysm as well as mitral and tricuspid valve disease. These are the usual causes of early death often in the forties.

The condition was first described in 1896[19] although one of Marfan's cases was certainly congenital contractural arachnodactyly.[20] The differential diagnosis is therefore important and includes homocystinuria and congenital contractural arachnodactyly.[21] Homocystinuria has only been described recently and can be differentiated from Marfan syndrome by the presence of widened epiphyses and metaphyses, frequent osteoporosis of the spine in particular, and an increased incidence of thromboembolism.[22] Arachnodactyly and scoliosis are less common in homocystinuria. Congenital contractural arachnodactyly is characterized by multiple joint contractures present at birth with elbow, knee, and ankle particularly affected whereas if contractures develop in Marfan syndrome they do so later. There is also the characteristic abnormality of the ears and there is no lens dislocation, heart disease, or ligament laxity.

In Marfan syndrome severe planovalgus feet are very common in association with the arachnodactyly of the digits (▶ Fig. 10.6). The prevalence rate of scoliosis in Marfan syndrome varies from about one-third to three-quarters in series of reasonable numbers of patients suggesting an average figure of about 50%.[23-28] The deformity is very similar to that in idiopathic scoliosis (lordoscoliosis). An increased prevalence rate is however readily explicable on the basis that the less strong soft tissue support for the spine increases the intrinsic load on the spine rendering it less able to resist buckling deformation (lordoscoliosis) or simple angular collapse (kyphosis). Of 35 patients reported by Winter and Moe in 1969,[25] 18 had a scoliosis with a curve size varying from 15 to 185 degrees. There were two typical curve patterns, right thoracic or thoracolumbar and double-structural—the latter giving rise to the typical flat-back appearance (▶ Fig. 10.7). Interestingly the curve was painful in five of their cases. The progression rate was similar to that in idiopathic scoliosis and treatment was along the same principles. In a later report of 35 cases of scoliosis in association with Marfan syndrome three-quarters were painful and almost half started in the infantile or juvenile periods.[28] There was no evidence, not surprisingly, that the 14 who were braced derived any benefit therefrom. The adolescent with Marfan syndrome can undergo precisely the same type of surgical correction as the idiopathic counterpart and there would appear to be no significant surgical risk from a delicate cardiac status. However, prior to surgery, cardiovascular assessment including ultrasonography of the heart valves and aorta should be undertaken, regularly in childhood anyway, and essentially before undertaking any major surgery in older children and teenagers. Aortic replacement with or without aortic valve replacement is frequently required and is best undertaken early because vascular complications are the usual cause of the premature death. In this regard hypotensive anesthesia is to be recommended.[6]

Whereas in Minneapolis, Louisville, Leeds, and Karlsbad, we have not encountered any surgical problems peculiar to Marfan syndrome rather than those of the late-onset idiopathic counterpart; some more recent reports seem to raise concern. Whereas in China, Li reported 12 consecutive cases with posterior segmental instrumentation correction and observed no significant complications,[29] a multicenter study from several orthopaedic centers in the United States suggested differences in outcome compared to similar adolescent idiopathic cases[30]; as did that of Zenner et al.[31] One of the differences observed by Gjolaj et al[30] was that many more patients with Marfan syndrome had a kyphosis of more than 50 degrees. One does find it slightly irritating to put it mildly that one still hears of kyphosis when we have published so many papers establishing that all structural scolioses are lordotic and what is being perceived as kyphosis is just a severely rotated lordoscoliosis (see Chapter 3). Yes, the spine is pointing backward but it is the front of the spine pointing backward and not the back of the spine (Chapters 2 and 3 as well should remove all reasonable doubt). These sizeable pseudokyphoses do indicate the need to go anteriorly with instrumentation as well as posteriorly if necessary, as with neurofibromatosis 1 (NF1) (▶ Fig. 8.7).

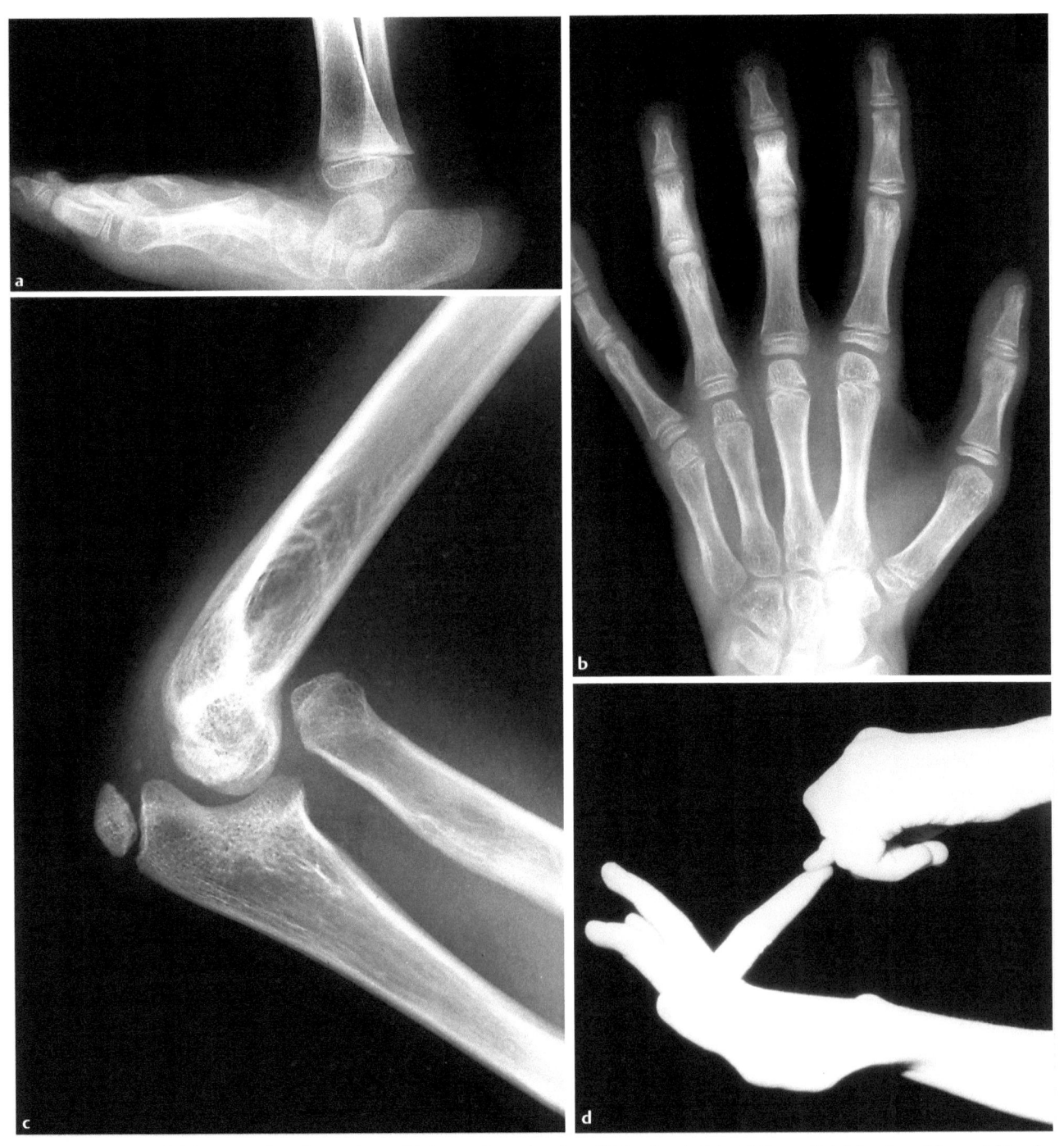

Fig. 10.6 The typical deformities of Marfan syndrome. **(a)** Severe planovalgus feet. **(b)** Arachnodactyly. **(c)** Congenital dislocation of the radial head. **(d)** Typical joint hypermobility in Marfan syndrome.

As multiple curve patterns are particularly prevalent in Marfan syndrome then lengthier instrumentations are bound to be required, but this is not a complication—rather, it is an idiopathic-type curve pattern seen more frequently in Marfan syndrome. There were three cerebrospinal fluid (CSF) leaks in the 34 Marfan patients with none in the idiopathic group. Dural ectasia has been reported in the Marfan syndrome[32] and there is no reason of course why the soft tissue of the dura should not be subject to the same Marfan soft tissue weakness (as with the cardiovascular system). The problem of "adding on" should be obviated with rigorous attention to LIV selection. In seven cases instrumentation was taken down into the pelvis, four primarily and three for revision, the need for which we simply cannot envisage. Unlike paralytic curves where maybe significant pelvic obliquity in both Marfan and idiopathic scoliosis L5 is always the robust LIV with immensely strong attachments to the pelvis via the iliolumbar and lumbosacral ligaments, as well as stronger bone than the pelvis.

Meanwhile Zenner et al[31] reported on 23 Marfan patients while using unnecessarily expressive language such as "the

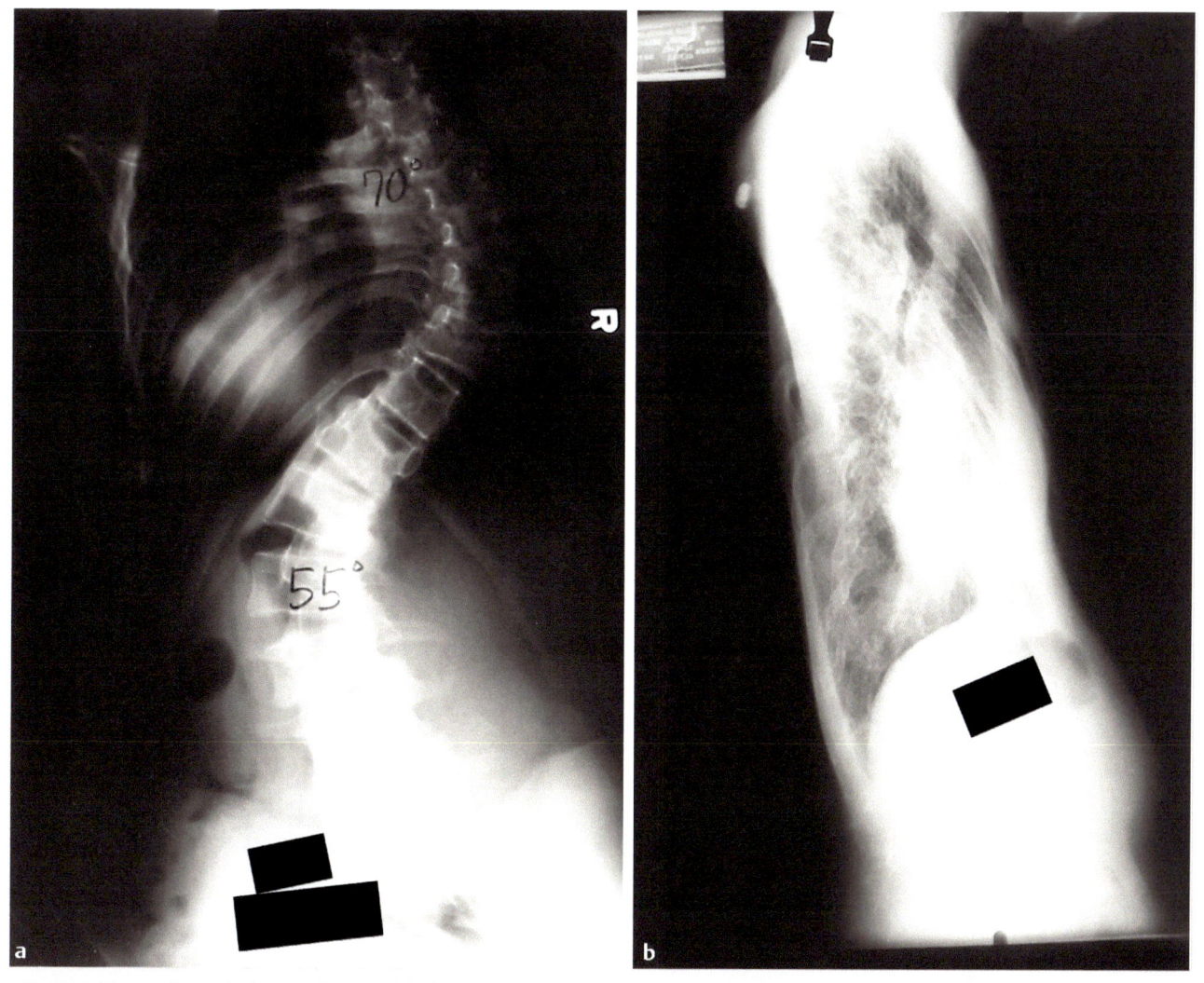

Miscellaneous Conditions Associated with Spine Deformities

Fig. 10.7 (a) PA radiograph showing the typical double-structural curve with Marfan syndrome. **(b)** Lateral radiograph showing the severe flat-back deformity of a double lordosis in Marfan syndrome.

individual challenges of the underlying desmogenic disorder" went on to demonstrate that excellent/good outcomes were noted overall in 80% of patients.

There is absolutely no reason why the Marfan patient should not be treated exactly as the idiopathic counterpart with the same excellent expectations.

Whereas scoliosis is less frequent than in homocystinuria it is important to make sure that the suspected Marfan case does not have homocystinuria (detectable in the urine by the nitroprusside test) because vascular damage leading to thrombosis would be a surgical contraindication.

10.1.3 Mucopolysaccharidoses

These disorders affect the skeleton by way of failure of the normal breakdown of complex carbohydrates which therefore accumulate in the tissues and appear in excess in the urine. The last several decades have seen knowledge of these conditions change from purely descriptive aspects to a more clear understanding of the biochemical defects involved.[7] There are two groups: mucopolysaccharidoses (MPS) and mucolipidoses. The dreadful prognosis of the latter makes them very unlikely to be encountered by orthopaedic surgeons. The incompletely broken down mucopolysaccharides accumulate in the lysosomes of cells and many tissues can therefore be affected (e.g., cartilage, bone, liver, central nervous system).

The typical deformity of the MPSs is a thoracolumbar kyphosis due to apical developmental wedge-shaped vertebrae. Although spinal surgeons are unlikely to encounter MPSs other than Morquio's syndrome, in MSII Hunter syndrome—which is milder physically and mentally than Hurler syndrome (MPS I)—there is again a thoracolumbar kyphosis with characteristic upper lumbar vertebral beaking (▶ Fig. 10.8).

10.1.4 MPS IV: Morquio's Syndrome

This condition was first described in 1929 by Morquio of Uruguay[33] who described four children, two girls and two boys, out of a family of five. At the same time in Birmingham, Brailsford published a case of Naughton Dunn's.[34] The condition is caused by a deficiency of the enzymes responsible for the degradation of keratan sulphate. The condition is autosomal recessive

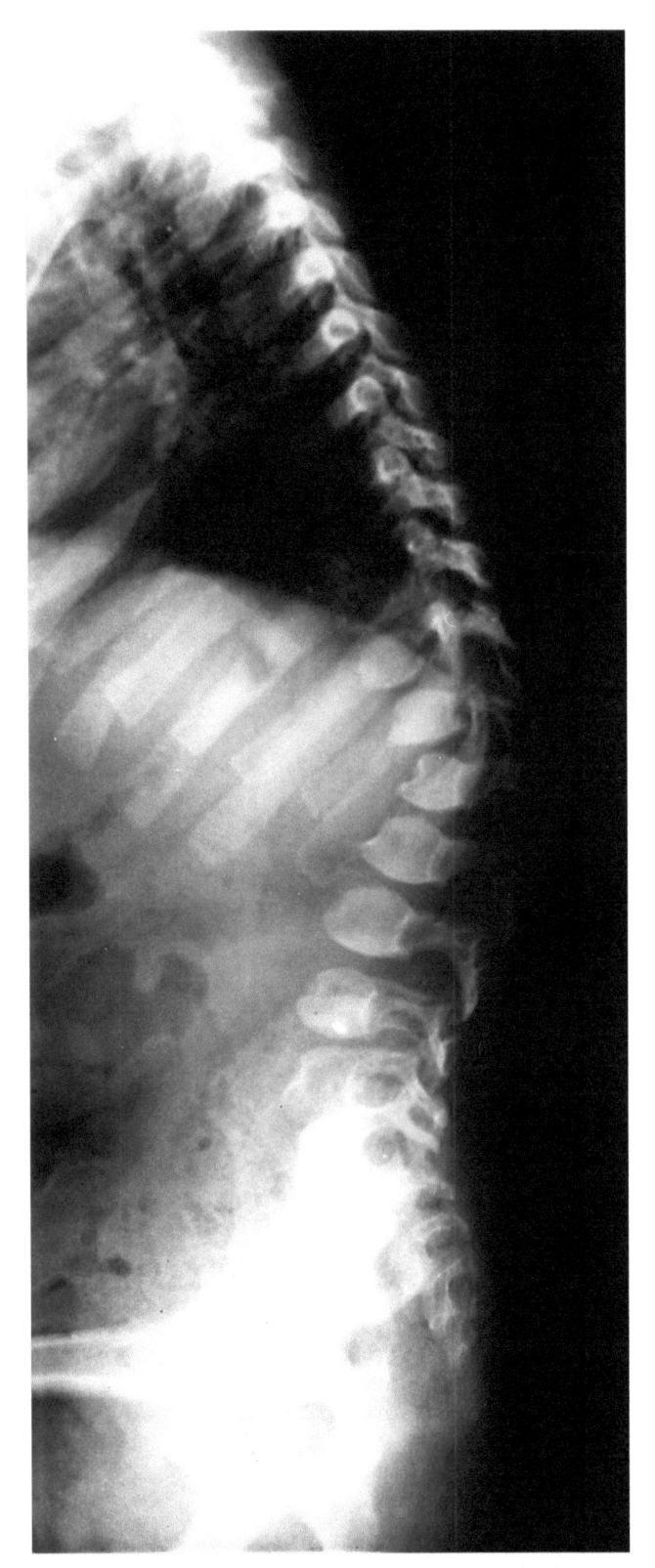

Fig. 10.8 Hurler's syndrome. Lateral radiograph showing the characteristic thoracolumbar kyphosis with the apical bullet-shaped vertebra.

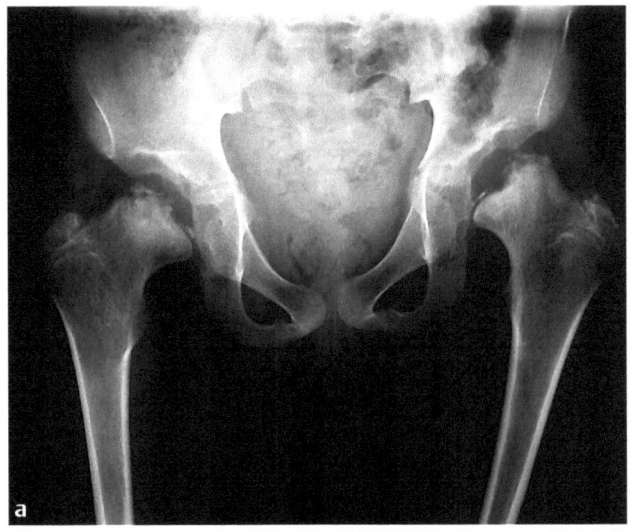

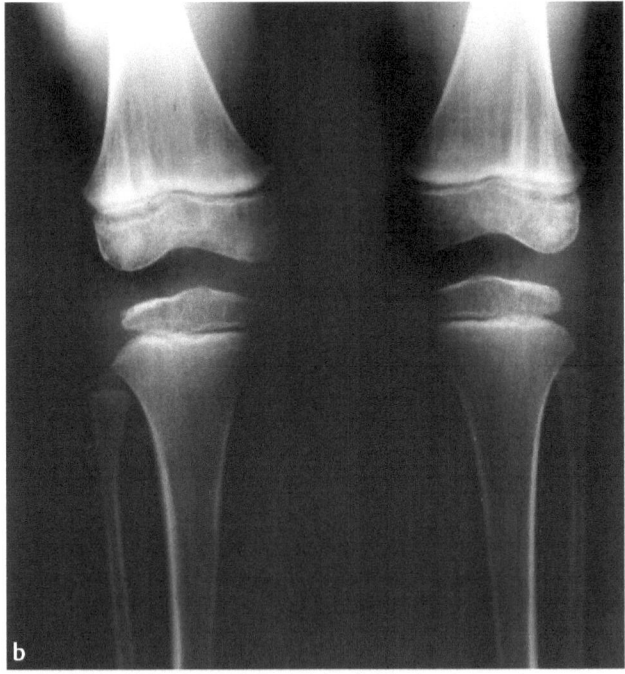

Fig. 10.9 Two characteristic skeletal features of Morquio's syndrome. (a) PA of the pelvis showing a hypoplastic pelvis with iliac flaring and a wine glass–shaped pelvis with marked dysplasia of the femoral capital epiphysis. (b) The characteristic radiographic appearances of the knees in Morquio's syndrome. There is deficient lateral ossification of the femoral and tibial epiphyses and metaphyses which leads to genu valgum.

with a normal intelligence and a variable severity of associated physical disability (▶ Fig. 10.9). The major problems are skeletal with deformity and short-trunk dwarfism—patients rarely achieving a height greater than 1.2 m. There is a flexed stance with genu valgum and there is often hyperextensibility of joints and skin as well as corneal clouding. The prognosis is variable and death often occurs early from cardiorespiratory failure or spinal cord compression.

As regards the spine there is an early thoracolumbar kyphosis with later platyspondyly and anterior vertebral beaking (▶ Fig. 10.10). There are two major problems: the thoracolumbar kyphosis and atlantoaxial instability as a result of a deficient odontoid (▶ Fig. 10.11). The thoracolumbar kyphosis is important because it is both common and dangerous from the point of view of spinal cord compression. Melzak reported two

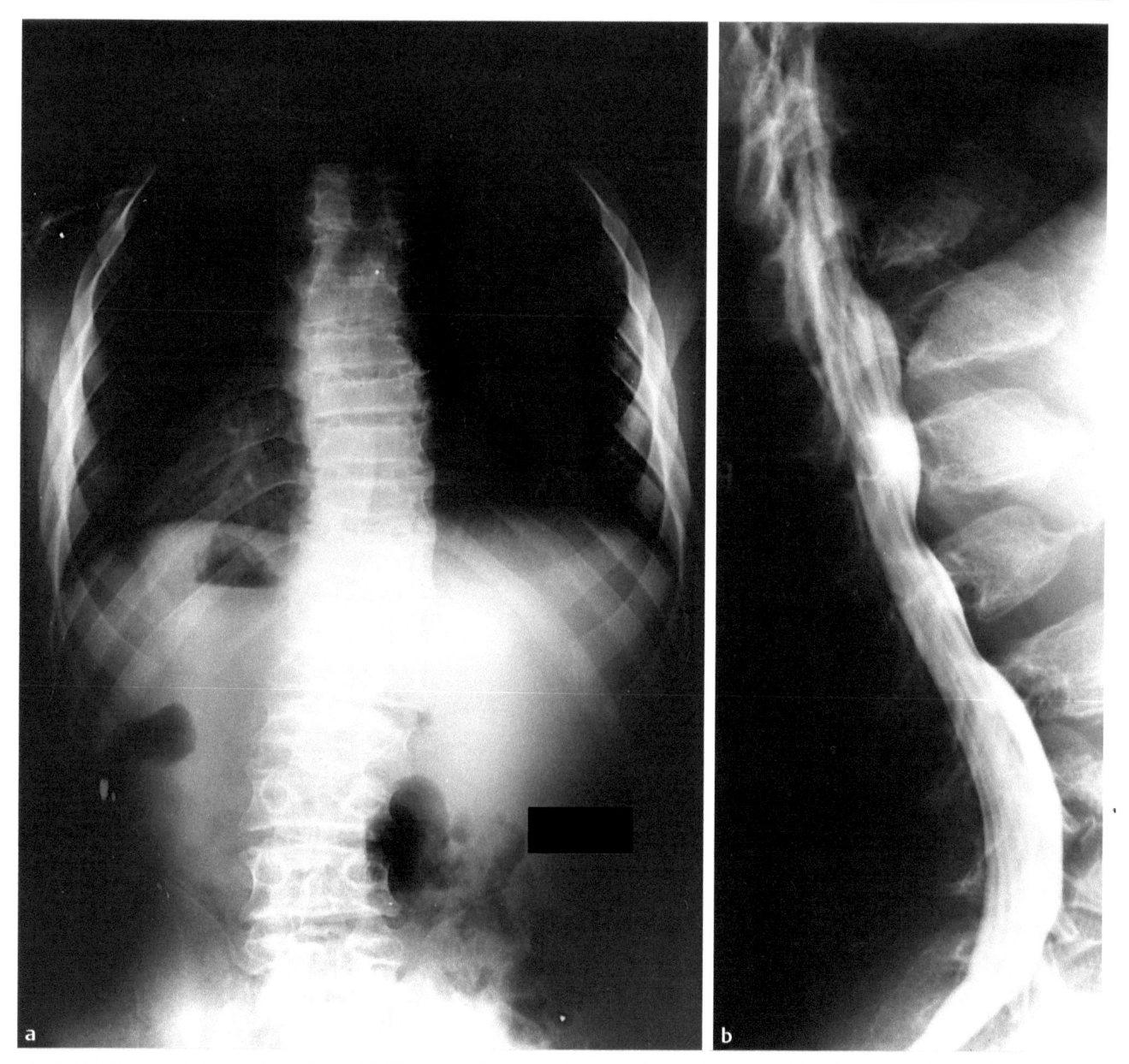

Fig. 10.10 The spine in Morquio's syndrome. (a) PA radiograph showing the severe degree of platyspondyly. (b) Lateral myelogram showing indentation of the dye column over the region of the kyphosis thought to be due to meningeal thickening. Note the apical vertebra hooked anteriorly.

sisters with Morquio's syndrome who both had spinal cord compression from thoracolumbar kyphoses.[35] More recently in a study of 80 dwarfs of various types, 18 were MPSs and 14 of these had a thoracolumbar kyphosis measuring between 14 and 53 degrees.[36] Thoracolumbar kyphosis is associated with a barrel-shaped chest, a prominent sternum above, and premature fusion of the sternal segments with an immobile chest which can lead to severe chest dysfunction resulting in early death.

For the thoracolumbar kyphosis bracing can be prescribed to prevent progression and can be, perhaps surprisingly, quite successful. Leatherman treated three siblings with Morquio's syndrome in extension braces for more than 5 years each with no progression (▶ Fig. 10.12). However, if there are neurological signs of impending spinal cord dysfunction then anterior apical wedge resection with spinal cord decompression, anterior strut grafting of the anterior and middle columns followed by tension band type posterior metalwork is the treatment of choice (see ▶ Fig. 10.20).

Scoliosis is seldom a serious problem and of Bethem's 18 MPS cases, only 8 had a scoliosis of more than 10 degrees, the biggest measuring only 38 degrees.[36]

The most worrying spinal aspect concerning Morquio's syndrome is the very high prevalence rate of neurological problems from atlantoaxial instability. This is due to a hypoplastic dens with associated ligamentous instability. Indeed this is a significant source of mortality as well as morbidity. In Kopits' first series of 29 dwarfs with odontoid dysplasia, 23 had atlantoaxial subluxation with associated myelopathy in 15.[37] Ten of these patients were Morquio's syndrome. In a later series

Miscellaneous Conditions Associated with Spine Deformities

including 18 Morquio's cases, Kopits described clearly the myelopathy picture.[38] There are often atypical signs with tiredness, weakness, vague leg pains, paroxysmal tachypnea, respiratory arrest, syncope, and gait abnormality. Furthermore the signs are often unilateral or predominantly so. Progression occurs due to chronic injury from repetitive minor trauma in the environment of instability and stenosis.[39] While it has been suggested that fusion should be offered if there is evidence of atlantoaxial instability, Kopits based upon his enormous experience clearly indicates that the problem of atlantoaxial instability in the Morquio patient is so important that a posterior C1/2 fusion should be performed in all cases prophylactically. This implies surgery in all cases by the age of 7 or 8 years.

Trying to assess surgically significant atlantoaxial instability radiographically is not easy although it is generally considered that an atlas-dens interval (ADI) of more than 5 mm is abnormal at any age with a 2 mm change on flexion/extension[39] although neurological symptoms and signs are known to occur with lesser measurements and reciprocally no neurological problems with greater measurements (▶ Fig. 10.13). A useful valid assessment is to consider the upper cervical spine as being divided into thirds—an anterior third for the odontoid, a posterior third for the cord, and the middle third which is called "the space available for the cord," or SAC. If the degree of displacement is such that the dens is only into the SAC then there should be no neurological concerns but when into the posterior third then neurological problems are inevitable. The indications for surgical treatment are the relief of neurological symptoms and signs along with restoration of a stable upper cervical spine. Although one tends to talk about C1/2 instability there is often a craniocervical junction compression with the C1 posterior arch lying within the foramen magnum. In addition the local C1 or C2 bone may not be user-friendly for fixation so rather than attempt a complex civil engineering project it is better to apply a halo vest in the reduced position and perform an on-lay bone

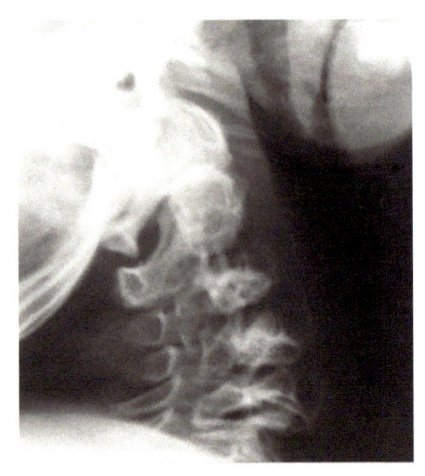

Fig. 10.11 Lateral radiograph of the upper cervical spine showing a deficient odontoid, the cause of atlantoaxial instability (AAI). The neck is extended and this reduces the AAS.

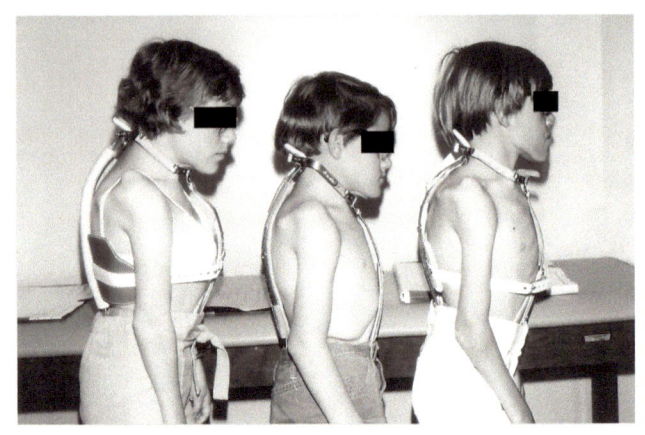

Fig. 10.12 Clinical photo of three Morquio siblings in extension braces.

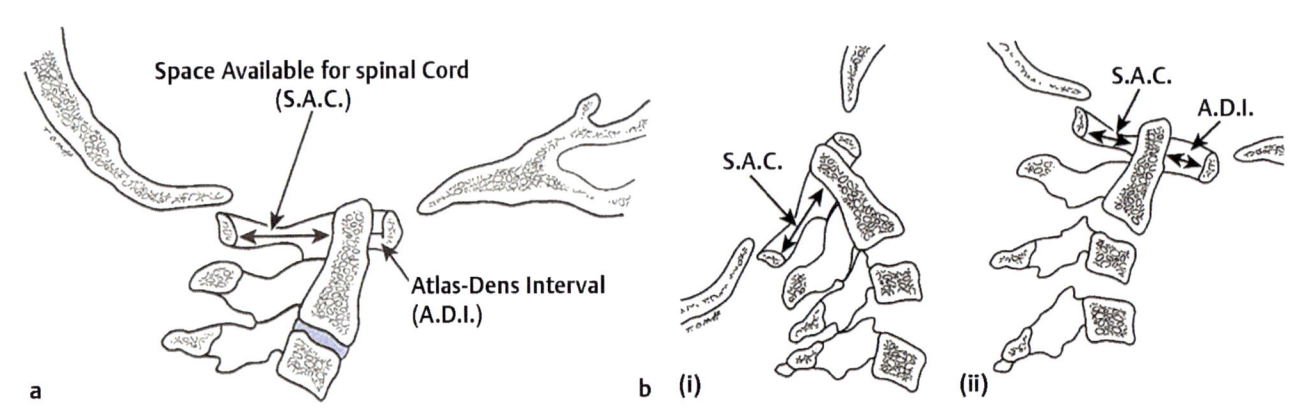

Fig. 10.13 (a) Diagram showing the lateral aspect of the craniocervical junction and in particular the relationship between the odontoid peg of the atlas and the arch of the atlas. In the normal position there is a potential space between the front of the top of the odontoid and the back of the anterior arch of the atlas called the atlas-dens interval (ADI). Behind the odontoid is what is referred to as the space available for the spinal cord (SAC). This is not really accurate because the spinal cord occupies the posterior half of the SAC and so there is a space in the middle third and that should be referred to as the SAC. (b) In extension the head and the atlas move backward, closing the ADI and maximizing the SAC. With ligament laxity on flexion the head and the atlas move forward on the odontoid with lengthening of the ADI and shortening of the SAC. As the spinal cord occupies only the posterior half of the SAC then the odontoid has to move backward through the middle third before it impinges upon the spinal cord. (Reproduced with the permission of Rothman-Simeone, The Spine, 6th Edition, Elsevier, USA. In Congenital Anomalies of the Cervical Spine, Bedi A, Hensinger RN, Chapter 30, Figs 30-4 and 30.5, p. 529.)

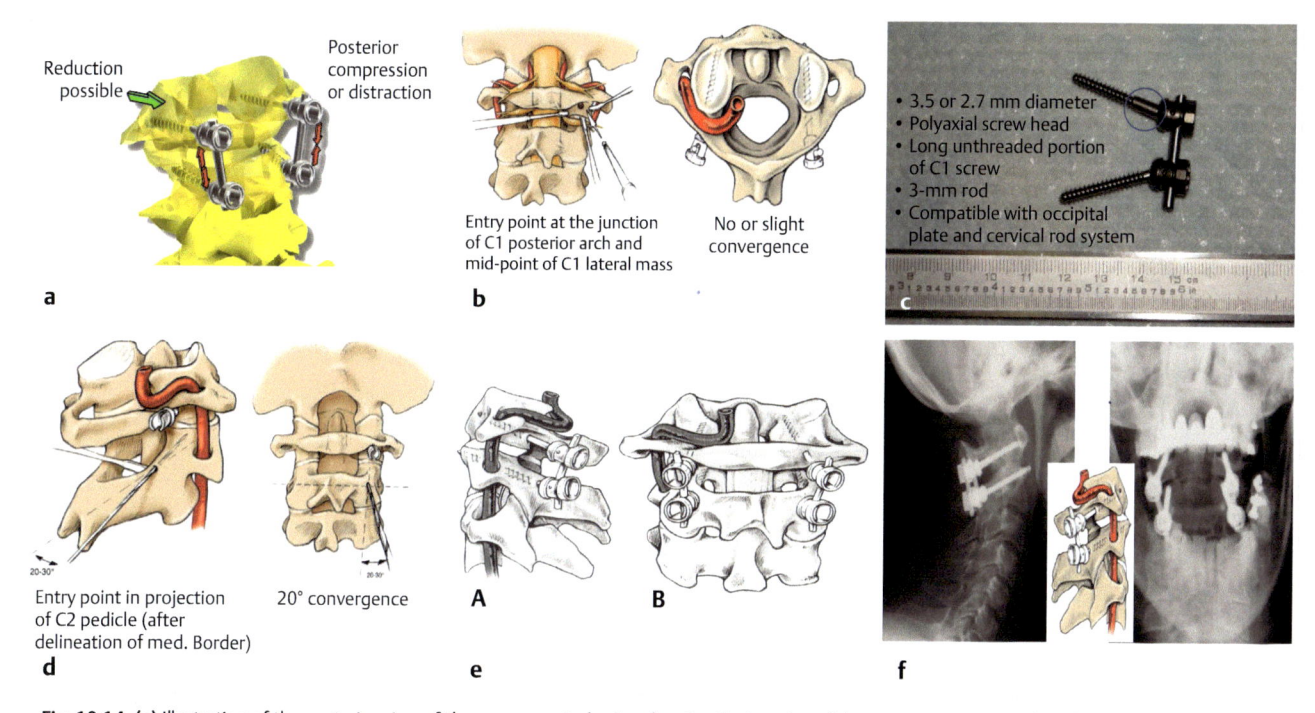

Fig. 10.14 (a) Illustration of the posterior view of the upper cervical spine showing the location of the entry point in C1 and C2 for screw placement in the polyaxial screw and rod fixation technique. (b) Superior view of the atlas showing polyaxial screws placed bicortically into the lateral mass. (c) Posterior C1/C2 fixation with polyaxial-head screws. (d) Entry point in projection of C2 pedicle (after delineation of medial border). (e) Upper cervical spine after C1–2 fixation by the polyaxial screw and rod fixation technique: (A) lateral view, (B) posterior view. (f) Lateral and PA views of the final construct.

grafting procedure. Old fashioned wiring techniques are anachronistic[40,41] but with an adequate bone mass, transarticular screws, lateral mass screws, pulley axial screws, and segmental fixation are all applicable. However, these screw techniques have all reported a high incidence of vertebral artery damage at between 4% and 8%.[42] In addition, screw insertion occurs after reduction of the problem and this can be difficult technically. However, in Karlsbad, we have developed a technique of C1/2 fixation with a very low risk of vertebral artery damage and allowing in situ reduction of C1/2 subluxation and fixation using 3.4 mm polyaxial screws and a 3-mm rod[43] (▶ Fig. 10.14a).

Practice Points

To avoid injury to the vertebral artery, computed tomography (CT) angiography is carried out preoperatively (▶ Fig. 6.28) and in 20% of cases it will be found that the vertebral artery passes more medially than normal as it goes toward the posterior atlanto-occipital membrane. Under general anesthesia, the patient is placed in the prone position with the head flexed and the torso inclined slightly downward (the anti-Trendelenburg position) to minimize venous bleeding. The position of the C1-C2 complex is verified by use of an image intensifier then the cervical spine is exposed subperiosteally from the inion to C3-C4 spinous processes. The insertions of rectus capitis posterior major and the inferior oblique muscles are incised sharply from the spinous process of the axis and then the C1-C2 complex is exposed by blunt soft tissue dissection using swabs out to the lateral border of the C1-C2 articulation. Bleeding commonly occurs from dissection near the epidural venous plexus around the ganglion of the second cervical nerve and the plexus around the C1-C2 joint. This is best controlled by a combination of bipolar cautery, gel foam with thrombin, and cotton pledgets. The C1-C2 joint is exposed and opened by dissection over the superior surface of the C2 pars interarticularis. This joint is a key anatomical landmark for accurate placement of the C1 lateral mass screw. The dorsal root ganglion of C2 is retracted in a caudal direction to expose the entry point for the C1 screw, which is in the middle of the junction of the C1 posterior arch and the midpoint of the posterior inferior part of the C1 lateral mass (▶ Fig. 10.14b). This entry point is marked with a 1 to 2 mm high speed bur to prevent slippage of the drill point. The pilot hole is then drilled in a straight or slightly convergent trajectory in an anteroposterior direction and parallel to the plane of the C1 posterior arch in the sagittal direction with the tip of the drill directed toward the anterior arch of C1. The drilling is accomplished with guidance from intraoperative landmarks, preoperative fine-cut axial CT images, and lateral fluoroscopic imaging. The hole is tapped and a 3.5-mm polyaxial screw of an appropriate length is inserted bicortically into the lateral mass of C1 (▶ Fig. 10.14b). Currently, the C1 screw is manufactured as a custom device, and the length of the screw used must be determined by depth gauge and preoperative CT. An 8-mm unthreaded portion of the C1 screw stays above the bony surface of the lateral mass, minimizing any chance of irritation of the greater occipital nerve and allowing the polyaxial portion of the screw to lie above the posterior arch of C1 (▶ Fig. 10.14c). The position of the screws is verified by an image intensifier.

A number 4 Penfield is used to delineate the medial border of the C2 pars interarticularis, and the entry point for placement of the C2 pedicle screw is marked with a high-speed bur. This is in the cranial and medial quadrant of the isthmus surface of C2 (▶ Fig. 10.14d). The pilot hole is prepared with a 2-mm drill bit, just perforating the opposite cortex. The direction of the bit is approximately 20 to 30 degrees in a convergent and cephalad direction, guided directly by the superior and medial surface of the C2 isthmus, respecting individual anatomic variations. The integrity of the pilot hole is verified with a blunt probe. The hole is tapped, and a 3.5 mm polyaxial screw of the appropriate length after depth gauge measurement is inserted bicortically.

If necessary, reduction of the C1 ring is performed by positioning the patient's head and/or directly manipulating C1 and C2 using the screws, followed by fixation to the rods to maintain the alignment (▶ Fig. 10.14e). Check X-rays are again taken, this time of the final construct (▶ Fig. 10.14f). If a definitive fusion is required, C1 and C2 are decorticated posteriorly, and cancellous bone taken from a small incision in the posterior iliac crest can be placed over the decorticated surfaces of C1 and C2. An intra-articular fusion can also be performed by decorticating the C1–2 joint surfaces under direct vision.

In selected cases, this technique can be used to obtain temporary stabilization without definitive fusion. Implant removal at an appropriate time will allow the patient to regain atlantoaxial motion. Patients are mobilized on the first postoperative day and wear a soft cervical collar for 2 to 3 weeks.

10.2 Skeletal Dysplasias

The skeletal dysplasias are a group of conditions—some not infrequent but most rare—with the common denominator that there is disordered development in growth of some part of the skeleton. Knowledge of these conditions is essentially descriptive but over the past four decades more knowledge has been added to these conditions and many new ones have emerged making classification important. Furthermore, although the skeletal involvement of a particular dysplasia may be indefinite and indescribable, it is often the case that the nonskeletal features alert the clinician to the likely diagnosis of a bone dysplasia. The great majority have disproportionate short stature (dwarfism) and, even if treatment is not deemed appropriate these families can have the benefit of increased knowledge by way of a more accurate medical and surgical prognostication and genetic counseling.[8]

The bone dysplasias are divided according to whether epiphysis, metaphysis, vertebra, or combinations of the above are predominantly involved, to which is added those with decreased or increased bone density.

10.2.1 Achondroplasia

This is a dysplasia with predominantly metaphyseal involvement. It is an autosomal dominant condition with the great majority arising as spontaneous mutations. The prevalence rate in Europe is approximately 2 or 3 per 100,000.[44] The condition has been recognized for thousands of years but was only described a century ago.[45] The typical appearance is that of short limbs with short podgy fingers on trident hands, a bulging cranium with low nasal bridge, a narrowed lumbar spinal canal with lordosis, and characteristic pelvic changes[46–49] (▶ Fig. 10.15). Skeletal growth is abnormal in achondroplasia with stunted bone formation. However, when height is plotted at regular intervals, the slope parallels that of the normal individual, although the achondroplast starts and stays well below the third percentile. The pathology has been likened to the proteolytic changes that occur when animals are injected with the enzyme papain. When the glycosaminoglycans and proteoglycans in achondroplastic cartilage were inspected the main problem appeared to be in the processes of maturation, hypertrophy, and degeneration of chondrocytes in the growth plate.[50]

The diagnosis is obvious at birth and these individuals achieve a standing height of just over 4 feet with a normal life expectancy and normal intelligence. The main differential diagnosis is from hypochondroplasia and pseudoachondroplasia, the former being less severe with no skull or pelvic changes and the latter being similar while the skull is normal but there are severe epiphyseal and vertebral changes (▶ Fig. 10.16). There is considerable clinical variation in both achondroplasia and hypochondroplasia such that at its most severe hypochondroplasia is not distinguishable from achondroplasia at its least severe.[48]

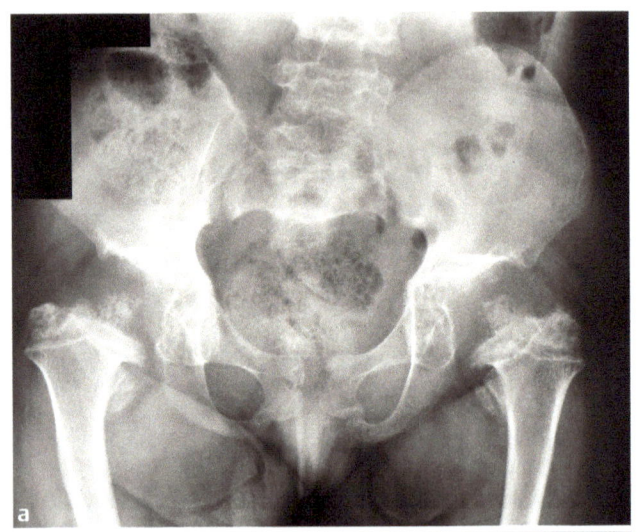

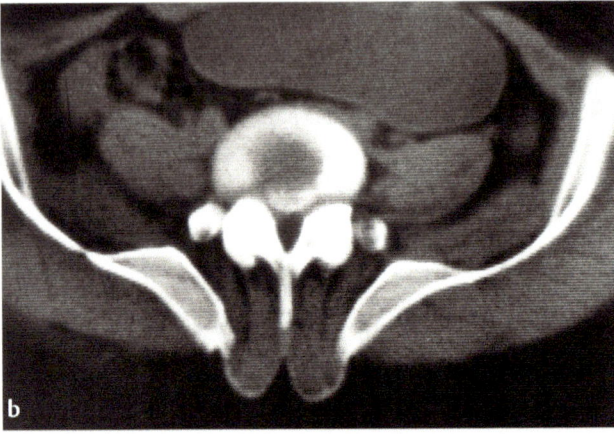

Fig. 10.15 (a) AP radiograph of the pelvis in an achondroplast showing poorly developed femoral capital epiphyses and medial femoral neck beaking. (b) Axial CT of the lower lumbar spine of an achondroplast showing grossly underdeveloped pedicles with concomitant stenosis. Observe also the massive paraspinal muscles bulging backward on each side of the spinous process.

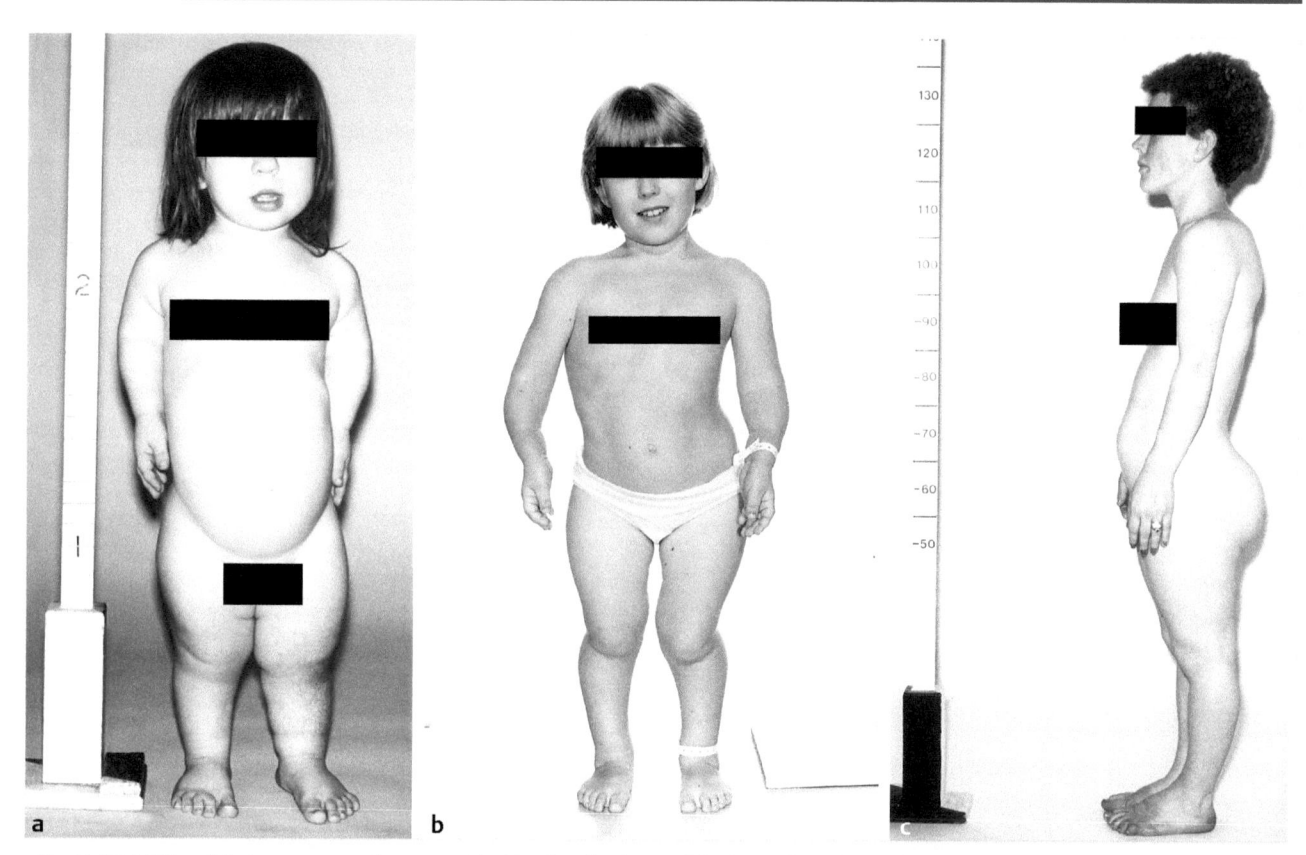

Fig. 10.16 (a) The clinical appearance of a young girl with achondroplasia. While the trunk is of normal length the limbs are short, particularly in the proximal segment. There is a prominent forehead with flat nasal bridge (measuring rule in feet: 1 foot equals 0.30 m). (b) Clinical appearance of a young girl with pseudo achondroplasia. The head and face are normal. (c) The clinical appearance of hypochondroplasia, similar to achondroplasia but less severe skull and pelvic changes and better height.

There are two important features with regard to the spine—spinal stenosis (▶ Fig. 10.17) and a thoracolumbar kyphosis (▶ Fig. 10.18)—both of which can give rise to neurological problems and the biggest risk is when stenosis and kyphosis coexist. As regards spinal deformity, Bailey reviewed the radiographs of 87 cases and found mild or moderate scoliosis in 12 cases and mild to moderate kyphoses in 7 cases.[49] A severe spinal deformity is rare in achondroplasia but the deformity of thoracolumbar kyphosis is important because of its neurological risk. Kopits reviewed 158 achondroplasts and only 1 had a scoliosis, a double structural curve of 40 degrees each, and of little consequence.[37] On a lateral radiograph of the thoracolumbar region there is concavity of the posterior vertebral borders and anterior wedging with a bullet-haped vertebra giving rise to an angular kyphosis. In 90% of cases this does not persist[51] with therefore only 10% progressing in a proper epidemiological survey of achondroplasts (▶ Fig. 10.18). On these figures it would be unwise to rush in if such a great proportion do not progress. A higher figure for the proportion with persisting kyphosis stems from Bethem's study of 30 achondroplasts, 18 of whom had a persistent thoracolumbar kyphosis, 2 of which required anterior decompression.[36] Beighton and Bathfield reported a thoracolumbar kyphosis in more than half their African patients with achondroplasia but in only 1 in 20 of their Europeans.[52] Meanwhile, Hensinger reports a severe kyphosis in more than a third of patients with achondroplasia, again a selected group.[53] Whatever the precise figure for a persistent thoracolumbar kyphosis it is probably much less than 20% and therefore it is important to bear in mind the age of the child at presentation, the likelihood of spontaneous resolution, but the need to observe for progression. While extension bracing can be prescribed its benefits are dubious. For those with a severe and persistent kyphosis with neurological signs of impending paraplegia there is only one certain method of decompressing the spinal cord and that is by anterior vertebral body resection so that the cord can be seen to be truly decompressed followed by anterior strut grafting and posterior segmental instrumentation.

A notorious aspect of achondroplasia is the characteristic stenosis of the lumbar spinal canal although the entire spine is stenotic—that is, cervical and thoracic regions also. It is in relation to this that neurological symptoms and signs in these patients have frequently been reported.[54-57] When Kahanovitz et al reviewed 47 cases of achondroplasia with a mean age of almost 30 years, they found that more than half their patients had either no symptoms or symptoms of low back pain only.[58] Only 17% had objective neurological findings in association with spinal claudication while as many had a history of claudication but no objective evidence. Only 6% had disk symptoms. He thought that thoracolumbar kyphosis and an increased lumbar lordosis below were important predisposing factors. Lutter et al looked at the anatomy of the achondroplastic lumbar canal and found a 40% reduction in transverse area at the first lumbar level and a 27% reduction at the L5 level.[59] Eisenstein indicates that it is the anteroposterior diameter that is significantly reduced in stenosis but the average limit of normal size is 15 mm and the lumbar spinal canal is already narrowest at the L2 to 4 levels.[60] Verbiest measured spinal dimensions at surgery and went even further by stating that the interpedicular distance and body size do not contribute to stenosis.[61] Of much greater importance were short pedicles and thickened laminae and articular processes (▶ Fig. 10.17). Several authorities recently put a definition to spinal stenosis and described it as "a condition involving any type of narrowing of the spinal canal, nerve root canals, or channels of intervertebral foraminae." That encountered in achondroplasia belongs to the developmental category. In Leeds a wide variety of presentation has been observed from no neurological signs to paraplegia despite the radiographic appearances.[54]

Four patterns of neurological deficit have emerged.[56] The first is a steadily progressive cauda equina syndrome associated with an increased thoracolumbar kyphosis which should be treated as already indicated. The second is a more typical spinal claudication picture and as the majority of these cases are low back pain with claudication or neurological symptoms and signs,[58] the goals of surgery in the achondroplast are the same as those with idiopathic degenerative stenosis, namely: (1) relief of pain and (2) restoration of neurological function.[62] Furthermore once severe symptoms of spinal stenosis have developed there is little likelihood that improvement would occur without surgical treatment. If the neurological problem is deemed by history, physical examination, plain radiography, and scanning to pertain to the central canal then more midline decompression is indicated. In the achondroplast the most common site for stenosis is the thoracolumbar or upper lumbar regions and for one level stenosis, only partial laminectomy is required; if only the medial half of the facet is removed or the pars interarticularis on one side then there is no question of instability arising postoperatively. Additionally, provided there is no spondylolisthesis present, it does not appear to matter how much bone is taken away for the purposes of decompression as there is only a 2% prevalence rate of subsequent instability whereas in the presence of degenerative spondylolisthesis this figure rises to 66%.[62] So if radiographs indicate preexisting

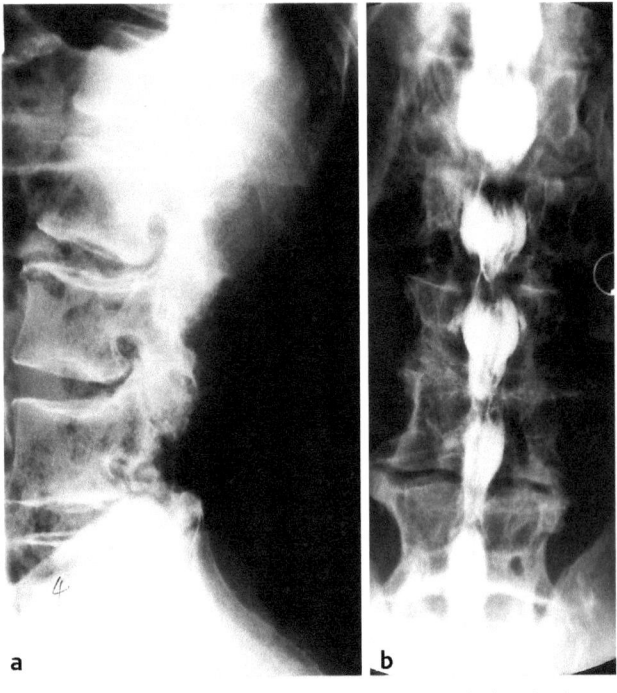

Fig. 10.17 The characteristic lumbar spinal stenosis of achondroplasia. (a) Lateral radiograph of the lower lumbar spine showing the very short pedicles and thickened laminae and articular processes. (b) AP myelogram showing gradual attenuation of the dye column from above down to the lumbosacral junction with complete blocks at the lower four levels.

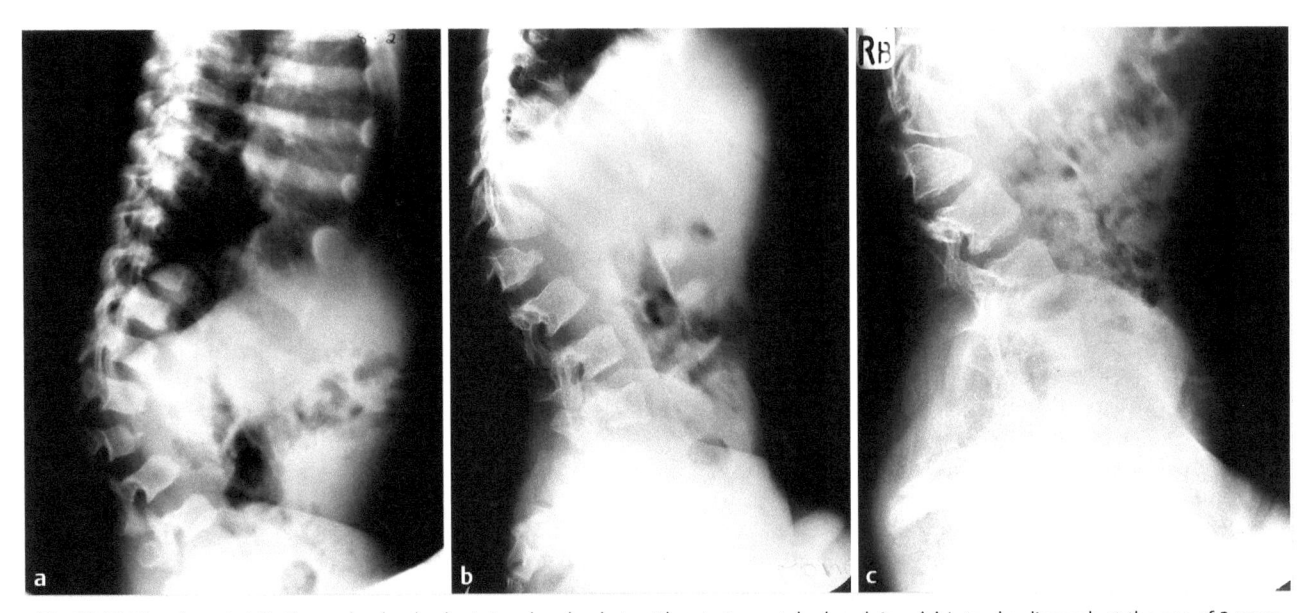

Fig. 10.18 The characteristic thoracolumbar kyphosis in achondroplasia with anterior vertebral wedging. (a) Lateral radiograph at the age of 3 years showing a pronounced kyphosis. (b) Lateral radiograph at the age of 6 years showing improvement. (c) Lateral radiograph at the age of 16 years showing a mature spine with no increase in the kyphosis during the adolescent growth spurt.

spondylolisthesis then either an anterior or preferably bilateral intertransverse fusion can be added. Kopits reported on nine cases who underwent wide decompressive posterolateral laminectomy and did not require fusion for instability.[37] The third type of presentation is that of a prolapsed intervertebral disk.[63] The condition should be treated as for any other prolapsed disk and if there is significant radicular pain with at least one objective neurological finding in the presence of a positive scan confirming diagnosis and level then microdiskectomy and removal of any sequestrated portion is the treatment of choice. If there is a more sudden presentation of a disk prolapse rather like the cauda equina syndrome in the normal spine it should also be treated as an emergency by immediate and wide decompression.

The fourth type involves the cervical spine which is not uncommonly involved in achondroplasia, although not as severely as with Morquio's syndrome. The problem results from occipitalization of C1 and together with stenosis of the foramen magnum can give rise to secondary atlantoaxial instability with neurological evidence of both root and canal stenosis. Extension of the atlantoaxial articulation reduces the subluxation and subsequent instability is halted by posterior atlantoaxial fusion which because of the atlantooccipital fusion can be continued to the occiput. This can be dealt with by posterior C1-C2 fusion with polyaxial screw and rod fixation as with Morquio's disease but should the bone be user-unfriendly or the anatomy too deformed, then on-lay graft is the technique of choice controlled by halo-cast external fixation.

In Leeds we have encountered a teenage girl with right thoracic idiopathic scoliosis with pseudoachondroplasia who successfully underwent the Leeds procedure, anterior multiple diskectomy, followed by posterior instrumentation (▶ Fig. 10.19).

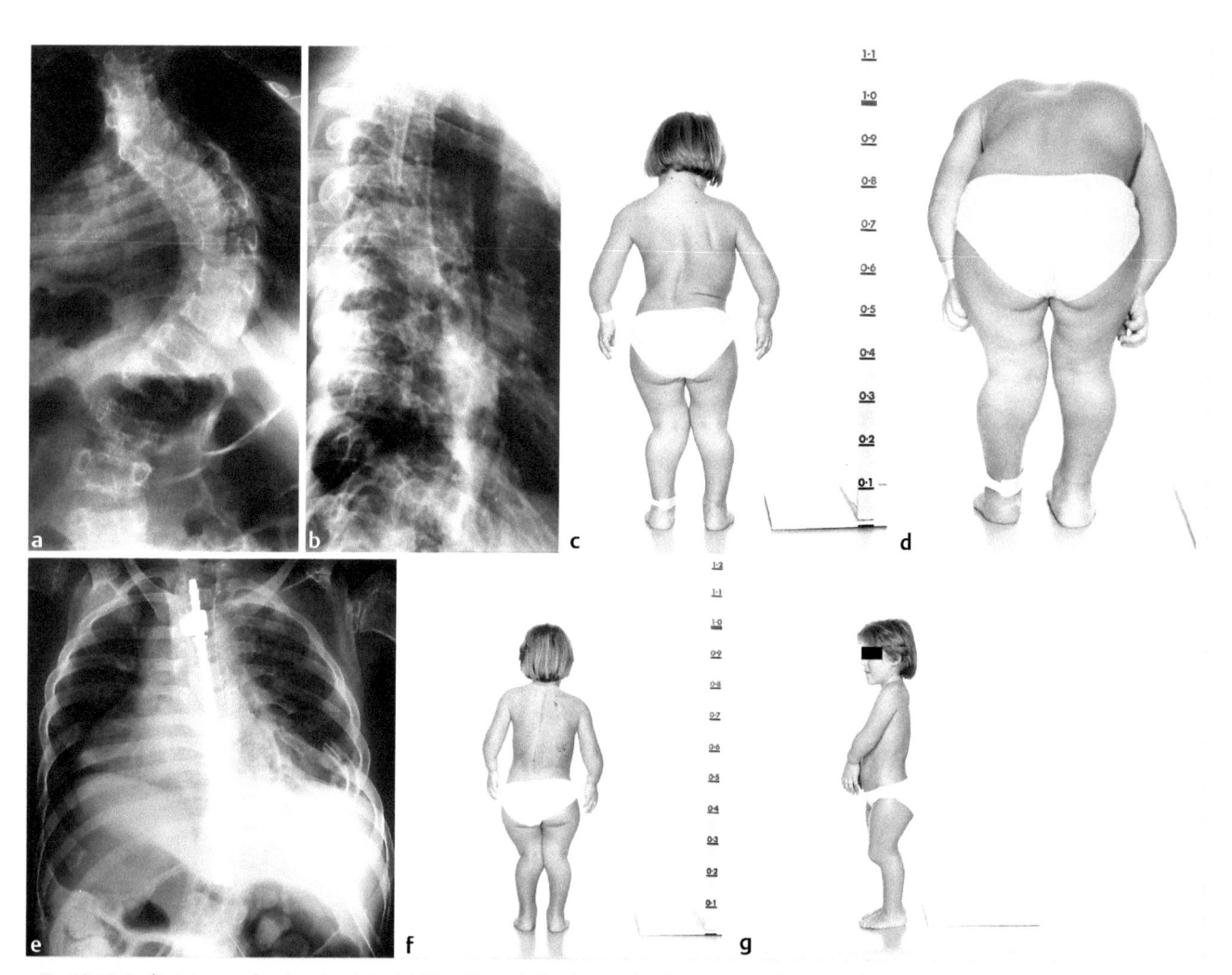

Fig. 10.19 Scoliosis in pseudoachondroplasia. (a) PA radiograph showing a right thoracic idiopathic curve. This curve had developed and progressed to this extent over the short course of a year. (b) Lateral radiograph of the thoracic radiograph showing that this, like all other scolioses with rotation, is lordotic. (c) Back view of this 13-year-old girl showing her right thoracic curve. (d) Forward-bending view showing the lordosis and the prominent right rib hump. (e) PA radiograph of the spine after two-stage procedure, Leeds procedure. In the first stage via thoracotomy the apical five disks were resected and then in the second stage the posterior fusion was performed along with division of the convex ribs to improve the rib hump appearance. In view of thoracic canal stenosis, it was not deemed advisable to add concave sublaminar wiring. (f,g) Back and side views of this girl showing the considerable improvement in her deformity, in particular the rib hump with the Leeds procedure.

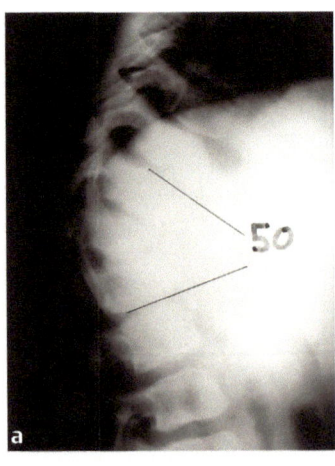

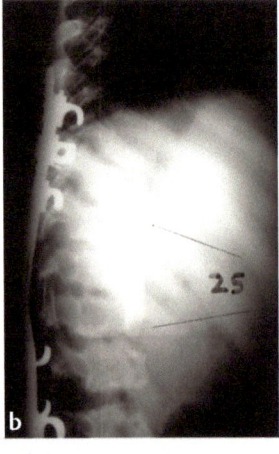

Fig. 10.20 (a) Lateral radiograph of a 12-year-old boy with the recessive form of spondyloepiphyseal dysplasia tarda showing a thoracolumbar kyphosis with anterior wedging of the apical vertebral body. Increasing signs of paraparesis had developed. (b) Lateral radiograph 1 year after AVR and anterior strut grafting and posterior instrumentation. There has been a good correction of the deformity and the neurological signs resolved rapidly.

10.2.2 Spondyloepiphyseal Dysplasia Tarda

This more benign late-onset variety of spondyloepiphyseal dysplasia was first clearly described by Maroteaux et al in 1957.[64] There is mild dysplasia of vertebrae and large joints and it is often confused with Morquio's syndrome.[65] The trunk is short and the overall stature reaches about 1.4 m. Sternal protrusion occurs along with the short trunk. The changes are typical.[66] The vertebrae are flat but are humped posteriorly which differentiates their appearance from those in multiple epiphyseal dysplasia and Morquio's syndrome. Even with deficient anterior ossification of the vertebral bodies significant kyphosis is allegedly not common. Hensinger[53] and Bethem et al[36] have encountered a Scheuermann's like appearance that has been treated successfully by extension bracing, rather like Scheuermann's disease proper. We have encountered two cases of the recessive tarda variety, both of whom had significant and progressive kyphoses. Both responded well to anterior strut grafting and posterior instrumentation (▶ Fig. 10.20).

References

Note: References in **bold** are Key References.

[1] Gray PHK. A case of osteogenesis imperfecta, associated with dentinogenesis imperfecta, dating from antiquity. Clin Radiol. 1970; 21(1):106–108
[2] Ekmann OJ. Descriptio et casus Aliquot Osteomalaciae. Upsaliae: J F Edman, 1788. Cited by McKusick VA. Heritable Disorders of Connective Tissue. 4th ed. St Louis: CV Mosby; 1972
[3] Looser E. On the difference between osteogenesis imperfecta congenital and tarda (so-called idiopathic osteopsathyrosis). Mittell Grenzgebeiten Med Chir. 1906; 15:161–207
[4] **King JD, Bobechko WP. Osteogenesis imperfecta. An orthopaedic description and surgical review. J Bone Joint Surg. 1971; 53B:72–89**
[5] Falvo KA, Root L, Bullough PG. Osteogenesis imperfecta: clinical evaluation and management. J Bone Joint Surg Am. 1974; 56(4):783–793
[6] **Bauze RJ, Smith R, Francis MJO. A new look at osteogenesis imperfecta. A clinical, radiological and biochemical study of forty-two patients. J Bone Joint Surg Br. 1975; 57(1):2–12**
[7] Cole WG. Bone, cartilage, and fibrous tissue disorders. In: Benson M, Fixsen J, Macnicol M, Parsch K, eds. Children's Orthopaedics and Fractures. 3rd ed. London: Springer; 2010:75–105
[8] Sillence DO, Senn A, Danks DM. Genetic heterogeneity in osteogenesis imperfecta. J Med Genet. 1979; 16(2):101–116
[9] Jones ET, Hensinger RN. Spinal deformity in idiopathic juvenile osteoporosis. Spine. 1981; 6(1):1–4
[10] Dent CE, Friedman M. Idiopathic juvenile osteoporosis. Q J Med. 1965; 34:177–210
[11] Hoek KJ. Scoliosis in osteogenesis imperfecta (sažetak). Proceedings of the Western Orthopaedic Association. J Bone Joint Surg (AM). 1975; 57:136
[12] **Benson DR, Donaldson DH, Millar EA. The spine in osteogenesis imperfecta. J Bone Joint Surg Am. 1978; 60(7):925–929**
[13] Anissipour AK, Hammerberg KW, Caudill A, et al. Behavior of scoliosis during growth in children with osteogenesis imperfecta. J Bone Joint Surg Am. 2014; 96(3):237–243
[14] Patel RM, Nagamani C, Cuthbertson D, et al. A cross-sectional multi-centre study of osteogenesis imperfecta in North America – results from the linked clinical research centres. Clin Genet. 2014. DOI: 10.1111/cge.12409Epubahe adofprint
[15] Yong-Hing K, MacEwan GD. Scoliosis associated with osteogenesis imperfecta. Results of treatment. J Bone Joint Surg Br. 1982; 64:36–43
[16] Waugh TR. The biomechanical basis for the utilisation of methylmethacrylate in the treatment of scoliosis. J Bone Joint Surg. 1971; 53A:194–195
[17] Herron LD, Dawson EG. Methylmethacrylate as an adjunct in spinal instrumentation. J Bone Joint Surg Am. 1977; 59(7):866–868
[18] Yilmaz G, Hwang S, Oto M, et al. Surgical treatment of scoliosis in osteogenesis imperfecta with cement-augmented pedicle screw instrumentation. J Spinal Disord Tech. 2014; 27(3):174–180
[19] Marfan AB. Un cas de déformation congénitale des quatre membres, plus prononcee aux extrémités, caractérisée par l'allongement des o saves un certain degré d'amincissement. Bull Mem Soc Med Hop Paris. 1896; 13:220–226
[20] Beals RK, Hecht F. Congenital contractural arachnodactyly. A heritable disorder of connective tissue. J Bone Joint Surg Am. 1971; 53(5):987–993
[21] Achard MC. Arachnodactylie. Bull Mem Soc Med Hop Paris. 1902; 19:834–840
[22] Field CMB, Carson NAJ, Cusworth DC, Dent CE, Neill DW. Homocystinuria, a New Disorder of Metabolism. Abstracts of the 10th International Congress of Pediatrics. Lisbon; 1962: 274
[23] Sinclair RJG, Kitchin AH, Turner RWD. The Marfan Syndrome. Q J Med. 1960; 29:19–46
[24] Wilner HI, Finby N. Skeletal manifestations in the Marfan syndrome. JAMA. 1964; 187:490–495
[25] Winter RB, Moe JH. Scoliosis and the Marfan syndrome. J Bone Joint Surg. 1969; 51A:204–205
[26] **Robins PR, Moe JH, Winter RB. Scoliosis in Marfan's syndrome. Its characteristics and results of treatment in thirty-five patients. J Bone Joint Surg Am. 1975; 57(3):358–368**
[27] Orcutt FV, DeWald RL. The special problems which the Marfan syndrome introduces to scoliosis. J Bone Joint Surg Am. 1974; 56A:1763
[28] Robins PR, Moe JH, Winter RB. Scoliosis in Marfan's syndrome. Its characteristics and results of treatment in thirty-five patients. J Bone Joint Surg Am. 1975; 57(3):358–368
[29] Li ZC, Liu ZD, Dai LY. Surgical treatment of scoliosis associated with Marfan syndrome by using posterior-only instrumentation. J Pediatr Orthop B. 2011; 20(2):63–66
[30] Gjolaj JP, Sponseller PD, Shah SA, et al. Spinal deformity correction in Marfan syndrome versus adolescent idiopathic scoliosis: learning from the differences. Spine. 2012; 37(18):1558–1565
[31] Zenner J, Hitzl W, Meier O, Auffarth A, Koller H. Surgical outcomes of scoliosis surgery in Marfan syndrome. J Spinal Disord Tech. 2014; 27(1):48–58
[32] Stern WE. Dural ectasia and the Marfan syndrome. J Neurosurg. 1988; 69 (2):221–227
[33] Morquio L. Sur une forme de dystrophie osseuse familiale. Arch Méd Enfants. 1929; 32:129–140
[34] Brailsford JF. Chondro-osteo-dystrophy: roentgenographic and clinical features of a child with dislocation of vertebrae. Am J Surg. 1929; 7:404–410
[35] Melzak J. Spinal deformities with paraplegia in two sisters with Morquio-Brailsford syndrome. Paraplegia. 1969; 6(4):246–258

[36] Bethem D, Winter RB, Lutter L, et al. Spinal disorders of dwarfism. Review of the literature and report of eighty cases. J Bone Joint Surg Am. 1981; 63(9):1412–1425

[37] Kopits SE. Orthopedic complications of dwarfism. Clin Orthop Relat Res. 1976(114):153–179

[38] Kopits SE, Perovic MN, McKusick V, Robinson RA. Congenital atlanto-axial dislocations in various forms of dwarfism. J Bone Joint Surg [Am]. 1972; 54-A:1349–1350

[39] Solanki GA, Lo WB, Hendriksz CJ. MRI morphometric characterisation of the paediatric cervical spine and spinal cord in children with MPS 1VA (Morquio-Brailsford syndrome). J Inherit Metab Dis. 2013; 36:329–337

[40] Brooks AL, Jenkins EB. Atlanto-axial arthrodesis by the wedge compression method. J Bone Joint Surg Am. 1978; 60(3):279–284

[41] Gallie WE. Fractures and dislocations of the cervical spine. Am J Surg. 1939; 46:494–499

[42] Magerl F, Seeman P. Stable posterior fusion of the atlas and axis by transarticular screw fixation. In: Kehr P, Weidner A, eds. Cervical Spine. New York: Springer Verlag; 1987:322

[43] **Harms J, Melcher RP. Posterior C1-C2 fusion with polyaxial screw and rod fixation. Spine. 2001; 26(22):2467–2471**

[44] Stevenson AC. Achondroplasia: an account of the condition in Northern Ireland. Am J Hum Genet. 1957; 9(1):81–91

[45] Parrot JMJ. Sur les malformations achondroplasiques et le Dieu. Path Bull Soc Anthrop. 1878; 1:296

[46] Caffey J. Achondroplasia of pelvis and lumbosacral spine; some roentgenographic features. Am J Roentgenol Radium Ther Nucl Med. 1958; 80(3):449–457

[47] Langer LO, Jr, Baumann PA, Gorlin RJ. Achondroplasia: clinical radiologic features with comment on genetic implications. Clin Pediatr (Phila). 1968; 7(8):474–485

[48] Wynne-Davies R, Walsh WK, Gormley J. Achondroplasia and hypochondroplasia. Clinical variation and spinal stenosis. J Bone Joint Surg Br. 1981; 63B(4):508–515

[49] Bailey JA, II. Orthopaedic aspects of achondroplasia. J Bone Joint Surg Am. 1970; 52(7):1285–1301

[50] Pedrini-Mille A, Pedrini V. Proteoglycans and glycosaminoglycans of human achondroplastic cartilage. J Bone Joint Surg Am. 1982; 64(1):39–46

[51] Wynne-Davies R, Hall CM, Apley AG. Atlas of Skeletal Dysplasias. 3rd ed. Edinburgh: Churchill Livingstone; 1985

[52] Beighton P, Bathfield CA. Gibbal achondroplasia. J Bone Joint Surg Br. 1981; 63-B(3):328–329

[53] **Hensinger RN. Kyphosis secondary to skeletal dysplasias and metabolic disease. Clin Orthop Relat Res. 1977(128):113–128**

[54] Nelson MA. Spinal stenosis in achondroplasia. Proc R Soc Med. 1972; 65(11):1028–1029

[55] Hancock DO, Philips DG. Spinal compression in achondroplasia. Paraplegia. 1965; 3(1):23–33

[56] Bergström K, Laurent U, Lundberg PO. Neurological symptoms in achondroplasia. Acta Neurol Scand. 1971; 47(1):59–70

[57] Lutter LD, Langer LO. Neurological symptoms in achondroplastic dwarfs—surgical treatment. J Bone Joint Surg Am. 1977; 59(1):87–92

[58] **Kahanovitz N, Rimoin DL, Sillence DO. The clinical spectrum of lumbar spine disease in achondroplasia. Spine. 1982; 7(2):137–140**

[59] Lutter LD, Longstein JE, Winter RB, Langer LO. Anatomy of the achondroplastic lumbar canal. Clin Orthop Relat Res. 1977(126):139–142

[60] Eisenstein S. The morphometry and pathological anatomy of the lumbar spine in South African negroes and Caucasoids with specific reference to spinal stenosis. J Bone Joint Surg. 1977; 59(2):173–180

[61] Verbiest H. Fallacies of the present definition, nomenclature and classification of the stenoses of the lumbar vertebral canal. Spine. 1976; 1:217–225

[62] Grabias S. Current concepts review. The treatment of spinal stenosis. J Bone Joint Surg. 1980; 62(2):308–313

[63] Schreiber F, Rosenthal H. Paraplegia from ruptured lumbar discs in achondroplastic dwarfs. J Neurosurg. 1952; 9(6):648–651

[64] Maroteaux P, Lamy M, Bernard J. La dysplasie spondylo-epiphysaire tardive; description clinique et radiologique. Presse Med. 1957; 65(51):1205–1208

[65] Diamond LS. A family study of spondyloepiphyseal dysplasia. J Bone Joint Surg Am. 1970; 52(8):1587–1594

[66] **Langer LO. Spondyloepiphyseal dysplasia tarda. Radiology. 1964; 82:833–839**

Chapter 11

Spondylolysis and Spondylolisthesis

11.1	Introduction	288
11.2	Etiology and Radiology	288
11.3	The Terminology and Measurement of Spondylolisthesis	293
11.4	The Marchetti and Bartolozzi (M-B) Classification	294
11.5	Mac-Thiong and Labelle's Classification	299
11.6	Clinical Features and Treatment	300
11.7	Practice Points	304
11.8	Intertransverse Fusion	304

11 Spondylolysis and Spondylolisthesis

11.1 Introduction

Spondylolisthesis was first described in 1782 by the Belgium obstetrician Herbiniaux, who reported severe obstetric difficulties due to an anteriorly displaced fifth lumbar vertebra.[1] Kilian considered the condition as a slow subluxation of the lumbosacral facet joints and accordingly coined the word spondylolisthesis.[2] In one of the early mechanical studies performed by Robert in 1855, he found that spondylolisthesis could not be produced unless there was a breach in the neural arch.[3] Lambl then recognized the cardinal importance of a neural arch defect (spondylolysis).[4] In 1882, Neugebauer[5] provided a clear description of how spondylolisthesis could occur due to L5/S1 facet joint aplasia with elongation of the pars interarticularis without a specific defect. This work, a century after Herbiniaux, was based upon many cases of obstetric problems that had occurred in Freiburg, Strasburg, Berlin, and Paris. Neugebauer's thoughts were that the etiology would be either congenital or acquired, with the former being failure of the normal development of the L5 articular processes with attenuation of the pars interarticularis and progressive rounding of the upper border of the sacrum—the classic features of dysplastic spondylolisthesis. He felt that the acquired form was due to a fracture of the posterolateral elements of L5. In 1931 Meyer-Burgdorff reported that there was always a fatigue fracture of the isthmus and this was due to lumbar spine hyperlordosis.[6]

The congenital theory had its proponents in Putti,[7] Le Double[8] and Willis[9] while Brailsford[9] and Brocher[10] proposed a dysplastic theory due to disturbance of the ossification of the vertebral arch during childhood very similar to developmental hip dysplasia. In 1963 Newman and Stone published their classification following a 15-year study of more than 300 cases and reported these five types: dysplastic, isthmic, degenerative, traumatic, and pathological.[11] Taillard gathered all these categories together into a final common pathway of rupture of the articular bolt safety mechanism.[13] Then in 1975 the International Society for the Study of the Lumbar Spine (ISSLS) put forward a classification based upon that of Newman and Stone, referred to as the Wiltse classification, which is still in use today[14] (▶ Table 11.1).

There have been other proposed classifications[15] but one of the most popular is that of Marchetti and Bartolozzi (M-B) in 1997.[16] However, like many classifications, such as idiopathic scoliosis (see Chapter 4), there are problems and, indeed, flaws.

Before considering the M-B classification it is necessary to go back to the Wiltse classification drawn up by access only to plain films and oblique views whereas nowadays we have both three-dimensional (3D) computed tomography (CT) and 3D magnetic resonance imaging (MRI) available, which we have used extensively, making the geometry of spondylolisthesis more readily visualized.

11.2 Etiology and Radiology

11.2.1 Dysplastic

This was the type reported by Herbiniaux[1] and Neugebauer[5] that so troubled obstetricians because only with this category does the L5 vertebra slip forward so far that it reduces the sagittal diameter of the pelvis to block the passage of the fetus.

This used to be referred to as congenital spondylolisthesis and although the basic pathology is congenital the deformity of spondylolisthesis may never occur or at least develops during subsequent growth. Hence the word dysplastic is deemed more appropriate and refers to congenital anomalies of the lumbosacral joint and, in particular, the L5/S1 facet joints (▶ Fig. 11.1). There is also an obligatory spina bifida occulta of L5 or S1.

There is then secondary deformation of the L5 vertebra being much more lordotic and the top of the sacrum becoming progressively more rounded. Finally, slippage can be so severe that the L5 vertebral body lies in front of the upper sacrum (spondyloptosis). Meanwhile the anteroposterior (AP) view shows a wide open sacrum and superimposition of the L5 vertebral body over the sacrum with the appearance of the upside-down Napoleon's hat (▶ Fig. 11.2). When slippage begins the whole of the L5 vertebra is intact but progressive slippage does not occur unless the pars elongates and eventually develops a secondary

Table 11.1 The 1976 classification

- Dysplastic
- Isthmic
   - Lytic-fatigue fracture of the pars
   - Elongated but intact pars
   - Acute pars fracture
- Degenerative
- Traumatic
- Pathological

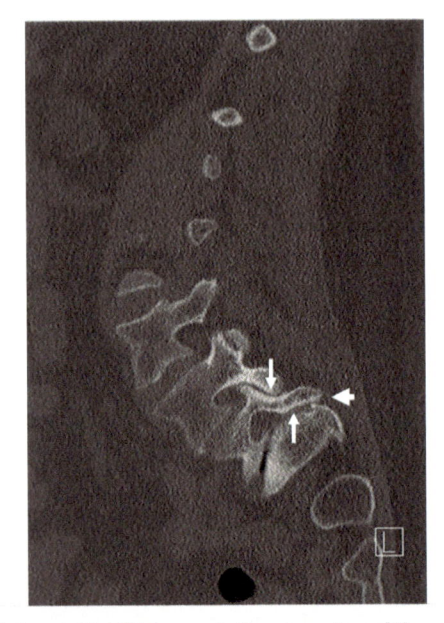

Fig. 11.1 Parasagittal CT demonstrating elongation of the pars (*arrows*) and hypoplasia of the facet joint (*large arrow*).

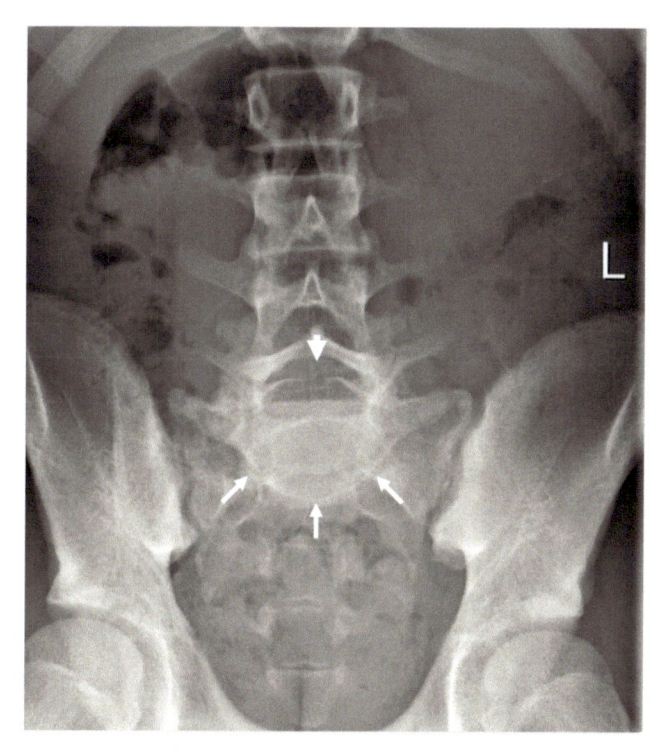

Fig. 11.2 AP radiograph of the lumbosacral region in a case of spondyloptosis giving the appearance of the upside-down Napoleon's hat (*arrows*). Note also the spina bifida occulta (*large arrow*).

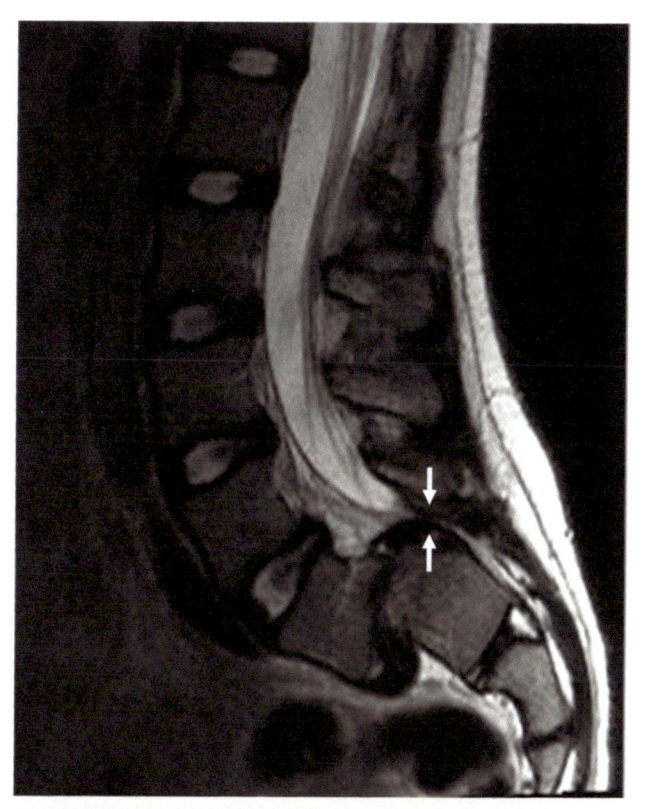

Fig. 11.3 Sagittal T2-weighted MRI of the lumbosacral region in a severe spondylolisthesis showing the upper back corner of the sacrum indenting the lower lumbar and sacral nerve roots (*arrows*).

spondylolysis. The top back corner of the body of the sacrum can appear to significantly indent into the local nerve roots (▶ Fig. 11.3) although clinical cauda equina problems are rare.

Originally it was thought that the secondary lysis in association with dysplastic spondylolisthesis might be difficult to distinguish radiographically from a straightforward lytic (stress fracture) spondylolisthesis but this is not so as the elongated attenuated dysplastic pars is readily recognizable (▶ Fig. 11.1) along with the other typical features (the lordotic L5 body, the rounding of the sacrum, and the spina bifida occulta). Dysplastic spondylolisthesis is also much less common. The more downward the L5 vertebral body on the sacrum the more it allows the body weight above to exert a more shearing effect, favoring progressive kyphosis.[17,18] Recently attention has been focused on what happens below the spine in the pelvis.

11.2.2 Isthmic

This was subdivided into the three categories[14] lytic, elongated but intact pars, and acute fracture.

This is by far the most prevalent variety (▶ Fig. 11.4) and cases have been, rarely, described in infants younger than a year of age.[3] By the time children get to the age of 7, the prevalence rate rises appreciably in the general population. However, certain sports during adolescence are considered to be an important contributing factor,[19] such as ballet dancing, gymnastics, trampolining, and fast bowling/pitching.

Jackson et al felt that the prevalence of pars defects was only about 2 to 3% in the general population but in gymnasts that rate was four times higher.[19] They reported on 14-year-old female volunteers and with X-rays that included oblique projections they showed that 11% had pars defects and 6% had a grade 1 spondylolisthesis (▶ Fig. 11.5). Lytic spondylolisthesis can occur at multiple levels but nearly always at the L5/S1 level. Interestingly, in Jackson's series, 38% had a spina bifida occulta at the bottom of the spine. Jackson emphasized that these girls were doing very hard gymnastic training with repetitive flexion-extension cycles of the lumbar spine. Just under 10% had positive isotope bone scans but no lysis on plain films suggesting a stress reaction. They also observed that many athletes were noted to have defects that healed as did Taillard.[12]

From around the world came reports on spondylolyses, in Japan in young athletes,[21] and in U.S. college football linemen.[22] The higher prevalence may be because now the search for lyses in young promising athletes includes the use of modern imaging techniques including MRI (▶ Fig. 11.6) and 3D CT and 3D MRI. In the UK it seems that every professional soccer player with a back problem, or indeed professional cricketer, comes to the clinical consultation along with their medical file that always includes an obligatory MRI scan. It would appear that some young athletes are denied a promising future purely on the basis of an MRI scan showing a lysis on one or both sides. Indeed, lyses and other defects are so common that the radiological reporting of them on plain films has already been cautioned against,[23] although seemingly not heeded.

Jackson et al[19] and Wynne Davies[24] also confirmed the very familial nature of spondylolysis in the general population. Interestingly it has been reported that the prevalence rate of neural arch defects in Alaskan natives is of the order of 50%.[25] With modern imaging techniques maybe all Alaskans have a spondylolysis! A study of 485 skeletons from South Africa demonstrated a 3.5% prevalence rate for spondylolysis but with no difference between races and genders.[26] A study of 400 schoolchildren demonstrated that in those with spondylolyses almost a third of parents had the same lesion.[27] One important etiological factor in the development of a spondylolysis is the orientation of the lumbar posterior facet joints with defects being much higher in those with coronally orientated facet joints (▶ Fig. 11.7).[28] Perhaps that is what is passed on in families and then the development of lyses modulated by physical activity.

Various authorities have felt that either repetitive extension or flexion or both are the main cause of these fatigue fractures.[29-33] Farfan believed that the pars defect was due originally to a single and not exceptional overload with repeated microfractures producing the lysis.[29] Others supported Farfan's mechanical theory.[30-32] Pfeil showed that it was the upright posture that was the cause of the lysis in age studies.[33]

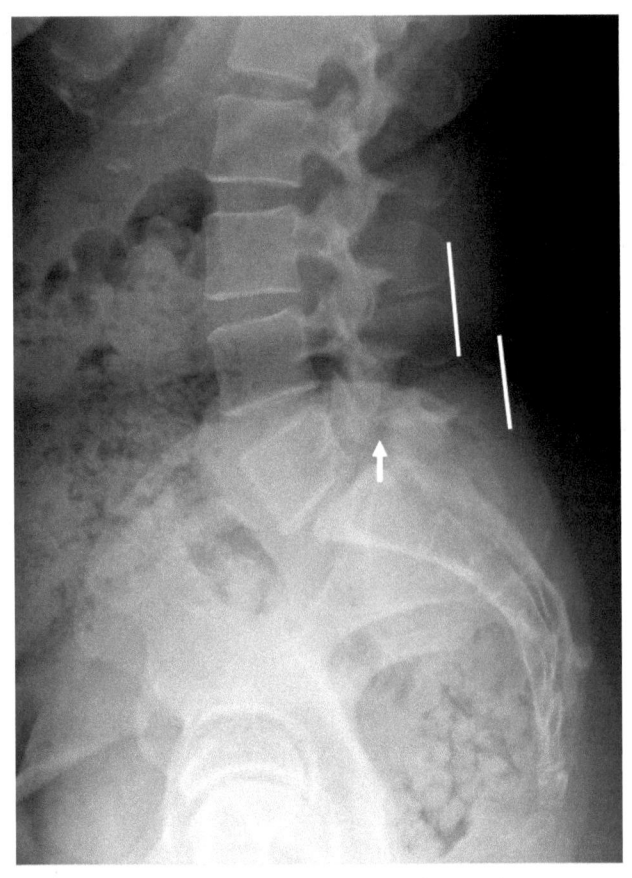

Fig. 11.4 Lateral radiograph of the lumbosacral region showing a grade 1 lytic spondylolisthesis. Note the defect of the pars (*arrow*). The L5 spinous process is no longer connected to the L5 vertebral body and is out of alignment with the L4 spinous process (*lines*).

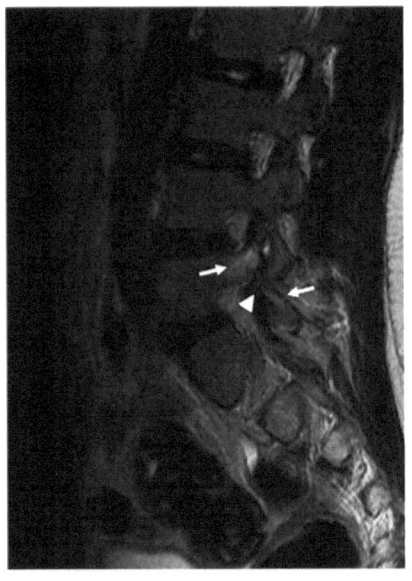

Fig. 11.6 Sagittal T2-weighted fat-saturated MRI. Unilateral spondylolysis. There is bone edematous change (*arrows*) on either side of a pars defect (*arrowhead*).

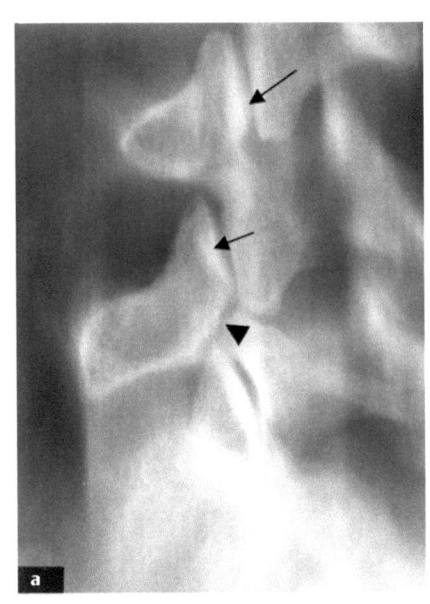

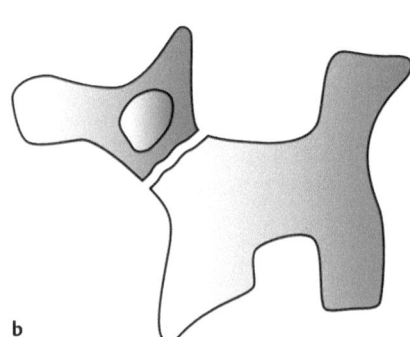

Fig. 11.5 (a) This is an oblique tomogram of the lower lumbar spine which shows the posterior facet joints (*arrows*) and the bone in between, the pars interarticularis. These oblique views are very helpful in identifying lyses (*arrowhead*). (b) The oblique lumbar spine appearance has been likened to that of a Scottie dog by La Chapelle.[20] If the Scottie dog has a collar (*arrowhead*) this is a spondylolysis. This oblique view is particularly helpful in identifying such a lesion. (Reproduced with the permission and copyright of The Medico-Legal Back: An Illustrated Guide, 2003, Cambridge Uniiversity Press. Dickson RA and Butt WP, fig 5.2.)

Severe slippage does not occur with lytic spondylolistheses seldom, if ever, beyond 50% and usually not more than 30%, principally because there is movement only in the sagittal plane in contrast to dysplastic spondylolisthesis which is effectively a progressive lumbosacral kyphosis.

Until maturity, which may, as far as the spine is concerned, be in the early 20 s,[34] the lysis is filled with a zone of endochondral ossification[12] and therefore it is quite probable that some spondylolyses heal and then develop in new cases keeping the overall prevalence pool at a relatively constant figure.[12,19] By contrast, lyses persisting in the more mature are established nonunions filled with hypertrophic callus and debris (▶ Fig. 11.8).

In the Wiltse classification[13] subtype (b) was elongation of the pars without separation but this does not occur with the so-called isthmic spondylolisthesis. Rather, elongation of the pars is part and parcel of the progressive development of slippage in the dysplastic form of spondylolisthesis (▶ Fig. 11.1). Elongation of the pars should therefore not belong to the isthmic variety but should be included as part of the radiological appearance of dysplastic spondylolisthesis.

Finally, subtype (c) of the old classification was an acute pars fracture and it has been shown quite categorically that the pars only cannot be broken by one discrete injury[31] nor do we ever see it clinically other than being part and parcel of more severe traumatic damage; it does not occur in isolation. Therefore, the acute pars fracture category (c) should belong to one of the classifications of thoracolumbar fractures and dislocations and not spondylolisthesis.

In contrast to the lysis that develops secondarily to stretching/thinning/attenuation of the dysplastic type, the lysis of isthmic spondylolisthesis is the essential component of slippage. As there is therefore only one type of isthmic spondylolisthesis, the primary lytic variety, then it could be renamed primary lytic spondylolisthesis.

11.2.3 Degenerative

The degenerative variety of spondylolisthesis is due to primary generalized osteoarthritis (OA) affecting the synovial posterior facet joints and this is particularly prevalent in females who much more commonly have the gene for OA (▶ Fig. 11.9). Indeed, when we were residents we were taught that if we had a youngish, under 60, male, with OA hip then when we looked at the AP pelvis X-rays we must also check the status of the sacroiliac joints looking for inflammatory/erosive disease, so much less common in males is the genetic expression.

This tends to occur at the L4/5 level and sometimes the level above, the L3/4 level. The L5/S1 level is seldom if ever involved. Yes, the L5/S1 level is commonly affected by degenerative disk disease but this is a completely different pathology to primary degenerative osteoarthritis of the posterior facet joints that is the cause of degenerative spondylolisthesis.

Degenerative spondylolisthesis was called pseudospondylolisthesis by Junghans,[35] but the preferred term is degenerative spondylolisthesis as proposed by Newman.[36] Rosenberg made a detailed study of this condition in 200 patients and 20 skeletons.[37] He found it to be four times more common in females and six to nine times more frequently encountered at the L4/5 level. The condition is not usually encountered under the age of 50 years and the degree of slip never exceeds 30%.

The destruction of the articular cartilage of these facet joints is thought to be the principal factor in rendering them incompetent mechanically and allowing slippage to occur although Farfan believed that the altered geometry was due to multiple small compression fractures of the inferior articular processes.[38] Harms recently studied the geometry of the degenerative spondylolisthetic level and compared 23 patients with

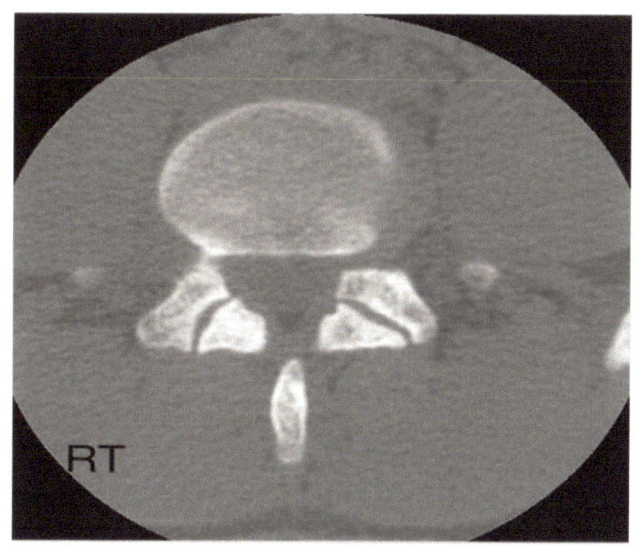

Fig. 11.7 Axial CT section through the L4/5 facet joints in a case of a left-sided L5 lysis. The left facet joint is more coronally orientated.

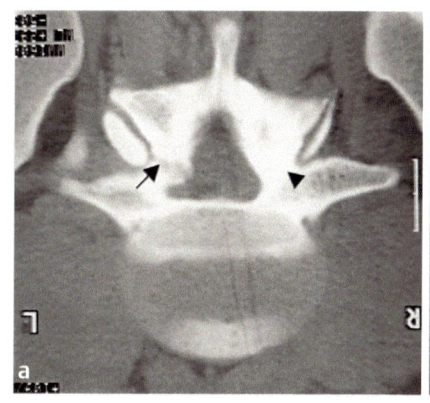

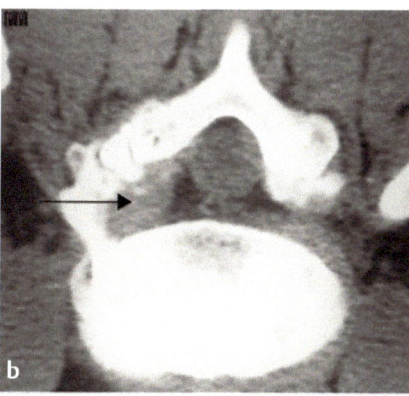

Fig. 11.8 (a,b) Axial CT scan through spondylolyses in a young adult showing the typical appearance of hypertrophic nonunions. The hypertrophy affects both sides of the lysis (arrows). **(a)** On the right side the pars is thickened due to reactive new bone formation (arrowhead).

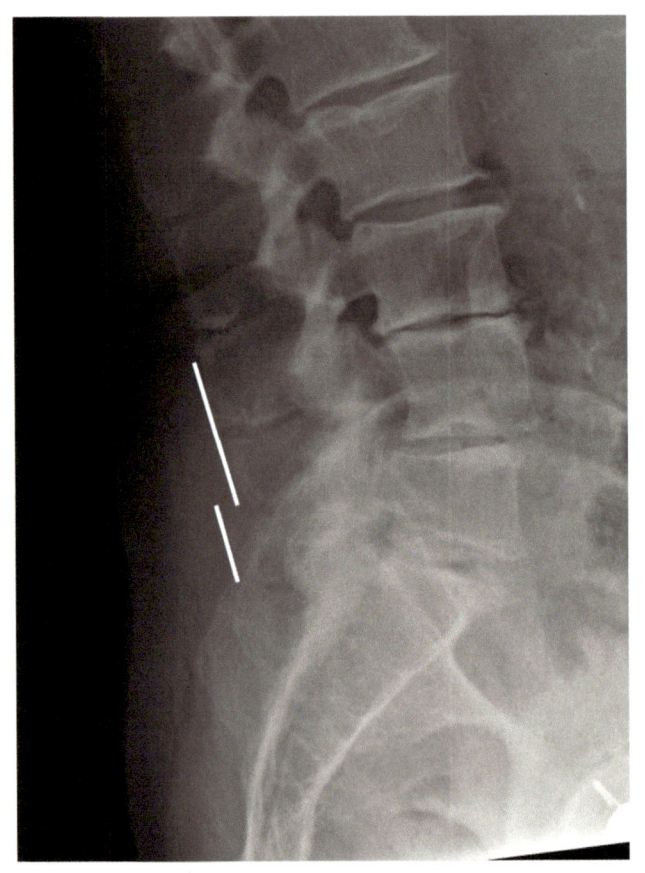

Fig. 11.9 Lateral radiograph of a 60-year-old woman with significant degenerative spinal disease. There is a degenerative spondylolisthesis at the usual L4/5 level. The L4 spinous process is connected to the L4 vertebral body and therefore moves forward out of alignment with the L5 spinous process (*lines*).

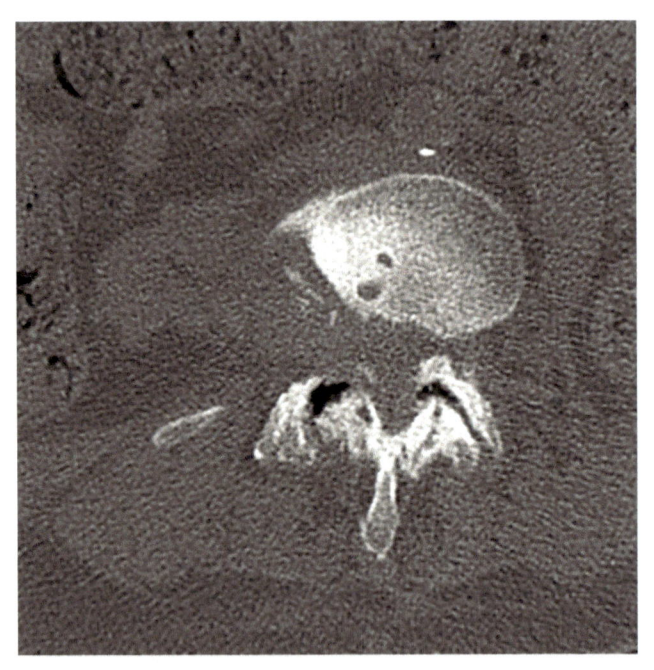

Fig. 11.10 Facet joint angulation is more sagittally orientated in degenerative spondylolisthesis.

degenerative spondylolisthesis with 40 age- and sex-matched controls.[39] Both CTs and MRIs were assessed. One of the more important findings was that the patients' facet joints were aligned in a more sagittal direction thus favoring slippage while the inclination of the vertebral end plates was more horizontal in the normal controls (▶ Fig. 11.10).

The same group looked at facet joint remodeling and came to the conclusion that the sagittal alignment of the facet joints was more likely due to secondary remodeling rather than a preexisting morphology.[40] We in Leeds have also noted a much more sagittal orientation of the facet joints in degenerative spondylolisthesis in contrast to the more coronal orientation in lytic spondylolisthesis.

Quite obviously the incompetence of the facet joints due to the degenerative process may not be equal on both sides and so the slippage is often rotational rather than strictly in the transverse plane producing a local degenerative scoliosis. Therefore the condition of degenerative spondylolisthesis should be thought of in all three dimensions often including a significant scoliotic component.

11.2.4 Traumatic

The traumatic subcategory refers to an acute injury that fractures in some part of the bony hook other than the pars and therefore really should not be part of the classification of spondylolisthesis at all; rather, it should belong to the classification of thoracolumbar spinal fractures and fracture-dislocations as with so-called acute pars fractures from the isthmic category.

11.2.5 Pathological

Finally, pathological spondylolisthesis refers to any pathological process whereby the pedicle, pars, or articular processes are weakened allowing forward thrust of the body weight above to produce slippage. These can be regarded as being generalized such as in Paget's disease (▶ Fig. 11.11), arthrogryposis, Albers-Schönberg, syphilis, and osteogenesis imperfecta[11–13] or can be localized whereby the segments adjacent to a very long fusion, as is occasionally seen with a fusion for idiopathic scoliosis years later, produce a spondylolysis and subsequent slippage (spondylolisthesis acquisita).[41] As these pathological processes increase in their own severity so images reveal the spondylolisthesis progressing pari passu with the underlying pathological process.

Therefore we propose that the Wiltse classification be reduced to four simple categories (▶ Table 11.2).

Spondylolysis and Spondylolisthesis

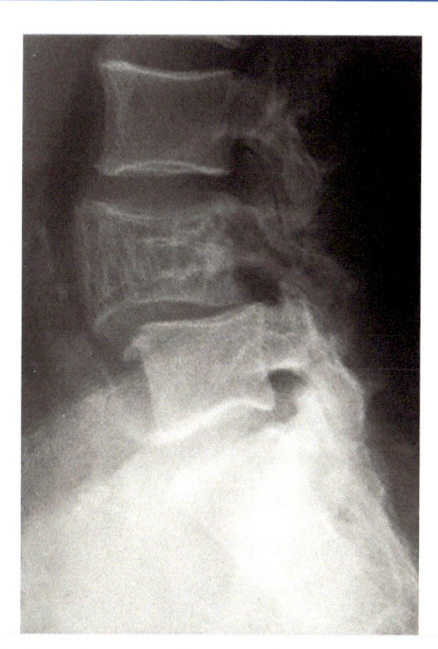

Fig. 11.11 Classically, Paget's disease produces its vertebra magna and a small amount of pathological spondylolisthesis.

Table 11.2 The Revised Wiltse/ISSLS classification

Dysplastic

- Isthmic
- Degenerative
- Pathological

11.3 The Terminology and Measurement of Spondylolisthesis

This has been usefully summarized in a review article by Wiltse and Winter.[42]

Anterior displacement has also been called anterior translation, slip, and olisthesis. The degree of this can be measured as recommended by Taillard,[43] expressing the degree of slip as a percentage of the AP diameter of the top of the first sacral vertebra (A/A' × 100) (▶ Fig. 11.12). Meyerding graded slip by simply dividing the top of S1 into quarters and noting how far L5 slips by, say, 0, 1, 2, etc.[44] (▶ Fig. 11.13).

Sacral inclination is also known as sacral tilt and refers to the angular relationship in the sagittal plane between the sacrum and the vertical plane (▶ Fig. 11.14).

The most important angular relationship in dysplastic spondylolisthesis is the angle of sagittal rotation also called sagittal roll, slip angle, or lumbosacral kyphosis. Dysplastic spondylolisthesis is of course a real lumbosacral kyphosis and is measured by the angle subtended by a line along the anterior border of L5 and a line along the posterior border of the first sacral vertebra (▶ Fig. 11.15).

As the fifth lumbar vertebra rotates round on the top of the sacrum there is rounding of the upper border of the sacrum and this can also be measured (▶ Fig. 11.16).

Then the fifth lumbar vertebra becomes progressively more lordotically shaped and wedging of the L5 vertebra can also be measured (▶ Fig. 11.17).

The angle of the lumbar lordosis can be measured by the angle subtended by the upper borders of the first and fifth lumbar vertebrae (▶ Fig. 11.18).

The sacro-horizontal angle, also called the sacral angle or Ferguson's angle, is the angular relationship between the upper border of the sacrum and a horizontal line (▶ Fig. 11.19).

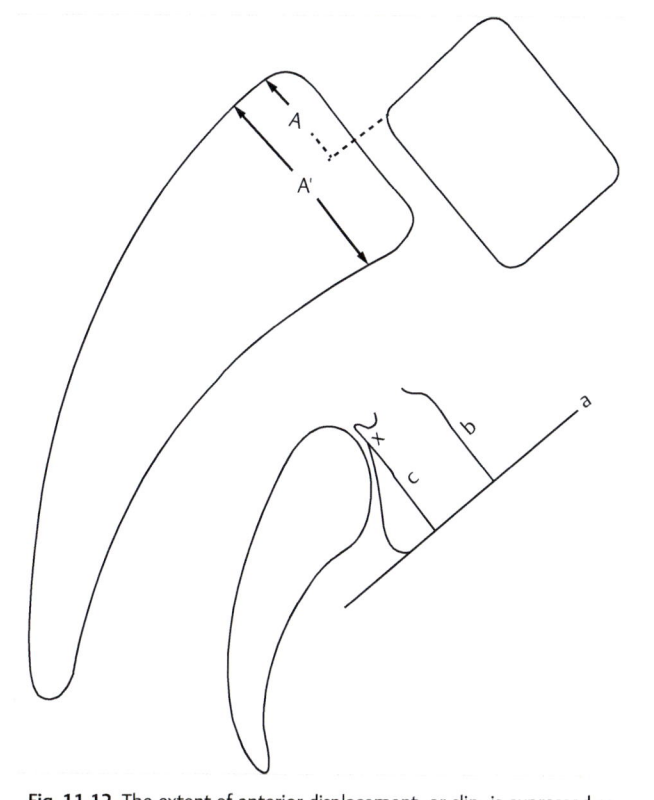

Fig. 11.12 The extent of anterior displacement, or slip, is expressed as a percentage obtained by dividing A, the amount of displacement (determined by the relationship of the posterior part of the cortex of the fifth lumbar vertebra to the posterior part of the cortex of the first sacral vertebra), by A, the maximum anteroposterior diameter of the first sacral vertebra, and multiplying by 100. The smaller drawing shows how to determine the posteroinferior tip of the body of the firth lumbar vertebra, which is often indistinct due to either hypoplasia or spur formation in this area (x on this drawing). Line a is drawn parallel to the front of the body of the fifth lumbar vertebra. Line b is drawn perpendicular to line a, to the posterosuperior tip of the body of the fifth lumbar vertebra (a point that usually is easily located). Line c is drawn parallel to line b and is exactly the same length as line b. The point at which line c intersects the inferior border of the body of the fifth lumbar vertebra is point x. Point x is the relative constant used in measuring the percentage of slip. (Reproduced with permission from L Wiltse, R Winter. Terminology and measurement of spondylolisthesis. Wolters Kluwer Health, Inc. 1983.)

The lumbosacral joint angle is the angle subtended by lines along the lower border of L5 and the upper border of S1 (▶ Fig. 11.20).

These measurements are all relevant to spondylolisthesis, anterior displacement being particularly relevant to isthmic spondylolisthesis and several of the others specifically to the dysplastic variety of which the sagittal roll angle is perhaps the most important, at least of those above the pelvis.

Spondylolysis and Spondylolisthesis

Fig. 11.13 Meyerding grading.

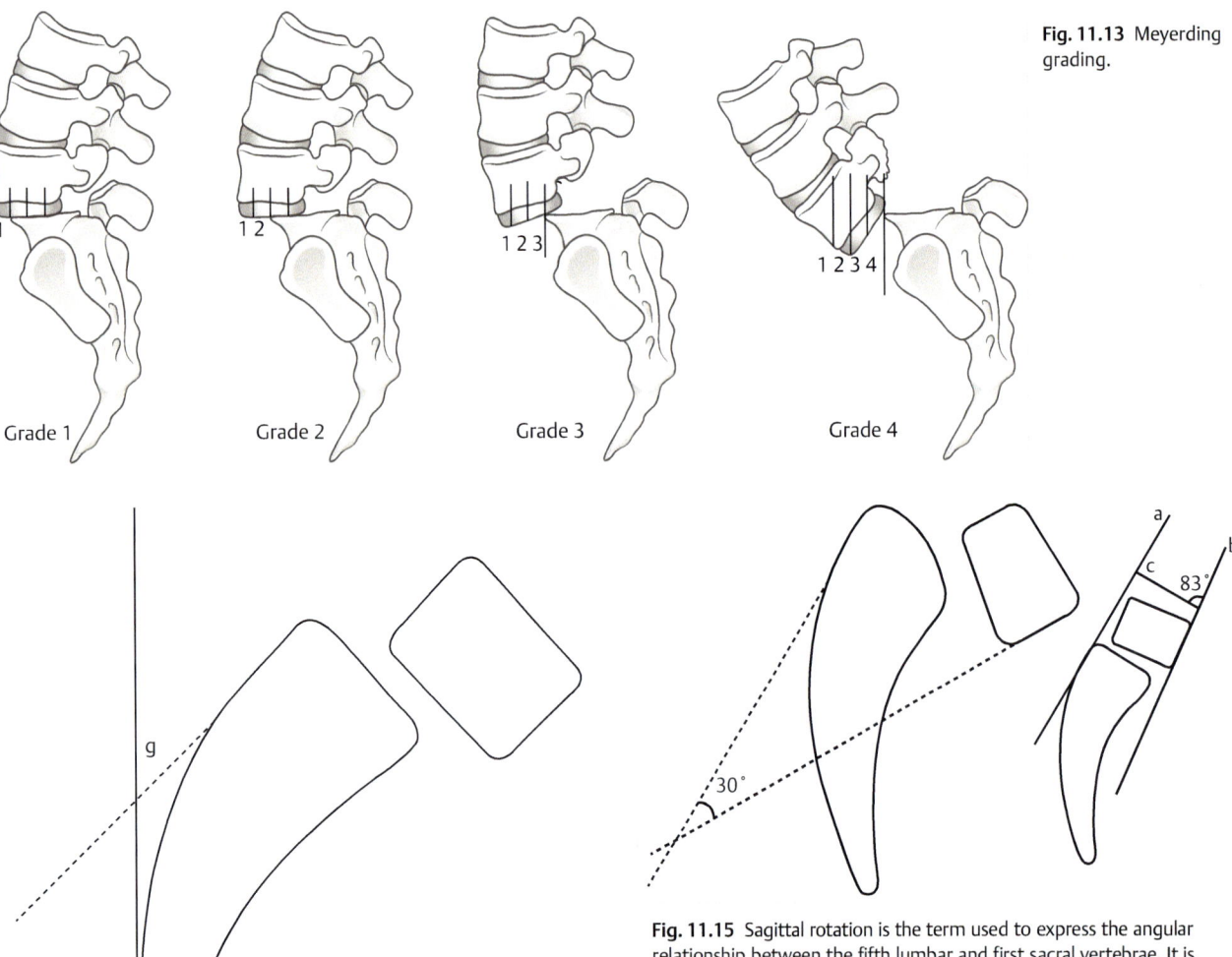

Grade 1   Grade 2   Grade 3   Grade 4

Fig. 11.14 Sacral incliniation, g, is determined by drawing a line along the posterior border of the first sacral vertebra and measuring the angle created by this line intersecting a true vertical line. (Reproduced with permission from L Wiltse, R Winter. Terminology and measurement of spondylolisthesis. Wolters Kluwer Health, Inc. 1983.)

Fig. 11.15 Sagittal rotation is the term used to express the angular relationship between the fifth lumbar and first sacral vertebrae. It is determined by extending a line along the anterior border of the body of the fifth lumbar vertebra until it intersects a line drawn along the posterior border of the body of the first sacral vertebra. The drawing on the right shows an alternative method of measuring sagittal rotation, to be used when the degree of olisthesis is small and lines a and b do not intersect. A third line, c, is added perpendicular to line a. Lines c and b intersect to form the angle of sagittal rotation. (Reproduced with permission from L Wiltse, R Winter. Terminology and measurement of spondylolisthesis. Wolters Kluwer Health, Inc. 1983.)

11.4 The Marchetti and Bartolozzi (M-B) Classification

This was originally published in 1982 in Italian but was revised in 1994 to introduce further elaboration of the developmental forms such as high and low dysplastic and in the acquired group the post-surgery, degenerative, and pathologic categories or subgroups (▶ Table 11.3).[15]

The difference between the use of the words congenital and dysplastic was then pointed out. They considered all developmental forms as essentially alike—that is, defects such as lysis, elongation, and those involving the bony hook, the L5 vertebra, and the upper border of the sacrum, along with spondyloptosis being determined by the same congenital cause—the distinguishing features of these forms being the degree to which the congenital defect has determined morphological alterations. Thus, their classification (M-B) proposed that the dysplastic and isthmic forms of spondylolisthesis in the original Wiltse classification be classified in a single developmental category, "disagreeing with the definition of isthmic spondylolisthesis by Wiltse as a separate entity," arguing that some forms must be classed as dysplastic. They were then able to argue that the category of developmental forms included the majority of cases of spondylolisthesis referred to them, somewhat surprisingly.

Meanwhile the spinal surgical world has always been quite comfortable with the dysplastic (▶ Fig. 11.1) and lytic (▶ Fig. 11.4) varieties of spondylolisthesis coming to the clinic being discrete entities, with the latter being far more prevalent than the former and the former being much more important than the latter. The problem arises when M-B tried to use the suffix "-lysis" for the stress fractures of the old isthmic form of spondylolisthesis as well as the secondary lysis that occurs with

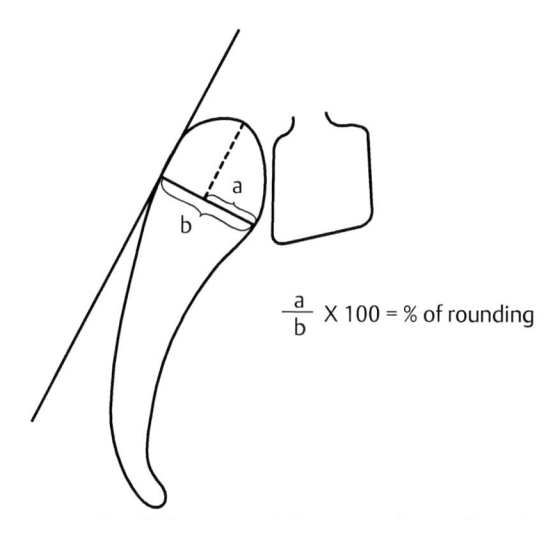

Fig. 11.16 Rounding of the top of the centrum of the first sacral vertebra is expressed as the relationship between lines a and b, drawn as shown. The result, when multiplied by 100, gives the percentage of rounding of the first sacral vertebra. (Reproduced with permission from L Wiltse, R Winter. Terminology and measurement of spondylolisthesis. Wolters Kluwer Health, Inc. 1983.)

$$\frac{a}{b} \times 100 = \% \text{ of rounding}$$

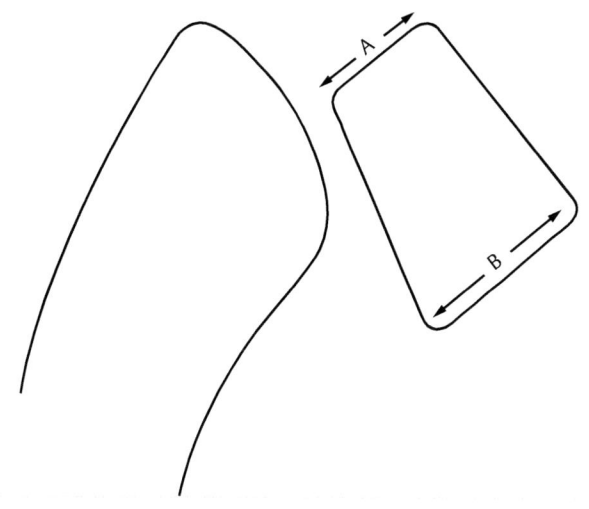

Fig. 11.17 Wedging of the olisthetic vertebra is expressed as a percentage determined by dividing line a by line b, drawn as shown, and multiplying by 100. (Reproduced with permission from L Wiltse, R Winter. Terminology and measurement of spondylolisthesis. Wolters Kluwer Health, Inc. 1983.)

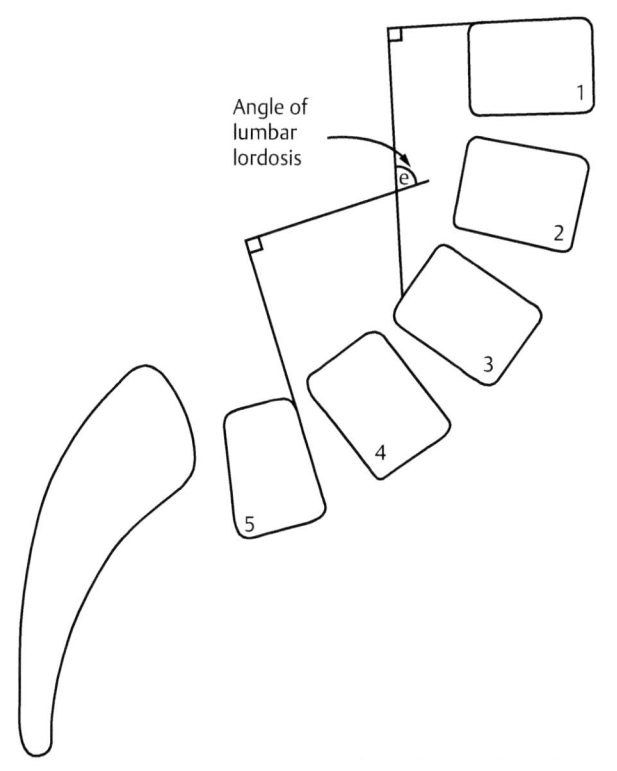

Fig. 11.18 The degree of lumbar lordosis is defined as angle c, as shown. With significant sagittal rotation of the fifth lumbar vertebra, there may be lordosis extending well up into the thoracic spine, in which case "total spinal lordosis" should be distinguished from "lumbar lordosis". (Reproduced with permission from L Wiltse, R Winter. Terminology and measurement of spondylolisthesis. Wolters Kluwer Health, Inc. 1983.)

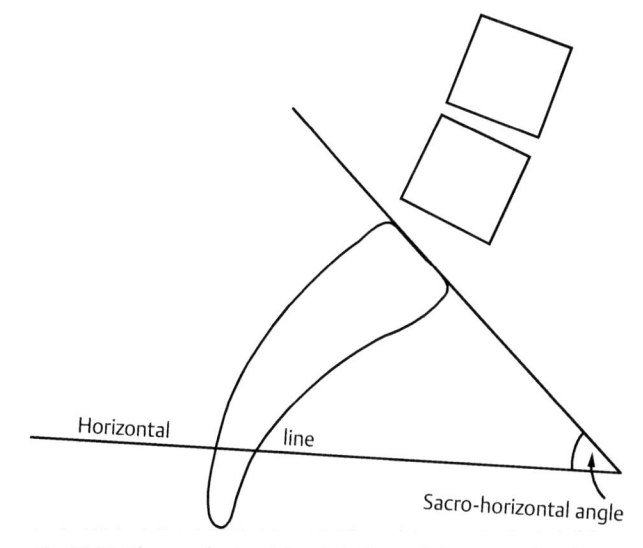

Fig. 11.19 The sacrohorizontal angle is the angle between a line drawn across the cranial border of the body of the first sacral vertebra and the horizontal. (Reproduced with permission from L Wiltse, R Winter. Terminology and measurement of spondylolisthesis. Wolters Kluwer Health, Inc. 1983.)

attenuation of the pars in the dysplastic form. The word lysis comes from the Greek word *lusis* meaning a loosening and in medical parlance a loosening, decomposition, or breaking down, clearly a precise event occurring over time and so secondary in that regard. Perhaps therefore we should reserve the phrase *secondary lysis* as pertaining to secondary disruption of the attenuated pars in dysplastic spondylolisthesis and reserve the term *primary lysis* for that which occurs with the isthmic form of our revised Wiltse/ISSLS classification (▶ Table 11.2). Then the tendency for confusion would be minimized and so presumably would be the desirability to lump all "lyses" into one category, regardless of origin. Notwithstanding, Marchetti and Bartolozzi considered that some forms of isthmic spondylolisthesis must be classed as dysplastic for reasons that are not abundantly clear from their descriptions.

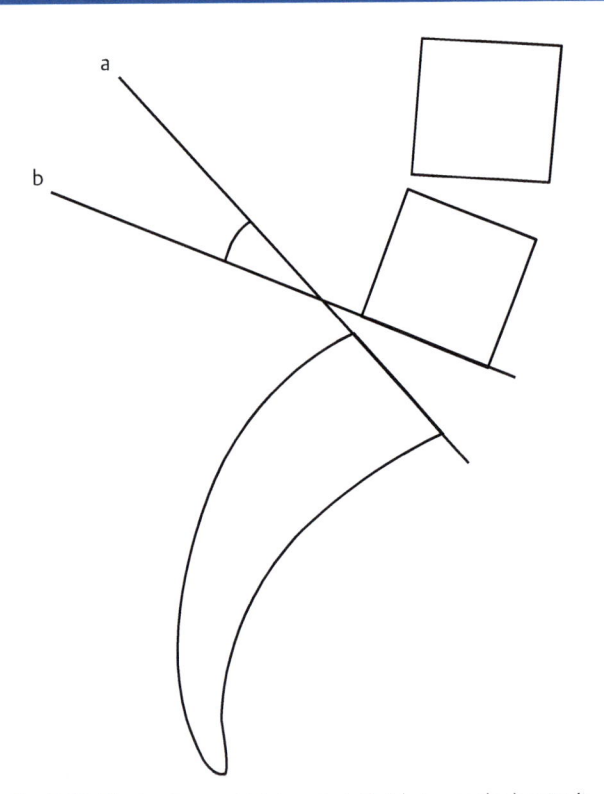

Fig. 11.20 The lumbosacral joint angle is that between the longitudinal axes of the bodies of the fifth lumbar and first sacral vertebrae. In the normal spine one can use lines across the caudal and cranial borders of the centra of these vertebrae. The angle between these two lines is the lumbosacral joint angle. (Reproduced with permission from L Wiltse, R Winter. Terminology and measurement of spondylolisthesis. Wolters Kluwer Health, Inc. 1983.)

Table 11.3 Classification of Marchetti-Bartolozzi

Developmental		
	High dysplastic	
		With lysis
		With elongation
	Low dysplastic	
		With lysis
		With elongation
Acquired		
	Traumatic	
		Acute fracture
		Stress fracture
		Post-surgery
		Direct surgery
		Indirect surgery
	Pathologic	
		Local pathology
		Systemic pathology
	Degenerative	
		Primary
		Secondary

Then in the dysplastic category they further subdivided lesions as high dysplastic or low dysplastic according to how much dysplasia is present. In the high dysplastic group they state that there are most invariably localized kyphosis and angulation of the axis of the two vertebrae and we would quite agree and would add that these are the chief criteria for differentiating dysplastic from isthmic spondylolisthesis. The high dysplastic would have further local problems such as the upper S1 body rounded. These vertebral body changes in L5 and the top of the sacrum are secondary mechanical growth alterations and not as a result of the primary dysplasia. If a secondary lysis develops in the attenuated pars of L5 then slippage can freely progress, again an attribute typical of dysplastic spondylolisthesis. Meanwhile M-B describe low dysplastic spondylolisthesis as demonstrating relatively intact rectangular forms of L5 or L4 (if the spondylolisthesis is at that level), good preservation of the upper end plate of S1 or L5, and a parallel alignment of adjacent vertebral end plates with no sacral verticalization or compensatory hyperlordosis, all the attributes of a typical isthmic spondylolisthesis. M-B state that "forms with lysis and very rarely with elongation are so similar that they can be described here as one item." Furthermore, in terms of progression, low dysplastic forms usually do not worsen, any slippage being invariably slow and displacement being translational rather than tilting, changes that are clearly not dysplastic, and so it is difficult to see why there should be high and low dysplastic forms when the latter appear to have no dysplastic elements at all.

Meanwhile for the past 10 to 20 years increasing emphasis has been placed upon the shape of the pelvis and spondylolisthesis.[45–50] In 1997 Schwab et al looked at X-rays of children/adolescents with spondylolisthesis with particular reference to sagittal plane pelvic rotation with the degree of slip over time.[45] They sought to determine whether the degree of standing sagittal offset of L5 with respect to the acetabulum correlated with slip progression and symptoms. A total of 52 patients with dysplastic spondylolisthesis were looked at, with serial standing lateral radiographs including the hips and lumbar spine, to measure the sagittal pelvic tilt index (SPTI) as the ratio of the relative distances from the center of S2 to the projection of L5 in the center of the femoral heads horizontal (▶ Fig. 11.21). The lower the SPTI the more vertical the sacrum and more anteriorly displaced the hip joint with more progression and imbalance. A total of 32 patients had spondylolisthesis and 20 spondylolysis. Slip progression occurred in 13 patients with spondylolisthesis along with a decrease in the SPTI. These patients had significant symptoms whereas those patients with a stable SPTI did not progress and remained symptom free. They therefore postulated that an abnormal SPTI was etiological in dysplastic spondylolisthesis and led to progressive displacement. In the normal and balanced patient L5 is centered above the hip joint whereas with an unbalanced patient the more anteriorly translated L5 facilitates a lumbosacral kyphosis to develop a compensatory lumbar lordosis above.

Then in 2002 Rajnics et al looked at 48 patients with isthmic spondylolisthesis and 30 healthy volunteers using digitized standing lateral spinal radiographs.[46] The lateral X-rays included both femoral heads. They measured the SFAC (the sacrofemoral anatomic constant or incidence) (▶ Fig. 11.22), the

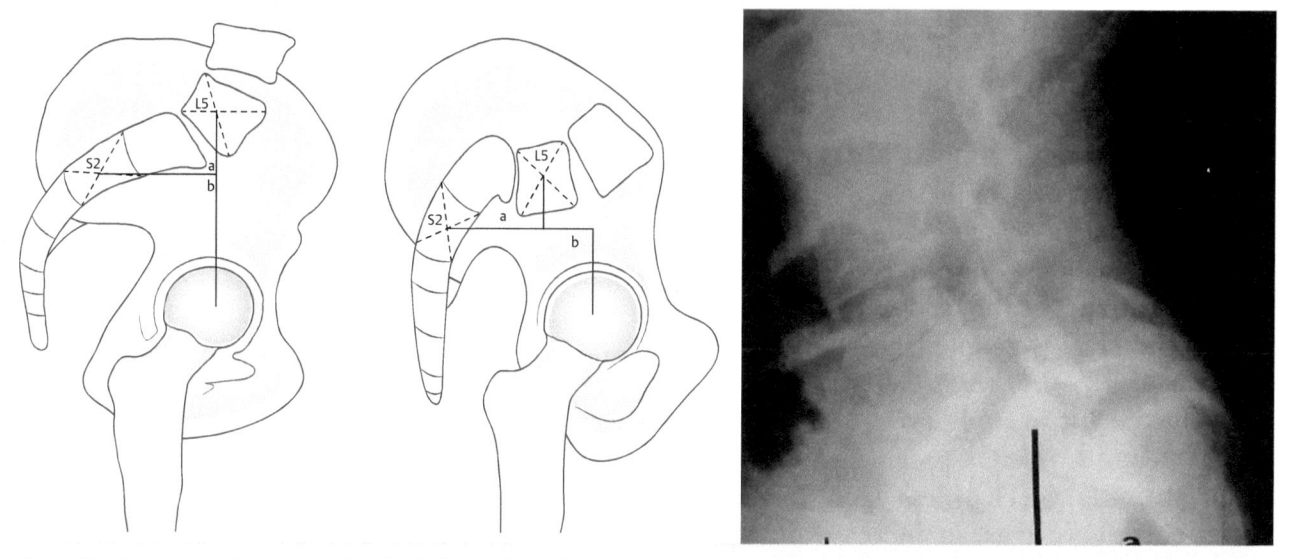

Fig. 11.21 The sagittal pelvic tilt index (SPTI) calculated *a/b*. **(a)** The SPTI is near 1 in this schematic. **(b)** The SPTI in this case would be near 0.6. Note the verticalization of the sacrum that occurs thus displacing the hip joint anteriorly increasing distance **(b)**. **(c)** Lateral standing radiograph demonstrating an imbalanced spondylolisthesis with an SPTI of approximately 0.5. (Reproduced with permission from Frank Schwab, Jean-Pierre Farcy, and David Roye. The Sagittal Pelvic Tilt Index as a Criterion in the Evaluation of Spondylolisthesis: Preliminary Observations. Spine (Phila Pa 1976). Oct 5, 0716;22(14):1661-7.)

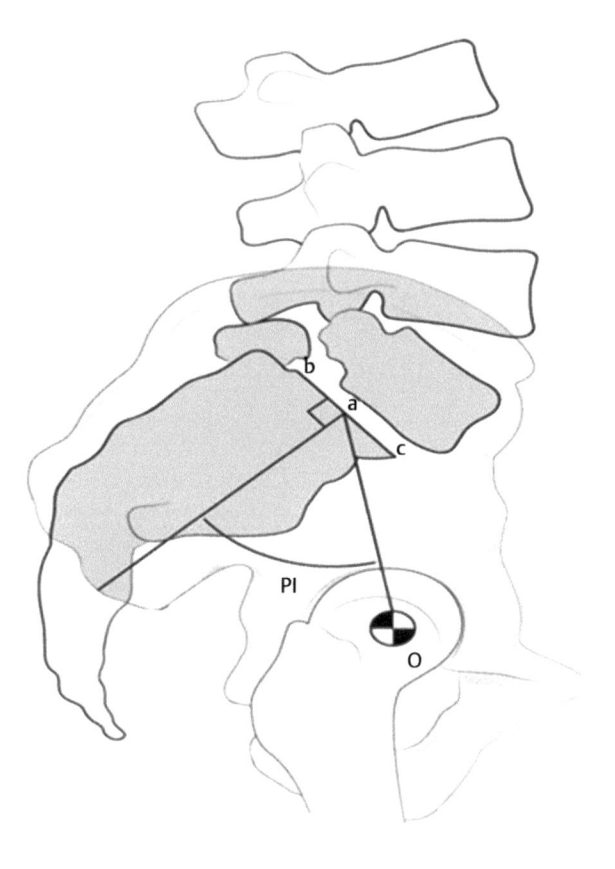

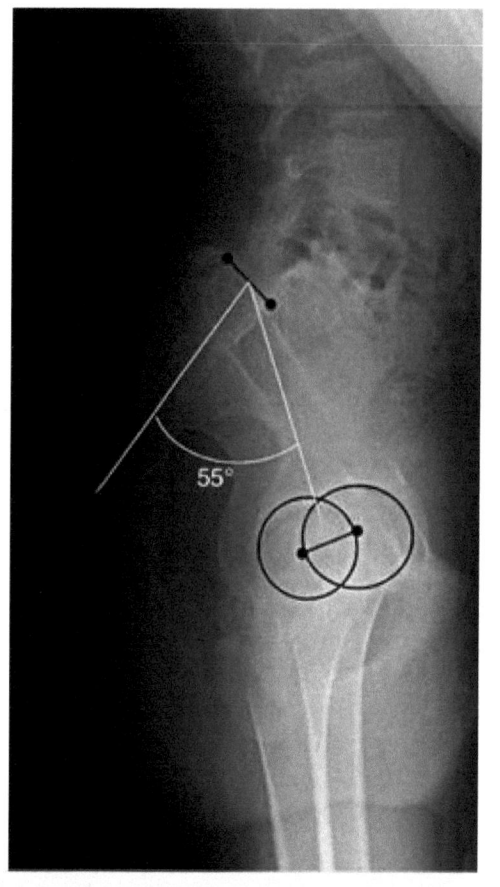

Fig. 11.22 Measuring the sacrofemoral anatomic constant (SFAC) or pelvic incidence (PI), a fixed anatomic parameter that is unique to each person. Standing lateral radiograph of the spine demonstrating a PI of 55 degrees. b= posterior margin of the sacral end plate. c= anterior margin of the sacral end plate. (Reproduced with permission from Ying Li, Timothy Hresko. Radiographic Analysis of Spondylolisthesis and Sagittal Spinopelvic Deformity. Wolters Kluwer Health, Inc.; 2012.)

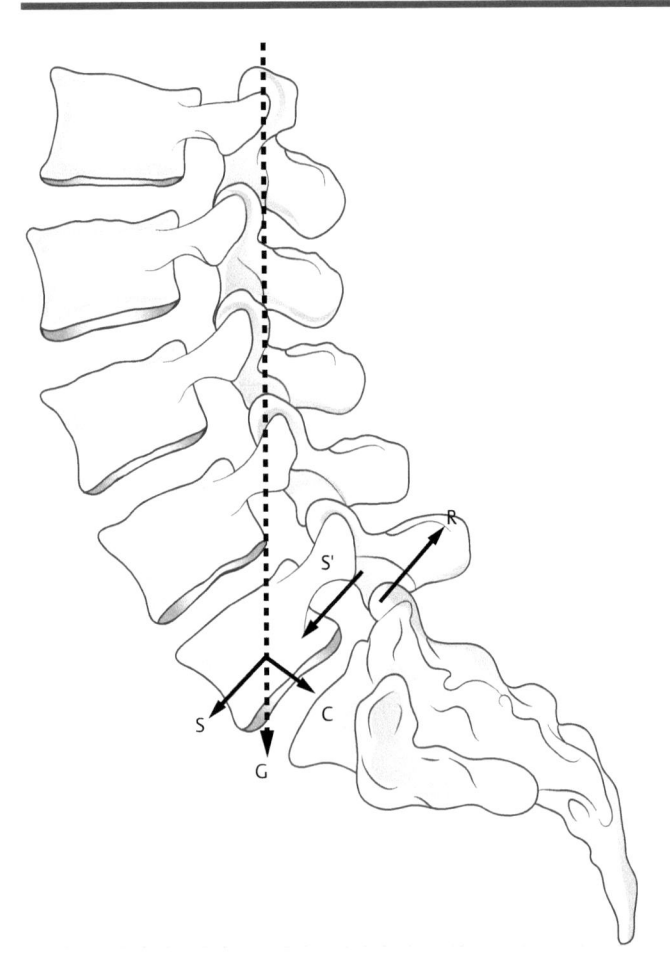

Fig. 11.23 With a horizontally positioned sacrum and hyperlordosis the shearing component of gravity is greater than the compressive force.

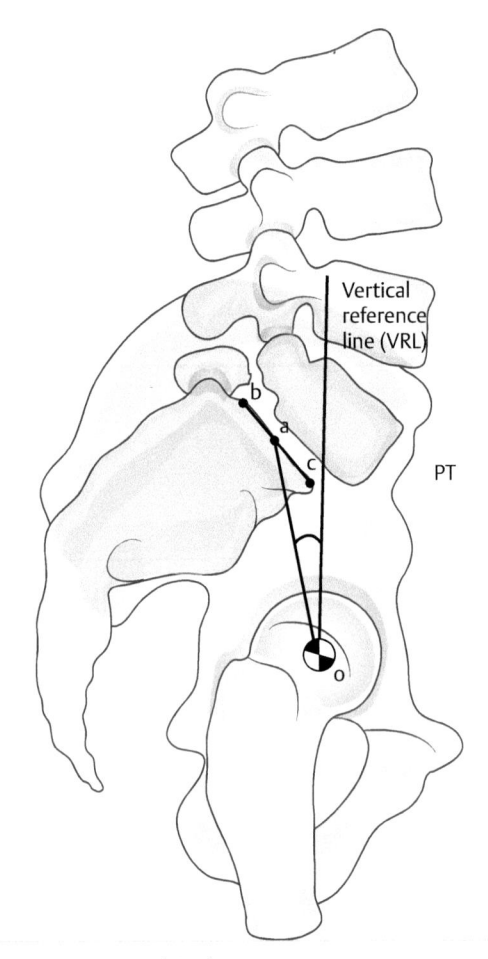

Fig. 11.24 Measuring pelvic tilt.

sacral slope (SS; already called the sacrohorizontal angle[41] (▶ Fig. 11.19), and L1 to L5 lordosis (▶ Fig. 11.18). These three measures were all greater in patients with isthmic spondylolisthesis than in the healthy volunteers. They postulated that the horizontally positioned sacrum and hyperlordosis caused the shearing component of gravity to be greater than the compressive force (▶ Fig. 11.23) and thus causes fracture of the interarticular part of the vertebra. The two acetabula were located well anterior to the lumbosacral junction giving rise to instability. The SFAC is a hereditary factor that correlates well with the degree of slipping.

In the same year Marty et al studied the relationship between the sacrum and the angle of incidence[17] and compared these parameters in three populations—young adults (44), infants before walking (32), and patients with spondylolisthesis (39). They argued that the incidence was strongly correlated with the sacral slip and lumbar lordosis and so ensured individuals an economical standing position. The angle of incidence had also been shown to depend partly on the sagittal anatomy of the sacrum which was established in childhood while learning to stand and walk. Hence the purpose of the study was to define the relationship between the sacrum and angle of incidence and to compare these parameters in the above three populations. All underwent sagittal standing spine radiography. A close relationship existed between the angle of incidence and the slip of spondylolisthesis and all parameters in young infants were less than adults. They concluded that the sagittal anatomy of the sacrum played a key role in spinal sagittal balance. The sacrum in the spondylolisthesis group differed from normal with a greater angle of incidence and sacral slope that could predispose to vertebral slip.

Hubert Labelle seems to have done more work on spinopelvic relationships than practically anybody else and as usual he is a good read. In 2005 he and his team from Montreal viewed the radiological measurements of spinopelvic balance in relationship to dysplastic spondylolisthesis which he referred to as developmental, tacitly accepting the M-B classification.[47] Again, lateral standing radiographs were studied with dedicated software calculating pelvic incidence, sacral slope, pelvic tilt (▶ Fig. 11.24), L5 incidence angle (▶ Fig. 11.25), lumbosacral angle, lumbar lordosis, thoracic kyphosis, and grade of spondylolisthesis. They compared these measures in patients to an adult and children reference population. Pelvic incidence, sacral slope, pelvic tilt, and lumbar lordosis were all found to be significantly greater in subjects with dysplastic spondylolisthesis while thoracic kyphosis was significantly less. The difference between patient and reference populations increased linearly when the degree of spondylolisthesis increased. Better surgical outcomes occurred with an improvement in L5 incidence angle and lumbosacral angle while those who faired less well had a higher preoperative grade.

Spondylolysis and Spondylolisthesis

11.5 Mac-Thiong and Labelle's Classification

Then Mac-Thiong from Labelle's department proposed a new surgical classification of lumbar spondylolisthesis, from a literature review.[48] Interestingly, it also showed the difference between balanced and unbalanced high grade dysplastic spondylolisthesis (▶ Fig. 11.26). Sagittal spinopelvic balance was assessed by measurement of pelvic incidence, sacral slope, and pelvic tilt (▶ Fig. 11.27). This in turn led to their own eight-part surgical classification of L5/S1 spondylolisthesis.

However, when Mac-Thiong and Hubert Labelle tested reliability of the classification in a group of spinal surgeons about dysplastic spondylolisthesis, the point that they were least clear about or could differentiate was the difference between the high and low dysplastic forms—to the point where they abandoned this subdivision.[49] This is extremely important because not only is the M-B classification unreliable but with dysplastic spondylolisthesis you either have dysplasia or you don't, as with the Wiltse classification, and that is where the M-B classification falls down. Quite sensibly they then reduced it to only six types (▶ Table 11.4). Also as you never have more than a grade 2 (50%) slip with isthmic spondylolisthesis then the isthmic form cannot be high grade.

Marchetti and Bartolozzi agreed that the isthmic lesions are readily explained by mechanical stress on the pars which offers less resistance when subjected to force—the stress lysis sustained by gymnasts and weightlifters seeming to beg to belong to the isthmic variety. Then under both high dysplastic and low dysplastic they have with lysis or with elongation. This seems difficult to reconcile because you do not see elongation in the isthmic form, only with the dysplastic category.

Then under acquired they agree that acute pars fractures are part and parcel of more severe trauma. Why then do they not suggest them being classified with other classifications of thoracolumbar spinal trauma? Post-surgery spondylolisthesis is also part and parcel of the SRS classification of spinal deformities (see Chapter 2, ▶ Table 2.1); so why suffer from classificationitis and clutter up the terminology of spondylolisthesis unnecessarily?

Notwithstanding, the M-B chapter is fascinating reading and goes on to discuss treatment of the different categories. It certainly would be inappropriate to be too critical of these distinguished authors who are honest enough at the end to state "although we do not claim to have had the last word on this

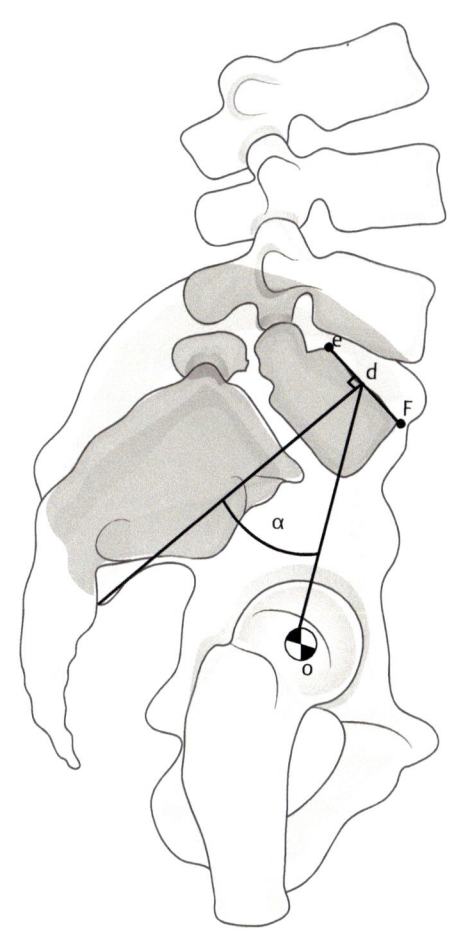

Fig. 11.25 The L5 incidence angle, measured in a similar manner as pelvic incidence.

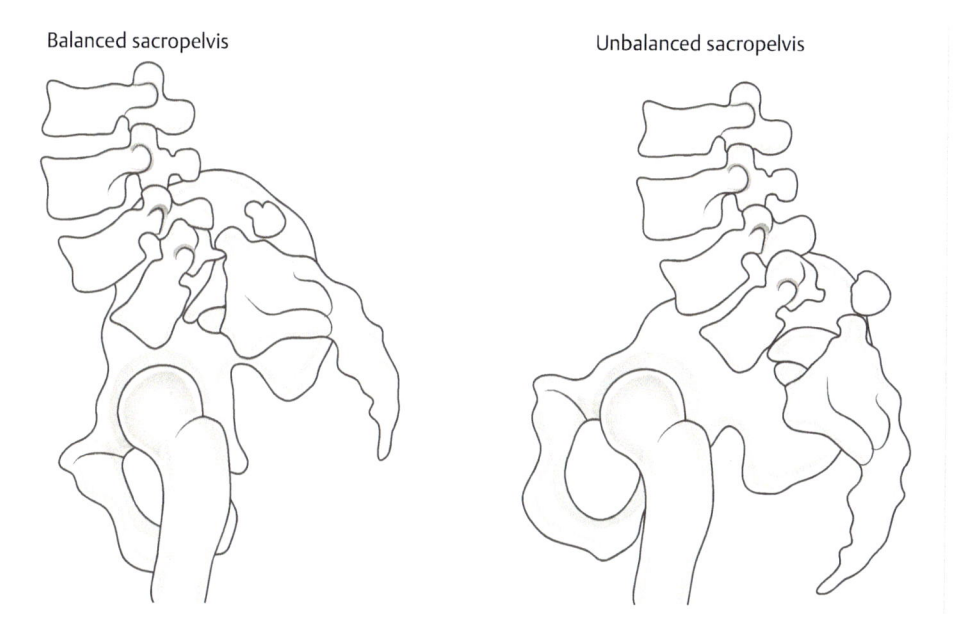

Balanced sacropelvis

Unbalanced sacropelvis

Fig. 11.26 Balanced and unbalanced spondylolistheses. When the hip joints are just below the lumbosacral junction the sacropelvis is balanced but when the hip joints are well in front then this produces an unbalanced sacropelvis.

Low-grade spondylolisthesis | High-grade spondylolisthesis

Low PI/low SS (nutcracker type) | High PI/high SS (shear type) | High SS/low PT (balanced pelvis) | Low SS/high PT (retroverted pelvis)

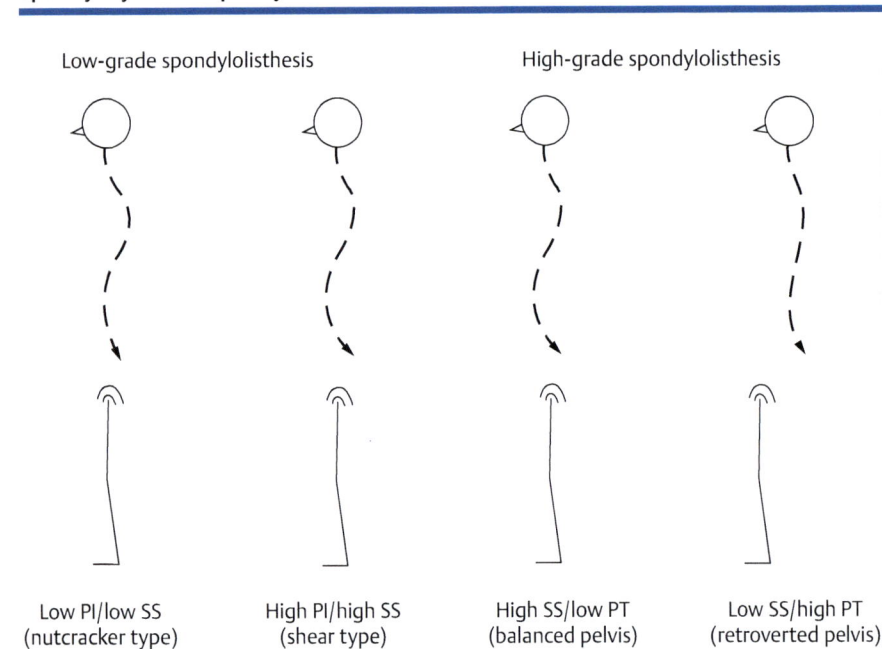

Fig. 11.27 Sacropelvic balance with low and high grade spondylolisthesis. For low-grade spondylolisthesis, the sagittal spinopelvic balance can be classified as low PI/low SS (*nutcracker type*) or high PI/high SS (*shear type*). For high-grade spondylolisthesis, it can be classified as high SS/low PT (*balanced pelvis*) or low SS/high PT (*retroverted pelvis*). (Reproduced with permission from Jean-Marc Mac-Thiong. A proposal for a surgical classification of pediatric lumbosacral spondylolisthesis based on current literature. Eur Spine J 2006;15(10):1425-1435.)

Table 11.4 Revised Mac-Thiong and Labelle's six-part classification of lumbosacral spondylolisthesis

Slip grade	Sacropelvic balance	Spinopelvic balance[a]	Spondylolisthesis type
Low grade (<50%)	Low PI (<45°)	-	1
	Normal PI (45–60°)	-	2
	High PI (≥60°)	-	3
High grade (≥50%)	Balanced (high SS/low PT)	-	4
	Unbalanced (low SS/high PT)	Balanced (C7 plumbline between femoral heads and sacrum)	5
		Unbalanced (C7 plumbline anterior to femoral heads or posterior to sacrum)	6

Abbreviations: PI, pelvic incidence; PT, pelvic tilt; SS, sacral slope.
[a]The spine is almost always balanced in patients with low- or high-grade spondylolisthesis with a balanced pelvis.

subject, we consider ourselves satisfied if we have managed to shed some light on the many unanswered questions about spondylolisthesis." That, indeed, they have accomplished.

This revised six-part classification (▶ Table 11.4) (Mac-Thiong et al[49]) is supported by the Spinal Deformity Study Group (SDSG) and is based on three important characteristics that can be assessed from preoperative imaging studies: grade of slip, the sacropelvic balance, and the global spinopelvic balance. To classify a patient first of all the degree of slip is Meyerding quantified low grade (grades 0, 1, 2, or less than 50% slip) or high grade (grades 3, 4, and spondyloptosis or more than 50% slip). Then sagittal balance is measured by determining through pelvic global spinopelvic balance, using the measurements of pelvic incidence (PI), sacral slip (SS), and pelvic tilt (PT) plus the C7 plumb line. The low grade is virtually always balanced and divided into three groups according to pelvic incidence and the high grade group divided into balanced and unbalanced types based on to the plumb line—that is, with the balanced group, the L5/S1 joint lies over the hips and in the unbalanced group the spine lies well behind.

Then more recently Li and Hresko emphasized the importance of global sagittal balance with spine and pelvis in patients with spondylolisthesis and reinforced the six-part classification of Mac-Thiong.[50]

Therefore while it is very important to stress, but not over stress (as many seem to do), the significance of the dysplastic form of spondylolisthesis, this really should not be confused with the straightforward primary stress fracture type of isthmic spondylolisthesis which is never high grade, so in a way we find ourselves back to the Wiltse classification, particularly in its more refined form (▶ Table 11.2). After all Wiltse, Newman, and McNab were not inexperienced spondylolisthesiologists having spent their collective working years of more than a century on this condition so they knew spondylolisthesis inside and out or should we say upside down to pay homage to the pelvis! Even their classification[13] really only reinforced the thoughts of Neugebauer[5] and Meyer-Burgdorff[5] a hundred years earlier. Is there anything new in orthopaedics?

11.6 Clinical Features and Treatment

11.6.1 Dysplastic Spondylolisthesis

This is the type of spondylolisthesis in children and adolescents that may well require surgical attention. Pain is of two types: musculoskeletal or, very uncommonly, radicular. The former is felt in the low back but can radiate to the buttocks and upper thighs but not below the knee.[51] Back pain is much more commonly the case with dysplastic spondylolisthesis than with the isthmic variety and again it is sclerotomal, initiated, or aggravated by strenuous activity—particularly, repetitive lower lumbar spine flexion and extension. Progression of the slip is also more common than with the isthmic variety and is in the form of progressive lumbosacral kyphosis. While symptoms may be intermittent and tolerable as slip progression passes through the lower grades, when the slippage gets into grade 4 and the L5 vertebra begins to tilt further and further over the anterosuperior angle of S1 then symptoms can sometimes be acute with severe low back pain combined with an incredible amount of low back musculoligamentous spasm to provide a deformity of bent knee, hip flexed with hamstring tightness, and severe limitation of straight leg raising described by the classic Phalen-Dickson paper,[52] also called the adolescent crisis (▶ Fig. 11.28). Indeed so severe can the hamstring tightness be that a straight leg cannot be lifted from the examining table—indeed, it may not be possible to lie supine with a straight leg. Above the L5/S1 level there is a hyperlordosis of the lumbar spine fixed by muscle spasm.

There is rarely any evidence of radicular symptoms or objective neurology in children/adolescents[53] although mature

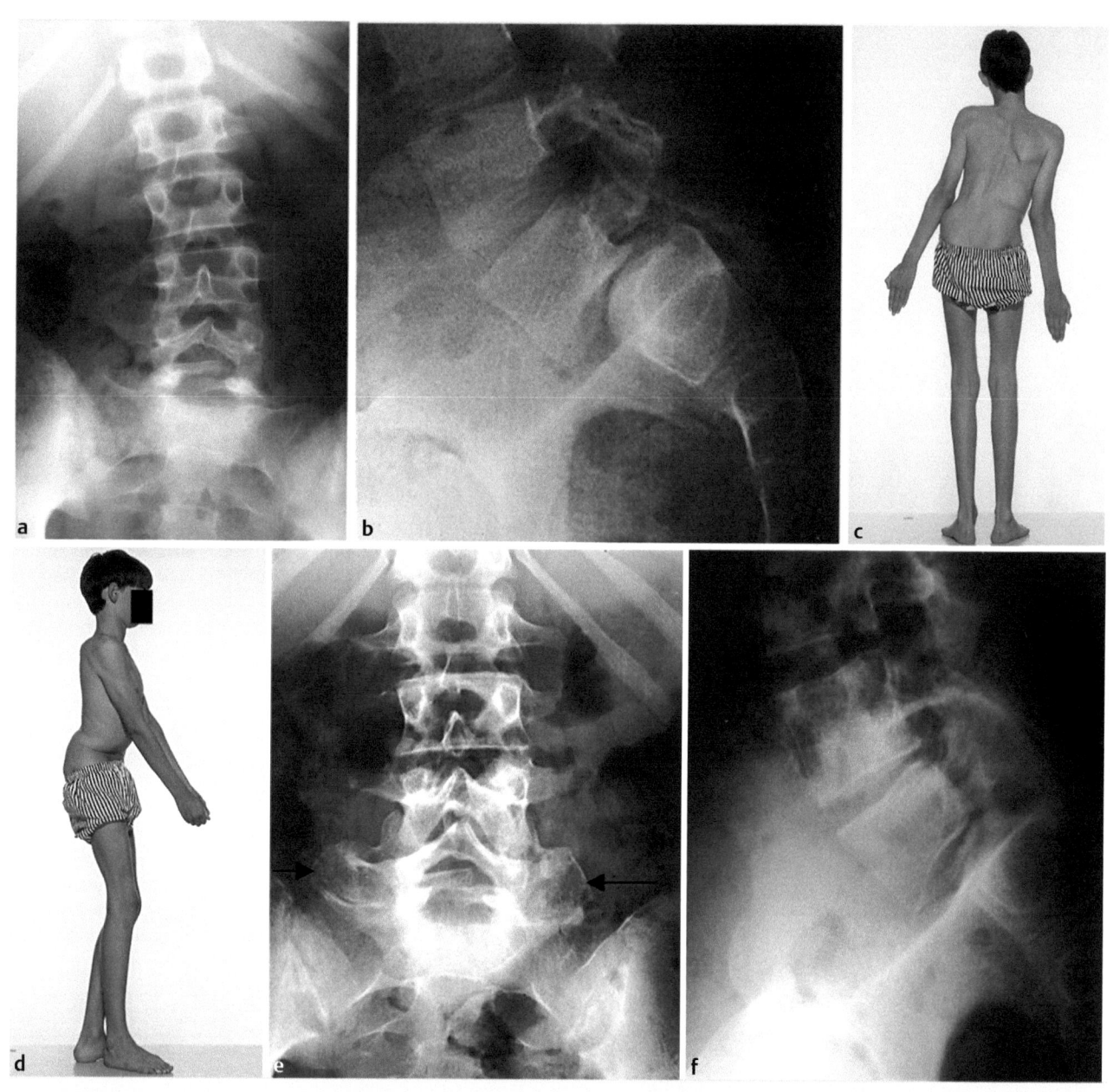

Fig. 11.28 (a,b) AP and lateral radiographs of a boy with dysplastic spondylolisthesis of about 50%. Note the list to the side on the frontal film due to muscle spasm. Note the obligatory spina bifida occulta of L5 which is a constant accompaniment of dysplastic spondylolisthesis. (c,d) Back and side view of this boy of 14 years. This deformity is entirely due to muscle spasm secondary to the pain of the spondylolisthesis. This is called the adolescent crisis. Note on the side view the lumbosacral kyphosis, the real deformity of dysplastic spondylolisthesis. (e,f) AP and lateral views 2 years after surgery showing a solid fusion (*arrows*) and a straight spine. This is what an intertransverse fusion should look like when performed by the technique illustrated in ▶ Fig. 11.32. There was no visible deformity at follow-up and the young man had actually grown 5 inches. (Reproduced with the permission and copyright of The Medico-Legal Back: An Illustrated Guide, 2003, Cambridge University Press. Eds Dickson RA and Butt WP, Fig 5.5.)

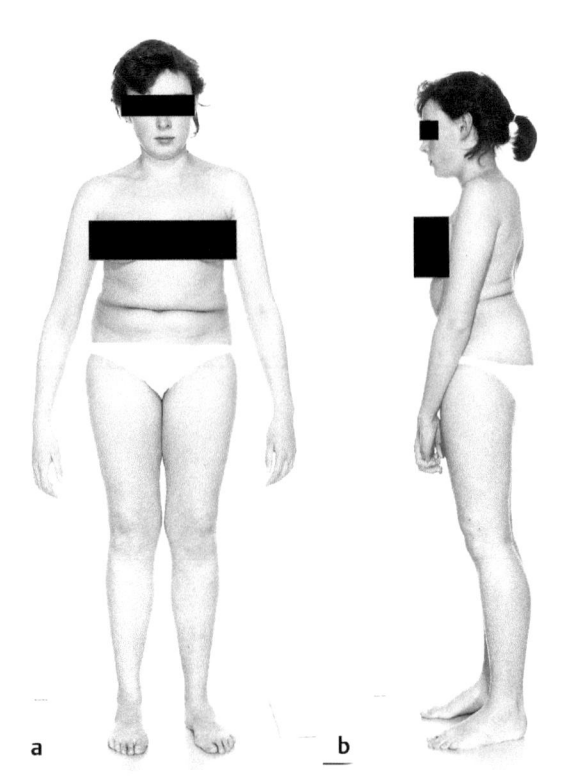

Fig. 11.29 Patient with spondyloptosis. (a) Front view with abdo crease. (b) Side view with flat pelvis.

patients can have L5 root irritation from hypertrophic callus around the lysis. A patient looked at from the side or front displays a transverse abdominal crease at the level of the umbilicus (▶ Fig. 11.29) and when viewed from the side the buttocks are flattened and there may be a prominent spinous process of L5. These clinical features are quite diagnostic of the dysplastic form of spondylolisthesis. These unfortunate children with severe dysplastic spondylolisthesis or even spondyloptosis do have a rather peculiar short stride and pelvic-waddling gait.[54]

When detected in the child or adolescent before the growth spurt then surgical treatment is recommended whether or not symptoms are present. Progression tends to occur during the growth spurt and is much less common after adolescence and if the degree of slippage is less than 50%. Slippage doesn't occur in adulthood when the condition stabilizes. Conservative management with physiotherapy stretching hamstrings and antilordotic bracing (full-time for all of 6 months) are frequently prescribed for the older adolescent along obviously with rest from sporting or other physical activities.[55,56] Good results from these programs tend to occur, not surprisingly, in those with lesser degrees of slippage and lumbosacral kyphosis.

Surgical intervention is generally accepted as the treatment of choice for high grade dysplastic spondylolisthesis. Whether reduction should be attempted and the extent of fusion have both been debated for years. Posterolateral fusion in situ from L4 to S1 has been recommended by many regardless of severity[57-62] but the pseudarthrosis rate is unacceptably high[58,60,63] with the sagittal alignment through the deformity remaining the same so that the deformity can progress by plastic deformation despite apparently solid fusion masses.[64-66] In addition, neurological compromise has been described as a late complication.[63,65,67] Clearly monosegmental fusion from L5 to S1 avoiding going up to L4 must be the desirable extent of fusion while reduction of the deformity would appear to be the ideal mechanical solution. As a sort of halfway house, partial reduction techniques have evolved and these have included pre- or perioperative casting, traction, and fusion by anterior, posterior, or combined approaches.[58,62-64,67-73]

However, complete reduction was reported to have an excessively high rate of L5 nerve root injury caused by distraction of these nerve roots.[71,72] Scaglietti was also concerned about the degree of correction obtained by longitudinal distraction and the risk of severe neurological complications and while recommending reduction felt that repositioning was more safely produced by serial preoperative plaster casts, the reduction position then being stabilized using instrumentation not dissimilar to that of Harrington followed by fusion.[73]

Indeed, posterior fusion and trying to reduce the deformity was reported in 1932 by Capener[74] and again by Jenkins.[75] La-Chapelle favored closed reduction but was disappointed with the results.[20] Harris in 1951 prescribed reduction by skeletal traction on the basis that improvement in the degree of slippage was desirable in severe cases.[53] Freebody in 1969 used an anterior transperitoneal approach for his fusions.[76] Harrington first used his instrumentation for the reduction of spondylolisthesis and although this could only alter the local anatomy by distraction vertically,[77] the technique was soon used by others.[78-80] In 1976 Harrington reported alterations to his original technique with the use of a sacral bar against which the distraction rods bore with the resultant A-frame configuration.[81] In the belief that an improvement in the sagittal component of the deformity could be achieved using pedicle screws attached to the distraction rods, he tried this but did not feel that they were in any way contributory. A posterior laminectomy was performed so that reduction could be visualized and the final position was stabilized by intertransverse fusion. Snijder adopted a different approach using wires attached to the spinous processes of L3 and L4 coupled to an external fixation device in an attempt to reduce the slip and then an interbody L5/S1 fusion was carried out.[82]

Verbiest, believing that intertransverse fusion was insufficient, reported anterior console lumbosacral fusion for severe degrees of spondylolisthesis or frank spondyloptosis.[83] After posterior laminectomy he removed the posterosuperior portion of S1 and performed his anterior approach as a second stage retroperitoneally with the patient in hyperextension. After obliteration of the disk space at the level of the slip, tibial cortical strut grafts were inserted from the front of S2 upward into the body of L5, or through it into L4. The space behind the strut grafts was filled with cancellous bone. Satisfactory results were reported in 11 cases with no significant complications other than strut graft collapse.

This approach of staged posterior then anterior surgery was adopted by others with some variations. Bradford used halo-femoral traction in extension followed by a posterior Gill procedure and lateral mass fusion followed by anterior fusion.[84] Patients were kept supine for 4 months postoperatively and spent a further 4 months in a cast. Of his 10 cases there were 6 with significant problems—three with L5 nerve root weakness, two with foot drop, and one with loss of correction. McPhee and O'Brien, using a method similar to Bradford's, reported one bilateral L5 neuropraxia and one loss of reduction.[85] DeWald et al first performed posterior Harrington distraction instrumentation and posterolateral fusion followed by anterior fusion,[86] but one case developed severe neurological problems and they did not recommend this technique for severe degrees of slip. To overcome objections to anterior surgery in teenagers (what's the problem?), Bohlman and Cook reported a one-stage decompression and posterolateral fusion with interbody fusion for spondyloptosis, all done through a posterior approach.[87] They used two fibular strut grafts on each side of the dural sac for the interbody L5/S1 fusion (▶ Fig. 11.30). We liked this anterior and posterior combined fusion through a single posterior approach for prophylactic fusion for dysplastic spondylolisthesis before significant slippage.

For irreducible spondyloptosis the Gaines procedure should be considered whereby L5 is resected and L4 placed upon S1.[88]

Because of conflicting results with these various techniques we devised a technique in Karlsbad where reduction and one-level fixation and fusion can both be achieved.[89]

We have carried out this procedure on 27 patients with severe dysplastic spondylolisthesis and all patients finished up with a solid bony fusion at a minimum follow-up of 2 years (▶ Fig. 11.31). A major concern in any reduction procedure of L5 on S1 is injury to the L5 nerve roots. In six patients who had L5 root symptoms in the early postoperative phase only one had persistent L5 sensory impairment which of course because of dermatomal overlap is only a very small area on the dorsum of the first interdigital cleft. There were no L5 motor problems. One patient had residual pain. The L5 nerve root is extremely delicate, much more so than the robust S1 root, and the L5/S1 roots must therefore be visualized during the entire reduction procedure. Importantly this procedure avoids interfering with a primarily healthy L4/5 segment particularly in these young persons.

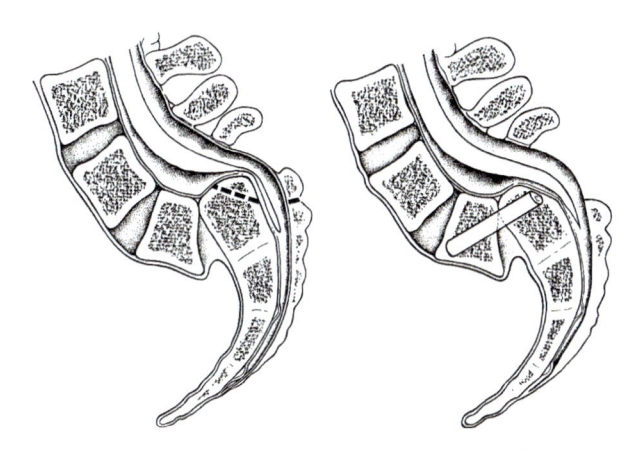

Fig. 11.30 Bohlman's procedure. An L5/S1 laminectomy is performed in order to gain access to the L5/S1 level anteriorly and to ensure protection of neural tissue. The top back corner of the body of S1 is removed to decompress the dura and two strut grafts are drilled across the L5/S1 disk. An alar-transverse fusion is added.

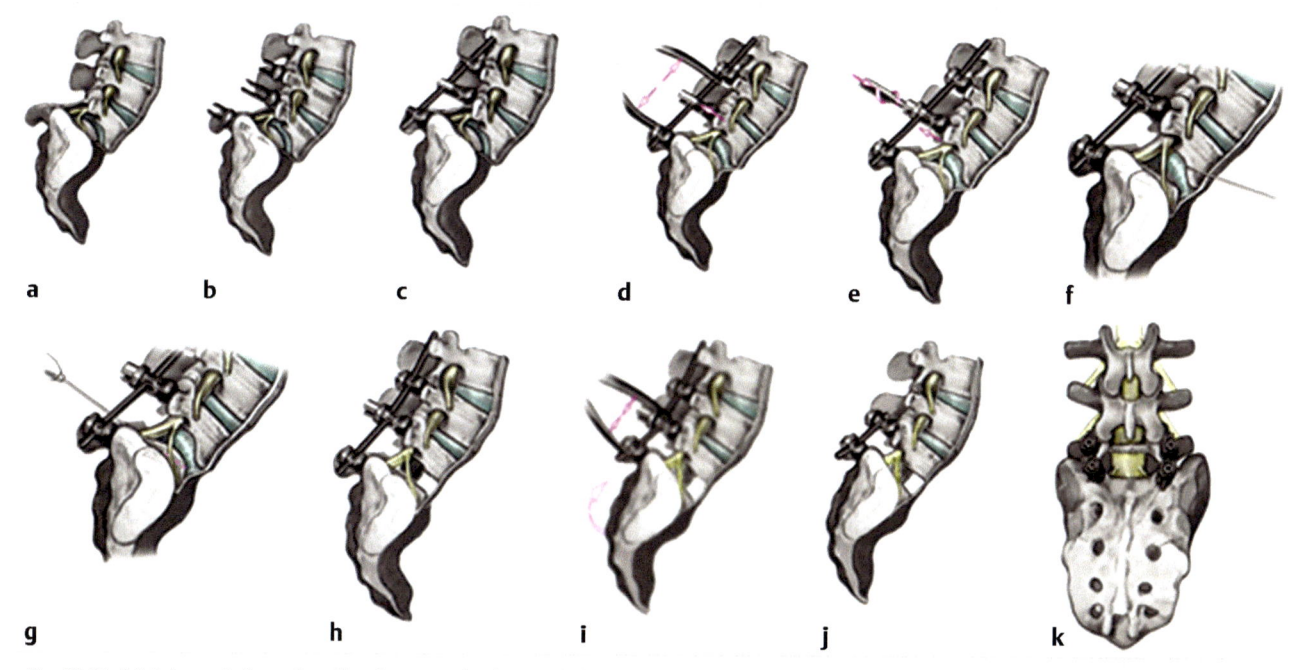

Fig. 11.31 (a) Schematic from the side of a severe lumbosacral dysplastic spondylolisthesis after L5 laminectomy. (b) After insertion of polyaxial pedicle screws into S1 on each side and long-head screws into the pedicles of L4 and L5. (c) The rod has been loosely inserted. (d) After tightening the screws at L4 and S1 distraction is applied to begin the reduction of the L5 vertebra by ligamentotaxis. (e) Further reduction is achieved by partially tightening the nuts over the L5 screw. (f) The L5/S1 disk is now removed bilaterally. (g) Osteotomizing the top of the sacrum. (h) Continuing the reduction of the L5 vertebral body. The amount of dome resection, the entry point, and angle of the osteotomy are monitored fluoroscopically. The L5/S1 disk space is then packed with cancellous bone and titanium cages. (i) Correction of the segmental kyphosis. (j) The L5 rods are cut above the L5 screws and the L4 screws removed leaving one level fixation. (k) Frontal view of the final construct.

11.7 Practice Points

11.7.1 Reduction, Fixation, and Fusion of Severe Dysplastic Spondylolisthesis

The lumbosacral junction is exposed posteriorly. The exposure is continued laterally out to the transverse processes of L4, L5, and the sacral alae. This procedure is usually more difficult at the L5 level because of the combined slippage and kyphosis. The inferior articular facets of L5 and superior facets of S1 are removed. A partial or complete resection of the lamina of L5 is performed with identification of the L5 nerve roots. The L5 nerve roots are exposed far laterally (▶ Fig. 11.31a). Polyaxial pedicle screws are inserted in S1 bilaterally. Specially designed, long-head screws are placed in the pedicles of L4 and L5 (▶ Fig. 11.31). The long heads of these screws facilitate insertion of straight or mildly prebent rods (▶ Fig. 11.31b,c).

The reduction is initiated by distraction between L4 and the sacrum. As the distance from L4 to the sacrum is increased, L5 reduces as a result of ligamentotaxis (▶ Fig. 11.31d,e). Placement of the L5 screw is often difficult because of severe slippage and kyphosis. In this situation, partial reduction via distraction of L4 from S1 through a contralateral rod is performed before insertion of the L5 screw. This process provides better visualization of the screw entry point at L5. Furthermore, distraction opens the L5/S1 foramina.

The disk at L5/S1 is removed via a bilateral approach (▶ Fig. 11.31f). The posterior longitudinal ligament is completely resected to avoid bulging in after reduction. The lateral and anterior annulus is thinned out to mobilize the segment. The dome-shaped end plate of S1 is osteotomized to create a flat surface perpendicular to the posterior wall (▶ Fig. 11.31g). To assess the amount of dome resection, the entry point and angle of the osteotomy are monitored fluoroscopically.

The second step in reduction of L5 is now performed. By tightening the nuts of the long-head screws in L5, its body is pulled posteriorly to the rod between L4 and the sacrum (▶ Fig. 11.31h). During reduction, the L5 roots are continually visualized and controlled to avoid any compression. The elongated flanges of the long-headed screws are then removed. Reduction of the anterior slippage of L5/S1 is now completed. However, lumbosacral kyphosis is still present.

The anterior part of the disk space of L5/S1 is then debrided and packed with cancellous bone, and disk spacers (titanium cages) are inserted in the posterior part (▶ Fig. 11.31h). These cages enhance considerably the friction between L5 and S1, hence, counterstretching the L5 roots and allowing reconstruction of lordosis. This part of the operation is performed either by a posterior (posterior lumbar interbody fusion) or by a second anterior approach (anterior lumbar interbody fusion).

The third step of reduction is the correction of the segmental kyphosis at L5/S1. This correction is achieved by posterior compression via the rods against the anterior pivot (cages). The sacral screw is loosened, and approximated to the fixed L4 and L5 screws (▶ Fig. 11.31i). Loosening the polyaxial head allows for change of the angulation, and the sacral retroversion is corrected. This procedure is supported by hyperextension of the hip joints via the operating table. The sacral screws are fixed again and further compression is applied between L5 and S1. Posterior instrumentation combined with compression loaded cages anteriorly results in a very stable, shear-resistant construct. The rods are cut above L5, and the L4 screws are removed (▶ Fig. 11.31j). In selected cases in which we believe that high traction and shear forces may lead to screw loosening, the L4 screws are left in for removal at 3 months after surgery. The PA schematic (▶ Fig. 11.31k) shows the final result, a one-level reduction and fusion.

11.8 Intertransverse Fusion

R. A. D. devised a useful technique for maximizing the recipient area in an intertransverse fusion to cover the entire intertransverse bare area while retaining a vascularized recipient bed.[90] This was based upon Hibb's posterior fusion technique for scoliosis whereby successive flaps of cortical bone are raised to expose subcortical healthy bleeding cancellous bone yet still remaining attached. The two adjacent transverse processes are denuded of soft tissue so there is nothing in between except the intertransverse membrane. Then, using a sharp osteotome, the posterior cortices of the transverse processes are split along their length and the upper and lower flaps are then turned upward and downward, respectively, so that these flaps fill the intertransverse gap. Then when the upper flap of the upper transverse process is turned upward, and vice versa for the lower transverse process, a vascularized base for the fusion is maximized (▶ Fig. 11.32). It is upon this large and healthy surface that bone grafts readily incorporate.

If the fusion is alar-transverse then a flap of corticocancellous bone is raised from the top of the ala and turned upward to meet the flap from the lower half of the transverse process of L5 which has been turned down to make a broad vascularized recipient surface upon which bone grafts are placed.

It is a simple procedure but it is a biological one with a definite solid fusion as the endpoint. You don't just put in some metalwork and then bung in a few thousand dollars' worth of granules of bone substitute and hope for the best!

Others thought they had invented this technique[91] until they were corrected.[92]

11.8.1 Spondylolysis

Spondylolyses can produce much the same symptoms as isthmic spondylolisthesis particularly if the lyses are bilateral. However, unilateral spondylolysis is a very difficult matter because with so many potential causes for back pain in the athletically physical growing individual it is very difficult if not impossible to localize pain to the spondylolysis itself. This is rather like trying to identify the painful level in the lumbar spine for someone with persistent back pain—MRI scanning and stress diskography being spectacularly unsuccessful,[93-95] yet continue to be relied upon. Rather like the conservative treatment for spondylolisthesis, rest from strenuous athletic sports particularly combined repetitive stresses, with physical therapy plus bracing, usually relieve symptoms and these are the mainstays of treatment. This phase of rest, in particular, can be very frustrating for all concerned—patients and therapists—because what these individuals want to do more than anything else is carry on their particular sport particularly if they may have already achieved a very high level. Pain, having first settled with rest and physical

Spondylolysis and Spondylolisthesis

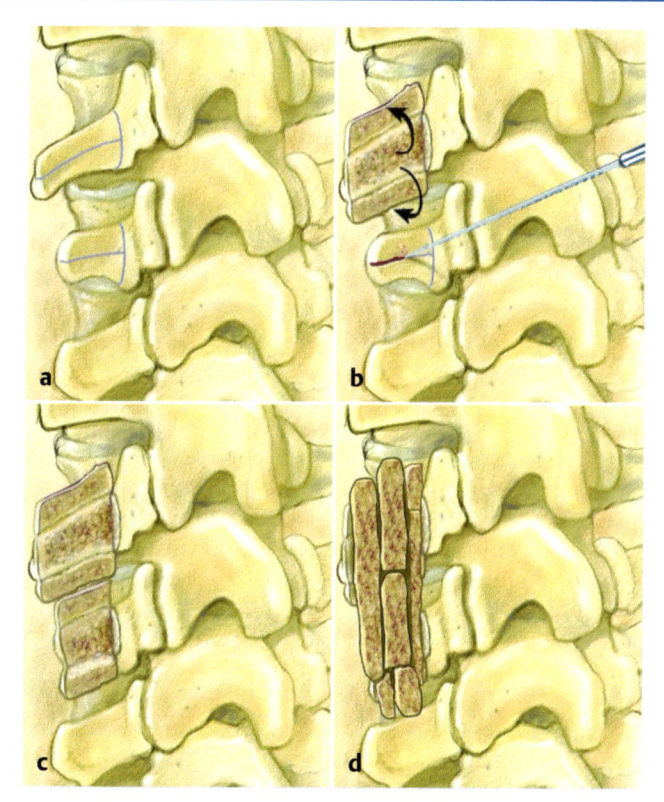

Fig. 11.32 (a) Indicating the osteotomy lines of the posterior cortex of the adjacent transverse processes. (b) With a sharp osteotome or fine bur these osteotomies are made in the transverse processes and then the upper and lower dorsal flaps so produced are turned upward and downward, respectively. (c) These flaps first of all conjoin over the intertransverse space and also extend upward and downward so as to maximize the vascularized recipient area. (d) Pieces of iliac crest bone graft are then laid on top of this recipient area so maximizing the fusion mass. (Reproduced with the permission of Deen JH, Open Book Technique, J Neurosurgery/Spine Vol 93, 2000, p 333.)

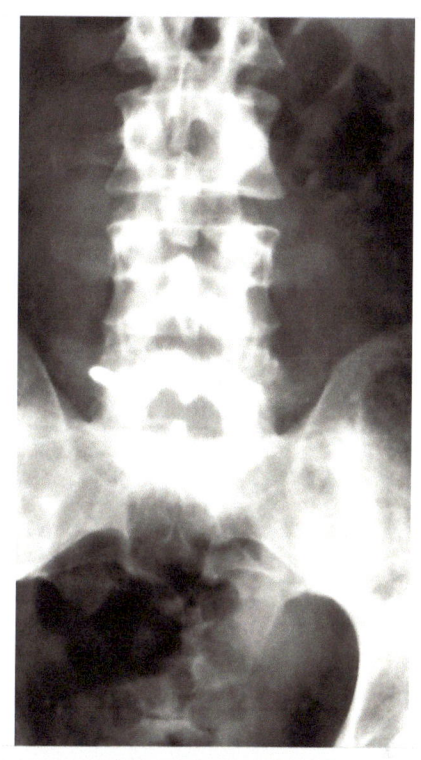

Fig. 11.33 PA radiograph of the lower lumbar spine of a young man who years earlier had undergone Buck fusions for bilateral lyses. He continued to complain of the same low back pain and stiffness as he did when he presented with is lyses. What's the diagnosis? Look again at the X-ray. He has got quite severe bilateral sacroiliitis indicative of ankylosing spondylitis. His clinical picture of pain and stiffness particularly in the early morning confirmed that diagnosis clinically. The Buck fusions were almost certainly unnecessary. When looking at lumbar spine films don't forget the sacroiliac joints and it is not a bad idea to look at them first so you never forget. We had removed the screws because the lyses had healed, but of course his symptoms remained.

therapy for a minimum period of 3 months, helps to prevent recurrent pain in the majority of cases but there is a hard minority whose symptoms reappear once sport is resumed. A further period of 3 months of rest and physical therapy with an antilordotic brace should be prescribed.[55] Modern day sports science, exercise physiology, and exercise physiotherapy make conservative treatment a much more structured and objective treatment regimen and that is why the results of nonoperative treatment can be so good.

For mature patients whose lyses are established nonunions, injecting with CT guidance the lysis with local anesthetic and steroids can be helpful both diagnostically and therapeutically and, rather like low grade isthmic spondylolisthesis, surgical treatment should be avoided and probably at all costs for the elite athlete.[56-58] Anyway, screw fixation across the lysis is probably the most popular method of surgical treatment and was first reported by Buck in 1970[96] (▶ Fig. 11.33) and then by Buring from Scandinavia in 1973.[97] Buck knew that placing the screw correctly was not always easy and it goes without saying that the defect should be transverse to the line of the screw and then in the middle portion of the pars. When you look carefully at CT scans of the lysis it is extraordinary how variable its position is—from being close to the pedicle at one extreme to being close to the lamina at the other. Only relatively few are central enough in the pars to be amenable to sound mechanical screw fixation and this is a very important matter for preoperative assessment.

One lysis is not an important piece of pathology and symptoms, if they are from that, will settle eventually if only surgeons desist from surgical treatment.

Surgical treatment should not be prescribed for the immature spine. The gap is filled with a zone of endochondral ossification that can do what it is supposed to do, namely ossify, if just left alone. It is for the established nonunion that surgical treatment has been carried out with varying results. In most reports the hypertrophic callus and debris have been removed and the opposing surface of the pars freshened up. Bone graft has then been applied. This is rather a strange philosophy in that while the lyses that developed with stretching of the pars in dysplastic spondylolisthesis are quite clearly atrophic nonunions, the nonunions of mature lyses that have not healed are typically hypertrophic. Treatment-wise, atrophic nonunions require bone while hypertrophic nonunions require compression which will then make the intervening nonunion material ossify, hopefully. The Nottingham Group described their surgical experience with 22 athletes, age range 15–34, many of whom were professional or elite athletes, with unilateral lyses only.[98] A total of 19 had screw fixation while 3 had the wiring technique described by Scott from Edinburgh.[99] The wire goes round the base of the transverse process above and the superior facet below and is tightened around the base of the spinous process. Again the lyses were curetted out of hypertrophic callus before grafting. All but one of the Buck's fusion patients returned to sport but the three wiring patients did not do well. This is in contrast to the Birmingham experience with Scott wiring where all 19 patients were under the age of 25 and had excellent or good results.[100] It was felt that degenerative disk disease with increasing age might be an important confounding symptomatic variable. Similar results were achieved for Scott wiring in Minneapolis.[101] Interestingly whether the lysis fused or not did not seem to relate to outcome. Meanwhile the majority of spinal surgeons do seem to favor direct screw repair. In 2014 the Miami group reported on 16 patients with no implant failures and only one failed fusion with all eight athletes returning to sport.[102] Again there was a suggestion that in an older age group degenerative disk disease might be the cause of back pain indistinguishable from that of a lysis (very convenient). The problem of course is trying to say with authority that the lysis or lyses is the cause of the patient's back pain or is it the stress reaction in the pars on the other side without the break which is commonly seen that is the cause of symptoms or, nearby disk degeneration or more probably, none of the above. Looking at ▶ Fig. 11.33 again this young man was on the list for removal of Buck screws from healed lyses as it was thought that they might be the cause of continuing low back pain and stiffness. Note the presence of quite severe bilateral sacroiliitis. His original symptoms in all probability were not related to his lyses but to his ankylosing spondylitis. Take a proper history and have a good look at the X-rays before contemplating lysis screws. The young man in ▶ Fig. 11.33 presented with low back pain and stiffness, still had low back pain and stiffness when he was scheduled for removal of screws and a diagnosis of ankylosing spondylitis made, still had his symptoms, was cancelled from the operating list, and at follow-up a year later still had low back pain and stiffness but had only recently started anti-inflammatory drugs from the rheumatologist.

Meanwhile in 1984 Morscher introduced his new method of treating pars defects with a special hook screw reporting on 12 patients, 10 of whom had good or excellent results.[80] Tokuhashi introduced a variation on the hook screw theme and reported on six patients[103] while Fan reported on the hook screw variation in 11 patients more on the biomechanical evaluation of the hook screw fixation but did say that excellent clinical results were achieved.[104] Chen reported on another hook screw variation on 21 patients focusing on bone union, displacement and intervertebral disk space height rather than pain and function.[105] Gillet[106] reported yet another type of rod–screw construct, reporting on their first 10 patients as regards everyday life and work rather than the Nottingham group who focused on athletes at the elite end of the spectrum and this is the crucially important patient group because a return to top level sport must be the only really excellent outcome from surgery and indeed the only acceptable result.

From the foregoing it can be said that wiring does not produce the same sort of results as either the Buck screw approach or the Morscher hook screw device. However many of the reports do not focus on the elite athlete and the evidence base does not need any more of these other sort of reports but more of the Nottingham-type elite athletes series. However for those with unilateral lesions surgery should be a last resort.

Our preferred treatment particularly for the high class sports person is to pursue proper nonoperative sports therapy for at least a year. In our experience more often than not the athlete's technique needs to be analyzed and there are now sophisticated computer techniques for this purpose. As the Nottingham group point out, a successful outcome also depends on motivation and no one is more motivated than the elite athlete. The great majority of individuals can be returned to top level physical activity by nonoperative treatment and that should be the primary goal. Patients need to earn their operation which should be regarded as failures of conservative treatment. It would be tempting to put a compression screw across the defect and see if the hypertrophic callus organizes and ossifies but top class athletes are not experimental models and so we would recommend removing redundant callus outside the lysis zone, compressing the lysis, and adding bone graft to decorticated local bone (▶ Fig. 11.33).

For those with L5 radicular irritation symptoms L5 nerve root injections should be successful to the point where removal of hypertrophic callus material should not be necessary, although surgical decompression can be prescribed for intractable L5 radicular symptoms (▶ Fig. 11.34).

11.8.2 Isthmic Spondylolisthesis

Isthmic spondylolisthesis caused by a primary stress fracture of the pars of the L5 vertebra is by far the most common type of spondylolisthesis we see in children and adolescents. It is a benign condition compared to the dysplastic form. With such a high prevalence rate it is quite clear that only a small fraction of those affected ever present clinically and the vast majority of these can be treated conservatively with surgery necessary for only a small percentage, the principal reason for which is relief of severe intractable pain. Slippage never goes beyond 50% and usually not more than about 30% so there is never a question of

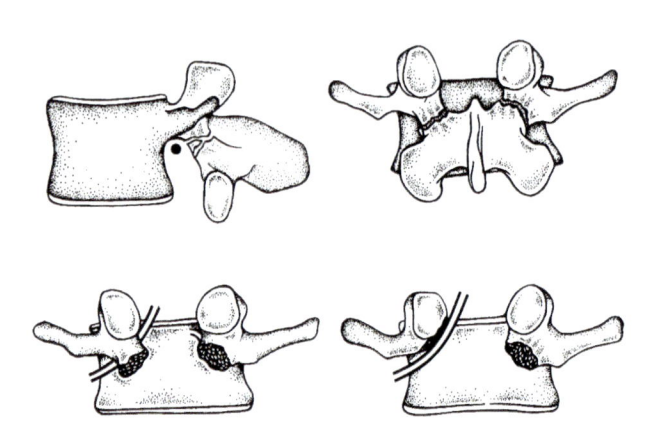

Fig. 11.34 Crock's procedure, named after the late Harry Crock, a well-known Australian senior figure in spinal surgery. He pointed out that Gill's procedure (removal of the loose fragment) would leave behind the hypertrophic callus on the pedicular side of the lysis and so was the pioneer of the extended Gill procedure.

significant deformity or worry about progression such as that which can occur with the dysplastic form, nor is reduction an issue. The pain in lytic spondylolisthesis is musculoskeletal sclerotomal and probably due to an abnormal drag on the ligaments and muscles at the back of the L5/S1 level and higher up as well.[51,56] The backache is a dull aching pain referred down the backs of the thighs, no further than the knees, and is clearly nonradicular. This is not accompanied by reflex or sensory changes in the legs neither is there muscle group weakness. Patients will often have a full range of forward flexion of the lumbar spine and normal straight leg raising. These are the typical features described by Wiltse and Hutchinson[51] who, if the pain did not settle conservatively, prescribed alar-transverse fusion using bone graft taken from the back of the pelvis harvested correctly and so not causing any donor site pain[56] (▶ Fig. 11.35) which begs the question as to the whether the seemingly much higher incidence of donor site pain and much greater disability nowadays is simply the result of not siting the approach correctly.

In the younger child or adolescent pars defects are filled with a zone of growing cartilage and therefore the L5 nerve roots that pass under the lyses are not affected and so radicular symptoms and neurological features should not be found in this age group. However in older adolescents and young adults the lysis is an established nonunion so the gap is filled with hypertrophic cartilage and debris which mass effect can irritate or compress the L5 nerve roots (▶ Fig. 11.8). Therefore an in depth history and examination are important to establish who needs surgical treatment and of what kind. To deal with the loose fragment only (Gill's procedure[107]) is of no value as the foramina through which the L5 nerve roots pass are not dealt with. To deal with the hypertrophic debris then the extended Gill procedure is required with decompression right back to the base of the pedicle[108] (▶ Fig. 11.34). As movement is also thought to be a possible provocative agent for symptoms then L5 nerve root decompression is accompanied by an alar-transverse fusion. There is no need to consider percentage slip here as progression is not a problem, nor is reduction and so an in situ fusion (▶ Fig. 11.36) is all that is required for a patient who almost certainly never knew he/she had the condition in the first place until painful activity cropped up followed by an X-ray (good or bad practice?). You can put metalwork in only if you insist. If done properly an alar-transverse fusion has a 100% fusion rate (▶ Fig. 11.36) but of course not a 100% pain success rate.

Lenke reported a series of 56 isthmic spondylolisthesis cases dealt with by in situ fusion in patients with back or leg pain

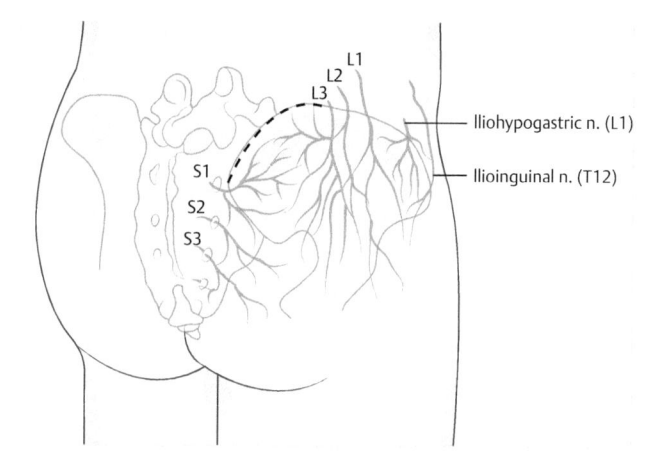

Fig. 11.35 Iliac crest incision. Note that the cluneal nerves come across the iliac crest about a handbreadth from the posterior spine. If the incision is kept well posterior and the area in front undermined, one can avoid cutting or damaging these. (Reproduced with permission from L. Wiltse, Robert Hutchinson. Surgical Treatment of Spondylolisthesis. Wolters Kluwer Health, Inc.. 2017.)

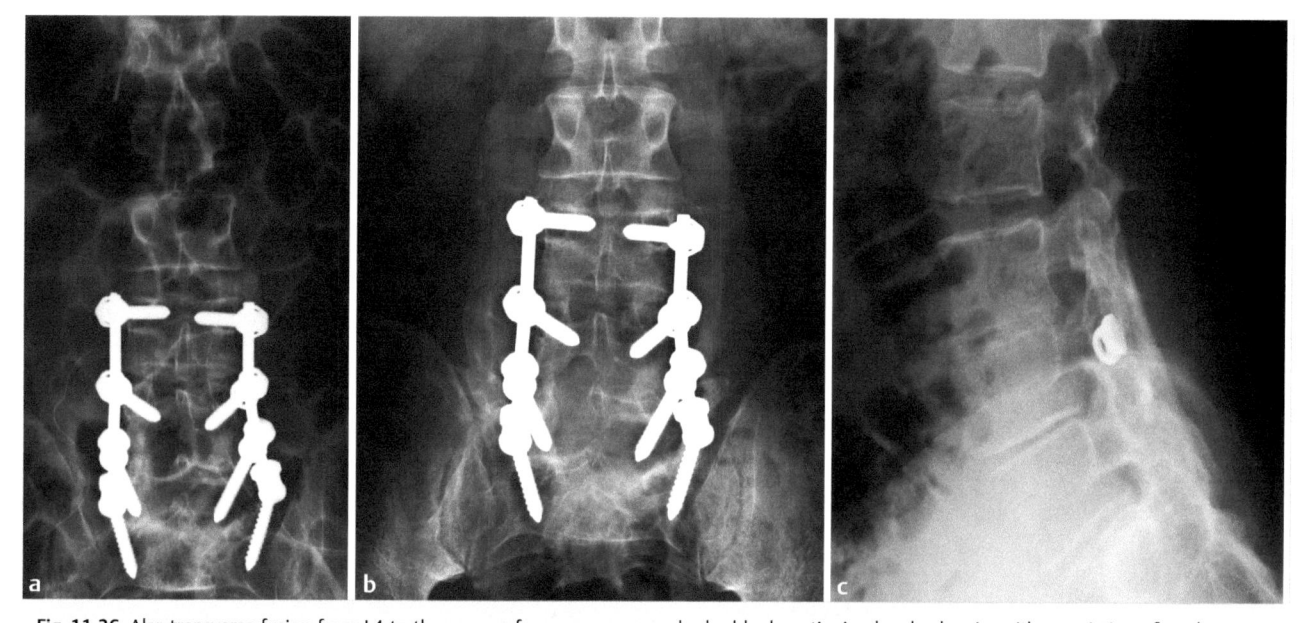

Fig. 11.36 Alar transverse fusion from L4 to the sacrum for a young man who had had continuing low back pain, with no sciatica, after three laminectomies with facet joint disruption. (a) Inclined frontal view just after the insertion of the pedicular screws and rods. (b) Inclined frontal view 4 years later showing solid intertransverse fusions from L4 to the sacrum. (c) Lateral radiograph confirming solid mass of bone from L4 to the sacrum. It was not possible to remove part of the previous metalwork construct. Mercifully, his back pain had resolved.

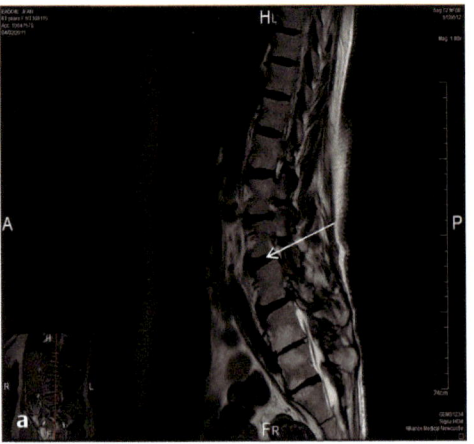

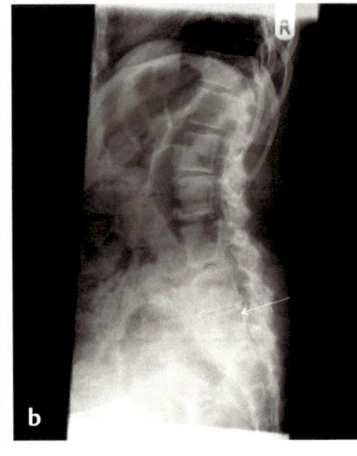

Fig. 11.37 a) MRI scan and b) xray showing an L4/5 degenerative spondylolisthesis (arrowed).

unresponsive to conservative treatment.[109] Some had severe hamstring tightness or neurological involvement and with an average age of 15.5 years would include a sample of older adolescents/young adults who might have L5 root problems and therefore included some dysplastic cases. Postoperative immobilization varied from casts to simple braces and in 47 patients followed for more than 2 years 70% had a fusion from L5 to S1 whereas 30% had a fusion from L4 to S1. These latter included some with a grade 4 slip and a kyphotic slip angle indicating that their defect was secondary to the attenuation of the pars in dysplastic spondylolisthesis and not strictly the primary stress fracture variety. At final follow-up a fifth of their patients did not have solid fusions with a slightly higher pseudarthrosis rate in the higher grade slips. It might be anticipated in the bizarre world of surgery for back pain that there is no clear relationship between failure of fusion and continuing symptoms and so it seems. Interestingly, in one series, half the successes had pseudarthroses while half the failures had sound unions![110] Discussing explanations for their lower than expected radiographic fusion rate Lenke pointed out that they used the Ferguson AP view rather than a standard AP view. This of course is very important as the Ferguson view or inclined frontal view is centered over the L5/S1 level and not the mid-lumbar region as for a standard AP of the lumbar spine (▶ Fig. 11.36). Of course a lateral view of the lumbosacral region can also confirm continuity and solidity of the fusion as in ▶ Fig. 11.36. They used the Wiltse bilateral approach[57] in most of their patients but a midline approach in a third which would be preferable for those who require laminectomy and extended Gill bilaterally.

However, hopefully with modern exercise physiology and physiotherapy approaches along with increased familiarity of this condition, surgery should be virtually preventable for this simplest form of spondylolisthesis.

11.8.3 Degenerative Spondylolisthesis

Low back pain in over 40-year-old women is very often associated with significant degenerative change in the posterior facet joints in the lumbar spine which on X-rays is found to be maximal at the L4/5 and less so at the L3/4 levels (▶ Fig. 11.37). The degenerative process itself can be painful and if the facet joints hypertrophy significantly, as is often the case, then there can be localized spinal stenosis. Commonly, however, the degenerative process in the facet joints plus their original more sagittal orientation, facilitates facet joint instability such that, at the L4/5 level, the L4 vertebra moves forward on L5 and its facet joints progressively dig into the spinal canal producing cauda equina type symptoms. Both the degree of degenerative change and the degree of cauda equina compression are well visualized on MRI scans. If symptoms are not too intrusive or neurologically concerning then conservative treatment with painkillers and physiotherapy can be useful in at least making symptoms tolerable. If, however, the pain is considerable and there are worrying cauda equina type symptoms then surgical decompression and fusion are necessary. The decompression requires complete or virtually complete removal of the L4/5 facet joints because these are the compressive agents and therefore that leaves an even more unstable articulation demanding concomitant monosegmental transpedicular fixation. When the facet joints are not so sagittally orientated instability can be seen in the frontal plane with a scoliosis apical at the L4/5 level. The cauda equina compression is therefore more on one side than the other but surgical treatment is the same—decompression and fusion and alignment of the rotated L4/5 level which not only alleviates symptoms but corrects the degenerative scoliosis.

11.8.4 Pathological Spondylolisthesis

This should also not belong to the classification of spondylolisthesis, rather slippage of one vertebra on the next is a natural accompaniment of the bone destructive process going on at that level. Treatment is therefore part and parcel of the treatment of the underlying pathological process.

References

Note: References in **bold** are Key References.

[1] Herbiniaux G. Traite sur Divers Accouchments Laborieux, et sur les Polypes de la Matrice. Bruxelles: JL DeBoubers; 1782
[2] Kilian HF. Schilderungen neuer Beckenformen und ihres Verhaltens in Leven. Mannheim: Verlag von Bassermann & Mathy; 1854
[3] Robert HLF. Eine eigenthümliche angeborene Lordose, wahrscheinlich bedingt durch eine Verschiebung des Körpers des letzten Lendenwirbels auf die vordere Fläche des ersten Kreuzbeinwirbels (Spondylolisthesis Kilian), nebst Bemerkungen über die Mechanik dieser Beckenformation. Monatschr Geburtsk FrauenKr Berl. 1855; 5:81–94
[4] Lambl W. Beitrage zur Geburtskunde und Gynackologie. Von FW v. Scanzoni, 1958

[5] Neugebauer FL. Aetiologie der sogenannten Spondylolisthesis. Arch Gynäk Munich. 1882; 35:375
[6] Meyer-Burgdorff H. Untersuchungen über das Wirbelgleiten. Leipzig: Thieme; 1931
[7] Putti V. Die angeborene Deformitäten der Wirbelsäule. Fortschr Rontgenstr. 1909; 14:284
[8] Le Double E. Traité des variations de la colonne vertébrale de L'homme et de leurs significations au point de vue de l'anthropologie zoologique. Paris: Vigot; 1912
[9] Willis TA. The separate neural arch. J Bone Joint Surg. 1931; 13:709–721
[10] Brailsford JF. Spondylolisthesis. British J Radiol. 1933; 6:666–684
[11] Brocher JEW. Die Wirbelverschiebung in der Lendengegend. Leipzig: Thieme; 1951
[12] Newman PH, Stone KH. The etiology of spondylolisthesis with a special investigation. J Bone Joint Surg. 1963; 45:39–59
[13] Taillard WF. Etiology of spondylolisthesis. Clin Orthop Relat Res. 1976 (117):30–39
[14] Wiltse LL, Newman PH, Macnab I. Classification of spondylolisis and spondylolisthesis. Clin Orthop Relat Res. 1976(117):23–29
[15] Herman MJ, Pizzutillo PD. Spondylolysis and spondylolisthesis in the child and adolescent: a new classification. Clin Orthop Relat Res. 2005 (434):46–54
[16] Marchetti PG, Bartolozzi P. Classification of spondylolisthesis as a guideline for treatment. In Bridwell KH, DeWald RL, eds. Textbook of Spinal Surgery. 2nd ed. Philadelphia: Lippincott-Raven; 1997:1211–1254
[17] Marty C, Boisaubert B, Descamps H, et al. The sagittal anatomy of the sacrum among young adults, infants, and spondylolisthesis patients. Eur Spine J. 2002; 11(2):119–125
[18] Vialle R, Schmit P, Dauzac C, Wicart P, Glorion C, Guigui P. Radiological assessment of lumbosacral dystrophic changes in high-grade spondylolisthesis. Skeletal Radiol. 2005; 34(9):528–535
[19] Jackson DW, Wiltse LL, Cirincoine RJ. Spondylolysis in the female gymnast. Clin Orthop Relat Res. 1976(117):68–73
[20] La Chapelle EH. Spondylolisthesis. Ned Tijdschr Geneeskd. 1939; 83:2005–2010
[21] Kono S, Hayashi N, Kashahara G, et al. A study on the aetiology of spondylolysis with reference to athletic activities. J Jap Orthop Assoc. 1975; 49(3):125
[22] Ferguson RJ, McMaster JH, Stanitski CL. Low back pain in college football linemen. J Sports Med. 1974; 2(2):63–69
[23] Roland M, van Tulder M. Should radiologists change the way they report plain radiography of the spine? Lancet. 1998; 352(9123):229–230
[24] Wynne-Davies R, Scott JHS. Inheritance and spondylolisthesis: a radiographic family survey. J Bone Joint Surg Br. 1979; 61-B(3):301–305
[25] Stewart TD. [The age incidence of neural-arch defects in Alaskan natives, considered from the standpoint of etiology]. J Bone Joint Surg Am. 1953; 35-A(4):937–950
[26] Eisenstein S. Spondylolysis. A skeletal investigation of two population groups. J Bone Joint Surg Br. 1978; 60-B(4):488–494
[27] Baker DR, McHollick W. Spondyloschisis and spondylolisthesis in children. J Bone Joint Surg. 1956; 38A:933–934
[28] Rankine JJ, Dickson RA. Unilateral spondylolysis and the presence of facet joint tropism. Spine. 2010; 35(21):E1111–E1114
[29] Farfan HF, Osteria V, Lamy C. The mechanical etiology of spondylolysis and spondylolisthesis. Clin Orthop Relat Res. 1976(117):40–55
[30] Kraus H. Effect of lordosis on the stress in the lumbar spine. Clin Orthop Relat Res. 1976(117):56–58
[31] Troup JDG. Mechanical factors in spondylolisthesis and spondylolysis. Clin Orthop Relat Res. 1976(117):59–67
[32] Shah JS, Hampson WGJ, Jayson MIV. The distribution of surface strain in the cadaveric lumbar spine. J Bone Joint Surg Br. 1978; 60-B(2):246–251
[33] Pfeil E. Spondylolysis und Spondylolisthesis bei Kindern. Z Orthop Ihre Grenzgeb. 1971; 109(1):17–33
[34] Bernick S, Cailliet R. Vertebral end-plate changes with aging of human vertebrae. Spine. 1982; 7(2):97–102
[35] Junghanns H. Spondylolisthesis ohne Spalt im Zwischengdenk-Stück. Arch Orthop Unfallchir. 1931; 29:118–127
[36] Newman PH. Spondylolisthesis, its cause and effect. Ann R Coll Surg Engl. 1955; 16(5):305–323
[37] Rosenberg NJ. Degenerative spondylolisthesis. Predisposing factors. J Bone Joint Surg Am. 1975; 57(4):467–474
[38] Farfan HF. The pathological anatomy of degenerative spondylolisthesis. A cadaver study. Spine. 1980; 5(5):412–418
[39] Berlemann U, Jeszenszky DJ, Bühler DW, Harms J. The role of lumbar lordosis, vertebral end-plate inclination, disc height, and facet orientation in degenerative spondylolisthesis. J Spinal Disord. 1999; 12(1):68–73
[40] Berlemann U, Jeszenszky DJ, Bühler DW, Harms J. Facet joint remodeling in degenerative spondylolisthesis: an investigation of joint orientation and tropism. Eur Spine J. 1998; 7(5):376–380
[41] Tietjen R, Morgenstern JM. Spondylolisthesis following surgical fusion for scoliosis: a case report. Clin Orthop Relat Res. 1976(117):176–178
[42] Wiltse LL, Winter RB. Terminology and measurement of spondylolisthesis. J Bone Joint Surg Am. 1983; 65(6):768–772
[43] Taillard W. Le spondylolisthesis chez l'enfant et l'adolescent. Acta Orthop Scand. 1954; 24(2):115–144
[44] Meyerding HW. Spondylolisthesis: surgical treatment and results. Surg Gynecol Obstet. 1932; 54:371–377
[45] Schwab FJ, Farcy JP, Roye DP, Jr. The sagittal pelvic tilt index as a criterion in the evaluation of spondylolisthesis. Preliminary observations. Spine. 1997; 22(14):1661–1667
[46] Rajnics P, Templier A, Skalli W, Lavaste F, Illés T. The association of sagittal spinal and pelvic parameters in asymptomatic persons and patients with isthmic spondylolisthesis. J Spinal Disord Tech. 2002; 15(1):24–30
[47] Labelle H, Roussouly P, Berthonnaud E, Dimnet J, O'Brien M. The importance of spino-pelvic balance in L5-s1 developmental spondylolisthesis: a review of pertinent radiologic measurements. Spine. 2005; 30(6) Suppl:S27–S34
[48] Mac-Thiong J-M, Labelle H. A proposal for a surgical classification of pediatric lumbosacral spondylolisthesis based on current literature. Eur Spine J. 2006; 15(10):1425–1435
[49] Mac-Thiong J-M, Labelle H, Parent S, Hresko MT, Deviren V, Weidenbaum M, members of the Spinal Deformity Study Group. Reliability and development of a new classification of lumbosacral spondylolisthesis. Scoliosis. 2008; 3:19–27
[50] Li Y, Hresko MT. Radiographic analysis of spondylolisthesis and sagittal spinopelvic deformity. J Am Acad Orthop Surg. 2012; 20:194–205
[51] Wiltse LL, Hutchinson RH. Surgical treatment of spondylolisthesis. Clin Orthop Relat Res. 1964; 35(35):116–135
[52] Phalen GS, Dickson JA. Spondylolisthesis and tight hamstrings. J Bone Joint Surg. 1961; 43(A):505–512
[53] Harris RI. Spondylolisthesis. Ann R Coll Engl. 1951; 8(4):259–297
[54] Newman PH. A clinical syndrome associated with severe lumbo-sacral subluxation. J Bone Joint Surg Br. 1965; 47:472–481
[55] Pizzutillo PD, Hummer CD, III. Nonoperative treatment for painful adolescent spondylolysis or spondylolisthesis. J Pediatr Orthop. 1989; 9 (5):538–540
[56] Steiner ME, Micheli LJ. Treatment of symptomatic spondylolysis and spondylolisthesis with the modified Boston brace. Spine. 1985; 10(10):937–943
[57] Wiltse LL, Jackson DW. Treatment of spondylolisthesis and spondylolysis in children. Clin Orthop Relat Res. 1976(117):92–100
[58] Boxall D, Bradford DS, Winter RB, Moe JH. Management of severe spondylolisthesis in children and adolescents. J Bone Joint Surg Am. 1979; 61 (4):479–495
[59] Peek RD, Wiltse LL, Reynolds JB, Thomas JC, Guyer DW, Widell EH. In situ arthrodesis without decompression for Grade-III or IV isthmic spondylolisthesis in adults who have severe sciatica. J Bone Joint Surg Am. 1989; 71 (1):62–68
[60] Seitsalo S, Osterman K, Hyvärinen H, Schlenzka D, Poussa M. Severe spondylolisthesis in children and adolescents. A long-term review of fusion in situ. J Bone Joint Surg Br. 1990; 72(2):259–265
[61] Boos N, Marchesi D, Zuber K, Aebi M. Treatment of severe spondylolisthesis by reduction and pedicular fixation. A 4-6-year follow-up study. Spine. 1993; 18(12):1655–1661
[62] Poussa M, Schlenzka D, Seitsalo S, Ylikoski M, Hurri H, Osterman K. Surgical treatment of severe isthmic spondylolisthesis in adolescents. Reduction or fusion in situ. Spine. 1993; 18(7):894–901
[63] Roca J, Ubierna MT, Cáceres E, Iborra M. One-stage decompression and posterolateral and interbody fusion for severe spondylolisthesis. An analysis of 14 patients. Spine. 1999; 24(7):709–714
[64] Molinari RW, Bridwell KH, Lenke LG, Ungacta FF, Riew KD. Complications in the surgical treatment of pediatric high-grade, isthmic dysplastic spondylolisthesis. A comparison of three surgical approaches. Spine. 1999; 24(16):1701–1711
[65] Seitsalo S, Osterman K, Hyvärinen H, Tallroth K, Schlenzka D, Poussa M. Progression of spondylolisthesis in children and adolescents. A long-term follow-up of 272 patients. Spine. 1991; 16(4):417–421

[66] Maurice HD, Morley TR. Cauda equina lesions following fusion in situ and decompressive laminectomy for severe spondylolisthesis. Four case reports. Spine. 1989; 14(2):214–216

[67] Schoenecker PL, Cole HO, Herring JA, Capelli AM, Bradford DS. Cauda equina syndrome after in situ arthrodesis for severe spondylolisthesis at the lumbosacral junction. J Bone Joint Surg Am. 1990; 72(3):369–377

[68] Molinari RW, Bridwell KH, Lenke LG, Baldus C. Anterior column support in surgery for high-grade, isthmic spondylolisthesis. Clin Orthop Relat Res. 2002(394):109–120

[69] Bradford DS, Boachie-Adjei O. Treatment of severe spondylolisthesis by anterior and posterior reduction and stabilization. A long-term follow-up study. J Bone Joint Surg Am. 1990; 72(7):1060–1066

[70] Ani N, Keppler L, Biscup RS, Steffee AD. Reduction of high-grade slips (grades III-V) with VSP instrumentation. Report of a series of 41 cases. Spine. 1991; 16(6) Suppl:S302–S310

[71] Bartolozzi P, Sandri A, Cassini M, Ricci M. One-stage posterior decompression-stabilization and trans-sacral interbody fusion after partial reduction for severe L5-S1 spondylolisthesis. Spine. 2003; 28(11):1135–1141

[72] Petraco DM, Spivak JM, Cappadona JG, Kummer FJ, Neuwirth MG. An anatomic evaluation of L5 nerve stretch in spondylolisthesis reduction. Spine. 1996; 21(10):1133–1138, discussion 1139

[73] Scaglietti O, Frontino G, Bartolozzi P. Technique of anatomical reduction of lumbar spondylolisthesis and its surgical stabilization. Clin Orthop Relat Res. 1976(117):165–175

[74] Carpenter N. Spondylolisthesis. Br J Surg. 1932; 19:374–386

[75] Jenkins JA. Spondylolisthesis. Br J Surg. 1936; 24:80–85

[76] Freebody D, Bendall R, Taylor RD. Anterior transperitoneal lumbar fusion. J Bone Joint Surg Br. 1971; 53(4):617–627

[77] Harrington PR, Tullos HS. Spondylolisthesis in children. Observations and surgical treatment. Clin Orthop Relat Res. 1971; 79(79):75–84

[78] Michel C. Réduction et fixation des spondylolisthesis et des spondyloptoses. Rev Chir Orthop. 1971; 57 Supplement 1:148–157

[79] Vidal J, Allieu Y, Fassio B, Adrey J, Goalard C. Le Spondylisthesis. Réduction par le matériel de Harrington. Rev Chir Orthop Repar Appar Mot. 1973; 59(1):21–41

[80] Morscher E. Zweizeitige Reposition und Stabilisation der Spondyloptose mit dem Harrington-Instrumentarium und vorderer interkorporeller Spondylodese. Arch Orthop Unfallchir. 1975; 83(3):323–334

[81] Harrington PR, Dickson JH. Spinal instrumentation in the treatment of severe progressive spondylolisthesis. Clin Orthop Relat Res. 1976(117):157–163

[82] Snijder JGN, Seroo JM, Snijder CJ, Schijvens AWM. Therapy of spondylolisthesis by repositioning and fixation of the olisthetic vertebra. Clin Orthop Relat Res. 1976(117):149–156

[83] Verbiest H. Spondylolisthesis: the value of radicular signs and symptoms. A study based on surgical experience and treatment. J Int Coll Surg. 1963; 39:461–481

[84] Bradford DS. Treatment of severe spondylolisthesis. A combined approach for reduction and stabilization. Spine. 1979; 4(5):423–429

[85] McPhee IB, O'Brien JP. Reduction of severe spondylolisthesis. A preliminary report. Spine. 1979; 4(5):430–434

[86] DeWald RL, Faut MM, Taddonio RF, Neuwirth MG. Severe lumbosacral spondylolisthesis in adolescents and children. Reduction and staged circumferential fusion. J Bone Joint Surg Am. 1981; 63(4):619–626

[87] Bohlman HH, Cook SS. One-stage decompression and posterolateral and interbody fusion for lumbosacral spondyloptosis through a posterior approach. Report of two cases. J Bone Joint Surg Am. 1982; 64(3):415–418

[88] Gaines RW, Nichols WK. Treatment of spondyloptosis by two stage L5 vertebrectomy and reduction of L4 onto S1. Spine. 1985; 10(7):680–686

[89] Ruf M, Koch H, Melcher RP, Harms J. Anatomic reduction and monosegmental fusion in high-grade developmental spondylolisthesis. Spine. 2006; 31(3):269–274

[90] Leatherman KD, Dickson RA. The Management of Spinal Deformities. London. John Wright; 1988

[91] Gordon Deen H. The "open book" technique for preparation of the lumbar transverse process for posterolateral fusion. J Neurosurg. 2000; 93(2) Suppl:332–334

[92] Dickson RA, Rao A. Letter to the Editor re The "open book" technique for preparation of the lumbar transverse process for posterolateral fusion. J Neurosurg (Spine 2) 2000;93:332–334. J Neurosurg Spine, Neurosurgical Forum, 2000;95:281

[93] Carragee EJ. Clinical practice. Persistent low back pain. N Engl J Med. 2005; 352(18):1891–1898

[94] Carragee EJ. The role of surgery in low back pain. Curr Orthopaedics. 2007; 21(1):9–16

[95] Pither C. Optimising non-operative care. Curr Orthop. 2007; 21(1):1–8

[96] Buck JE. Direct repair of the defect in spondylolisthesis. Preliminary report. J Bone Joint Surg Br. 1970; 52(3):432–437

[97] Buring K, Fredensborg N. Osteosynthesis of spondylolysis. Acta Orthop Scand. 1973; 44:91–92

[98] Debnath UK, Freeman BJ, Grevitt MP, Sithole J, Scammell BE, Webb JK. Clinical outcome of symptomatic unilateral stress injuries of the lumbar pars interarticularis. Spine. 2007; 32(9):995–1000

[99] Scott JHS. The Edinburgh repair of isthmic (Group II) spondylolysis. J Bone Joint Surg Br. 1987; 69:491

[100] Johnson GV, Thompson AG. The Scott wiring technique for direct repair of lumbar spondylolysis. J Bone Joint Surg Br. 1992; 74(3):426–430

[101] Bradford DS, Iza J. Repair of the defect in spondylolysis or minimal degrees of spondylolisthesis by segmental wire fixation and bone grafting. Spine. 1985; 10(7):673–679

[102] Snyder LA, Shufflebarger H, O'Brien MF, Thind H, Theodore N, Kakarla UK. Spondylolysis outcomes in adolescence after direct screw repair of the pars interarticularis. J Neurosurg Spine. 2014; 21(3):329–333

[103] Tokuhashi Y, Matsuzaki H. Repair of defects in spondylolysis by segmental pedicular screw hook fixation. A preliminary report. Spine. 1996; 21(17):2041–2045

[104] Fan J, Yu GR, Liu S, Zhao J, Zhao WD. Direct repair of spondylolysis by TSRH's hook plus screw fixation and bone grafting: biomechanical study and clinical report. Arch Orthop Trauam Surg. 2010; 130(2):209–215

[105] Chen XS, Zhou SY, Jia LS, Gu XM, Fang L, Zhu W. A universal pedicle screw and V-rod system for lumbar isthmic spondylolysis: a retrospective analysis of 21 cases. PLoS One. 2013; 8(5):e63713

[106] Gillet P, Petit M. Direct repair of spondylolysis without spondylolisthesis, using a rod-screw construct and bone grafting of the pars defect. Spine. 1999; 24(12):1252–1256

[107] Gill GG, Manning JG, White HL. Surgical treatment of spondylolisthesis without spine fusion; excision of the loose lamina with decompression of the nerve roots. J Bone Joint Surg. 1955; 37A:493

[108] Crock HV. Normal and pathological anatomy of the lumbar spinal nerve root canals. J Bone Joint Surg. 1983; 65A:768–772

[109] Lenke LG, Bridwell KH, Bullis D, Betz RR, Baldus C, Schoenecker PL. Results of in situ fusion for isthmic spondylolisthesis. J Spinal Disord. 1992; 5(4):433–442

[110] Flynn JC, Hoque MA. Anterior fusion of the lumbar spine. End-result study with long-term follow-up. J Bone Joint Surg Am. 1979; 61(8):1143–1150

Index

Note: Page numbers set **bold** or *italic* indicate headings or figures, respectively.

A

AAI, *see* Atlantoaxial instability (AAI)
Achondroplasia 30, *280*, **280**, *281–283*
Adjacent segment degeneration, in late-onset idiopathic scoliosis 81
Age, bone 21
Aneurysmal bone cyst 266
Anterior cerebral artery 177
Anterior communicating artery 177
Anterior inferior cerebellar artery 177
Anterior instrumentation, in history of spinal deformity surgery *8*, **8**
Anterior longitudinal ligament, in idiopathic scoliosis 42, *42*
Anterior multiple diskectomy, *see* Anterior release
– in late-onset idiopathic scoliosis **102**, *114–115*, **115**, *116*
–– with posterior instrumentation **122**, *123–124*, **124**, *125*
– in Scheuermann's disease **146**, *147–148*
Anterior release, *see* Anterior multiple diskectomy, Leeds procedure
– as term 9
– in cerebral palsy 221
– in Leeds procedure 56, 83
– in Scheuermann's disease **143**, *151*
– pedicle screws and 102
Anterior spinal artery 177
Apert's syndrome **199**, *201*
Apical vertebral resection (AVR)
– in congenital scoliosis **170**, *172–175*, *177*
– in late-onset idiopathic scoliosis **104**, *106–107*
– in Scheuermann's disease **149**, *151*
Arachnodactyly 70
Arnold-Chiari syndrome 196
Arthrogryposis **225**
Atlantoaxial instability (AAI), in Morquio's syndrome **277**, *278*

B

Basilar artery 177
Becker muscular dystrophy **226**
Body mass index (BMI), late onset idiopathic scoliosis aid 71, *72*
Bone age measurement 21
Bone anomaly(ies)
– congenital **159**, *160–178*
–– *See also* Congenital deformities
– congenital scoliosis as **160**, *161–178*
– formation failure in 159
– kyphosis in 160
– lordotic 160
– segmentation failure in 159
– types of 159
Bone dysplasias 26, 30, 32
Boston brace 77
Bracing, *see* Boston brace, Milwaukee brace
– in late-onset idiopathic scoliosis 75, *76*, 77
– in Morquio's syndrome **277**, *278*
– in poliomyelitis 222
– in Scheuermann's disease *140–141*, **141**
– in spondylolisthesis 302
Brittle bone syndrome, *see* Osteogenesis imperfecta (OI)
Butterfly vertebra 158, *159*, 184

C

Carotid sinus 175
Casts
– elongation derotation flexion *76*, *110*, **110**
– Minerva 2
CD, *see* Cotrel-Dubousset (CD) instrumentation
Center sacral line (CSL) 73–74
Center sacral vertical line (CSVL) 73, *73*, 74
Centile charts **23**, *25*
Cerebral palsy (CP)
– anterior release in 221
– causes of 216
– classification of 216
– defined 216
– gait in 217
– Galveston technique in **220**, *220*
– Harrington technique in 218
– hemiplegia in 216
– Luque segmental L-rod instrumentation in *219*, 220
– orthopaedic principles in **217**, *218*
– osteotomies in 221
– pedicle screws in 221
– spinal dysraphism vs. 193
– spine in **218**, *219*
– Zielke procedure in 218
Cervical spine deformities, in neurofibromatosis **247**, *249*
– *See also* Atlantoaxial instability (AAI)
Charcot-Marie-Tooth disease **225**, 229
Circle of Willis 177
Classification
– of cerebral palsy 216
– of congenital kyphosis **184**, *184*
– of late-onset idiopathic scoliosis **71**, *72*, *73–74*
– of neuromuscular disorders 216
– of spinal deformities **26**, **127**
– of spondylolisthesis **288**, *291*, **294**, *296*, *297–299*, **299**, *300*
Cobb angle 16, *18*, 53–54
– in late-onset idiopathic scoliosis 70, 80
– in thoracic insufficiency syndrome 199
– in treatment conceptualizations 53, 56
– measurement of 15, *18*, 80
Common carotid artery 175
Community, scoliosis in 64
Congenital cord deformities **187**, *190–194*
Congenital deformities
– as structural deformities 26, **28**, *30–31*
– case gallery *204*, **204**, *205–210*
– clinical spectrum of 159
– developmental basis of **154**, *156*
– etiology of **154**, *155–159*
– failure of formation in *30*, *156*, **156**, *157*, 159
– failure of segmentation in *156–157*, **157**, 159, 181
– genetics in **203**
– notochord anomalies in *157*, *158–159*
– of bone **159**, *160–178*
– pathogenesis of *156*, **156**, *157–159*
– syndromes with *197*, **197**, *198–202*
– treatment concepts in 59
Congenital kyphosis **180**, *183–193*
– butterfly vertebra in 184
– classification of **184**, *184*
– natural history in **181**, *184–186*
– of myelomeningocele **191**, *192–193*
Congenital lordosis 191
Congenital muscular dystrophy **227**
Congenital myopathies **227**
Congenital scoliosis
– formation failures in 162
– growth spurts and 160
– hemivertebra resection and posterior instrumentation in **176**, *180–183*
– in spinal cord deformities **188**, *189–191*
– natural history in **160**, *161–162*
– progression potential in 160–161
– sagittal plane in **161**, *162–163*
– segmentation failure in 160, *162*
– thoracic spine in 163
– treatment of **163**, *166–179*
– unilateral anomalies in 160
Connective tissue disorders **270**, *270*, *271–279*
Contralateral bar **170**, *172*, *206*, **206**
Coronal plane 14, *14*
Costs, of screening 65
Cotrel-Dubousset (CD) instrumentation
– in history of spinal deformity surgery *7*, **7**
– in neurofibromatosis 242
– in Scheuermann's disease **143**, *145*
CP, *see* Cerebral palsy (CP)
Crankshaft phenomenon 47
Crouzon's syndrome **199**, *201*
CSL, *see* Center sacral line (CSL)
CSVL, *see* Center sacral vertical line (CSVL)
Curve characteristics **15**, *18–25*, *188–190*
Curve patterns **17**, *22–25*
– in late-onset idiopathic scoliosis **80**, *82*, *83–101*
Curve size **15**, *18–19*

D

Decompensation 19, *23*, 57
Definitions
– in early-onset scoliosis screening **65**, *65*, *66*
– in spinal deformities generally **14**
Déjérine-Sottas disease **225**
Development, normal **20**, *25*, *46*, **154**, *155–156*

Diastematomyelia 192
– *See also* Spinal dysraphism
Diplomyelia 158
DMD, *see* Duchenne muscular dystrophy (DMD)
Double curves, in late-onset scoliosis **93**, *94–101*, **127**, *127*
– thoracic **94**, *95–96*
– thoracolumbar **96**, *98–100*, **128**, *128*, *129*
Duchenne muscular dystrophy (DMD) **226**, **227**, *231–232*, **232**
Dwyer procedure
– in history of spinal deformity surgery *8*, **8**
– in poliomyelitis **223**, *223*
Dysraphism, *see* Spinal dysraphism

E

Early-onset idiopathic scoliosis (EOIS)
– as structural deformity **24**, *28*
– case gallery *115*, **115**, *116–130*
– clinical features of 88, **106**, *108*, *108–109*
– elongation derotation flexion casts in *110*, **110**
– etiology of 108
– gender in 108
– growing rods in **111**, *112–113*
– infantile *107–108*
– juvenile 108
– natural history in **66**, *67–68*
– operative treatment of *111*, **111**, *112–114*
– pain in 68
– progression of, curve size and **66**, 68
– rib vertebra angle difference in 109
– Risser sign in 67
– screening for **65**, *65*, *66*, *67*
– treatment concepts in 58
– vertebral body expandable prosthetic titanium rib in *114*, **114**
– vertebral body stapling in **113**, *114*
Eating disorders 71, *72*
Ectoderm *154–155*, *155*
Ehlers-Danlos syndrome 30
Elongation derotation flexion (EDF) casts *76*, *110*, **110**
Embryonic adhesions 156
Endoderm 155, *156*
EOIS, *see* Early-onset idiopathic scoliosis (EOIS)
Eosinophilic granuloma **266**, *266*
Etiology
– in idiopathic scoliosis **38**, *38*
– of congenital deformities **154**, *155–159*
– of idiopathic scoliosis 38, *38*, 40, *41*, **42**, *43*, 44, *44–47*
–– early-onset 108
– of spondylolisthesis *288*, **288**, *289–293*
– treatment and *53–59*
Euler's law 38, 45, 47, 66
Experimental models *47*, *48–52*
External carotid artery 175
Extradural tumors 32, *254*, **260**, *262–264*

311

Index

F

Facial artery 175
Facioscapulohumeral myopathy 227
Familial dysautonomia 227
Ferguson's angle 293, 295
Formation failure, in congenital deformities 30, 156, **156**, *157*, 159, 162
Forward bend test 42
Freeman-Sheldon whistling face syndrome 201
Friedrich's ataxia 193, **225**, **226**, 229

G

Gait
- in cerebral palsy 217
- in idiopathic scoliosis 70

Galveston technique, in cerebral palsy 220, *220*
Gender
- in early-onset idiopathic scoliosis 108
- spinal dysraphism and 192

Genetics
- in Scheuermann's disease in 136, *136*
- in spinal muscular atrophy 224
- in spinal shape 46, *47*

Genetics, in congenital deformities 203
Giant cell tumor 263, *264–265*
Goldenhar syndrome 199, *201*
Gower's sign 227, *227*
Grafts, rib, in Scheuermann's disease 145
Growing rods
- in early-onset idiopathic scoliosis 111, *112–113*
- in spinal muscular atrophy 228

Growth, spinal 20, *25*, 46, 154, *155–156*

H

Harrington technique
- in cerebral palsy 218
- in history of spinal deformity surgery 3, *4*
- in poliomyelitis 222

Hemifacial dysplasia 199, *201*
Hemiplegia, in cerebral palsy 216
Hemivertebra 205
- dorsal 28, *30*
- fetal detection of 163, *164*
- in case study 204, **204**, *205–206*, **206**
- in congenital scoliosis 160
- in pathogenesis of congenital vertebral malformations 156, *157*
- multiple 204, **204**, *205*
- notochord and *157*
- rotation and 14, *17*
- with contralateral bar 206, **206**

Hemivertebra resection and posterior instrumentation, in congenital scoliosis 176, *180–183*
History, of spinal deformity surgery
- anterior instrumentation in 8, *8*
- early days of 2, *3*
- posterior instrumentation in 3, *4–6*

Holt-Oram syndrome 199
Homocystinuria 30
Hunter's syndrome 30

Hurler's syndrome 30
Hypertrophic polyneuritis 225
Hysterical scoliosis 36

I

Iatrogenic deformities 30
Idiopathic deformities 24, *28–29*
Idiopathic kyphosis 28, *29*
Idiopathic scoliosis
- anterior longitudinal ligament in 42, *42*
- as structural deformity 24, *28*
- differential diagnosis of 129, *130*
- early-onset
-- as structural deformity 24, *28*
-- case gallery 115, **115**, *116–130*
-- clinical features of 88, 106, 108, *108–109*
-- elongation derotation flexion casts in 110, *110*
-- etiology of 108
-- gender in 108
-- growing rods in 111, *112–113*
-- infantile 107–108
-- juvenile 108
-- natural history in 66, *67–68*
-- operative treatment of *111*, **111**, *112–114*
-- pain in 68
-- progression of, curve size and 66, *68*
-- Risser sign in 67
-- screening for 65, **65**, *66*, 67
-- treatment concepts in 58
-- vertebral body expandable prosthetic titanium rib in 114, **114**
-- vertebral body stapling in 113, *114*
- essential lesion in 42, 44
- etiology of 38, *38*, 40, *41*, *42*, *43*, 44, *44–47*
-- early-onset 108
- imaging of 44, 70, *79*
-- in community 64
-- kyphosis in 44
- late-onset
-- adjacent segment deterioration in 81
-- anterior diskectomy with posterior instrumentation in 122, *123–124*, **124**, *125*
-- anterior instrumentation only in 116, *117*, **117**, *118–120*
-- anterior multiple diskectomy in 102, *114–115*, **115**, *116*
-- apical vertebral resection in 104, *106–107*
-- as structural deformity 25, *28*
-- classification of 71, *72*, *73–74*
-- clinical presentation of 68, *69–70*, *72*
-- Cobb angle in 70, 80
-- curve patterns in 80, *82*, *83–101*
-- differential diagnosis of 69, *69*
-- double curves in 93, *94–101*, 127, **127**
--- thoracolumbar 96, *98–100*, 128, **128**, *129*
-- eating disorders and 71, *72*
-- epidemiology of 64, **64**
-- evaluation of 68, *69–70*, *72*
-- imaging of 70, *79*
-- in screening 65

-- intraoperative traction in 101
-- large curves in, in adolescents 99
-- lowest instrumented vertebra in 83, *85–86*, 91
-- lumbar curves in 91, *92–93*
-- magnetic resonance imaging in 79
-- Marfan syndrome vs. 70
-- neurofibromatosis vs. 70
-- nonoperative treatment of 75, *76*, *77*
-- osteotomies in 102, *103–104*, *106–107*
-- pain in 69
-- pedicle subtraction osteotomy in *104*, **104**
-- Ponte osteotomy in 103, *104*
-- posterior instrumentation only in 121, **121**, *122*, **122**
-- pseudokyphosis in 75
-- shoulder balance in *85*, 90
-- single curves in 83, **83**, *84–93*
-- Smith-Peterson osteotomy in 102, *103*
-- surgical treatment of 78
-- thoracic curves in 83, **83**, *84–91*
--- double 94, *95–96*
-- thoracolumbar curves in 91, *92–93*, **124**, *126*
--- double curves in 96, *98–100*
-- treatment of 75, *76*, *77*
-- triple curves in 97
-- tumor vs. 69, *69*
-- upper instrumented vertebra in 90, *91*
- sagittal plane in 45
- screening 46
- spinal growth and 46
- spinal lengths and 42–43
- thoracic lordosis in 44, 47, 53
- vertebral body heights in 43–44

Imaging
- of idiopathic scoliosis 44, 70
-- late-onset 79
- of intradural tumors 255, *258*
- of neurofibromatosis 239, *240*, 243
- of osteoid osteoma 263
- of Scheuermann's disease 139
- of spondylolisthesis 288, **288**, *289–293*

Implants, in history of spinal deformity surgery 2
Indices of maturity 20, *25*
Infection, deformity due to 26, *32*, *34*
Internal carotid artery 175, *177*
Intersegmental rotation 58, *59*
Intradural tumors 32, 195, 254, **254**, **254**, 255, *256*, *257*, *258*
Intraoperative traction, in late-onset idiopathic scoliosis 101
Intraspinal lipoma 192
Intratransverse fusion, for spondylolisthesis 304, *305–307*
Irritative lesions 36

K

King classification 72–73
Klippel-Feil syndrome 197, **197**, *198*
Kyphosis
- congenital 180, *183–193*
-- butterfly vertebra in 184
-- classification of 184, *184*
-- natural history in 181, *184–186*

-- of myelomeningocele 191, *192–193*
- in achondroplasia 281, *282*
- in bone anomalies 160
- in idiopathic scoliosis 44
- in Morquio;s syndrome 277
- in neurofibromatosis 240, **245**, *246*, *249*, *250*
- in normal growth 45, *45*, 46
- in Scheuermann's disease 136, *136*
-- See also Scheuermann's disease
- in spinal deformity classification 26
- in spondylolisthesis 293, *294*
- in treatment 54, *55*
- postlaminectomy 260, *261*
- pseudokyphosis measurement 17

L

Labyrinthine artery 177
Larsen's syndrome 199, *201*
Late-onset idiopathic scoliosis (LOIS)
- acceptable deformity in 71
- adjacent segment deterioration in 81
- anterior diskectomy with posterior instrumentation in 122, *123–124*, **124**, *125*
- anterior instrumentation only in 116, *117*, **117**, *118–120*
- anterior multiple diskectomy in 102, *114–115*, **115**, *116*
- apical vertebral resection in 104, *106–107*
- as structural deformity 25, *28*
- classification of 71, *72*, *73–74*
- clinical presentation of 68, *69–70*, *72*
- Cobb angle in 70, 80
- curve patterns in 80, *82*, *83–101*
- differential diagnosis of 69, *69*
- double curves in 93, *94–101*, 127, **127**
-- thoracolumbar 96, *98–100*, 128, **128**, *129*
- eating disorders and 71, *72*
- epidemiology of 64, **64**
- evaluation of 68, *69–70*, *72*
- imaging of 70, *79*
- in screening 65
- intraoperative traction in 101
- larger curves in, in adolescents 99
- lowest instrumented vertebra in 83, *85–86*, 91
- lumbar curves in 91, *92–93*
- magnetic resonance imaging in 79
- Marfan syndrome vs. 70
- nonoperative treatment of 75, *76*, *77*
- osteotomies in 102, *103–104*, *106–107*
- pain in 69
- pedicle subtraction osteotomy in *104*, **104**
- Ponte osteotomy in 103, *104*
- posterior instrumentation only in 121, **121**, *122*, **122**
- pseudokyphosis in 75
- shoulder balance in *85*, 90
- single curves in 83, **83**, *84–93*
- Smith-Peterson osteotomy in 102, *103*
- surgical treatment of 78
- thoracic curves in 83, **83**, *84–91*
-- double 94, *95–96*

Index

- – thoracolumbar curves in 91, *92–93*, **124**, *126*
- – – double curves in **96**, *98–100*
- – – treatment of **75**, *76*, 77
- – – triple curves in **97**
- – – tumor vs. 69, *69*
- – – upper instrumented vertebra in 90, *91*
- Leatherman two-stage wedge resection, in history of spinal deformity surgery 8, *8*, *166*
- Leeds procedure
- – and etiology of scoliosis 43
- – development of 54
- – in history of spinal deformity surgery 3, *6*
- – in pseudoachondroplasia 283
- – results with 88
- Lenke classification 73–74
- Limb girdle muscular dystrophy **227**
- Lingual artery *175*
- Lipoma, intraspinal 192
- LOIS, *see* Late-onset idiopathic scoliosis (LOIS)
- Lordosis
- – congenital **191**
- – in congenital deformities 160
- – in neurofibromatosis 241
- – thoracic
- – – in idiopathic scoliosis 44, 47, 53
- – – natural 14, *15*
- Lumbar agenesis **201**, *202*
- Lumbar curves, in late-onset idiopathic scoliosis 91, *92–93*
- Lumbosacral joint angle 293, *296*
- Lumbosacral kyphosis 293, *294*
- Luque segmental L-rod instrumentation
- – in cerebral palsy *219*, 220
- – in history of spinal deformity surgery 3, *5*

M

- Mac-Thiong-Labelle classification 299, **299**, *300*
- Magnetic resonance imaging (MRI)
- – intradural tumors in **255**, *258*
- – late-onset idiopathic scoliosis 79
- – vertebral rotation measurement in 21
- Malignant hyperpyrexia **227**
- Mandibulofacial dysostosis 199
- Marchetti-Bartolozzi classification **294**, *297–299*
- Marfan syndrome 30, *32*, 70, **272**, *273–275*
- Maroteaux-Lamy syndrome 30
- Maxillary artery *175*
- Medial striate artery *177*
- Meningocele **208**, *209*
- Mesenchymal disorders 26, **30**, *32*
- Mesoderm 154, *155*
- Middle cerebral artery *177*
- Milwaukee brace 2, 76–77, 222
- Minerva cast 2
- Moe method 16, *20*
- Morquio's syndrome 30, **275**, *276–279*
- MPSs, *see* Mucopolysaccharidoses (MPSs)
- MRI, *see* Magnetic resonance imaging (MRI)

- Mucopolysaccharidoses (MPSs) 30, **250**, **275**, *276*
- Muscular dystrophies **226**, *227*
- Myelodysplasia 31
- Myelomeningocele, congenital kyphosis of **191**, *192–193*

N

- Natural history, in early-onset idiopathic scoliosis **66**, 67–68
- Neurofibromatosis
- – as structural deformity **29**, 31
- – axial skeletal lesions in *239*, **239**
- – case gallery **249**, *250*
- – cervical spine deformities in **247**, *249*
- – diagnosis of 238–239, *239*
- – forms of 238
- – imaging of 239, *240*, 243
- – in classification 26
- – kyphosis in 240, **245**, *246*, **249**, *250*
- – late-onset idiopathic scoliosis vs. 70
- – lordosis in 241
- – management of spinal deformities in **242**, *244–246*
- – neurological involvement in 241
- – scoliosis in **242**, *244–245*
- – spinal deformities in **239**, *240*
- – treatment concepts in 58
- Neuromuscular deformities
- – case gallery *232*, **232**
- – classification of 216
- – disorders in 216
- – in classification 26, **29**, 31
- – muscular dystrophies in **226**, *227*
- – peripheral neuropathies in *161*, **226**
- Nonoperative treatment, of late-onset idiopathic scoliosis **75**, *76*, 77
- Nonstructural deformities **36**
- – in classification 26
- – in hysterical scoliosis **36**
- – in irritative lesions **36**
- – structural vs. 14, *16–18*
- Normal development 20, *25*, 46, **154**, *155–156*
- Normal spinal shape 38, *39*
- Not 155
- Notochord
- – anomalies, in congenital deformities **157**, *158–159*
- – in development 154, *156*

O

- OA, *see* Osteoarthritis (OA)
- Occipital artery *175*
- OI, *see* Osteogenesis imperfecta (OI)
- Osteoarthritis (OA)
- – idiopathic scoliosis and 68, 81
- – in spondylolisthesis 291
- Osteogenesis imperfecta (OI) 30, 47, **270**, *270*, **271–272**, *274*
- Osteoid osteoma 36, 69, **260**, *262*
- Osteotomies
- – apical vertebral resection
- – – in late-onset idiopathic scoliosis **104**, *106–107*
- – – in Scheuermann's disease 149, *151*
- – in cerebral palsy 221
- – in late-onset idiopathic scoliosis **102**, *103–104, 106–107*

- – pedicle subtraction, in late-onset idiopathic scoliosis **104**, *104*
- – Ponte
- – – in late-onset idiopathic scoliosis **103**, *104*
- – – in Scheuermann's disease 145
- – Smith-Peterson, in late-onset idiopathic scoliosis **102**, *103*
- Oxford Cobbometer 18

P

- Pain
- – in early-onset idiopathic scoliosis 68
- – in late-onset idiopathic scoliosis 69
- – in Scheuermann's disease 138–139
- Pedicle screws
- – in cerebral palsy 221
- – in Scheuermann's disease 143, 145
- Pedicle subtraction osteotomy, in late-onset idiopathic scoliosis **104**, *104*
- Pedriolle's protractor 16, *21*
- Pelvic obliquity
- – causes of 191
- – in cerebral palsy 29, *31*, 220–221
- – in Duchenne muscular dystrophy 230, *231–232*
- – in myelodysplasia 31
- – in poliomyelitis 31, 222
- – in scoliosis 188
- – in spinal muscular atrophy 229
- – suprapelvic 188
- – transpelvic 188
- – windswept deformity and 217, *218*
- Pelvic tilt scoliosis 26, **36**
- Peripheral neuropathies **225**, *226*
- Peroneal muscular atrophy **225**
- PL 14
- Plain radiography
- – in idiopathic scoliosis 44, 70, *79*
- – in neurofibromatosis 239, *240*, 243
- Plan d'élection view 15, *19*
- Planes 14, *14*
- Poliomyelitis 31
- – abduction deformity in 222
- – bracing in 222
- – defined 221
- – Harrington instrumentation in 222
- – pelvic obliquity in 222
- – phases of 221
- – spinal dysraphism vs. 193
- – spine in 222, *223*
- Ponte osteotomy
- – in late-onset idiopathic scoliosis **103**, *104*
- – in Scheuermann's disease 145
- Pontine arteries *177*
- Posterior auricular artery *175*
- Posterior cerebral artery *177*
- Posterior communicating artery *177*
- Posterior inferior cerebellar artery *177*
- Posterior instrumentation
- – in congenital scoliosis **176**, *180–183*
- – in history of spinal deformity surgery 3, *4–6*
- – in neurofibromatosis 242–243
- Posterior wedge resection, in congenital scoliosis 166
- Primitive streak 154
- Pseudoachondroplasia 283
- Pseudokyphosis
- – in late-onset idiopathic scoliosis 75
- – measurement 17

- Pterygium syndrome 199

R

- Rabbit models *49*, 50
- Rat models *52*, 53
- Refsum's disease 225
- Rib grafts, in Scheuermann's disease 145
- Rib vertebra angle difference (RVAD) 16, 109
- Rib vertebra angles (RVAs) 16
- Risser sign 20, *25*, 67
- Rods, growing, in early-onset idiopathic scoliosis **111**, *112–113*
- RVA, *see* Rib vertebra angles (RVAs)
- RVAD, *see* Rib vertebra angle difference (RVAD)

S

- Sacral agenesis **201**, *202*
- Sacral angle 293, *295*
- Sacral tilt 293, *294*
- Sacro-horizontal angle 293, *295*
- Sagittal curvatures 38, *41*
- Sagittal plane 14, *14*, 45
- Sagittal roll 293, *294*
- Scheuermann's disease **28**, *29*
- – Anterior multiple diskectomy in 146, *147–148*
- – apical vertebral resection in 149, *151*
- – bracing in 141
- – combined anterior-posterior fusion in 143
- – combined thoracoscopic anterior release with posterior fusion in 144
- – complications of spinal fusion in 146
- – conservative treatment of *140–141*, **141**
- – Cotrel-Dubousset instrumentation in 143, *145*
- – diagnosis of **137**, *138–139*
- – imaging of 139
- – in families *136*, **136**
- – kyphosis in *136*, **136**
- – management of *140–141*, **141**, *143–145*, *147–151*
- – nonoperative treatment of 76
- – pain in 138–139
- – pathogenesis of **136**, *137*
- – pedicle screws in 143, 145
- – Ponte osteotomy in 145
- – prevalence of 136
- – rib grafts in 145
- – spinal cord integrity in 149
- – surgical treatment of **142**, *143–145, 147–151*
- Scoliosis, *see* Congenital scoliosis, Idiopathic scoliosis
- Screening, for early-onset idiopathic scoliosis 46, 65, **65**, *66*, 67
- Segmentation failure, in congenital deformities *156–157*, **157**, *159–160*, *162*, 181
- Silver's syndrome 199
- Single curves, in late-onset scoliosis 83, **83**, *84–93*
- Situs inversus 38, *39*
- Skeletal dysplasias **280**, **280**, *281–284*

313

Index

Slip angle 293, *294*
SMA, *see* Spinal muscular atrophy (SMA)
Smith-Peterson osteotomy, in late-onset idiopathic scoliosis 102, *103*
Spina bifida 158, *167*, 187, *188*, 196
- *See also* Congenital cord deformities, Spinal dysraphism
Spinal balance 19, *23*
Spinal cord deformities, congenital 187, *190–194*
Spinal deformities
- classification of 26, **127**
- experimental models of 47, *48–52*
- nonstructural **36**
-- in classification 26
-- in hysterical scoliosis **36**
-- in irritative lesions **36**
-- structural vs. 14, *16–18*
- structural **24**
-- congenital 26, **28**, *30–31*
-- idiopathic **24**, *28–29*
-- in classification 26
-- in infection 26, **32**, *34*
-- in mesenchymal disorders 26, **30**, *32*
-- in neurofibromatosis 26, **29**, *31*
-- neuromuscular 26, **29**, *31*
-- nonstructural vs. 14, *16–18*
-- traumatic 26, **30**, *33*
-- with tumors 26, **32**, *33–34*
Spinal deformity classification 26, **127**
Spinal dysraphism 192, *194–196*
Spinal fusion, in Scheuermann's disease 144, *146*
Spinal growth 20, *25*, 46, **154**, *155–156*
Spinal lengths 42–43
Spinal muscular atrophy (SMA) 224, **224**, 228
Spinal shape
- in families 46, *47*
- normal 38, *39*
Spinocutaneous fistula 192, *195*
Spondyloepiphyseal dysplasia tarda 30, **284**, *284*
Spondylolisthesis **34**, *35*
- anterior displacement in 293, *293–294*
- bracing in 302
- classification of 288, 291, **294**, 296, *297–299*, **299**, *300*
- degenerative 291, *292*, 308
- dysplastic 288, **288**, *289*, **300**, *301–303*

- etiology of *288*, **288**, *289–293*
- Ferguson's angle in 293, *295*
- history of 288
- imaging of 288, **288**, *289–293*
- in classification 26
- intratransverse fusion for **304**, *305–307*
- isthmic **289**, *290–291*, **306**, *307*
- kyphosis in 293, *294*
- lumbosacral joint angle in 293, *296*
- measurement of 293, **293**, *294–296*
- pathological **292**, 293, *293*, **308**
- posterior fusion for 302
- reduction, fixation, and fusion of *303*, **304**
- sacral angle in 293, *295*
- sacral tilt in 293, *294*
- sacro-horizontal angle in 293, *295*
- sagittal roll in 293, *294*
- slip angle 293, *294*
- terminology in 293, **293**, *294–296*
- traumatic 292
- treatment 301–303, **304**, *305–307*
Spondylolysis **304**, *306*
Spondylothoracic dysplasia (STD) 198
- *See also* Thoracic insufficiency syndrome
Sprengel's elevated scapula 197, *198*
Structural deformities **24**
- congenital 26, **28**, *30–31*
-- *See also* Congenital deformities
- idiopathic **24**, *28–29*
- in classification 26
- in infection 26, **32**, *34*
- in mesenchymal disorders 26, **30**, *32*
- in neurofibromatosis **29**, *31*
- neuromuscular 26, **29**, *31*
- nonstructural vs. 14, *16–18*
- traumatic 26, **30**, *33*
- with tumors 26, **32**, *33–34*
Subclavian artery 175
Superficial temporal artery 175
Superior cerebral artery *177*
Superior thyroid artery 175
Suspension casting 2
Syringomyelia 32, **256**, *258*, *260–261*
Syrinx *34*

T

Tenotomy 2
Terminology 14, *14*
Tethered conus 192, *194*, **196**

Thoracic curves, in late-onset idiopathic scoliosis 83, **83**, *84–91*
- double **94**, *95–96*
Thoracic insufficiency syndrome 198, *199–200*
Thoracic lordosis
- in idiopathic scoliosis 44, 47, 53
- natural 14, *15*
Thoracic meningocele 208, *209*
Thoracolumbar curves, in late-onset idiopathic scoliosis 91, *92–93*, **124**, *126*
- double **96**, *98–100*
Traction, intraoperative, in late-onset idiopathic scoliosis 101
Transverse plane
- defined *14*
- deformities in 51
- in scoliosis 51, *51*
- in situs inversus *39*
- vertebral shape in 38, *39*
Traumatic deformities 26, **30**, *33*
Traumatic spondylolisthesis 292
Treacher Collins syndrome 199
Treatment
- etiology and 53–59
- of congenital scoliosis 163, *166–179*
- of early-onset idiopathic scoliosis *111*, **111**, *112–114*
- of intramedullary tumors 255
- of late-onset idiopathic scoliosis 75, *76*, 77
- of neurofibromatosis-associated scoliosis 243, *244–245*
- of Scheuermann's disease **140–141**, *141*, *143–145*, *147–151*
- of spondylolisthesis 301–303, **304**, *305–307*
Triple curves, in late-onset scoliosis 97
Tumor-like lesions 266, *266*
Tumors
- deformities due to 26, **32**, *33–34*
- extradural 32, *254*, **260**, *262–264*
- intradural 32, *195*, 254, *254*, **254**, 255, *256*, **257**, *258*
- late-onset idiopathic scoliosis vs. 69, *69*
- syringomyelia 32, **256**, *258*, *260–261*

U

Unilateral bar *157*, 160

V

VACTERL 198
Vascular anatomy 175
VBS, *see* Vertebral body stapling (VBS)
VCR, *see* Vertebral column resection (VCR)
VEPTR 199, *199–200*
Vertebrae
- named, in curve characteristics 15, *18*
- shapes of 38, *39*
Vertebral artery 175, *177*, 263
Vertebral body expandable prosthetic titanium rib (VEPTR), in early-onset idiopathic scoliosis **114**, *114*
Vertebral body heights, in idiopathic scoliosis 43–44
Vertebral body shape, spinal deformity and 46, *46*, 56
Vertebral body stapling (VBS), in early-onset idiopathic scoliosis **113**, *114*
Vertebral column resection (VCR), in congenital scoliosis 170
Vertebral resection, apical, in late-onset idiopathic scoliosis **104**, *106–107*
Vertebral rotation 16, *20–22*
Von Recklinghausen's disease *31*, 58
- *See also* Neurofibromatosis

W

Whistling face syndrome 201
Windswept deformity 217, *218*

X

X-ray, *see* Plain radiography

Z

Zielke procedure
- in cerebral palsy 218
- in history of spinal deformity surgery 9, *9*
- in poliomyelitis *219*, 223

"Winking owl" sign 69